Prescription for NUTRITIONAL HEALING

Prescription for
NUTRITIONAL HEALING

JAMES F. BALCH, M.D. • PHYLLIS A. BALCH, C.N.C.

AVERY PUBLISHING GROUP INC.
Garden City Park, New York

Cover Designers: Rudy Shur and Martin Hochberg
In-House Editors: Cynthia J. Eriksen, Karen Price, Nancy Marks Papritz, and Diane Lebow
Typesetters: Graphic Connections, Bethpage, NY

Library of Congress Cataloging-in-Publication Data

Balch, James F., 1933–
    Prescription for nutritional healing.

    Includes bibliographical references.
        1. Nutrition—Popular works. 2. Diet therapy
—Popular works. 3. Vitamins—Therapeutic use.
4. Herbs—Therapeutic use. I. Balch, Phyllis A.,
1930–   . II. Title.
RA784.B248 1990   615.8'54   90–452
ISBN 0-89529-429-X

Printed in the United States of America

20 19 18 17 16 15 14 13 12 11 10

Contents

Appendix

Preface

"A wise man should consider that health is the greatest of human blessings."

—*Hippocrates*

Socrates once said, "There is only one good, knowledge, and one evil, ignorance." This statement should guide us in all of our actions, especially where our health is concerned. Too many of us do not have the slightest idea of how to maintain good health. When illness strikes, we rely on our doctors to cure us. What we fail to realize is that "the cure" comes from within. Nature has provided us with a wondrous immune system, and all we have to do is take proper care of this inner healing force.

Does this sound too simple? Basically, it is simple; our modern lifestyles have gotten us off the right track with fast foods, alcohol abuse, drug dependencies, a polluted environment, and high-tech stress. Nature intended to fuel our inner healing force with the right natural substances in order for the body to function at its fullest potential. Nature's resources—whole foods, vitamins, minerals, enzymes, amino acids, and other natural bounties—are designed for use in our immune systems. However, because most of us have a profound "lack of knowledge" as to what our bodies need to function properly, we find ourselves out of balance and susceptible to all sorts of illnesses.

All individuals should take an active part in the maintenance of their health and in the treatment of their disorders with the guidance of a health care professional. The more we take it upon ourselves to learn about nutrition, the better prepared we will be to take that active role. Attitude is also an important factor in the processes of health maintenance and healing. We must have a positive state of mind in order to bring harmony to the body. The realization that body (lifestyle), spirit (desire), and mind (belief) must come together is the first step to better health.

This book has taken over ten years of study, work, and research to put together. It is intended to provide you and your health care professional with a more natural approach to healing, which may be used in conjunction with your current medical treatment. A number of the suggestions offered, such as intravenous therapy, can be administered only by or under the supervision of a licensed physician. Also, because our body chemistries differ, some of us may have allergic reactions to certain supplements. Before taking any nutrient in question, check with your health care professional regarding its appropriateness. Should you experience an allergic reaction to any supplement, immediately discontinue use of the supplement. No one should attempt to treat himself without professional counseling.

The supplementation programs recommended in this book should be followed for three to twelve months, depending upon the needs of the individual and the recommendations of the attending physician or health care professional. Always decrease supplement dosages gradually so that the body has a chance to adjust.

Individuals following a nutrition program for longer than a year should change brands so that they do not build up an intolerance to an ingredient of one supplement. Test the supplements one at a time to find out if you have a reaction to any of them. Remember, we can develop an intolerance to the ingredients in vitamins and other supplements the same as we can to foods. Learn to listen to your body. Given time, you will notice changes in your body and be able to identify their cause. If you do not notice an improvement after a month, consult your doctor. You may suffer from malabsorption.

No statement in this publication should be construed as a claim for cure, treatment, or prevention of any disease. It is also important to point out that you should not reject mainstream medical methods. Learn about your condition, and don't be afraid to ask questions. Feel free to get second and even third opinions from qualified health professionals. It is a sign of wisdom, not cowardice, to seek more knowledge through your active participation as a patient, not a victim.

All information in this book has been carefully researched, with data being reviewed and updated throughout the production process. Because this body of knowledge promises to continue growing and changing, we suggest that when questions arise, you refer to other current sources of information to verify textual material. We will strive to keep abreast of new scientific information, treatments, and supplements, and make this information available to you in future editions of this book.

Over eight hundred years ago, Maimonides said, "The physician should not treat the ailment, but the patient who is suffering from it." This book was designed to meet the differing needs of individuals and to help each person create his own nutrition program.

James F. Balch, Jr., M.D.
Phyllis A. Balch

How to Use This Book

This is a comprehensive in-home guide that will help you achieve and maintain the greatest level of health and fitness through careful dietary planning and nutritional supplementation. Even those who are free from so-called disorders will benefit from this book, because advice is given on how to achieve optimum health, build the immune system, and increase energy levels. Written by a medical doctor and a certified nutritionist, the book blends the latest scientific research with traditional nonsurgical treatments. This guide provides all the information needed for you to design your own personal nutrition program. In addition to giving advice on vitamin and mineral supplementation for optimum health, the authors also offer traditional and up-to-date home remedies and suggest healthful modifications in diet and lifestyle.

It is important to stress that the suggestions offered in this book are not intended to replace appropriate medical investigation and treatment. The supplements and medications recommended for a particular disorder should be approved and monitored by your medical doctor or trained health care professional.

The book is divided into three parts: Part One explains and lists the various types of nutrients, food supplements, and herbs found in health food shops and drugstores; Part Two alphabetically lists common disorders from acne to cancer to yeast infection, discusses how to identify the symptoms, and suggests how to correct the disorder through dietary guidelines and a supplementation program; and Part Three offers a listing of traditional therapies and conventional treatments that can be used in conjunction with a nutritional program. In addition, there are insets throughout the book providing in-depth coverage of important topics and self-diagnostic tests in Part Two to help you determine whether you have a particular illness. The ramifications of different drug therapies are discussed and the latest medical updates are provided.

Also included in an appendix are a recommended reading list, a list of health organizations and their addresses or phone numbers where they can be reached for information, and a list of hospitals, clinics, and the services they provide. A glossary is provided for easy reference.

PART ONE

UNDERSTANDING THE ELEMENTS OF HEALTH

INTRODUCTION

Think of the body as being composed of millions of tiny little engines. Some of these engines work in unison, some work independently; they all are on call twenty-four hours a day. In order for the engines to work right, they require specific fuels. When the type of fuel given is the wrong blend, the engine will not perform to its maximum capacity. When the fuel is of a poor grade, the engine may sputter and hesitate, creating a loss of power. When the engine is given no fuel, it will stop.

For us, much of the fuel we give our engines comes directly from the things we eat. The foods we eat contain nutrients. These nutrients come in the form of vitamins, minerals, hydrocarbons, water, enzymes, amino acids, and fats. And it is these nutrients that allow us to sustain life by providing us with the basic materials our body needs to carry on its daily functions.

Each nutrient differs in form, function, and amount needed by the body; however, they are all vital to our needs. While the actions that involve these nutrients take place on microscopic levels, the specific processes differ greatly. Nutrients are involved in all body processes from combating infection to repairing tissue to thinking. Although these nutrients function on different levels, their common goal is to keep us going.

When we do not give ourselves the proper nutrients, we can cause great harm to the body by impairing its normal functions. The problem with most of us is that we do not get what we need from our "modern diet." Even if you are not sick, you may not necessarily be healthy. It simply may be that you are not yet exhibiting any overt symptoms of illness. By understanding the principles of wholistic nutrition, and knowing what nutrients we need, we can improve the state of our health, stave off disease, and maintain a harmonious balance in the way nature intended.

The following sections should provide you with a clear understanding of the vitamins and minerals you need as well as important information on natural food supplements, products, and herbs that enhance nutrient function.

VITAMINS

THE FUNCTION OF VITAMINS

Vitamins are essential to life. They contribute to good health by regulating the metabolism and assisting the biochemical processes that release energy from digested food. They are considered micronutrients because the body needs them in relatively small amounts compared with other nutrients such as carbohydrates, proteins, fats, and water.

Enzymes are essential chemicals that are the foundation of human bodily functions. They are catalysts (activators) in the chemical reactions that are continually taking place within the body. Vitamins work with these enzymes as coenzymes, thereby allowing all the activities that occur within the body to happen quickly and accurately.

Of the major vitamins, some are water soluble and some are oil soluble. Water-soluble vitamins must be taken into the body daily as they cannot be stored and are excreted within one to four days. These include vitamin C and the B-complex vitamins. Oil-soluble vitamins can be stored for longer periods of time in the body's fatty tissue and the liver. These include vitamins A, D, E, and K. Both types of vitamins are needed by the body for proper functioning.

RDA VERSUS ODA

The *Recommended Daily Allowance* (RDA) was instituted over forty years ago by the U.S. Food and Nutrition Board to determine what daily amount of vitamins were necessary to prevent disease. Unfortunately, what they came up with only gives us the bare minimum to ward off such diseases as beri beri, rickets, scurvy, and night blindness. What it does not account for is the amount needed to maintain maximum health rather than borderline health. Current scientific studies indicate that larger dosages of these vitamins help our bodies work better. By providing an *Optimum Daily Allowance* (ODA) of vitamins, we can enhance our own health. This entails taking a larger percentage of what the RDA recommends. By using each dosage properly, a vitamin program can be designed that is custom-tailored for the individual. The RDAs are too generalized and cannot easily be obtained from today's foods.

BALANCE AND SYNERGY

Taking vitamins and minerals in their proper balance is important to the proper functioning of all vitamins. Scientific research has proven that an excess of an isolated vitamin or mineral can produce the same symptoms as a deficiency of that vitamin or mineral. For example, high doses of isolated B vitamins are proven to cause depletion of other B vitamins. Zinc must also be taken in the proper amounts. When taken in excess, this mineral causes symptoms of zinc deficiency.

Synergy is the combination of two or more vitamins in order to create a stronger vitamin function. For example, in order for bioflavanoids to work properly (they prevent bruising and bleeding gums), they must be taken along with vitamin C.

In addition, there are certain substances that block the absorption and effects of vitamins. For example, because the absorption of vitamin C is greatly reduced while taking antibiotics, more supplementation is necessary at this time.

Vitamins and minerals should be taken with meals unless specified otherwise: oil-soluble vitamins should be taken before meals, and water-soluble ones should be taken between or after meals.

CHEMICAL VERSUS NATURAL

Synthetic vitamins are vitamins produced in a laboratory from isolated chemicals that mirror their counterparts found in nature. Although there are no major chemical differences between a vitamin found in food and one created in a laboratory, natural supplements do not contain other unnatural ingredients. Supplements that are not labeled natural may include coal tars, artificial coloring, preservatives, sugars, starch, as well as other additives. The buyer should beware of such harmful elements. However, the shopper should also note that a "natural vitamin" bottle may contain vitamins that have not been extracted from a natural food source.

Studies have shown that protein bonded supplements are absorbed, utilized, and retained in the tissues better than supplements that are not protein bonded. Vitamins and minerals in food are bonded to proteins, lipids, carbohydrates, and bioflavonoids. Dr. Abram Hoofer explains:

> Components [of food] do not exist free in nature; nature does not lay down pure protein, pure fat, or pure carbohydrates. Their molecules are interlaced in a very complex three-dimensional structure which even now has not been fully described. Intermingled are the essential nutrients such as vitamins and minerals, again not free, but combined in complex molecules.

Using a natural form of vitamins and minerals in nutritional supplements is the objective of the protein bonding process. Taking the supplements with meals will supply the missing nutrients needed for better assimilation as well.

WHAT'S ON THE SHELVES

Over-the-counter vitamins come in various forms, combinations, and amounts. They are available in tablet, capsule, powder, sublingual, lozenge, and liquid form. In most cases, it is a matter of personal preference as to how they are taken; however, due to slight variations in how rapidly the supplements are absorbed and assimilated into the body, we will sometimes recommend one form over another. These recommendations are listed throughout the book.

Vitamin supplements are usually available as isolated vitamins or in combination with other nutrients. It is important to select your vitamins based upon what you really need. (*See* NUTRITION, DIET, AND WELLNESS in Part One.)

The amount you take should be based upon your own requirements. A program designed for health maintenance would be different from one designed to overcome a specific disorder. If you find one supplement that meets your needs, remember to take it daily. If it does not contain a large enough quantity of what you want, you may consider taking more than one. Just make sure that you are aware of the increased dosage of the other nutrients it may contain. If there is no single supplement that provides you with what you are looking for, consider taking a combination of different supplements.

Because the potency of most vitamins may be decreased by sunlight, make sure that the container holding your vitamins is dark enough to shield its contents properly. Some people may be sensitive to plastic, and may need to purchase glass containers. Vitamins should be kept in a cool, dark place.

VITAMINS FROM A TO Z

Vitamin A (Beta-Carotene)

This supplement prevents night blindness and other eye problems as well as some skin disorders such as acne. It enhances immunity, may heal gastrointestinal ulcers, protects against pollution and cancer formation, and is needed for epithelial tissue maintenance and repair. It is important in the formation of bones and teeth, aids in fat storage, and protects against colds, influenza, and infections. Vitamin A acts as an antioxidant, which helps protect the cells against cancer and other diseases. This important vitamin also slows the aging process. Protein cannot be utilized by the body without this supplement.

When food containing beta-carotene is consumed, it is converted to vitamin A in the liver. Beta-carotene aids in cancer prevention, according to recent reports. No vitamin overdose can occur with beta-carotene, although the skin may turn slightly yellow-orange in color.

Sources

Vitamin A can be found in fish liver oils, animal livers, and green and yellow fruits and vegetables. Foods that contain significant amounts include alfalfa, apricots, asparagus, beets, broccoli, cantaloupe, carrots, Swiss chard, dandelion greens, fish liver oil and liver, garlic, kale, mustard, papayas, parsley, peaches, red peppers, sweet potatoes, spinach, spirulina, pumpkin and yellow squash, turnip greens, and watercress.

Warnings

Vitamin A should not be taken in large amounts in pill form or as cod liver oil by those suffering from liver disease. Pregnant women should avoid amounts of vitamin A over 25,000 IU. Children taking vitamin A for more than one month should avoid amounts over 18,000 IU. Antibiotics, laxatives, and some cholesterol-lowering drugs interfere with vitamin A absorption.

Diabetics should avoid beta-carotene as should hypothyroid individuals, because they cannot convert beta-carotene to vitamin A.

Vitamin B Complex

The B vitamins help to maintain healthy nerves, skin, eyes, hair, liver, and mouth, as well as muscle tone in the gastrointestinal tract. B-complex vitamins are coenzymes involved in energy production and may be useful for depression or anxiety. The B vitamins should always be taken together, but up to two to three times more of one B vitamin than another can be taken for a particular disorder. Although the B vitamins are a team, they will be discussed individually.

Vitamin B₁ (Thiamine)

Thiamine enhances circulation and assists in the production of hydrochloric acid, blood formation, and carbohydrate metabolism. Thiamine affects energy, growth disorders, and learning capacity, and is needed for normal muscle tone of the intestines, stomach, and heart.

Sources

Food sources of thiamine include dried beans, brown rice, egg yolks, fish, organ meats (liver), peanuts, peas, pork, poultry, rice bran, soybeans, wheat germ, and whole grains. Other sources are asparagus, beans, broccoli, Brussels sprouts, most nuts, oatmeal, plums, dried prunes, and raisins.

Warnings

Antibiotics, sulfa drugs, and oral contraceptives may decrease thiamine levels in the body. A high-carbohydrate diet increases the need for thiamine. Beriberi, a nervous system disease, is caused by a thiamine deficiency.

Vitamin B₂ (Riboflavin)

Riboflavin is necessary for red blood cell formation, antibody production, cell respiration, and growth. It alleviates eye fatigue and is important in the prevention and treatment of cataracts. It aids in the metabolism of carbohydrates, fats, and proteins. When used with vitamin A, it maintains and improves the mucous membranes in the digestive tract. Riboflavin also facilitates oxygen use by the body tissues (skin, nails, hair), eliminates dandruff, and helps the uptake of iron and vitamin B_6. Vitamin B_2 is important during pregnancy because a lack of this vitamin may damage the fetus even though the mother may be unaware of a deficiency. B_2 is needed for the metabolism of tryptophan, which is converted to niacin in the body. Carpal tunnel syndrome may benefit from a treatment program that includes riboflavin and B_6.

Deficiency symptoms include cracks and sores at the corner of the mouth.

Sources

Vitamin B_2 is found in the following food products: beans, cheese, eggs, fish, meat, milk, poultry, spinach, and yogurt. Other sources include asparagus, avocados, broccoli, Brussels sprouts, currants, and nuts.

Warnings

Factors that increase the need for riboflavin include use of oral contraceptives and strenuous exercise. This B vitamin is easily destroyed by light, cooking, antibiotics, and alcohol.

Vitamin B₃ (Niacin, Niacinamide, Nicotinic Acid)

Vitamin B_3 is needed for proper circulation and healthy skin. B_3 aids in the functioning of the nervous system, in the metabolism of carbohydrates, fats, and proteins, and in the production of hydrochloric acid for the digestive system. Niacin lowers cholesterol and improves circulation. B_3 is also effective in the treatment of schizophrenia and other mental illnesses.

Sources

Niacin and niacinamide are found in beef, broccoli, carrots, cheese, corn flour, eggs, fish, milk, pork, potatoes, tomatoes, and whole wheat.

Warnings

A flush, usually harmless, may occur after ingestion of niacin; a red rash will appear on the skin and a tingling sensation may be experienced as well. High amounts should be used with caution by those who are pregnant and those suffering from gout, peptic ulcers, glaucoma, liver disease, and diabetes.

Pantothenic Acid (B₅)

Known as the "antistress" vitamin, pantothenic acid plays a role in the production of the adrenal hormones and formation of antibodies, aids in vitamin utilization, and helps to convert fats, carbohydrates, and proteins into energy. This vitamin is needed to produce vital steroids and cortisone in the adrenal gland, and is an essential element of coenzyme A. It is required by all cells in the body and is concentrated in the organs. It is also needed for normal functioning of the gastrointestinal tract and may be helpful in treating depression and anxiety.

Sources

The following foods contain pantothenic acid: beans, beef, eggs, salt-water fish, mother's milk, pork, fresh vegetables, and whole wheat.

Warnings

No side effects have been documented to date.

Vitamin B₆ (Pyridoxine)

Pyridoxine is involved in more bodily functions than any other single nutrient. It affects both physical and mental health. It is beneficial if you suffer from water retention. It is necessary in the production of hydrochloric acid and the absorption of fats and protein. Pyridoxine also aids in maintaining sodium and potassium balance, and promotes red blood cell formation. It is required by the nervous system, and is needed for normal brain function and for the synthesis of RNA and DNA (nucleic acids), which contain the genetic instructions for the reproduction of all cells and for normal cellular growth. It activates many enzymes and aids in B_{12} absorption, immune system function, and antibody production. Vitamin B_6 has a role in cancer immunity and arteriosclerosis. It inhibits the formation of a toxic chemical called homocysteine, which attacks the heart muscle and allows the deposition of cholesterol around the heart muscle. B_6 may also be useful in preventing oxalate kidney stones and acts as a mild diuretic. It reduces the symptoms of premenstrual syndrome and is helpful in the treatment of allergies, arthritis, and asthma. Carpal tunnel syndrome is linked to a B_6 deficiency.

Sources

All foods contain small amounts of vitamin B_6; however, the following foods have the highest amounts: brewer's yeast, carrots, chicken, eggs, fish, meat, peas, spinach, sunflower seeds, walnuts, and wheat germ. Other sources not quite as rich in B_6 include avocado, bananas, beans, blackstrap molasses, brown rice and other whole grains, cabbage, and cantaloupe.

Warnings

Antidepressants, estrogen, and oral contraceptives may increase the need for vitamin B_6 in the body.

Vitamin B₁₂ (Cyanocobalamin)

Vitamin B_{12} is needed to prevent anemia. It aids in cell formation and cellular longevity. This vitamin is also required for proper digestion, absorption of foods, protein synthesis, and metabolism of carbohydrates and fats. In addition, vitamin B_{12} prevents nerve damage, maintains fertility, and promotes normal growth and development.

A vitamin B_{12} deficiency can be caused by malabsorption, which is most common in the elderly and in those with digestive disorders. Vegetarians are also more likely to have a B_{12} deficiency. Deficiency symptoms include abnormal gait, memory loss, hallucinations, eye disorders, anemia, and digestive disorders.

Sources

The largest amounts of vitamin B_{12} are found in blue cheese, cheese, clams, eggs, herring, kidney, liver, mackerel, milk, seafood, and tofu. B_{12} is not found in vegetables; it is available only from animal sources.

Warnings

Anti-gout medications, anticoagulant drugs, and potassium supplements may block absorption of B_{12} in the digestive tract. Vegetarians need this supplement because it is found mostly in animal sources.

Biotin

Biotin aids in cell growth, in fatty acid production, in the metabolism of carbohydrates, fats, and proteins, and in the utilization of the B-complex vitamins. Sufficient quantities are needed for healthy hair and skin. Biotin may prevent hair loss in some men. Biotin also promotes healthy sweat glands, nerve tissue, and bone marrow.

A deficiency of this B vitamin is rare because it can be produced in the intestines from foods.

Sources

Biotin is found in cooked egg yolk, salt-water fish, meat, milk, poultry, soybeans, whole grains, and yeast.

Warnings

Raw egg whites contain a protein called ovidin, which combines with biotin in the intestinal tract and depletes the body of this needed nutrient. A dry, scaly scalp and/ or face in infants, called seborrheic dermatitis, may indicate a deficiency. Consuming rancid fats or saccharin inhibits biotin absorption. The use of sulfa drugs and antibiotics threatens the availability of biotin.

Choline

Choline is needed for nerve transmission, gallbladder regulation and liver function, and lecithin formation. It minimizes excess fat in the liver, aids in hormone production, and is necessary in fat and cholesterol metabolism. Without choline, brain function and memory are impaired. Choline is beneficial for disorders of the nervous system such as Parkinson's disease and tardive dyskinesia. A deficiency may result in fatty build-up in the liver.

Sources

The following foods contain a significant amount of choline: egg yolks, legumes, meat, milk, and whole grain cereals.

Warnings

No side effects have been documented to date.

Folic Acid

Considered a brain food, folic acid is needed for energy production and the formation of red blood cells. Functioning as a coenzyme in DNA synthesis, it is important for healthy cell division and replication. It is involved in protein metabolism and has been used in the prevention and treatment of folic acid anemia. This nutrient may also help depression and anxiety and may be effective in the treatment of uterine cervical dysplasia. Folic acid helps regulate embryonic and fetal development of nerve cells, vital for normal growth and development. Folic acid works best when combined with vitamin B_{12}.

A sore, red tongue is one sign of a deficiency.

Sources

The following foods contain significant quantities of folic acid: barley, beans, beef, bran, brewer's yeast, brown rice, cheese, chicken, dates, green leafy vegetables, lamb, lentils, liver, milk, oranges, organ meats, split peas, pork, root vegetables, salmon, tuna, wheat germ, whole grains, whole wheat, and yeast.

Warnings

Oral contraceptives may increase the need for folic acid. High doses for extended periods should be avoided by anyone with a hormone-related cancer or convulsive disorder.

Inositol

Inositol is vital for hair growth. It helps prevent hardening of the arteries and is important in lecithin formation and fat and cholesterol metabolism. It also helps remove fats from the liver.

Sources

Inositol is found in fruits, vegetables, whole grains, meats, and milk.

Warnings

Drinking heavy amounts of caffeine may cause a shortage of inositol in the body.

PABA (Para-Aminobenzoic Acid)

PABA is one of the basic constituents of folic acid and also helps in the utilization of pantothenic acid. This antioxidant helps protect against sunburn and skin cancer, acts as a coenzyme in the breakdown and utilization of protein, and assists in the formation of red blood cells. Supplementing the diet with PABA may restore gray hair to its original color if the graying was caused by stress or a nutritional deficiency.

Sources

Foods that contain PABA are kidney, liver, molasses, and whole grains.

Warnings

Sulfa drugs may cause a deficiency of PABA.

Vitamin C (Ascorbic Acid)

Vitamin C is an antioxidant that is required for tissue growth and repair, adrenal gland function, and healthy gums. It protects against the harmful effects of pollution, prevents cancer, protects against infection, and enhances immunity. It also may reduce cholesterol levels and high blood pressure, and prevent atherosclerosis. Essential in the formation of collagen, vitamin C protects against blood clotting and bruising, and promotes the healing of wounds and the production of antistress hormones. It also aids in interferon production, and is needed for the metabolism of folic acid, tyrosine, and phenylalanine.

New evidence indicates that vitamin C and vitamin E work synergistically, that is, when they work together, they have a greater effect than when they work separately. Vitamin E scavenges for dangerous oxygen radicals in the cell membrane, while vitamin C breaks the free radical chain in biologic fluids. Both these vitamins greatly extend antioxidant activity.

Ester C polyascorbate is a breakthrough in vitamin C, especially for those suffering from chronic illnesses such as cancer and AIDS. This form of vitamin C (esterified) was first researched by Jonathan Wright, M.D. Dr. Wright proved that white blood cell ascorbate levels are increased four times more with ester C than with the average vitamin C or ascorbic acid, and only one-third of the amount is excreted through the urine. Because the body cannot manufacture vitamin C, it must be obtained through the diet or in the form of supplements. Most vitamin C intake is lost in the urine. When larger amounts of vitamin C are required due to illness, it is more effective to take vitamin C intravenously than to take high doses orally. Do so only under the advisement and supervision of your doctor. Ester C enters the bloodstream and tissues four times quicker and into the blood cells more efficiently. This is a big step for the immune system.

Ester C has naturally chelated (bonded) minerals that allow faster absorption. It comes in calcium, magnesium, potassium, zinc, and sodium forms. These polyascorbate pH balanced forms are manufactured according to exact specifications.

Sources

Vitamin C is found in green vegetables, berries, and citrus fruits. It is found in asparagus, avocados, beet greens, broccoli, Brussels sprouts, cantaloupe, collards, currants, grapefruit, kale, lemons, mangos, mustard greens, onions, oranges, papayas, parsley, green peas, sweet peppers, persimmons, pineapple, radishes, rose hips, spinach, strawberries, Swiss chard, tomatoes, turnip greens, and watercress.

Warnings

Aspirin, alcohol, analgesics, antidepressants, anticoagulants, oral contraceptives, and steroids may reduce levels of vitamin C in the body. Diabetic (diabinase) and sulfa drugs may not be as effective when taken with vitamin C. Large amounts may cause a false negative reading when testing for blood in the stool. Pregnant women should use amounts no larger than 5,000 milligrams daily. Infants may become dependent on this supplement and develop scurvy.

Vitamin D

Vitamin D is required for calcium and phosphorus absorption and utilization. It is necessary for growth, and is especially important for normal growth and development of bones and teeth in children. It is important in the prevention and treatment of osteoporosis, rickets, and hypocalcemia, and it enhances immunity.

The vitamin D that we get from food or supplements is not fully activated. It requires conversion by the liver, and then by the kidney before it becomes fully active.

People with liver or kidney disorders are at a higher risk for osteoporosis.

Because the sun's ultraviolet rays can be converted to vitamin D, exposing the face and arms to the sun three times a week is effective.

Sources

Fish liver oils, fatty salt-water fish, dairy products fortified with vitamin D, and eggs all contain vitamin D. It is found in alfalfa, butter, cod liver oil, egg yolk, halibut, liver, milk, oatmeal, salmon, sardines, sweet potatoes, tuna, and vegetable oils. Vitamin D can be converted from the action of sunlight on the skin.

Warnings

Toxicity may occur from amounts over 65,000 IU over a period of years. Vitamin D should not be taken without calcium. Intestinal disorders and liver and gallbladder malfunctions interfere with absorption of vitamin D. The use of some cholesterol-lowering drugs, antacids, mineral oil, or steroid hormones (cortisone) also interferes with absorption. Thiazide diuretics disturb the calcium/vitamin D ratio.

Vitamin E

Vitamin E is an antioxidant that prevents cancer and cardiovascular disease. This supplement improves circulation, repairs tissue, and is useful in treating fibrocystic breasts and premenstrual syndrome. It also promotes normal clotting and healing, reduces scarring from some wounds, reduces blood pressure, aids in preventing cataracts, improves athletic performance, and aids leg cramps. Vitamin E also prevents cell damage by inhibiting lipid peroxidation and the formation of free radicals. It retards aging and may prevent age spots as well.

The body needs zinc in order to maintain the proper levels of vitamin E in the blood.

Sources

Vitamin E is found in the following food sources: cold-pressed vegetable oils, whole grains, dark green leafy vegetables, nuts and seeds, and legumes. Significant quantities of this vitamin are also found in dry beans, brown rice, cornmeal, eggs, dessicated liver, milk, oatmeal, organ meats, sweet potatoes, and wheat germ.

Warnings

Do not take iron at the same time that you take vitamin E. Those suffering from diabetes, rheumatic heart disease, or an overactive thyroid should not use high doses.

Those suffering from high blood pressure should start with a small amount and increase slowly to the desired amount.

Vitamin K

Vitamin K is needed for blood clotting and may play a role in bone formation. It may also prevent osteoporosis. In addition, vitamin K converts glucose into glycogen for storage in the liver.

Sources

Vitamin K is found in alfalfa, broccoli, dark green leafy vegetables, and soybeans. Other foods that contain vitamin K include blackstrap molasses, Brussels sprouts, cabbage, cauliflower, egg yolks, liver, oatmeal, oats, rye, safflower oil, and wheat.

Warnings

When synthetic vitamin K is used in large doses during the last few weeks of pregnancy, it may result in a toxic reaction in the newborn. Megadoses can accumulate and cause flushing and sweating. Antibiotics interfere with the absorption of vitamin K.

Bioflavonoids

Although bioflavonoids are not true vitamins in the strictest sense, they are sometimes referred to as vitamin P. Bioflavonoids enhance absorption of vitamin C, and they should be taken together. There are many products and mixtures of different bioflavonoids including hesperetin, hesperidin, eriodictyol, quercetin, quercetrin, and rutin. The human body cannot produce bioflavonoids, which must be supplied in the diet. They are used extensively in athletic injuries because they relieve pain, bumps, and bruises. They also reduce pain located in the legs or across the back and lessen symptoms associated with prolonged bleeding and low serum calcium. Bioflavonoids act synergistically with vitamin C to protect and preserve the structure of capillary blood vessels. In addition, bioflavonoids have an antibacterial effect and promote circulation, stimulate bile production, lower cholesterol levels, and treat and prevent cataracts. When taken with vitamin C, bioflavonoids also reduce the symptoms of oral herpes.

Quercetin, found in blue-green algae and available as a supplement, may effectively treat and prevent asthma symptoms. Bromelin and quercetin are synergists, and should be taken in conjunction to enhance absorption. Take 1,000–2,000 milligrams of quercetin daily in 3–6 divided doses for asthma or allergies.

Sources

The white material just beneath the peel of citrus fruits,

peppers, buckwheat, and black currants contain bioflavonoids. Sources of vitamin F include apricots, cherries, grapefruit, grapes, lemons, oranges, prunes, and rose hips.

Warnings

Extremely high doses may cause diarrhea.

Coenzyme Q$_{10}$

Coenzyme Q$_{10}$ is a vitamin-like substance that resembles vitamin E, but which may be an even more powerful antioxidant. It is also called ubiquinone. There are ten common coenzyme Qs, but coenzyme Q$_{10}$ is the only one found in human tissue. Coenzyme Q$_{10}$ declines with age and should be supplemented in the diet. It plays a crucial role in the effectiveness of the immune system and in the aging process. The New England Institute reports that coenzyme Q alone is effective in reducing mortality in experimental animals afflicted with tumors and leukemia. Clinical tests are being used along with chemotherapy to reduce the side effects of the drugs.

In Japan, it is used in the treatment of heart disease and high blood pressure, and is also used to enhance the immune system. Research has revealed that use of coenzyme Q$_{10}$ benefits allergies, asthma, and respiratory disease, and it is used to treat the brain for anomalies of mental function such as those associated with schizophrenia and Alzheimer's disease. It is also beneficial in aging, obesity, candidiasis, multiple sclerosis, periodontal disease, and diabetes. AIDS is a primary target for research on coenzyme Q$_{10}$ because of its immense benefits to the immune system. Early research in Japan has shown coenzyme Q$_{10}$ to protect the stomach lining and duodenum. It may help heal duodenal ulcers. Coenzyme Q$_{10}$ has the ability to counter histamine and is valuable to allergy and asthma sufferers. The use of coenzyme Q$_{10}$ is a major step forward in the prevention and control of cancer.

Be cautious when purchasing coenzyme Q$_{10}$. Not all products will offer it in its purest form. Its natural color is bright yellow and has very little taste in the powdered form. It should be kept away from heat and light. Pure coenzyme Q$_{10}$ will deteriorate in temperatures above 115°F.

Sources

Mackerel, salmon, and sardines contain the largest amounts of coenzyme Q$_{10}$.

Warnings

No side effects have been documented to date.

NUTRITION, DIET, AND WELLNESS

In order to maintain proper health and well-being, many nutrients are needed by the body. The Food and Drug Administration (FDA) formulated what is referred to as the RDA (Recommended Daily Allowance), but, as discussed in VITAMINS in Part One, this allowance does not account for the amount needed to maintain maximum health rather than borderline health. Therefore, the average adult individual who is not suffering from any specific disorder, should increase the overall amount of nutrients he is obtaining from food sources and/or from supplements. The following chart should be used as a guideline. Although the amounts listed are safe (will not cause toxicity), they should be varied according to size and weight.

People who are active and exercise regularly need higher dosages of nutrients. Those who are under great stress, on restricted diets, mentally or physically ill, women who take oral contraceptives, those on medication, those recovering from surgery, and smokers and alcoholics also need higher amounts of vitamins and minerals.

In addition to a proper diet, exercise and a positive attitude are two important elements that are needed to prevent sickness and disease. If your lifestyle accounts for each of these, you will feel good and have more energy—something we all deserve.

NUTRIENTS AND DOSAGES
FOR MAINTAINING GOOD HEALTH

The nutrients listed below are recommended for good health. Daily dosages are suggested; however, before using any supplements, you should consult with your physician. Dosages will vary according to age and weight.

Vitamins	Daily Dosages	
Beta-carotene	15,000	IU
Vitamin A	10,000	IU
Vitamin D	400	IU
Vitamin E	600	IU
Vitamin K (alfalfa)	100	mcg
Vitamin C with the mineral ascorbates	3,000	mg
Bioflavonoids	500	mg

Vitamins	Daily Dosages	
Hesperidin	100	mg
Rutin	25	mg
Folic acid	400	mcg
Thiamine (B$_1$)	50	mg
Riboflavin (B$_2$)	50	mg
Niacin	100	mg
Niacinamide	100	mg
Pantothenic acid (B$_5$)	100	mg
Vitamin B$_6$ (pyridoxine)	50	mg
Vitamin B$_{12}$ (cyanocobalamin)	300	mcg
Biotin	300	mcg
Choline	100	mg
Inositol	100	mg
PABA (Para-aminobenzoic acid)	25	mg
Vitamin F (unsaturated fatty acids)		

Minerals	Daily Dosages	
Calcium (chelate)	1,500	mg
Chromium (GTF)	150	mcg
Copper	3	mg
Iodine (kelp)	225	mcg
Iron*	18	mg
Magnesium	750	mg
Manganese	2	mg
Molybdenum	30	mcg
Potassium	99	mg
Selenium	200	mcg
Zinc	30	mg

Optional Supplements	Daily Dosages	
Coenzyme Q$_{10}$	30	mg
Garlic (Kyolic)		
Germanium Ge-132	60	mg
L-Carnitine	100	mg
L-Cysteine	50	mg
L-Lysine	50	mg
L-Methionine	50	mg
L-Tyrosine	100	mg
Lecithin	200–500	mg
Pectin	50	mg
RNA-DNA	100	mg
Silicon		
Superoxide dismutase (SOD)		

*Iron should be taken separately, but may be omitted if no deficiency exists. Do not take iron in a multisupplement formula.

Other supplements that you may wish to take for increased energy are:

- Bee pollen.
- Bio-Strath.
- Floradix formula.
- Free form amino acids.
- Kyo-Green (Kyolic).
- Octacosanol.
- Siberian ginseng.
- Spirulina.

SYNERGY AND DEFICIENCY

All vitamins and minerals are synergistic. This means that there is a cooperative action between certain vitamins and minerals. They act as catalysts, promoting the absorption and assimilation of other vitamins and minerals. Correcting a vitamin or mineral deficiency requires the addition of other vitamins and minerals, not simply replacing the one in which you are deficient. Taking a single vitamin or mineral may be ineffective and dangerous. Always add a balanced vitamin and mineral preparation. The following table indicates what vitamins and minerals are necessary for certain deficiencies.

Vitamin Deficiency	Supplements Needed for Assimilation
Vitamin A	Choline, vitamins C, D, E, and F, zinc
Biotin	Folic acid, pantothenic acid (B$_5$), B complex, vitamins B$_{12}$ and C
Choline	B complex, inositol, vitamin B$_{12}$, folic acid
Inositol	B complex, vitamin C
Niacin	B complex, vitamin C
PABA	B complex, folic acid, vitamin C
Pantothenic acid	B complex, vitamins A, C, and E
Riboflavin (B$_2$)	B complex, vitamin C
Thiamine (B$_1$)	B complex, vitamins C and E, manganese
Vitamin B complex	Calcium, vitamins C and E
Vitamin B$_6$ (pyridoxine)	B complex, vitamin C, potassium
Vitamin C	Bioflavonoids, calcium, magnesium
Vitamin D	Calcium, choline, phosphorus, vitamins A, C, and F
Vitamin E	Inositol, manganese, selenium, vitamins A, B$_1$, C, and F
Vitamin F	Vitamins A, C, D, and E
Vitamin K	Use natural sources (i.e., alfalfa, green leafy vegetables)

Mineral Deficiency	Supplements Needed for Assimilation
Calcium	Iron, magnesium, manganese, phosphorus, vitamins A, C, D, and F
Copper	Folic acid and cobalt, iron, zinc
Iodine	Iron, manganese, phosphorus
Magnesium	Calcium, phosphorus, potassium, vitamins B$_6$, C, and D
Manganese	B complex, calcium, iron, vitamin E
Phosphorus	Calcium, iron, manganese, sodium, vitamin B$_6$ (pyridoxine)
Silicon	Iron, phosphorus
Sodium	Calcium, potassium, sulfur, vitamin D
Sulfur	Biotin, pantothenic acid, potassium, vitamin B$_1$
Zinc	Calcium, copper, phosphorus, vitamin B$_6$ (pyridoxine)

A recent study revealed that 43 percent of the people surveyed by the U.S. Department of Agriculture consumed a diet containing only 60 percent of the RDA of each of ten selected nutrients. This means that more than half of the population suffers from a deficiency in at least one important nutrient. In addition, a poll of 37,000 people conducted by Food Technology (1981) indicates that half of the population is deficient in vitamin B$_6$ (pyridoxine), 42 percent does not consume sufficient amounts of calcium, 39 percent has an insufficent iron intake, and 25–39 percent does not obtain the needed amounts of vitamin C.

Additional research has shown that a vitamin deficiency may not affect the whole body, but may weaken only specific cells. Those who smoke may suffer from vitamin deficiency, but only in the lung area.

THE HAZARDS OF OVERCOOKED FOODS

If you cook food for too long, especially over a charcoal grill, it will brown and burn. When ingested, overcooked foods have proven to be potentially highly carcinogenic. Bread crust and other toasted material that has been browned and burned will contain a variety of agents that may cause cancer. In fact, many chemicals that produce cancer in animals have been isolated from cooked protein.

The amount of overcooked foods that are ingested varies from person to person, but some may consume many grams daily. By comparison, a half gram of this same dangerous burned material is inhaled by someone smoking two packs of cigarettes a day. Smokers have readily detectable levels of these carcinogens in their urine as compared to nonsmokers. Similarly, nitrogenous substances are consumed by people who eat fried pork or bacon. When the fat, protein, and other organic compounds contained in the animal are cooked at extreme temperatures, changes in chemical structure occur. These toxic chemical changes in the overcooked foods, when ingested into the human body, put the individual at risk for cancer.

FOODS TO AVOID

Soybean products and peanuts contain certain enzyme inhibitors and should be consumed in moderation. Too many legumes, such as beans, in the diet can sometimes cause excessive gas and discomfort. Most illnesses accompany digestive problems. Therefore, foods that cause difficult digestion should be eaten only occasionally.

Nuts that are in showcases or exposed to air and light should be avoided. Nuts must be fresh, not roasted. Rancid nuts contain rancid oils, which cause many diseases.

PROTEIN REQUIREMENTS

The daily protein requirement of a 170-pound man doing light work is 25 to 30 grams. A bowl of pea or bean soup, a slice of whole grain bread, and a vegetable salad supplies all the protein he needs. The salad dressing should consist of pure apple cider vinegar, cold-pressed olive oil or safflower oil (or canola oil for those with high cholesterol), garlic, herbs, and a small amount of barley malt or honey for a touch of sweetness.

Complete proteins are necessary for sustenance of life. They provide the structure for all living things and participate in the chemical processes enabling life to go on. The following food combinations add up to a complete protein. Although each food lacks one or more of the necessary amino acids (see AMINO ACIDS in Part One), together they are a complete protein and a good substitute for meat.

Beans combined with any one of the following:

> Cheese
> Corn
> Nuts (all)
> Rice
> Sesame seeds
> Seeds (all)
> Wheat

Brown rice combined with the following:

> Beans
> Cheese
> Nuts
> Sesame seeds
> Wheat

In addition, cornmeal fortified with the amino acid L-lysine makes a complete protein. A combination of any grain, all nuts and seeds, legumes (such as beans, peanuts, and peas), and a variety of mixed vegetables will also make a complete protein.

By adding any of the above combinations to meals, the body will not require animal protein. Two dishes that you can add to a meal to meet the protein requirements are veggie chili and beans over brown rice. Eat bread with nut butters or add nuts and seeds to meals. Strict vegetarians must remember that they require vitamin B_{12} supplementation, as this vitamin is found almost exclusively in meat.

The protein content of the following fruits is one percent or more: apricots, avocados, bananas, cherries, figs, grapes, olives, papayas, and tomatoes.

All soybean products such as tofu and soybean milk are complete proteins. The availability of foods that are complete proteins when eaten alone is limited. Soybean products, however, contain the essential amino acids plus several other nutrients and are used to complement the meatless diet. Soy oil, soy flour, imitation meat products, cheese, and many other soy products are available in health food stores.

Yogurt is the only high quality source of protein that is derived from animals. Yogurt is made from milk that has been fermented using a mixture of yeast bacteria. The fermentation process gives yogurt its custard-like texture. *Lactobacillus acidophilus* and other "friendly" bacteria are necessary for the digestion of foods and the prevention of many disorders, including candidiasis and thrush. The digestive tract contains certain bacteria that are beneficial to the body. These bacteria aid in the digestion of food and are necessary in the production of certain vitamins, especially the B vitamins. These bacteria are responsible for maintaining a normal flora in the digestive tract, and also prevent the growth of pathogens (undesirable microorganisms that can cause disease). Yogurt contains these beneficial bacteria. Yogurt also contains vitamins A and D, as well as the B complex.

Do not use artificially sweetened and flavored yogurt containing added sugar and preservatives from the supermarket. Sugar feeds unwanted bacteria. Instead, you can either purchase fresh natural yogurt from a health food store or make it yourself. A yogurt maker is relatively inexpensive, easy to use, and available at most health food stores.

THE BENEFITS OF FRESH, RAW FOODS

Fresh fruits and vegetables contain more vitamins and enzymes than overripe fruits and vegetables or ones that have been stored for any length of time. The longer a food is kept, the more nutrients it will lose.

The healthiest foods are those that have been grown organically. These foods are grown without the use of insecticides, herbicides, artificial fertilizers, or growth-stimulating chemicals. Organically grown food can be found in select health food stores. Check with your local store.

All foods must be thoroughly washed before they are eaten to rid them of any insecticides or other residue. Use a soft vegetable brush to scrub the foods, and then let them soak in water for ten minutes. You can also clean the food with nontoxic rinsing preparations, which are available in reputable health food stores. However, if the food is obtained from an organic source, water and a vegetable brush are probably all that are necessary.

Although most people are used to eating almost all cooked foods, fruits and vegetables should be eaten raw as much as possible. Vitamins and enzymes are extremely sensitive to heat and are destroyed in the cooking process. If raw foods are unavailable, frozen foods can be used as a substitute; however, do not use processed, canned, or boxed foods. If you find it difficult to eat raw foods, steam them slightly or use a wok.

Most fruits and vegetables should be eaten in their entirety, as they have valuable nutrients in all of their parts. Except for citrus fruits, eat the skins and rinds as well as the flesh. Eat the white part inside the skin of the citrus fruit for its vitamin C and bioflavonoid content. Except for lemons, however, keep the ingestion of citrus fruits to a minimum. Lemon juice is an effective healing agent. Add to a cup of warm water first thing every morning.

WHEN DINING OUT

When eating in a restaurant, order only broiled fish or chicken, steamed or baked vegetables, and tossed vegetable salads. Avoid all fried and processed foods. Many restaurant foods are frozen and loaded with salt, animal fat, sulfites, and preservatives. During your meal, drink water with fresh lemon juice to aid in digestion and detoxification.

COOKING UTENSILS

Do not use aluminum cooking utensils. Aluminum salts are soluble in water and are also easily assimilated into the body. These aluminum salts have no known beneficial effect on the body. Foods cooked in aluminum produce a chloride poison, neutralize the digestive juices, and produce acidosis and ulcers. The unwanted aluminum is deposited in the brain and nervous system tissues, and will continue to accumulate there. Excessive amounts of aluminum have been implicated in

Alzheimer's disease. (*See* ALUMINUM TOXICITY and ALZHEIMER'S DISEASE in Part Two.) Use only pyrex glassware, stainless steel, and iron cookware. Avoid coated cookware as these plastics and metals can also deposit in the food.

SALT IS NOT THE SPICE OF LIFE

Common table salt (sodium chloride) is detrimental to the body in countless ways. In high concentrations, it causes the delicate fluid and mineral balance of the body to change. Too much salt in the system can cause excessive fluid build-up and create high hydrostatic pressure in the tissues. This can lead to high blood pressure and, ultimately, to severe heart disease and stroke. Salt does not allow the blood to circulate properly either. The blood is responsible for carrying nutrients and oxygen to all the cells of the body. The blood also transports metabolic waste for excretion by the body. This function is extremely important in any disease state. The increase of water in the tissues due to salt intake makes this essential process of waste excretion more difficult.

SIMPLE VERSUS COMPLEX CARBOHYDRATES

The ingestion of refined carbohydrates (sugar) can lead to many disorders. Sugar intake is a factor in many diseases. This sweet substance stimulates the pancreas to produce insulin, which is needed to metabolize simple carbohydrates. The pancreas must produce additional insulin with the ingestion of more simple carbohydrates. High intake of simple carbohydrates results in an overstimulation of the pancreas that "wears out" this important gland. When the pancreas cannot handle the sugar intake, diabetes results. (*See* DIABETES in Part Two.)

The pancreas is one of the most important organs utilized by the body to prevent disease. Too much protein (especially from an animal source) causes excess pancreatic enzyme excretion. These enzymes are extremely important in cancer prevention. In addition to excessive consumption of simple carbohydrates, an overindulgence in animal proteins leads to pancreatic deterioration.

The ingestion of refined simple carbohydrates can also lead to a condition, called hypoglycemia, in which the body is no longer able to metabolize the sugar properly (*see* HYPOGLYCEMIA in Part Two). The inability of the pancreas to metabolize simple carbohydrates sufficiently leads to fatigue, dizziness, confusion, headache, restlessness, and ultimately to other diseases such as collapse of the adrenal glands. Proper functioning of the adrenal glands is necessary in order to handle stress. When hypoglycemia is present, the body is under stress.

If you suffer from hypoglycemia, it is important that you do not put added stress on the body.

In addition, a meal that is high in both fats and simple carbohydrates will make you feel tired and lessen your ability to think properly because the tissues are not receiving enough oxygen. Blood cells will normally repel each other, as well as other cells, in order to prevent themselves from clumping together and forming clots. Like rubber bands, blood cells bend and twist as they migrate through hundreds of miles of blood vessels. This action maintains efficient blood flow. A meal high in fat, however, will change this normal process. When the fat enters the bloodstream through the intestinal wall, it coats the blood cells and causes them to clump together. This makes it difficult for the blood cells to get through the tiny capillaries, which decreases the oxygen supply to the tissues and leads to fatigue and disease. Because of their reactions in the body, fats should be reduced and simple carbohydrates should be eliminated to prevent disease and aid in healing.

Although simple carbohydrates should be eliminated from the diet, complex carbohydrates are beneficial and should be included. These are found in fresh fruits and vegetables, beans, and natural whole grains. They provide dietary fiber and have only one-third the calories found in fat and simple carbohydrates. Protein and carbohydrates are about equal in calories. Carbohydrates in the form of starch contain a good amount of vitamins and minerals. Carbohydrates can be converted into fat and provide the body with energy and warmth. A constant flow of energy is supplied by complex carbohydrates in contrast to the short-lived "rush" derived from simple carbohydrates.

Cravings for sweets can and should be satisfied with fresh fruit. Many fruits are sweet to the taste and are easy to digest. They also contain valuable nutrients that are necessary for good health. Fruits should be eaten by themselves, preferably first thing in the morning for a cleansing effect. It is important to remember that although sorghum and honey contain vitamins in the nitriloside group and beneficial minerals, they are also carbohydrates and can create "sugar problems."

It has been proven that adequate fiber and bulk are important in the diet. Fiber- and bulk-producing foods contain substances that pass through the digestive tract without being absorbed, have an intestinal cleansing action, and keep the digestive tract clean. Foods that are high in fiber move through the digestive tract due to the peristaltic action of the alimentary canal, and take with them many toxic substances that would otherwise become lodged. If these harmful substances are not excreted by the body, disease results. Whole foods such as fruits and vegetables, nuts, seeds, and whole grains contain bulk and fiber. Oat bran and rice bran are wise additions to the diet for added fiber.

Keep in mind that nothing in the universe stays at peak performance at all times. This includes the body. Everything and everyone has cycles—we all experience highs and lows. We must constantly work to maintain high performance levels and to avoid feeling low. This can be accomplished by adhering to the following basic program.

Basic Nutritional Guide

A nutritional diet is the key to good health. Use the following table as a guide when deciding which types of food to include in the diet and which ones to avoid in order to maintain good health.

Types of Food	Foods to Avoid	Acceptable Foods
Beans	Canned pork and beans, canned beans with salt or preservatives, frozen beans.	All beans cooked without animal fat or salt.
Beverages	Alcohol, coffee, cocoa, pasteurized and sweetened juices, fruit drinks, sodas, tea (except herb tea).	Herb teas, fresh vegetable and fruit juices, a coffee substitute made from cereal grains instead of coffee beans, mineral or distilled water.
Dairy Products	All soft cheeses, all pasteurized cheese products with orange coloring, ice cream.	Raw goat (light) cheese, nonfat cottage cheese, kefir, unsweetened yogurt, goat milk, raw or skim milk, buttermilk, all soy products.
Eggs	Fried or pickled.	Boiled or poached (limit to four weekly).
Fish	All fried fish, all shellfish, salted fish, anchovies, herring, fish canned in oil.	All fresh-water white fish, salmon, broiled or baked fish, water-packed tuna.
Fruits	Canned, bottled, or frozen fruits with sweeteners added.	All fresh, frozen, stewed and dried fruits without sweeteners, unsulfured fruits, home-canned fruits.
Grains	All white flour products, white rice, spaghetti and macaroni, crackers, overly processed oatmeal and hot or cold cereals.	All grains and products containing grains, cereals, breads, muffins, whole grain crackers, Cream of Wheat/Rye cereal, buckwheat, millet, oats, brown rice, wild rice. (Limit yeast breads to three times per week.)
Meats	Beef; all forms of pork; hot dogs; luncheon meats; smoked, pickled, and processed meats; corned beef; duck; goose; spare ribs; gravies; organ meats.	Skinless turkey and chicken, lamb. (Consume meat only three times per week.)
Nuts	Peanuts, all salted or roasted nuts.	All fresh raw nuts (except peanuts).
Oils (Fats)	All saturated fats, hydrogenated margarine, refined processed oils, shortenings, hardened oils.	All cold-pressed oils: corn, safflower, sesame, olive, soybean, sunflower, and canola oils; margarine from these oils; eggless mayonnaise.
Seasonings	Black or white pepper, salt, hot red peppers, white vinegar, all artificial vinegar.	Garlic, onions, dried parsley, Spike, all herbs, chives, cayenne, dried vegetables, apple vinegar, tamari, miso, seaweed, sea salt, dulse.
Soups	Canned with salt or preservatives (MSG), fat stock, or creamed.	Homemade (salt and fat free) bean, lentil, pea, vegetable, barley, brown rice, onion.
Sprouts and Seeds	Seeds cooked in oil or salt.	All slightly cooked sprouts (except alfalfa), wheatgrass, and all raw seeds.
Sweets	White, brown, or raw sugar, corn syrups, chocolate, sugar candy, fructose, all syrups except pure maple syrup, all sugar substitutes, jams and jellies with sugar.	Barley malt or rice syrup, small amounts of raw honey, pure maple syrup, unsulfured blackstrap molasses.
Vegetables	All canned and frozen with salt or additives.	All raw, fresh, frozen (no additives), or home-canned. (Undercook vegetables slightly.)

Minerals

THE FUNCTION OF MINERALS

Like vitamins, minerals function as coenzymes, enabling the body to quickly and accurately perform its activities. They are needed for the proper composition of body fluids, the formation of blood and bone, and the maintenance of healthy nerve function.

Minerals are naturally occurring elements found in the earth. Rock formations are made up of mineral salts. As rock and stone are broken down into tiny fragments by millions of years of erosion, dust and sand accumulate, forming the basis of soil. Besides these tiny crystals of mineral salts, the soil is teeming with microbes that utilize them. The minerals are then passed from the soil to plants, which are then eaten by herbivorous animals. Man, in turn, obtains these minerals for use by the body by consuming these plants or herbivorous animals.

Minerals belong to two groups: macro (bulk) minerals and micro (trace) minerals. Bulk minerals include calcium, magnesium, sodium, potassium, and phosphorus. These are needed in larger amounts than trace minerals. Although only minute quantities of trace minerals are needed, they are important for good health. Trace minerals include zinc, iron, copper, manganese, chromium, selenium, and iodine. Because minerals are stored primarily in the body's bone and muscle tissue, it is possible to overdose on minerals if an extremely large dose is taken. However, toxic amounts will accumulate only if massive amounts are taken for a prolonged period of time.

WHAT'S ON THE SHELVES

Bulk and trace minerals are often found in vitamin supplements and multivitamin formulas. Check to see whether the label lists the desired mineral supplements. Minerals can also be sold as a single supplement. These are available in tablet, capsule, powder, and liquid forms.

IMPROVING MINERAL ABSORPTION

Some mineral supplements are available in chelated form, which means that the minerals are attached to a protein molecule that transports them to the bloodstream in order to enhance their absorption. When mineral supplements are taken with a meal, they are usually automatically chelated in the stomach during digestion. There is controversy over which type of mineral to take, but we prefer to use the chelated preparations.

Mineral asporotate (orotate) preparations work in the same way. Dr. Hans Nieper from the Sibersee Hospital in Hanover, West Germany, has developed a theory related to mineral transportation. He found that orotates (a form of chelates) or orotic acid chelates are the most effective, since they have an affinity for and travel to the inner layer of the outer cell membrane. However, the Food and Drug Administration (FDA) has called for the removal of the orotates from the market. This decision is particularly disheartening. Our experience with the mineral orotates, like Dr. Nieper's, has shown them to be the most effective.

Once a mineral is absorbed, it must be carried by the blood to the cells and then transported across the cell membrane in a form that can be utilized by the cell. After the mineral enters the body, it must compete with other minerals for absorption; therefore, minerals should always be taken in balanced amounts. For example, too much zinc can deplete the body of copper and an excessive calcium intake can affect magnesium absorption. Always use a balanced mineral supplement. Anything else will not be effective.

In addition, fiber decreases the body's absorption of minerals. Therefore, take supplemental fiber and minerals at different times.

THE ABC'S OF MINERALS

Boron

Boron is needed in trace amounts for calcium uptake and healthy bones. Most people are not deficient in boron. However, the elderly will benefit from 2–3 milligrams daily because they have a greater problem with calcium absorption.

The latest study conducted by the U.S. Department of Agriculture indicated that within eight days of supplementing the diet with 3 milligrams of boron, a test group of postmenopausal women lost 40 percent less calcium, one-third less magnesium, and slightly less phosphorus through their urine.

Sources

Boron is found in leafy vegetables, fruits, nuts, and grains.

Warnings

Do not take more than 3 milligrams daily.

Calcium

Calcium is vital in the formation of strong bones and teeth and is also important in the maintenance of regular heartbeat and the transmission of nerve impulses. It is needed for muscle growth and contraction and for the prevention of muscle cramps. This important mineral is also essential in blood clotting and helps prevent colon cancer. It may lower blood pressure and prevent bone loss associated with osteoporosis as well. Calcium provides energy and participates in the protein structuring of RNA and DNA. It is also involved in the activation of several enzymes including lipase. The amino acid lysine is needed for calcium absorption.

Calcium protects the bones and teeth from lead by inhibiting absorption of this toxic metal. If there is a calcium deficiency, lead will be absorbed by the body and deposited in the teeth and bones. This may account for the higher levels of lead in children who have a higher incidence of cavities.

A calcium deficiency may result in the following symptoms: muscle cramps, nervousness, heart palpitations, brittle nails, eczema, hypertension, aching joints, increased cholesterol levels, rheumatoid arthritis, tooth decay, insomnia, rickets, and numbness in the arms and/or legs.

Calcium is more effective when taken in smaller doses spread throughout the day and before bedtime. When taken at night, it also promotes a sound sleep. This mineral works less effectively when taken in a single megadose.

Female athletes and women experiencing menopause need greater amounts of calcium due to lower estrogen levels. Estrogen protects the skeletal system by promoting the deposit of calcium in bone.

Sources

Sources of calcium include dairy foods, salmon (with bones), sardines, seafood, and green leafy vegetables. It is found in almonds, asparagus, blackstrap molasses, brewer's yeast, broccoli, buttermilk, cabbage, carob,

cheese, collards, dandelion greens, dulse, figs, filberts, goat's milk, kale, kelp, mustard greens, oats, parsley, prunes, sesame seeds, tofu, turnip greens, whey, and yogurt.

Warnings

Oxalic acid (found in soybeans, kale, spinach, rhubarb, beet greens, almonds, cashews, chard, and cocoa) interferes with calcium absorption by binding with calcium in the intestines and producing insoluble salts that cannot be absorbed. Casual consumption of foods with oxalic acid should not pose a problem, however overindulgence inhibits absorption of calcium.

Calcium supplements should not be taken by those suffering from kidney stones or kidney disease. Calcium may interfere with the effects of Verapamil, a calcium channel blocker for the heart. Tums, as a source of calcium, neutralizes the stomach acid needed for calcium absorption. Calcium taken with iron reduces the effect of both minerals. Too much calcium can interfere with absorption of zinc, just as excess zinc can interfere with calcium absorption. A hair analysis can determine the levels of these two minerals if needed.

Insufficient vitamin D intake or excess phosphorus and magnesium hinders the uptake of calcium. Although heavy exercising also hinders calcium uptake, moderate exercising contributes to its uptake. A diet that is high either in protein, fat, or sugar also affects calcium uptake. The average American diet of meats, refined grains, and soft drinks (high in phosphorus) leads to increased bone loss in adults. Foods such as vegetables, fruits, and whole grains, which contain significant amounts of calcium but lower amounts of phosphorus, should be consumed.

Several vitamin companies use D_1-calcium-phosphate, but do not list it on the label. This form of calcium interferes with the absorption of the nutrients in a multisupplement.

Test your brand of calcium to assure absorption. Place the calcium pill in a glass of warm water and shake. If the calcium does not dissolve within twenty-four hours, change to another brand or form.

Chromium (GTF)

Because it is involved in the metabolism of glucose, chromium (glucose tolerance factor or GTF) is needed for energy. It is also vital in the synthesis of cholesterol, fats, and protein. This essential mineral maintains stable blood sugar levels through proper insulin utilization in both the diabetic and the hypoglycemic. Low plasma chromium levels are an indication of coronary artery disease.

The average American diet is chromium deficient. Researchers estimate that two out of every three Americans are either hypoglycemic, prehypoglycemic, or diabetic. The ability to maintain normal blood sugar levels is jeopardized by the lack of chromium in our soil and water supply and by a diet high in refined white sugar, flour, and junk foods.

Sources

Chromium is found in the following food sources: beer, brewer's yeast, brown rice, cheese, meat, and whole grains. It may also be found in dried beans, cheese, chicken, corn and corn oil, dairy products, calves' liver, mushrooms, and potatoes.

Warnings

No side effects have been found to date.

Copper

Among its many functions, copper aids in the formation of bone, hemoglobin, and red blood cells, and works in balance with zinc and vitamin C to form elastin. It is involved in the healing process, energy production, hair and skin coloring, and taste sensitivity. This mineral is also needed for healthy nerves.

One of the early signs of copper deficiency is osteoporosis. Copper is essential for the formation of collagen, which makes up the connective tissue of the bone matrix.

Sources

Besides its use in cookware and plumbing, copper is also widely distributed in foods. Its food sources include almonds, avocados, barley, beans, beet roots, blackstrap molasses, broccoli, dandelion greens, garlic, lentils, liver, mushrooms, nuts, oats, oranges, organ meats, pecans, radishes, raisins, salmon, seafood, soybeans, and green leafy vegetables.

Warnings

Copper levels in the body are reduced if high amounts of zinc or vitamin C are taken. If copper intake is too high, the levels of vitamin C and zinc will drop.

Germanium (Ge-132)

This important trace mineral was recently discovered and researched by a Japanese scientist, Kazuhiko Asai. He found that an intake of 100–300 milligrams of germanium a day improved many illnesses including rheu-matoid arthritis, food allergies, elevated cholesterol, candidiasis, chronic viral infections, cancer, and AIDS. Germanium is also a fast-acting pain killer. Germanium works by attaching itself to molecules of oxygen, which are carried into the body to improve cellular oxygenation. The body needs oxygen to keep the immune system functioning properly as oxygen helps rid the body of toxins and poisons. Dr. Asai believes all diseases are caused by an insufficient oxygen supply to the area of the body where it is needed. Researchers have shown that organic germanium is an effective way to increase tissue oxygenation because it acts as a carrier in the same way as hemoglobin.

Ge-132 is expensive because the amount found in plants is so minute, and a large number of plants are needed to obtain a small amount of this mineral. At present there is only one factory in Japan that is producing germanium.

For more information on germanium (Ge-132), contact: Global Marketing, 435 Brannan Street, San Francisco, CA 94107; (415) 459-8524.

Sources

The following foods contain germanium: aloe vera, comfrey, garlic, ginseng, shiitake mushrooms, onions, and the herb suma.

Warnings

No side effects have been found to date.

Iodine

Needed in only trace amounts, iodine helps to metabolize excess fat and is important in physical and mental development. Iodine is also needed for a healthy thyroid gland and in the prevention of goiter. Mental retardation may result from an iodine deficiency in children. In addition, an iodine deficiency has recently been linked to breast cancer.

Sources

Foods that are high in iodine include iodized salts, seafood, salt-water fish, and kelp. It may also be found in asparagus, dulse, white deep-water fish, garlic, lima beans, mushrooms, sea salt, sesame seeds, soybeans, spinach (see warnings below), summer squash, Swiss chard, and turnip greens.

Warnings

Some foods block the uptake of iodine into the thyroid gland when eaten raw in large amounts. These include

Brussels sprouts, cabbage, cauliflower, kale, peaches, pears, spinach, and turnips. If a hypothyroid disorder is present, limit these foods in the diet. Excess iodine (over thirty times the RDA) produces a metallic taste and sores in the mouth, swollen salivary glands, diarrhea, and vomiting.

Iron

Perhaps the most important of its functions is its production of hemoglobin and oxygenation of red blood cells. Iron is the mineral found in the largest amounts in the blood. This mineral is essential for many enzymes, and is important for growth in children and resistance to disease. Iron is also required for a healthy immune system and for energy production. Vitamin C can increase iron absorption as much as 30 percent.

Iron deficiency symptoms include brittle hair, nails that are spoon-shaped or that have ridges running lengthwise, hair loss, fatigue, pallor, dizziness, and anemia.

Sufficient hydrochloric acid (HCl) must be present in the stomach in order for the iron to be absorbed. Copper, manganese, molybdenum, vitamin A, and the B-complex vitamins are also needed for complete iron absorption.

According to *Journal of Orthomolecular Medicine*, iron utilization is impaired by rheumatoid arthritis and cancer and will result in anemia despite adequate amounts of iron stored in the liver, spleen, and bone marrow. The journal also states that iron deficiency is more prevalent in those suffering from candidiasis and chronic herpes infections.

Excess iron build-up in the tissues has been associated with a rare disease know as hemochromatosis, a disorder that causes bronze skin pigmentation, cirrhosis, diabetes, and heart disorders.

Sources

Iron is found in eggs, fish, liver, meat, poultry, green leafy vegetables, whole grains, and enriched breads and cereals. Other food sources include almonds, avocados, beets, blackstrap molasses, brewer's yeast, dates, dulse, egg yolks, kelp, kidney and lima beans, lentils, millet, parsley, peaches, pears, dried prunes, pumpkins, raisins, rice and wheat bran, sesame seeds, and soybeans.

Warnings

Excessive amounts of zinc and vitamin E interfere with iron absorption. Those who engage in strenuous exercise and who perspire heavily deplete iron from the body. Because iron is stored in the body, high iron intake can cause problems. Increased iron in the tissues and organs leads to the production of free radicals and

increases the need for vitamin E, an important antioxidant (free radical scavenger).

An iron deficiency may result from intestinal bleeding, excessive menstrual bleeding, a diet high in phosphorus, poor digestion, a long-term illness, ulcers, prolonged use of antacids, excess coffee or tea consumption, and causes other than a nutrient deficiency. A doctor should investigate these symptoms before prescribing iron supplements. In some cases, doctors have discovered that a vitamin B_6 or B_{12} deficiency is the underlying cause of the anemia.

According to a 1988 issue of *Journal of Orthomolecular Medicine*, you should not take extra iron if you have an infection. Because bacteria require iron for growth, the body stores iron and does not utilize it when there is an infection.

Magnesium

Magnesium is vital to enzyme activity. It assists in calcium and potassium uptake. A deficiency interferes with the transmission of nerve and muscle impulses, causing irritability and nervousness. Supplementing the diet with magnesium helps prevent depression, dizziness, muscle weakness, twitching, heart disease, and high blood pressure, and also aids in maintaining the proper pH balance. This essential mineral protects the arterial lining from stress caused by sudden blood pressure changes, and plays a role in the formation of bone and in carbohydrate and mineral metabolism. With vitamin B_6, magnesium helps reduce and dissolve calcium phosphate stones.

Sources

Magnesium is found in most foods, especially dairy products, fish, meat, and seafood. Other rich food sources include apples, apricots, avocados, bananas, blackstrap molasses, brewer's yeast, brown rice, figs, garlic, kelp, lima beans, millet, nuts, peaches, black-eyed peas, salmon, sesame seeds, tofu, tourla, green leafy vegetables, wheat, and whole grains.

Warnings

Consumption of alcohol, use of diuretics, diarrhea, the presence of fluoride, and high amounts of zinc and vitamin D all increase the body's need for magnesium. Magnesium combined with vitamin B_6 (pyridoxine) may prevent calcium oxalate kidney stones.

Large amounts of fats, cod liver oil, calcium, vitamin D, and protein decrease magnesium absorption. Foods high in oxalic acid, such as almonds, chard, cocoa, rhubarb, spinach, and tea, also inhibit magnesium absorption.

Manganese

Minute quantities of manganese are needed for protein and fat metabolism, healthy nerves, and healthy immune system and blood sugar regulation. It is used for energy production and is required for normal bone growth and reproduction. Manganese is essential for iron-deficient anemics and is also needed for the utilization of thiamine (B_1) and vitamin E. Manganese works well with the B-complex vitamins to give an overall feeling of well-being. It aids in the formation of mother's milk and is a key element in the production of enzymes needed to oxidize fats and to metabolize purines.

Sources

The largest quantities of manganese are found in avocados, nuts and seeds, seaweed, and whole grains. This mineral may also be found in blueberries, egg yolks, legumes, dried peas, pineapples, spinach, and green leafy vegetables.

Warnings

No side effects have been found to date.

Molybdenum

This essential mineral is needed in extremely small amounts for nitrogen metabolism, which enables the body to use nitrogen. It aids in the final stages of conversion of purines to uric acid. It promotes normal cell function, and is part of the enzyme system of xanthine oxidase. Molybdenum is found in the liver, bones, and kidneys. A low intake is associated with mouth and gum disorders and cancer. Those whose diets are high in refined and processed foods are at risk of having a deficiency. A molybdenum deficiency may cause sexual impotence in older males.

Sources

This trace mineral is found in beans, cereal grains, legumes, peas, and dark green leafy vegetables.

Warnings

Heat and moisture may change the action of the mineral. Massive intake of over 15 milligrams daily may produce gout. High intake of sulfur may decrease molybdenum levels. Excess amounts of molybdenum may interfere with copper metabolism.

Phosphorus

Phosphorus is needed for bone and tooth formation, cell growth, contraction of the heart muscle, and kidney function. It also assists the body in the utilization of vitamins and the conversion of food to energy. A balance of magnesium, calcium, and phosphorus should always be maintained. If one of these is present in excess or insufficient amounts, it will have adverse effects on the body.

Sources

A deficiency of phosphorus is rare because it is found in most foods, especially soda. Significant amounts of phosphorus are contained in asparagus; bran; brewer's yeast; corn; dairy products; eggs; fish; dried fruit; garlic; legumes; nuts; sesame, sunflower, and pumpkin seeds; meats; poultry; salmon; and whole grains.

Warnings

Excessive amounts of phosphorus interfere with calcium uptake. A diet consisting of junk food is a common culprit.

Potassium

This mineral is important for a healthy nervous system and a regular heart rhythm. It helps prevent stroke, aids in proper muscle contraction, and works with sodium to control the body's water balance. Potassium is important for chemical reactions within the cells and aids in maintaining stable blood pressure and in transmitting electrochemical impulses. It also regulates the transfer of nutrients to the cells.

Sources

Food sources of potassium include dairy foods, fish, fruit, legumes, meat, poultry, vegetables, and whole grains. It is specifically found in apricots, avocados, bananas, blackstrap molasses, brewer's yeast, brown rice, dates, figs, dried fruit, garlic, nuts, potatoes, raisins, winter squash, tourla, wheat bran, and yams.

Warnings

Use of diuretics, kidney disorders, diarrhea, and laxatives all disrupt potassium levels. Although potassium is needed for hormone secretion, hormones secreted as a result of stress cause a decrease in the potassium-sodium ratio both inside and outside the cell.

Selenium

Selenium is a vital antioxidant, especially when combined with vitamin E. As an antioxidant, selenium protects the immune system by preventing the formation of free radicals, which can damage the body. (*See also* ANTIOXIDANTS in Part One and the free radical inset in RADIATION POISONING in Part Two.) Selenium and vitamin E act synergistically to aid in the production of antibodies and to help maintain a healthy heart. This trace element is needed for pancreatic function and tissue elasticity. A selenium deficiency is linked to cancer and heart disease.

Because New Zealand soils are low in selenium, its cattle and sheep have suffered a breakdown of muscles, including the heart muscle. However, human intake of selenium is adequate because of imported Australian wheat.

Sources

Depending on the soil content, selenium can be found in meat and grains. It can also be found in Brazil nuts, brewer's yeast, broccoli, brown rice, chicken, dairy products, garlic, liver, molasses, onions, salmon, seafood, tourla, tuna, vegetables, wheat germ, and whole grains.

Warnings

No side effects have been found to date.

Silicon (Silica)

Silicon is necessary for bone and connective tissue (collagen) formation, for healthy nails, skin, and hair, and for calcium absorption in the early stages of bone formation. It is needed to maintain flexible arteries, and plays a major role in preventing cardiovascular disease. Silicon counteracts the effects of aluminum on the body and is important in the prevention of Alzheimer's disease and osteoporosis. Silicon levels decrease with aging and, therefore, are needed in larger amounts by the elderly.

Boron, calcium, magnesium, manganese, and potassium aid in efficient utilization of silicon.

Sources

Foods that contain silicon include alfalfa, beets, brown rice, horsetail grass (an herb), mother's milk, bell peppers, soybeans, leafy green vegetables, and whole grains.

Warnings

No side effects have been found to date.

Sodium

Sodium is necessary for maintaining the proper water balance and blood pH. It is also needed for stomach, nerve, and muscle function. Although a sodium deficiency is rare, its symptoms include confusion, low blood sugar, weakness, dehydration, lethargy, and heart palpitations. Because a balance of potassium and sodium is necessary for good health but most people overindulge in sodium intake, potassium is typically needed in greater amounts.

Sources

Virtually all foods contain some sodium.

Warnings

Excess sodium intake results in edema, high blood pressure, potassium deficiency, and liver and kidney disease. Sodium intake may lead to heart disease when not properly balanced with potassium.

Sulfur

An acid-forming mineral that is part of the chemical structure of methionine, cysteine, taurine, and glutathione, sulfur disinfects the blood, resists bacteria, and protects the protoplasm of cells. It aids in oxidation reactions, stimulates bile secretions in the liver, and protects against toxic substances. Because of its ability to protect against the harmful effects of radiation and pollution, sulfur slows down the aging process and extends life span. It is found in hemoglobin and all body tissues and is needed for the synthesis of collagen, which prevents dryness and maintains elastin in the skin.

Sources

The following foods contain sulfur: Brussels sprouts, dried beans, cabbage, eggs, fish, garlic, horsetail (herb), kale, meats, onions, soybeans, turnips, wheat germ, and the amino acids L-cysteine, L-lysine, L-cystine, and L-methionine. DaVinci Laboratories supply sulfur in tablet and powdered form.

Warnings

Moisture and heat may destroy or change the action of sulfur in the body.

Vanadium

Vanadium is needed for cellular metabolism and in the formation of bones and teeth. It plays a role in growth and reproduction, and inhibits cholesterol synthesis. A vanadium deficiency may be linked to cardiovascular and kidney disease, impaired reproductive ability, and increased infant mortality. Vanadium is not easily absorbed.

Sources

Vanadium is found in fish, vegetable oils, and olives. It may also be found in snap beans, dill, meat, radishes, and whole grains.

Warnings

There may be an interaction between vanadium and chromium. Take extra chromium at a different time. Tobacco decreases uptake of vanadium.

Zinc

This essential mineral is important in prostate gland function and the growth of the reproductive organs. It is required for protein synthesis and collagen formation and promotes a healthy immune system and the healing of wounds. Zinc also allows acuity of taste and smell and protects the liver from chemical damage.

Sufficient intake and absorption of zinc is needed to maintain the proper concentrations of vitamin E in the blood.

Sources

Zinc is found in the following food sources: fish, legumes, meats, oysters, poultry, seafood, and whole grains. Significant quantities of zinc are found in brewer's yeast, egg yolks, lamb chops, lima beans, liver, mushrooms, pecans, pumpkin seeds, sardines, seeds, soy lecithin, soybeans, sunflower seeds, and tourla.

Warnings

Daily dosages of more than 100 milligrams of zinc can depress the immune system while dosages under 100 milligrams can enhance immune response. Zinc levels may be lowered by diarrhea, kidney disease, cirrhosis of the liver, diabetes, and fiber. The phylates found in grains and legumes bind with zinc so that it cannot be absorbed.

The proper copper and zinc balance should be maintained. Consumption of hard water can upset zinc levels.

WATER

INTRODUCTION

The human body is composed of approximately 70 percent water. In fact, the body's water supply is responsible for and involved in nearly every body process including digestion, absorption, circulation, and excretion. Water is also the primary transporter of nutrients throughout the body and is necessary for all building functions in the body. Water helps maintain a normal body temperature and is essential for carrying waste material out of the body. Therefore, replacing the water that is continually lost through daily sweat and elimination is very important. It is essential for the proper functioning of the body to drink at least eight glasses of quality water each day. Remember that while the body can survive without food for about five weeks, the body cannot survive without water for longer than five days.

It would seem relatively easy to use or purchase water that meets our particular needs; however, due to the numerous types of classifications given water, the average consumer can be easily confused about what is available. Water is usually classified either by its source (spring, spa, geyser, public water supply, etc.), by its mineral content (containing at least 500 parts per million of dissolved solids), or by the system of treatment it has gone through (purified, deionized, fluoridated, steam-distilled, etc.). Because there is a lot of overlap in the criteria used to group water, some water appears in more than one classification. In addition, most states have no rules governing appropriate labeling, so a number of bottled water claims may be misleading or incorrect. The following is a guide to understanding what the most commonly used classifications of water mean and how these varying waters may help or harm the body.

HARD VERSUS SOFT WATER

Hard water, found in varying parts of the country, contains the minerals calcium and magnesium, which prevent soap from lathering and deposit a sediment film on hair, clothing, pipes, dishes, and wash tubs. Although hard water can be annoying, studies show that deaths from heart disease are lower in areas where the drinking water is hard. However, we believe that the calcium found in hard water is not good for the heart, arteries, or bones. Unfortunately, hard water deposits its calcium and other minerals on the *outside* of these structures while it is the calcium found *within* these structures that is beneficial to the body.

Soft water can be naturally soft or it may be hard water that has been treated with sodium in order to remove the calcium and magnesium. The problem with artificially softened water is that it is more likely than hard water to dissolve the lining of pipes. This poses a significant threat where lead pipes are used. In addition, plastic and galvanized pipes are composed of cadmium, posing another threat of toxic poisioning. Although these two types of pipe are now rarely used, today's copper pipes can lead to dangerous levels of copper, iron, zinc, and arsenic entering the body through the use of soft water. (*See* ENVIRONMENTAL TOXICITY in Part Two.)

DEIONIZED OR DEMINERALIZED WATER

When the electric charge of an atom or molecule has been neutralized by removing or adding electrons, the resulting water is called deionized or demineralized. The deionization process removes nitrates and the minerals calcium and magnesium from water, in addition to the heavy metals cadmium, barium, lead, and some forms of radium.

FILTERED WATER

Water filtration is the means by which water is made pure, clean, uncontaminated, and better tasting. There are many different types of filtered water and ways in which water can be treated. Nature filters water by running water through streams. As this water passes over the rocks in the stream, the bacteria in the water leeches onto the rocks and is replaced with minerals such as calcium and magnesium.

In addition to nature, there are man-made ways of filtering water such as distillation, the granular activated carbon process, and reverse osmosis. (*See* DISTILLATION under its own heading in this section.)

The granular activated carbon process typically uses a solid, absorbent material that picks up the water's organic contaminants as the water passes through it. This process reduces the chlorine taste of the water.

Reverse osmosis is considered a good way in which

to filter water. It uses a special semipermeable membrane filter to strain impurities out of the water. However, we believe that no filter can prevent bacteria or viruses from passing through. Each pore of the finest filter is large enough for millions of germs to permeate.

FLUORIDATED WATER

For years now controversy has raged over whether fluoride should be added to drinking water. Proponents say that fluoride occurs naturally and helps develop and maintain strong bones and teeth. Opponents to fluoridation contend that toxic levels of fluorine, the poisonous substance that fluoride is derived from, build up in the body, causing irreparable harm to the immune system.

Today, more than half the cities in the United States fluoridate their water supplies. Although many ailments and disorders have been linked to fluoridated water such as Down's syndrome, mottled teeth, and cancer, fluoridation has become the standard rather than the exception.

Should your tap water contain fluoride, and you wish to remove it, you can use a reverse osmosis or distillation system to eliminate almost all of the fluoride from your water.

MINERAL WATER

Mineral water is natural spring water usually coming from Europe or Canada. The water must flow freely from the source, cannot be pumped or forced from the ground, and must be bottled directly at the source. Depending on where the source is, the water will contain varying minerals. If you are suffering from a deficiency in certain minerals and are drinking mineral water for therapeutic reasons, you must be aware of which minerals are in the particular brand of water you are drinking. If you are drinking mineral water containing minerals that you do not lack, then you could be doing more harm than good.

NATURAL SPRING WATER

Natural water means that the mineral content has not been altered, but it may or may not have been filtered or otherwise treated. Spring water rises naturally to the earth's surface from underground reservoirs. This water is unprocessed, and flavor or carbonation may be added.

STEAM-DISTILLED WATER

Distillation involves the process of vaporizing water by boiling it. The steam rises, leaving behind most bacteria, viruses, chemicals, minerals, and pollutants from the water. The steam is then moved into a condensing chamber where it is cooled and condensed to become distilled water.

Once consumed, steam-distilled water leaches inorganic minerals rejected by the cells and tissues out of the body. We believe that only steam-distilled water should be consumed.

One way in which flavor can be added to the water is to add one to two tablespoons of raw apple cider vinegar (obtained from a health food store) to one gallon of the distilled water. Vinegar is an excellent solvent and aids in digestion. For added minerals, you can also put Concentrace mineral drops by Trace Minerals Research Laboratories in steam-distilled water. Add two tablespoons of mineral drops to every five gallons of water.

TAP WATER

Water that comes out of household taps or faucets is obtained from surface water, that is, water that has run off from ponds, creeks, streams, rivers, and lakes. However, rainwater can wash pollutants into these bodies of water, causing our drinking water to be contaminated. Fertilizer and insecticide residue can easily be washed into surface water as can lead from automobile and factory exhausts. In addition, in order to purify drinking water, chemicals such as alum, carbon, chlorine, fluorine, lime, phosphates, soda ash, and sodium aluminates are often added. These chemicals are used to kill the bacteria found in water, but are now believed to cause cancer. Other toxic substances that may be found in tap water are arsenic, asbestos, cadmium, and cyanides, which can combine with the other chemicals to form carcinogenic substances.

Not all of these toxic substances are found in all drinking water. Some cities rate higher in water safety than others. In addition, not all cities and towns add chemicals or filter their water supplies in any way. Other cities and towns add chemicals to their water to kill bacteria, while still other cities and towns filter their water. It is up to the individual to find out how the drinking water is treated in order to determine how safe the water is that is coming out of his tap.

The taste of tap water can be improved in several ways. Boiling tap water will kill bacteria. However, the water must then be refrigerated if it is to be used for drinking. The taste can also be improved by keeping the water in an uncovered pitcher for several hours. In this way, the heavy chlorine taste and odor will dissipate. Water can also be aerated in a blender to remove chlorine and other chemicals. Nevertheless, none of these methods will improve the quality of the water—only the taste.

WATER ANALYSIS

The EPA has defined pure water as "bacteriologically safe" water, and it recommends—but does not require—that the water have a pH between 6.5 and 8.5. This allows a great deal of leeway for what passes as acceptable water. If you are concerned about what type of water is coming out of your tap, you can contact your local water officials or local health department, which may test your tap water free of charge. In some cases, you may have to contact your state's water supply or health department.

Typically, these agencies test the water only for bacteria levels, not for toxic substances. Therefore, you might want to contact a commercial laboratory or local state university laboratory to test your water for chemical content. Should you have any questions about the various types of water or methods of water treatment, you may contact the Water Quality Association at P.O. Box 606, Lisle, IL 60532.

If you find that your tap water is unacceptable either because of its taste or because of its toxic chemical content, you may choose to use one of the alternative water supplies described in this section.

AMINO ACIDS

THE FUNCTION OF AMINO ACIDS

Amino acids are the chemical units or the "building blocks," as they are popularly called, that make up proteins. Protein could not exist without the proper combination of amino acids. To understand how vital amino acids are, you must understand how essential proteins are to life. It is protein that provides the structure for all living things. Each organism from the largest animal to the tiniest microbe is composed of protein. And in its various forms, it is protein that participates in the vital chemical processes that enable us to sustain life.

In the human body, protein substances make up the muscles, ligaments, tendons, organs, glands, nails, hair, and body fluids (except for bile and urine). Proteins are essential for the growth of bones. Enzymes, hormones, and genes are also comprised of various proteins. Next to water, protein makes up the greatest portion of our body weight. Consequently, it is easy to see why meeting our body's protein requirements is so important to good health.

In order for a protein to be complete, it must contain all of its particular amino acids. Amino acids may be linked together almost indefinitely to form more than 50,000 different proteins and 20,000 known enzymes. Because each type of protein is composed of different amino acids, each being tailored for a specific need, they are not interchangeable. Amino acids contain about 16 percent nitrogen. This distinguishes them from carbohydrates and fats in the body.

The central nervous system cannot function without amino acids, which act as neurotransmitters or as precursors to the neurotransmitters. They are necessary in order for the brain to receive and send messages. Unless all of the amino acids are present together, almost anything can go wrong with the transmission of the message. A meal high in protein will temporarily increase alertness (see DEPRESSION in Part Two for more information).

There are approximately twenty-nine commonly known amino acids that account for the hundreds of different types of proteins present in all living things. In the human body, the liver produces about 80 percent of the amino acids we need. The remaining 20 percent must be obtained from outside sources. The amino acids that must be obtained from the diet are called *essential amino acids.* The essential amino acids that enter the body through diet are arginine, histidine, isoleucine, leucine, lysine, methionine, phenylalanine, threonine, tryptophan, and valine. Other amino acids that the body seems to be able to manufacture from other sources are alanine, arginine, aspartic acid, asparagine, glutamic acid, glutamine, glycine, proline, and serine.

Most of the amino acids (excluding glycine) can appear in two forms—one being the mirror image of the other. These are called the D- and L-series. Because amino acids in the L-series are in the same natural form as amino acids found in living plant or animal tissue, they are considered to be more compatible to human biochemistry. The ones that make up a protein are all of the L-configuration, except phenylalanine, which can also appear as DL-phenylalanine.

The process of assembling amino acids to make proteins or breaking down proteins into individual amino acids for the body's use is continuous. When we need more enzyme proteins, the body produces more enzyme proteins; when we need more cells, the body produces more proteins for cells. These different types of proteins are produced as the need arises. Should the body deplete itself of its reserves of any of the essential amino acids, it would not be able to produce those proteins requiring such amino acids. The resulting protein shortage could easily lead to any number of disorders.

How could such a deficiency occur? Easier than you might think. If the diet is improperly balanced, that is, contains inadequate amounts of the essential amino acids, physical disorders will arise. Other symptoms will appear if an individual suffers from a protein deficiency stemming from his inability to digest food properly. In order to avoid such problems, we can make sure we eat a properly balanced diet, or we can take supplements containing essential amino acids.

In addition to their other vital functions, amino acids enable vitamins and minerals to perform their jobs properly. Even if the vitamins and minerals are absorbed and assimilated rapidly, they will not be effective unless amino acids are present.

WHAT'S ON THE SHELVES

Amino acids are available in combination with various multivitamin formulas, as protein mixtures, in a wide variety of food supplements, and in a number of amino acid formulas. They can be purchased as capsules, tablets, and powders. Most amino acid supplements are derived from egg protein, yeast protein, or animal protein. The crystalline free form amino acids are generally extracted from a variety of grain products. Brown rice bran is a prime source, although cold-pressed yeast and milk proteins are also used. Amino acids in the free form are the purest. Free form amino acids can be taken for rapid absorption. These white crystalline amino acids are stable at room temperature and decompose when heated to temperatures between 350° F and 660° F (180° C and 350° C).

THE ABC'S OF AMINO ACIDS

Each amino acid has specific functions and is needed to prevent various symptoms from developing. The many functions and deficiency symptoms of twenty-eight amino acids are described below. When taking amino acids individually for healing purposes, take them on an empty stomach to avoid competition with other amino acids for absorption. Amino acids compete with each other for entry to the brain.

L-Alanine

L-Alanine is the amino acid that aids in the metabolism of glucose, a simple carbohydrate that the body uses for energy.

L-Arginine

L-Arginine causes retardation of tumors and cancer, aids in liver detoxification, assists in the release of growth hormones and maintenance of a healthy immune system, detoxifies ammonia, increases sperm count in males, and aids in kidney disorders and trauma. Scar tissue that forms during wound healing has a high arginine content. This amino acid is needed for protein synthesis and for optimum growth. An increase in muscle mass and a reduction of body fat occurs in the presence of L-arginine. It also helps increase production of collagen, and is good for liver disorders such as cirrhosis of the liver and fatty liver. L-Arginine should be avoided if pregnant or lactating.

L-Asparagine

L-Asparagine is needed to maintain balance in the cen-tral nervous system, preventing you from being overly nervous or overly calm.

L-Aspartic Acid

Because L-aspartic acid increases stamina, it is good for fatigue. Chronic fatigue may result from low levels of aspartic acid due to lowered cellular energy. This amino acid also protects the liver by aiding in the removal of excess ammonia from the body. L-aspartic acid combines with other amino acids to form molecules that absorb toxins and remove them from the bloodstream. It aids cell function and RNA/DNA formation.

L-Carnitine

L-Carnitine helps to transport long-chain fatty acids. By preventing fatty build-up, this amino acid aids in weight loss, decreases the risk for heart disease, and improves athletic ability. Carnitine can be manufactured in the body if sufficient amounts of lysine, B_1, B_6, and iron are available. Vegetarians are more likely to be deficient in carnitine due to a diet that is low in lysine.

Carnitine also enhances the effectiveness of antioxidant vitamins E and C.

L-Citrulline

L-Citrulline promotes energy, stimulates the immune system, metabolizes to L-arginine, and detoxifies ammonia, which damages living cells.

L-Cysteine

L-Cysteine has a high sulfur content. This amino acid is formed from L-methionine in the body; however, vitamin B_6 is necessary for this conversion. L-Cysteine helps to detoxify harmful toxins, thereby protecting and preserving the cells. Cysteine is a precursor to L-glutathione. One of the best free radical destroyers, it works best when taken with selenium and vitamin E. In addition to protecting the cells from the harmful effects of radiation, it protects the liver and brain from damage due to alcohol and cigarette smoke. Supplementation with L-cysteine is recommended in the treatment of rheumatoid arthritis. L-Cysteine has a chelating effect, removing excess copper from the body. This amino acid also promotes the burning of fat and the building of muscle.

Because of its ability to break down mucus in the respiratory tract, L-cysteine is often beneficial in the treatment of bronchitis, emphysema, and tuberculosis.

Cysteine is very unstable and is easily converted to L-cystine. You may purchase either L-cysteine or L-cystine supplements; each will offer the same benefits.

L-Cystine

Like L-Cysteine, L-cystine has a high sulfur content. It aids in the formation of skin and is important in detoxification. By reducing the body's absorption of copper, cystine protects against copper toxicity. This amino acid is necessary for the healing of burns and wounds after surgery. It promotes healing in respiratory disorders such as bronchitis, and plays an important role in the activity of the white blood cells, which fight disease. It assists in the supply of insulin to the pancreas, which is needed for assimilation of sugars and starches.

Gamma-Aminobutyric Acid

Gamma-aminobutyric acid (GABA) inhibits cells from overfiring. GABA can be taken to calm the body in much the same way as valium, librium, and other tranquilizers without the fear of addiction. Take 750 milligrams of this amino acid for its tranquilizing effect. GABA is being recommended in place of many drugs. With niacinamide and inositol, it prevents anxiety and stress-related messages from reaching the motor centers of the brain by filling its receptor site. GABA functions as a neurotransmitter in the central nervous system by decreasing neuron activity.

L-Glutamic Acid

L-Glutamic acid (or glutamate) increases firing of neurons in the nervous system. It metabolizes sugars and fats, and detoxifies ammonia when used with L-glutamine. This amino acid also helps correct personality disorders. Besides glucose, glutamic acid is the only compound used for brain fuel. The brain converts glutamic acid to a compound that regulates brain cell activity.

L-Glutamine

L-Glutamine is important in alcoholism, craving for sugar, mental ability, impotence, fatigue, epilepsy, senility, schizophrenia, mental retardation, peptic ulcers, and maintenance of a healthy digestive tract. It is converted to glutamic acid in the brain, which is essential for cerebral function, and increases the amount of GABA needed. Do not substitute glutamic acid for glutamine in the treatment of alcoholism; it does not work as well.

L-Glutathione

L-Glutathione is a powerful antioxidant that inhibits the formation of free radicals. It protects against damage from cigarette smoking and radiation, helps reduce the side effects of chemotherapy and x-rays, and combats alcohol poisoning. As a detoxifier of metals and drugs, it aids in the treatment of blood and liver disorders.

L-Glycine

L-Glycine retards muscle degeneration by supplying additional creatine. It is necessary for central nervous system function and a healthy prostate. Its inhibitory action helps prevent epilepsy. This amino acid has been used in the treatment of bipolar depression. L-Glycine is needed by the immune system for the synthesis of the nonessential amino acids. Too much of this amino acid can displace glucose in the metabolic chain and cause fatigue. The proper amount produces more energy.

L-Histidine

L-Histidine is significant in growth and repair of tissues, ulcers, hyperacidity, digestion, and gastric juices. It is needed for the treatment of allergies, rheumatoid arthritis, anemia, and in the production of red and white blood cells. Histamine is formed from histidine, and is released by the cells usually as an immune response. Both histamine and L-histidine can chelate trace elements like copper from the body.

L-Isoleucine

L-Isoleucine is needed for hemoglobin formation and also stabilizes and regulates the blood sugar and energy levels. It is metabolized in muscle tissue. Always take with the correct balance of leucine and valine. A deficiency of L-isoleucine can lead to symptoms similar to those for hypoglycemia.

L-Leucine

L-Leucine lowers elevated blood sugar levels. It must be taken in balance with isoleucine and valine. This important amino acid promotes the healing of bones, skin, and muscle tissue. This is a recommended supplement for those recovering from surgery. Leucine must be taken in moderation, otherwise hypoglycemia may result.

L-Lysine

As an essential building block for all protein, the amino acid L-lysine is needed for proper growth and bone development in children. It helps calcium absorption and maintains nitrogen balance in adults. Among the many functions of this amino acid is its ability to fight cold sores and herpes viruses; to aid in the production of antibodies, hormones, and enzymes; and to help in collagen formation and in the repair of tissue. Because it helps to build muscle protein, it is especially important for those recovering from surgery and sports injuries. It lowers high serum triglycerides as well.

Deficiencies result in loss of energy, inability to concentrate, irritability, bloodshot eyes, hair loss, anemia, retarded growth, and reproduction disorders.

L-Methionine

L-Methionine is not synthesized in the body, and must be obtained from food sources or from dietary supplements. In addition to being a good source of sulfur, L-methionine is important in the treatment of rheumatic fever and toxemia resulting from pregnancy. It assists in the breakdown of fats, preventing the build-up of fat in the liver and arteries, which obstructs blood flow to the brain, heart, and kidneys. This amino acid helps the digestive system, interacts with other substances to detoxify harmful agents, aids muscle weakness, helps to prevent brittle hair, and is beneficial for allergic chemical sensitivities and osteoporosis. Cysteine and taurine may rely on methionine for synthesis in the body.

Because the body uses L-methionine to derive a brain food called choline, it would be wise to supplement the diet with choline or lecithin (which is high in choline) so that the supply of L-methionine is not depleted.

L-Ornithine

L-Ornithine helps release a growth hormone that metabolizes excess body fat when combined with L-arginine and L-carnitine. It is necessary for immune system and liver function. This amino acid also detoxifies ammonia and promotes healing. Do not give this supplement to children unless prescribed by your physician.

L-Phenylalanine

L-Phenylalanine is often used to treat depression. It produces neurotransmitters, is used by the brain to manufacture norepinephrine, and aids in memory, learning, and obesity. Because of its action in the central nervous system, this amino acid elevates moods, enables the individual to overcome depression, and decreases the pain associated with migraines, menstruation, and arthritis.

L-Phenylalanine should not be used by pregnant women or those with high blood pressure, PKU (phenylketonuria), or with preexisting pigmented melanoma (a type of cancer).

DL-Phenylalanine

DL-Phenylalanine is very effective in the control of pain, especially in those with arthritis. It functions as a building block of all amino acids, increases mental alertness, suppresses the appetite, and aids in Parkinson's disease. Use with caution if you are pregnant or diabetic, or if you have high blood pressure.

L-Proline

L-Proline improves skin texture by aiding in the production of collagen, heals cartilage, and strengthens joints, tendons, and the heart muscle.

L-Serine

L-Serine is needed for proper metabolism of fats and fatty acids, muscle growth, and a healthy immune system, and it aids in the production of immunoglobulins and antibodies.

L-Taurine

High concentrations of L-taurine are found in the heart muscle, white blood cells, skeletal muscle, and central nervous system. This amino acid aids in fat digestion, heart disorders, hypoglycemia, artherosclerosis, hypertension, and edema, and acts as a building block of all the amino acids. It is a key component of bile, which is needed for the digestion of fats, the absorption of fat-soluble vitamins, and the control of serum cholesterol levels. Epilepsy, anxiety, hyperactivity, and poor brain function are related to L-taurine deficiency.

L-Taurine is not found in most animal proteins; therefore, synthesis by the body is crucial. Taurine may be synthesized from cysteine, but requires vitamin B_6 for this conversion.

L-Threonine

L-Threonine helps to maintain protein balance in the body. It is important for the formation of collagen and elastin, and aids liver and lipotropic function when combined with L-aspartic acid and L-methionine. L-Threonine is present in the heart, central nervous system, and skeletal muscle. This important amino acid helps to control epileptic seizures.

L-Tryptophan

L-Tryptophan is necessary for the production of niacin. It cures insomnia, helps stabilize moods, and is used by the brain to produce serotonin, a necessary neurotransmitter that transfers nerve impulses from one cell to another and is responsible for normal sleep. It helps control hyperactivity in children, alleviates stress, is good for the heart, aids in weight control, and enhances the release of growth hormones necessary for the production of vitamin B_6 (pyridoxine). A sufficient amount of vitamin B_6 is necessary for the formation of tryptophan, which, in turn, is required for the formation of serotonin.

In November of 1989, the Centers for Disease Control (CDC) reported evidence linking L-tryptophan supplements to a blood disorder called eosinophilia-myaglia syndrome (EMS). This illness, which is characterized by an elevated white blood cell count, has been reported in 475 cases as of November 27 and has resulted in at least one death. Common symptoms of EMS are muscular pain, fatigue, and respiratory ailments such as difficult breathing and coughing. Victims may also experience painful swelling (edema) of the extremities and/or a rash.

After the CDC established an association between the blood disorder and products containing L-tryptophan in New Mexico, the Food and Drug Administration warned consumers to stop taking L-tryptophan supplements. The FDA has since recalled all products in which L-tryptophan is the sole or major component. The cause of EMS is still unknown.

L-Tyrosine

L-Tyrosine is important in the treatment of anxiety, depression, allergies, and headaches. It aids in the production of melanin (pigment of the skin and hair) and in the functions of the adrenal, thyroid, and pituitary glands. Low plasma levels of tyrosine have been associated with hypothyroidism. It acts as a mood elevator, suppresses the appetite, and reduces body fat. It is involved in the initial breakdown of phenylalanine in the liver. L-Tyrosine can be produced from L-phenylalanine. A lack of tyrosine triggers a deficiency of the hormone norephinephrine at a specific brain location, which results in depression and mood disorders. In addition to being a precursor for norepinephrine, L-tyrosine is also used to synthesize epinephrine and dopamine. It has been used for withdrawal from drugs.

L-Valine

L-Valine has a stimulant effect. A deficiency results in negative hydrogen balance of the body. For better muscle metabolism, tissue repair, and nitrogen balance, use valine with leucine and isoleucine.

ANTIOXIDANTS

INTRODUCTION

There is a group of vitamins, minerals, and enzymes called *antioxidants* that help protect our body from the formation of free radicals. *Free radicals* are atoms or groups of atoms that can cause damage to our cells, impairing our immune system and leading to infections and various degenerative diseases. There are three known free radicals—the superoxide, the hydroxyl, and peroxide. (*See also* RADIATION POISONING in Part Two for an inset on free radicals.) They may be formed by exposure to radiation and toxic chemicals, overexposure to the sun's rays, or through the action of various metabolic processes, such as the use of stored fat molecules for energy.

The way in which free radicals are normally kept in check is by the action of *free radical scavengers* that occur naturally in the body. These scavengers neutralize the free radicals. Certain enzymes serve this vital function. Four important enzymes that neutralize free radicals naturally are superoxide dismutase (SOD), methione reductase, catalase, and glutathione peroxidase. The body makes these as a matter of course. In addition, the work of these scavenger enzymes can be supplemented by a diet rich in antioxidants such as vitamins A, E, and C, the mineral selenium, and other nutrients. These antioxidants are also scavengers, gobbling up the free radical particles.

THE ANTIOXIDANTS

If the diet is inadequate or lacking the appropriate anti-oxidants, or if the system is overwhelmed by free radicals, you can take the following supplements to aid the body in destroying free radicals.

Vitamin A

Vitamin A is necessary for healthy mucous cells and promotes germ-killing enzymes. Beta-carotene and vitamin A destroy carcinogens (cancer-producing substances).

Vitamin C

In addition to increasing interferon production, vitamin C is a potent stimulator of T-effector cell activity and is also a very powerful antioxidant. Vitamin C reduces lipid production in the brain and spinal cord, which frequently incur free radical damage. These sites can be protected by significant amounts of vitamin C, which is needed to cross the blood-brain barrier. Vitamin C acts as a more potent free radical scavenger in the presence of a bioflavonoid called hesperidin.

Vitamin E

Vitamin E is a powerful antioxidant that prevents fat and cell membrane rancidity and protects the coating around each cell. Vitamin E improves oxygen utilization and enhances immune response. New evidence suggests that zinc is needed to maintain normal blood concentrations of vitamin E.

Gamma-Linoleic Acid (GLA)

GLA is a key regulator of T-lymphocyte function in the body. GLA can be made from linoleic acid, which is found in vegetable oils, but if zinc, magnesium, and vitamins C, B_6 (pyridoxine), B_3 (niacin), and A are deficient, the conversion may be blocked. Hydrogenated vegetable oils, margarine, or a high-fat diet can also inhibit this important conversion to GLA. Evening primrose oil, black currant seed oil, and borage oil are the main sources of pre-formed GLA.

L-Cysteine

This sulphur-containing amino acid is needed to produce glutathione. It is used by the liver and the lymphocytes to detoxify chemicals and germ poisons. Cysteine is a powerful detoxifier of alcohol, tobacco smoke, and environmental pollutants, all of which are immune suppressors.

L-Glutathione

This powerful antioxidant rids the body of free radicals, protecting it from the harmful effects of metals, drugs, cigarette smoke, and alcohol.

Selenium

A partner/synergist with vitamin E, selenium is essential for the key enzyme, glutathione peroxidase (each enzyme molecule contains four selenium atoms). It stimulates increased antibody response to germ infection.

Superoxide Dismutase (SOD)

SOD is an enzyme. A health body produces nearly 5 million units of SOD and its partner catalase daily. SOD revitalizes the cells and reduces the rate of cell destruction. It removes the most common free radical, superoxide. SOD also aids in the body's utilization of zinc, copper, and manganese. Free radical production increases with aging, while SOD levels are reduced. The potential of SOD to slow the aging process is currently being explored. The SOD supplement in pill form must be enteric coated, that is, coated with a protective substance that allows the SOD pill to pass intact through the stomach acid into the small intestines to be absorbed. A supplement should be able to provide a daily amount of about 5 million units or higher. SOD naturally occurs in barley grass, broccoli, Brussels sprouts, cabbage, wheatgrass, and most green plants.

AOX/PLX From Biotec Foods

This product contains large amounts of antioxidants to aid the body in destroying free radicals.

ENZYMES

WHAT ARE ENZYMES?

Found in all living plant and animal matter, enzymes are essential for maintaining proper function of the body, digesting food, and aiding in the repair of tissue. Made up of protein, the thousands of known enzymes play a role in virtually all body activities. In fact, life could not be sustained without enzymes, despite the presence of sufficient amounts of vitamins, minerals, water, and proteins. Scientists are unable to manufacture enzymes synthetically.

Each enzyme has a specific function in the body that no other enzyme can fulfill. The shape of a particular enzyme is so specialized that it will initiate a reaction in only certain substances. The substance that is altered in the presence of the enzyme is called the substrate. The enzyme grasps, holds, and binds the substrate with other molecules, increasing its rate of reaction with these substances. Most reactions in cells are catalyzed (initiated) by these essential proteins, whose mineral component allows the reaction to take place. Because enzymes are needed for numerous body functions, it is important that they not be overloaded. For example, if the body must produce sufficient amounts of enzymes for digestive function, then production of enzymes for proper metabolic function may be lacking.

While the body manufactures a supply of enzymes, it can also obtain enzymes from food. Unfortunately, enzymes are extremely sensitive to heat. Low degrees of heat will destroy enzymes in food, so in order to obtain enzymes from the diet, the food must be eaten raw. Cooked foods will be depleted of all enzymes. Those who do not eat raw foods or supplement their diets with enzymes put undue strain on the supply of enzymes in their bodies. Because enzymes are the only nutrients that can supply the body with energy needed for its activities, overuse can impair the functioning capacity of the body, making it susceptible to cancer, obesity, cardiovascular disease, and a host of other illnesses.

To ease the burden of the enzymes manufactured in the body, it is helpful to eat raw foods. Not only will they supply enzymes for use by the body, but they will also inhibit the release of enzymes by the body that occurs with the consumption of cooked foods. This enables the body's supply of enzymes to work at a higher capac-

ity when needed. Avocados, bananas, and mangos are rich in enzymes, but sprouts are its highest source. If cooked and raw foods are eaten at the same meal, take one to three enzyme supplements during the meal—not afterward. Enzyme capsules can be opened and sprinkled on the food.

THE FUNCTION OF ENZYMES

Enzymes assist in practically all body functions. In hydrolysis, digestive enzymes break down food particles for storage in the liver or muscles. This stored energy is later converted by other enzymes for use by the body when necessary. Enzymes also utilize food ingested by the body to construct new muscle tissue, nerve cells, bone, skin, or glandular tissue. For example, one enzyme can take dietary phosphorus and convert it to bone.

These important nutrients also aid in elimination of toxins by the colon, kidneys, lungs, and skin. One enzyme, for instance, initiates the formation of urea, which is excreted in the urine, while another enables the elimination of carbon dioxide from the lungs.

In addition to its other functions, enzymes decompose poisonous hydrogen peroxide and liberate healthful oxygen from it. Iron is concentrated in the blood due to the action of enzymes, which also help the blood to coagulate in order to stop bleeding. These vital proteins promote oxidation, a process in which oxygen is united with other substances. Energy is created in the oxidation process. They also protect the blood from dangerous waste materials by converting these substances to forms that are easily eliminated by the body.

WHAT'S ON THE SHELVES

Over-the-counter enzymes are available in tablet, capsule, powder, and liquid forms. They may be sold in combination with each other or as separate items. Some enzymatic products may also contain garlic to help digestion. Most commercial enzyme products are made from animal enzymes such as pancreatin and pepsin. These supplements help in the digestion of food once it has reached the lower stomach and the intestinal tract. Some products make their supplements from plant enzymes (aspergillus), which begin their predigestive work in the upper stomach. This reduces the amount of work the body has to perform, thus saving the body's much needed enzymes.

All forms of enzymes should be kept in a reasonably cool area to insure potency. Tablets and liquids can be stored in the refrigerator. However, powder and capsule forms should not be refrigerated because they are susceptible to moisture; they should be stored in a cool, dry place.

The majority of commercially available enzymes are digestive enzymes; that is, they are specifically involved in the digestive process. The rest are metabolic enzymes that deal with other various phases of the life processes. All of the body's organs, tissues, and cells are run by the metabolic enzymes. They are the workers that build the body from proteins, carbohydrates, and fats.

Commercially Available Enzymes

There are three types of digestive enzymes available: amylase, protease, and lipase. Amylase and protease are the two most effective digestive enzymes that are secreted in high concentrations by the human body. Amylase, found in saliva, breaks down carbohydrates, while protease, found in the stomach juices, helps to digest protein. In addition, pancreatic and intestinal juices contain both enzymes.

The third type of enzyme, lipase, aids in fat digestion. Lipase is most beneficial when it is allowed to work in successive stages. Whereas pancreatic lipase digests fat in a highly alkaline environment, lipases found in food fats work in a more acidic environment. If the fat in food is exposed only to pancreatic lipase, it does not experience the sequence of substrate changes it would undergo had it first been worked on by a food lipase in the cardiac portion of the stomach (where the stomach is connected to the esophagus). Enzymes with diverse optimal pH characteristics working successively on substrates are more effective and may produce a more favorable product, which may be manifested in their future metabolism. The interaction of fat with lipase from food sources takes place every day in the upper part of the digestive tracts of billions of animals.

A healthy body produces nearly 5 million units of the enzymes superoxide dismutase (SOD) and its partner, catalase, daily. SOD revitalizes the cells and reduces the rate of cell destruction. It removes the most common free radical, superoxide. This antioxidant also aids in the body's utilization of zinc, copper, and manganese. With aging, free radical production increases, while SOD levels are reduced.

If the SOD supplement is in pill form, it must be enteric coated—that is, coated with a protective substance that allows the SOD pill to pass intact through the stomach acid into the small intestines to be absorbed. A supplement should be able to provide a daily amount of about 5 million units or higher. SOD naturally occurs in the following food sources: barley grass, broccoli, Brussels sprouts, cabbage, wheatgrass, and most green plants.

Plant enzymes differ substantially from animal enzymes. Pancreatin, derived from secretions of an animal pancreas, functions best in the alkaline media of the small intestine. This enzyme is important in cancer research.

Unripe papaya, pineapples, and the aspergillus plant are excellent sources of enzymes. The enzymes extracted from papaya and pineapple, papain and bromelin respectively, are proteolytic enzymes. These work on proteins exclusively, breaking them down into smaller peptones by hydrolysis. Other examples of proteolytic enzymes include pepsin, trypsin, rennin, pancreatin, and chymotrypsin. The enzyme pepsin is found in the gastric juice, and is responsible for the breakdown of protein into smaller peptides.

Beneficial results have been obtained by utilizing proteolytic enzymes as anti-inflammatory agents. These enzymes are used for sports injuries, diseases of the respiratory tract, laryngitis, bronchitis, pneumonia, emphysema, viral diseases, cancer, and most types of degenerative diseases. Proteolytic enzymes are available through Nature's Plus and Miller Pharmacal Group. See APPENDIX for how to contact these companies.

Aspergillus plants have different strains that allow protease, amylase, and lipase to be extracted from them, assuring proper digestion. The enzyme supplement you choose should contain all the enzyme groups to ensure maximum benefit for digestion of any cooked food.

Inflazyme Forte

American Biologics designed Inflazyme Forte, a specific combination of enzymes and antioxidants, for people requiring supplemental digestive enzymes to aid in the breakdown of proteins, fats, and carbohydrates. Research has shown that the combination of enzymes and antioxidants provided in Inflazyme Forte may also be beneficial in clinical applications concerning chronic and acute inflammation.

The recommended dosage for Inflazyme is one to three tablets following each meal. If using Inflazyme Forte for clinical purposes other than as a digestive aid, then take three to six tablets one hour before meals. Inflazyme Forte may be taken by those on a sodium restricted diet.

One microgranulated tablet of Inflazyme Forte contains the following:

Pancreatin N.F.	800.0 mg
Bromelin	125.0 mg
Papain	120.0 mg
Trypsin	120.0 mg
Chymotrypsin	2.5 mg
L-Cysteine	10.0 mg
Lipase	35.0 mg
Amylase	35.0 mg
Rutin	85.0 mg
Zinc	2.6 mg
Catalase	50.0 IU
Superoxide Dismutase	100.0 IU

Natural Food Supplements

INTRODUCTION

Natural food supplements include a wide variety of products. Almost all health food stores carry them, and a number of enlightened drug stores and supermarkets are beginning to stock them on their shelves as well. In general, natural food supplements are products composed of, derived from, or by-products of foods that provide a multitude of health benefits. In some cases, health benefit claims made by manufacturers are based upon a supplement's use in traditional healing; in other cases, they are based on modern research and development.

Food supplements can be high in certain nutrients, contain active ingredients that aid our digestive or metabolic processes, or provide a combination of nutrients and active ingredients. It is important to point out that some unscrupulous manufacturers make false promises. It is therefore vital to be an informed consumer. It is also necessary to be aware that many conservative "watchdog" organizations point to these few unsubstantiated products, and label the whole industry as unreliable. This occurs in spite of the fact that many of these products have been known to work for years, and these products are only medically endorsed when they are "discovered" by researchers deemed acceptable by these groups. Such recent discoveries include the positive effects of garlic, aloe vera, fiber, fish oils, and bran—products that have been used for centuries in other countries.

WHAT'S ON THE SHELVES

Food supplements come in every shape and form—tablets, capsules, powders, liquids, jellies, creams, biscuits, wafers, granules, etc. Product packaging depends entirely on the nature of the food supplement's composition. Potencies of these products vary. Because they are made up of perishable foods, food derivatives, or food by-products, their potency may be affected by the length of time they sit on a shelf, or the temperature they are kept in. If you don't understand how a product is to be used, ask questions or read the available literature on the particular supplement.

If you have never used such a product, please remember that you may be uncomfortable about buying and using it for the first time. This is very normal. Once you become familiar with its use and benefits, you won't give the idea of using it a second thought.

The following is a list of food supplements that have been recommended for use in dealing with the various disorders discussed in Part Two of this book.

Acidophilus (*Lactobacillus Acidophilus*)

Soured products such as buttermilk, yogurt, acidophilus milk, kefir, cheese, and acidophilus work by assisting in the digestion of proteins, a process in which lactic acid, hydrogen peroxide, enzymes, antibiotic substances that inhibit pathogenic organisms, and B vitamins are produced.

According to the *Colon Health Handbook*, the healthy colon should contain at least 85 percent *lactobacillus* and 15 percent *coliform* bacteria. However, the typical colon bacteria count is the reverse, resulting in excessive gas, bloating, intestinal and systemic toxicity, constipation, and malabsorption of nutrients, which leads to an overgrowth of *Candida*.

Acidophilus may help to detoxify harmful substances. Factors that contribute to candidiasis are recurrent use of antibiotics, oral contraceptives, aspirin, corticosteroids, poor diet, sugar, yeast, and stress. These all cause an imbalance of the "friendly" bacteria. The good flora bind with some of the unwanted substances, causing them to be excreted.

Acidophilus also has an antibacterial effect. Excess zinc and iron should be avoided because zinc promotes the growth of *Candida* and iron cannot be absorbed until the candidiasis is healed. (*See* CANDIDIASIS in Part Two.)

The acidophilus contained in various products can die at high temperatures. Keep the product in a cool, dry place—refrigerate, but do not freeze. It is not advisable to buy a combination product. One organism may be antagonistic to another. A single strain product with a count of at least one billion per gram or higher is often better than combinations.

Take acidophilus on an empty stomach in the morning and one hour before meals. If taking antibiotics, do not take the antibiotics and acidophilus simultaneously. These products come in tablet, capsule, and powdered forms. We recommend the powdered form placed in a glass of distilled water at room temperature.

There are nondairy acidophilus products such as DDS Acidophilus, Kyo-Dophilus from Wakunaga of America Company, Primadophilus from Nature's Way Products, and Neo-Flora from New Moon Extracts. These are best for those suffering from food allergies (milk), and they work well against *Candida*. Natren carries quality products that are very high in numbers of organisms.

Kyo-Dophilus is a milk-free product that remains stable at high temperatures. It contains the acidophilus strain known to populate the digestive system. It is currently being used in over 100 university medical centers and 30,000 hospitals. Kyo-Dophilus is a synergistic combination of three beneficial bacteria that normally live in a healthy intestinal tract. It is an ideal supplement for favorable intestinal flora.

Acidophilus, Maxidophilus, Megadophilus, and the nondairy forms of acidophilus all have antifungal properties, reduce blood cholesterol levels, aid digestion, and enhance absorption of nutrients.

Alfalfa

One of the richest mineral foods, its roots grow as much as 130 feet into the earth. Alfalfa comes in liquid form and is good to use while fasting because of its chlorophyll and nutrient content. Alfalfa contains calcium, magnesium, phosphorus, potassium, plus all known vitamins. The minerals are in a balanced form, which promotes absorption. These minerals are alkaline, but have a neutralizing effect on the intestinal tract.

For those who need a mineral supplement, this is a wise choice. It has helped many arthritis sufferers. Alfalfa, wheatgrass, barley, and spirulina, which all contain chlorophyll, have been found to aid in the healing of intestinal ulcers, gastritis, liver disorders, eczema, hemorrhoids, asthma, high blood pressure, anemia, constipation, body and breath odor, bleeding gums, infections, reduction in pus formation, burns, athlete's foot, and cancer.

Aloe Vera

This plant is known for its healing effect and is used in many cosmetic and hair products. There are over 200 different species that grow around the world in dry regions.

Aloe vera is commonly known as a skin healer, moisturizer, and softener. It is used on cuts, burns, insect stings, bruises, acne and blemishes, poison ivy, welts, ulcerated skin lesions, eczema, and sunburns. It is known to aid in the healing of stomach disorders, ulcers, constipation, hemorrhoids, rectal itching, colitis and all colon problems. Aloe vera is helpful in infections, varicose veins, skin cancer, and arthritis.

We have had excellent results with Aerobic's and George's Aloe Vera Juice. George's needs no refrigeration and tastes like plain water. Used with Aerobic Bulk Cleanse (ABC), a colon cleanser from Aerobic Life Products, and juice, it is not only good for its healing effect, but if constipation or diarrhea is present, it will return the stools to normal. It takes a few weeks to cleanse the colon, but continued use keeps it clean.

We have also found this combination to be good for food allergy and colon disorder sufferers. ABC keeps the folds and pockets in the colon free of toxic material that gathers there. However, certain individuals, especially diabetics, may develop an intolerance to aloe vera juice.

Barley Grass

Barley grass is high in calcium, iron, all the essential amino acids, vitamin C, the flavonoids, vitamin B_{12}, and many minerals plus enzymes. Dr. Kubota from Tokyo believes that this food heals stomach and duodenum disorders and pancreatitis, and is an ideal anti-inflammatory substance.

Bee By-Products

See BEE POLLEN AND HONEY, BEE PROPOLIS, and ROYAL JELLY.

Bee Pollen and Honey

Pollen is a fine powderlike material produced by the anthers of flowering plants, and gathered by the bee. Bee pollen contains the B-complex vitamins, vitamin C, amino acids, polyunsaturated fatty acids, enzymes, carotene, calcium, copper, iron, magnesium, potassium, manganese, sodium, and protein (10–35 percent). Bee pollen, bee propolis, and honey have an antimicrobial effect. Honey is produced by the bee when plant nectar, which is a sweet substance secreted by flowers, is mixed with bee enzymes.

Honey varies in color and taste depending on the origin of the flower and nectar. It contains 35 percent protein (one-half of all the amino acids), and is considered to be a complete food. It is a highly concentrated source of essential nutrients, containing large amounts of carbohydrates (sugars), the B-complex vitamins, vitamins C, D, and E, and some minerals. It is used to promote energy and healing. Two tablespoons daily is sufficient. It is twice as sweet as sugar and, therefore, not as much is needed. Only unfiltered, unheated, un-processed honey should be purchased.

Diabetics and hypoglycemics should be careful when consuming honey and its by-products. The blood sugar reacts to these substances as it would to refined sugars. However, tupelo honey contains more levulose than any other honey and is absorbed at a slower rate so some hypoglycemics can use this type sparingly. If you are hypoglycemic, check with your health care provider.

Do not feed honey to infants under one year of age, as they are more prone to develop botulism.

Bee Propolis

Propolis is a resinous substance collected from various plants by bees; it is not made by bees. It is used together with beeswax in the construction of hives. As a supplement, it is an excellent aid against bacterial infections. A Soviet scientist stated that bee propolis stimulates phagocytosis, which helps the white blood cells to destroy bacteria. Soviet surgeons often feed honey to their patients before surgery as a precaution against infection.

Bee propolis is also good as a salve and for abrasions and bruises because of its antibacterial effect. Reports proclaim good results against inflammation of the mucous membranes of the mouth and throat, dry cough and throat, halitosis, tonsillitis, ulcers, and acne, and for the stimulation of the immune system.

Be sure that all products from the bee are fresh and tightly sealed. It is best to purchase these products from a manufacturer who specializes in bee products. When used for allergies, it is best to obtain bee products that are produced within a ten-mile radius. This way, those with allergies get a minute dose of pollen to desensitize them to the local pollen in the area.

Brewer's Yeast

See YEAST.

CamoCare

CamoCare contains chamomile and other active ingredients. It relieves pain associated with a variety of ailments involving the muscles and joints such as backache and arthritis and pain from inflamed joints. Chamomile acts similarly to cortisone, but without the side effects. Rub this cream onto the affected parts four times a day for best results.

Cellulose

See FIBER.

Chlorella

Chlorella requires additional factory processing to break down its hard cell walls. The Japanese have found a way to protect the cell walls. The chlorophyll in chlorella can help speed the cleansing of the bloodstream. Chlorella is very high in RNA and DNA, and has been found to protect against the effects of ultraviolet radiation.

Chlorophyll

See CHLORELLA, KYO-GREEN, and GREEN MAGMA.

Corn Germ

Corn germ has a longer shelf life than wheat germ and is higher in some nutrients, especially zinc. Corn germ contains ten times the amount of zinc found in wheat germ. You can use corn germ to bread chicken or fish. It is also good when added to cereals and used as a topping.

Desiccated Liver

Desiccated liver is a concentrated form of dried liver that is put into powdered or tablet form. This form of liver contains the vitamins A, D, C, and B complex and the minerals calcium, copper, phosphorus, cholesterol, and iron. Desiccated liver is good for anemia and aids in building healthy red blood cells. It is known to increase energy, to aid in liver disorders, and to help relieve stress in the body. Use liver derived only from Argentine beef that is raised organically.

Essential Fatty Acids (Vitamin F)

Those fatty acids that cannot be made by the body and which must be supplied through the diet are called essential fatty acids (EFAs), also referred to as vitamin F. These essential fatty acids are also known as polyunsaturates, and are recommended in order to lower cholesterol and blood pressure and to reduce the risks of heart disease and stroke.

Fortified flax is rich in omega-3 factors, magnesium, potassium, and fiber. It is also a good source of the B vitamins, protein, and zinc. Fortified flaxseed is low in saturated fats and calories, and contains no cholesterol. It has a nutty taste and can be mixed with water or any fruit or vegetable juice. It can also be added to salads, soups, yogurt, and cereals.

The most essential of the fatty acids is linoleic acid. The daily requirement for essential fatty acids is satisfied by consuming an amount of vitamin F equivalent to 10 to 20 percent of total calorie intake. The natural form is found in many vegetables and vegetable oils (except coconut or palm kernel oils). If such oils are heated or hydrogenated (processed), the linoleic acid is converted to trans fatty acids, which are not essential substances and cannot be utilized.

Primrose oil and black currant oil contain high amounts of linoleic acid. Salmon, mackerel, menhaden, herring, and sardines, found in cold deep water, are good sources of fish oil because they have the highest fat content and provide more omega-3 factors than other fishes. For instance, four ounces of salmon can contain 3,600 milligrams of omega-3 fatty acids, while four ounces of cod (a low-fat fish) contains only 300 milligrams. Although diabetics should not take fish oil supplements, they should consume the fish for its essential fatty acids.

Carlson Laboratories has a good salmon oil (Norwegian) that we recommend. We also recommend Kyolic from Wakunaga of America Company and Cardiovascular's Essential Fatty Acid Complex. Cod liver oil from Norway is the most commonly used and is more mild tasting. Author Dale Alexander claims it is excellent for arthritis. He has marketed an oil containing 13,800 IU vitamin A and 1,380 IU vitamin D per tablespoon. Do not exceed this dose on a regular basis. Don't rely on cod liver oil to obtain the essential fatty acids. You would have to overdose on vitamins A and D to obtain the amount of fatty acids needed.

These essential fatty acids have desirable effects on many disorders. They reduce blood pressure, aid in the prevention of arthritis, reduce the growth rate of breast cancer, lower cholesterol and triglyceride levels, and help eczema, psoriasis, and arteriosclerosis. Found in high concentrations in the brain, EFAs aid transmission of nerve impulses and are needed for normal brain function. Essential fatty acids are also needed in the treatment of candidiasis and coronary heart disease, and to minimize blood clot formation.

Research done by Dr. William E. Connor, professor of medicine at Oregon Health Sciences University, indicates that dietary omega-3 fatty acids are essential for normal function and development of the brain. Japanese researchers concur that a deficiency of essential fatty acids leads to an impaired ability to learn and recall information.

Evening Primrose Oil

Evening primrose oil contains the highest amount of vital gamma-linoleic acid (GLA) of any food substance. GLA is an essential fatty acid. The body does not manufacture GLA; it must be supplied through the diet. This fatty acid is known to help prevent hardening of the arteries, heart disease, premenstrual syndrome, multiple sclerosis, and high blood pressure. It has a positive effect on sex hormone response including the hormones estrogen and testosterone, aids in lowering cholesterol levels, and is important in treating cirrhosis of the liver. Research also demonstrates that primrose oil helps relieve pain and inflammation. A lack of GLA may lead to a dysfunctional level of prostaglandins.

Those suffering from breast cancer that is estrogen related should avoid or limit their intake of primrose oil. Black currant oil is a good substitute.

Fiber

Found in many foods, fiber helps to lower the blood cholesterol level and stabilize blood sugar levels. It helps prevent colon cancer, constipation, hemorrhoids, obesity, and many other disorders. Because the refining process has removed much of the natural fiber from our foods, the American diet is lacking in fiber. There are more than 85,000 cases of colon cancer diagnosed in our country each year and the number is growing.

There are seven forms of fiber: pectin, bran, cellulose, hemicellulose, lignin, gums, and mucilages. Each form has its own function. Start with small amounts of fiber and gradually increase your intake until stools are the proper consistency. Those suffering from Crohn's disease should avoid supplemental fiber and consume natural fiber foods.

Pectin

Because it slows the absorption of food after meals, pectin is good for diabetics. It also removes unwanted metals and toxins, is valuable in radiation therapy, helps lower cholesterol, and reduces the risk of heart disease and gallstones. Pectin is found in apples, carrots, beets, bananas, cabbage, the citrus family, dried peas, and okra.

Cellulose

Cellulose is a nondigestible carbohydrate found in the outer layer of vegetables and fruits. It is good for hemorrhoids, varicose veins, colitis, and constipation, and for the removal of cancer-causing substances from the colon wall. It is found in apples, pears, lima beans, carrots, broccoli, peas, whole grains, Brazil nuts, green beans, and beets.

Hemicellulose

Hemicellulose is an indigestible complex carbohydrate that absorbs water. It is good for weight loss, constipation, colon cancer, and controlling carcinogens in the intestinal tract. Hemicellulose is found in apples, beets, whole grain cereals, cabbage, bananas, beans, corn, peppers, greens, and pears.

Lignin

This form of fiber is good for lowering cholesterol levels and preventing gallstone formation by binding with the bile acids. It is beneficial for those with diabetes or colon cancer. Lignin is found in carrots, green beans, peas, whole grains, Brazil nuts, peaches, tomatoes, strawberries, and potatoes.

Gums and Mucilages

Both gums and mucilages help to regulate blood glucose levels, aid in lowering cholesterol, and help in the removal of toxins. They are found in oatmeal, oat bran, sesame seeds, and dried beans.

One of the following should be part of daily meal planning:

- **Oat and Rice Bran.** Helps to lower cholesterol. This is the broken coat of the seed of cereal grain, which has been separated from the flour or meal by sifting or bolting.
- **Aerobic Bulk Cleanse (ABC).** An excellent fiber that contains psyllium seed husks, licorice, and hibiscus (herbs). Add it to a half aloe vera juice and half fruit juice combination. Be sure to take it on an empty stomach first thing in the morning. Stir it well and drink it down quickly so that it does not thicken. This therapeutic drink aids in healing and cleansing of the colon. It is excellent for diarrhea and constipation.
- **Glucomannan.** Derived from the tuber amorphophallis plant. It picks up and removes fat from the colon wall. This substance is good for diabetes and obesity because it is a fat mobilizer. It has been recognized for normalizing blood sugar and is good for the hypoglycemic. Glucomannan expands to sixty times its own weight, thereby helping to curb the appetite. Take 2–3 capsules with a large glass of water thirty minutes before meals. This will help reduce allergic reactions and some symptoms associated with high and low blood sugar disorders. Do not take fiber with any medications or other supplements. Not only will it lessen the strength and effectiveness of the fiber substances, but harmful substances may be absorbed by the body in addition to beneficial ones due to the absorbent properties of the fiber substances. Glucomannan is tasteless and odorless, and can be added to foods to help normalize the blood sugar after eating.
- **Guar Gum.** Good for the treatment of diabetes and for curbing the appetite. It should not be used by those who have difficulty swallowing or who have had gastrointestinal surgery. Some persons with colon disorders may have trouble using guar gum. This root also has the ability to reduce cholesterol, triglyceride, and low–density lipoprotein levels. It also binds toxic substances and carries them out of the body.
- **Psyllium Seed.** A good intestinal cleaner and stool softener. This is one of the most popular fibers used. It thickens very quickly and must be consumed immediately. The ABC colon cleanser contains blond psyllium seed husk, licorice, and hibiscus. Some doctors recommend Metamucil, which contains psyllium hydrophilic mucilloid, as a laxative and fiber supplement. It contains psyllium seed. We prefer less processing and all natural products.
- **Fennel Seed.** Helps rid the intestinal tract of mucus.

It is best to rotate the supplemental fiber. There are many to choose from besides the ones mentioned above, including corn, brown rice, apple bran, apple pectin, flaxseed, and agar agar. These are good for removing certain toxic metals. Kelp is also good and helps in weight control.

The correct diet should have fiber in it. Add these foods to the diet: whole grain cereals and flours, brown rice, all kinds of bran, apricots, dried prunes, apples, fruits (except oranges, which are too acidic, bad for arthritis, and highly allergenic), nuts, seeds, beans, lentils, peas, and vegetables. Eat several of these foods daily. Leave the skin on apples and potatoes. Coat chicken in corn bran or oats for baking. Add extra bran to cereals and breads.

Laxatives are habit-forming and irritating to the colon. Periodic internal cleansing and a liquid diet for 1–3 days can promote good health. Diabetics should not fast on liquids, but can benefit from a raw foods diet. Hypoglycemics do well on a liquid fast using spirulina. It contains vitamins, minerals, chlorophyll, and the protein needed to stabilize the blood sugar.

For weight loss, fiber and exercise should be part of the program. Find the fiber that works the best for you. A quarter cup of aloe vera juice, added to morning juice and before bed, works wonders. Unsalted, unbuttered popcorn is also excellent for added fiber.

Today's diet is lacking in fiber, but excessive amounts may decrease the absorption of zinc, iron, and calcium. Take fiber separately from other minerals and vitamins.

Garlic

Garlic is one of the most valuable foods on this planet. It has been used since Biblical times, and is found in the literature of the ancient Hebrews, Greeks, Babylonians, Romans, and Egyptians. Pyramid builders ate garlic daily for endurance and strength.

Garlic lowers the blood pressure through the actions of one of its components, methyl allyl trisulfide, which dilates vessel walls. Garlic thins the blood by inhibiting platelet aggression, and this reduces the risk of blood clots and aids in preventing heart attacks. It also lowers serum cholesterol levels and aids in digestion. Garlic is used for many diseases and illnesses including cancer. It is a potent immune system stimulant. The Russians call garlic a natural antibiotic. It should be consumed daily.

Garlic contains an amino acid derivative, allium. When garlic is consumed, an allinase enzyme that converts allium to allicin is released. Allicin has an antibiotic effect; its antibacterial action is equivalent to one percent that of penicillin. Because of its properties, garlic was used to treat wounds and infections and to prevent gangrene during World War I.

Garlic is also an antifungal agent effective against candidiasis, athlete's foot, vaginal yeast infections, and most pathogenic fungi. Two microbiologists from Brigham Young University report that the extract of garlic will destroy certain viruses such as those associated with fever, blisters, genital herpes, a form of the common cold, smallpox, and a type of influenza with a respiratory virus.

Garlic oil is good for the heart and colon, and is effective in the treatment of arthritis, candidiasis, and circulation problems. Add garlic cloves to one quart of olive or canola oil. Keep refrigerated. This mixture will keep for up to a month before you need to replace with fresh oil. Garlic can be used for sautéing, in salad dressings, or for a variety of other uses. If the odor is too strong after eating garlic, chew some sprigs of parsley, mint caraway, or fennel seeds.

An alternative to garlic is Kyolic from Wakunaga of America Company. Kyolic is an odorless garlic product, and is available in tablet, capsule, and oil extract.

Ginseng

Ginseng is used throughout the Orient as a tonic for general weakness and extra energy. There are many types of ginseng: *Eleuthrococcus senticosus* (Siberian ginseng), *Panax quinquifolium* (American ginseng), *Panax ginseng* (Chinese or Korean ginseng), and *Panax japonicum* (Japanese ginseng). Panax ginseng is the most widely used species.

Ginseng contains thirteen different ginsenosides (triterpenoid saponins). The most important constituents include: panacaene, B-elemene and panaxinol, low-molecular weight starches, pectin, vitamins (B_1, B_2, B_3, B_5, B_{12}, and biotin), choline, minerals, simple sugars, traces of germanium, and flavonoids.

The American Indians were familiar with ginseng. They called it gisens and used it for stomach and bronchial disorders, asthma, and neck pain.

Russian scientists claim that the ginseng root stimulates both physical and mental activity, improves endocrine glandular function, and has a positive effect on the sex glands. Today it is being used for fatigue because ginseng spares glycogen utilization in muscle by increasing the use of fatty acids as an energy source. It is also used to enhance athletic performances, to rejuvenate and to increase longevity, and to detoxify and normalize the entire system.

Many supplement combinations add ginseng to their products, but they contain such low amounts that it may not be effective. Lower doses of ginseng seem to raise blood pressure, while higher amounts lower the blood pressure. Research suggests that higher amounts may be effective for inflammatory diseases such as rheumatoid arthritis, without the side effects of steroids, and they also protect against the harmful effects of radiation. The hypoglycemic should avoid using large amounts of ginseng. Ginseng will benefit the diabetic, however, because it decreases serum cortisol levels. (Cortisol antagonizes insulin.)

We advise following the Russian approach: use ginseng for 15–20 days, followed by a rest period of two weeks. Avoid long-term usage of high amounts of ginseng, even though studies have shown no side effects. The root is sold in many forms: as a whole root, root pieces, or tails, which are either untreated or blanched; as a powder or powdered extract; as a liquid extract or concentrate; in granules for instant tea; as a tincture, in an oil base, and in tablets and capsules. These products should not contain sugar or added color, and should be pure ginseng.

Wakunaga of America Company distributes several high-quality Korean and Siberian ginseng products:

- ENAX PG1. High quality Korean ginseng that is processed according to the ancient method.
- ENAX EG1. Siberian ginseng powder made from wild, fully matured plants that have been harvested in a remote pollution-free northern Pacific island.
- ENAX EG2. Siberian ginseng extract and powder made from the same high quality plants as ENAX EG1, but of greater potency.

Green Magma

Green Magma, available from Green Foods Corporation, is a pure natural juice of young barley leaves. It is 100 percent organically grown in Japan and is pesticide free. The enzymes, proteins, vitamins (such as B_{15} and vitamins K and P), minerals, chlorophyll, and nutrients contained in the barley leaves are protected because they are processed at low temperatures and dried with a spray that does not contain chemicals.

Brown rice is added, which is a rich source of vitamins B_1 and B_2 and nicotinic and linoleic acids. Green Magma also contains thousands of enzymes, which play an important role in the metabolism of the body (*see* ENZYMES in Part One). A high concentration of superoxide dismutase (SOD) is found in Green Magma. The powdered product may be added to juice or quality water. There is also a product on the market called Barley Green. This product contains barley juice and kelp, and is manufactured by the same company.

Kelp

Kelp is a type of seaweed that can be eaten raw, but it is usually dried, granulated, or ground into powder. Granulated and powdered kelp are used as condiments or for flavoring. Kelp is a rich source of vitamins, minerals, and many trace elements, and has been used in the treatment of thyroid problems because of its iodine content. Kelp is recommended as a daily supplement in the diet and can be used as a salt substitute. It can be purchased in a health food store in tablet form if the taste is unappealing.

Kyo-Green

Kyo-Green is a highly concentrated natural source of chlorophyll, amino acids, vitamins and minerals, carotene, and enzymes. It is a unique combination of barley, wheatgrass, kelp, and the green algae chlorella. The barley and wheatgrasses are organically grown. Chlorella is a rich natural source of vitamin A, and kelp supplies iodine and other valuable minerals.

Kyo-Green is produced by a leading Japanese pharmaceutical company. This nutritious drink was developed after many years of research. It contains no preservatives, artificial color, or other additives. Kyo-Green offers the benefits of barley grass, chlorella, kelp, wheatgrass, and much more in one healthful drink. This product is distributed by Wakunaga of America Company.

Kyolic-EPA

Kyolic-EPA is a blend of the most potent aged garlic extract and fish oil. It is distributed by Wakunaga of America Company in soft gel capsules not only for convenience, but also for synergetic health benefits. The fish oil is derived from northern Pacific sardines. Kyolic-EPA is high in omega-3 polyunsaturated fatty acids, and is unesterified and cholesterol free.

Lactobacillus Bifidus (Eugalan Forte)

The *Lactobacillus bifidus* preparation, Eugalan Forte, aids synthesis of the B vitamins by creating a healthy intestinal flora. *L. bifidus* is the predominant organism in the intestinal flora and establishes a healthy environment for the manufacture of the B-complex vitamins and vitamin K.

When taking antibiotics, the "friendly" bacteria are destroyed along with the harmful bacteria. Supplementing with Eugalen Forte helps maintain a healthy intestinal flora. An unhealthy flora can lead to the liberation of large quantities of ammonia, which irritates the intestinal membranes. The ammonia can be absorbed into the bloodstream and cause nausea, a decrease in appetite, vomiting, and other toxic reactions.

The product Eugalan Forte was designed to support and maintain the growth of the *Lactobacillus bifidus* in the intestinal tract. Undigested food can stagnate or lead to constipation and gas. The putrefactive bacteria that is produced from undigested food may produce excessive histamine, causing an allergic reaction and additional toxic build-up.

Yeast infections of the vaginal tract respond very favorably to douching with Eugalan Forte. The lactobacillus bifidus microorganisms destroy the pathogenic organisms. When used as an enema, *L. bifidus* also helps establish a healthy intestinal environment. It improves bowel function by aiding peristalsis and results in the production of a softer, smoother stool. Harmful bacteria are kept in check, and waste toxins that have accumulated in the intestines are destroyed.

Eugalan Forte has proved useful in the treatment of cirrhosis of the liver and chronic hepatitis. Many people who do not respond to *L. acidophilus* react positively to *L. bifidus*. Eugalan Forte can be found in your local health food store.

Lecithin

Lecithin is needed by every living cell in the human body. Cell membranes, which regulate which nutrients may leave or enter the cell, are largely composed of lecithin. Without lecithin, the cell membranes would harden. Its structure protects the cells from damage by oxidation. The protective sheaths surrounding the brain are composed of lecithin, and the muscles and nerve cells also contain this essential fatty substance. Lecithin, which is largely composed of the B vitamin choline, also contains linoleic acid and inositol. Although lecithin is a fatty substance, it acts as an emulsifying agent.

It is especially important that the elderly obtain this nutrient because it helps prevent arteriosclerosis, protects against cardiovascular disease, increases brain function, and aids in the absorption of thiamine by the liver and vitamin A by the intestine. Lecithin is also known to promote energy and is needed to help repair the damage to the liver caused by alcoholism.

Lecithin would be a wise addition to anyone's diet. Two tablespoons of lecithin granules can be sprinkled on cereals and soups or added to juices or breads. Lecithin also comes in capsule form. Taking one capsule before meals helps the digestion of fats and absorption of the fat-soluble vitamins. Those taking niacin for high serum cholesterol and triglycerides need to include lecithin in their program. Lecithin enables fats, such as cholesterol and other lipids, to be dispersed in water and removed from the body. The vital organs and arteries are protected from fatty build-up with the inclusion of lecithin in the diet.

Most lecithin is derived from soybeans, but recently egg lecithin has become popular. This type is made from the yolk of fresh eggs. A liquid form is available by Source Naturals, who claim the emulsifying can actually be observed while blending or stirring the "Eggs-Act." This mixture will spoil within an hour, so drink it right away. Egg lecithin may hold promise for those suffering from AIDS, herpes, chronic Epstein Barr virus, and immune disorders associated with aging. Other sources of lecithin include brewer's yeast, grains, legumes, fish, and wheat germ.

Octacosanol

Octacosanol is derived from wheat germ. Although it is possible to extract octacosanol from whole wheat, ten pounds of wheat would be needed to obtain 1,000 micrograms of octacosanol. Studies indicate octacosanol is superior for improving endurance. Therefore, this substance would greatly benefit those who experience muscle pain after exercise or who have a lowered endurance level.

This naturally derived wheat germ oil concentrate has been clinically proven to increase oxygen utilization when exercising. Octacosanol also reduces blood cholesterol, muscular dystrophies, and other neuromuscular disorders. Wheat germ has long been known for its many benefits. Today, extracts of wheat germ weighing 2,000 micrograms are known to improve glycogen storage in muscle and endurance and reaction time, to reduce high altitude stress, and to aid in tissue oxygenation. Wheat germ should be included in the active person's program.

Royal Jelly

The thick, milky substance that is secreted from the pharyngeal glands of a special group of young nurse bees between their sixth and twelfth days of life is called royal jelly. When honey and pollen are combined and refined within the young nurse bee, royal jelly is naturally created. It contains all of the B-complex vitamins including a high concentration of pantothenic acid (B_5) and pyridoxine (B_6), and is the only natural source of pure acetylcholine. Royal jelly also contains minerals, vitamins A, C, D, and E, enzymes, hormones, eighteen amino acids, and antibacterial and antibiotic components. This product must be combined with honey to preserve its potency. Royal jelly is known to aid in bronchial asthma, liver disease, pancreatitis, insomnia, stomach ulcers, kidney disease, bone fractures, and skin disorders, and is a potentiator of the immune system. Royal jelly spoils easily. Keep it refrigerated and make sure it is tightly sealed when purchased.

Shiitake

Shiitake are Japanese mushrooms that contain a virus and which can be made to produce interferon. Their effectiveness in treating cancer has been reported in a joint study by the Medical Department of Koibe University and Nippon Kinoko Institute. This mushroom is considered a delicacy and is entirely edible.

There are two types of shiitake. Reishi mushrooms have been popular for at least 2,000 years in the Orient. There are six kinds of reishi. Both the shiitake and the reishi mushrooms have a delicate texture and strong stems with well-defined undersides and stoma. They are both attractive and have amazing properties.

The reishi mushroom was rated number one on ancient Chinese lists of superior medicines and touted as a substance that would give one eternal youth and longevity. Both shiitake and reishi mushrooms have long been used to treat a variety of disorders and to promote vitality. These mushrooms are used to prevent high blood pressure and heart disease, to control and lower cholesterol, to build resistance against viruses and disease, and to treat fatigue and viral infections. Now they are known for their effectiveness in treating cancer. Dried mushrooms can be purchased and added to soups. Shiitake are now cultivated in the United States.

Spirulina

Recognized the world over as the most promising of all microalgae, spirulina is being considered as an immediate food resource. Spirulina thrives in hot sunny climates and in alkaline waters around the world. It represents a breakthrough in the production of food, producing twenty times the amount of protein as that of soybeans on an equal land area.

Spirulina contains concentrations of nutrients unlike any other single grain, herb, or plant. It contains gamma-linolenic acid (GLA), linoleic and arachidonic acids, high amounts of B_{12} needed (especially by the vegetarian) for healthy red blood cells, high iron content, 60–70 percent protein content, the essential amino acids, RNA and DNA nucleic acids, chlorophyll, and a blue pigment (phycocyanin) found only in blue-green algae, which increased the survival rate of mice with liver cancer in laboratory experiments.

Spirulina is a naturally digestible food that aids in protecting the immune system, in cholesterol reduction, and in mineral absorption. Spirulina is beneficial while fasting. It supplies the nutrients needed to help cleanse and heal, while also curbing the appetite. The hypoglycemic individual may benefit by using this food supplement between meals because its high protein content helps stabilize the blood sugar.

Sub-Adrene

Sub-Adrene from American Biologics is a highly concentrated whole adrenal cortical extract of bovine origin. Its formula has been specifically designed for maximum absorption through sublingual administration. It has a peppermint taste and offers an effective and complete balance of natural steroids, which many people lack.

Sub-Adrene comes in plastic dropper bottles and contains 3,000 micrograms of pure adrenal cortical extract. The usual dose is five drops each day, which can be taken at one time.

Wheat Germ

Wheat germ rapidly becomes rancid. If wheat germ is purchased separately from the flour, make sure the product is fresh. The product should be vacuum packed or refrigerated with a packing date or a label stating the date before which the product should be used. Toasted wheat germ has a longer shelf life, but the raw product is better because no processing is used. Use wheat germ oil capsules or wheat germ that has been tightly sealed.

Wheatgrass

Wheatgrass is a rich nutritional food discovered by Dr. Ann Wigmore. She claims that wheatgrass contains the greatest variety of vitamins, minerals, and trace elements, and that 15 pounds of fresh wheatgrass is equal in nutritional value to 350 pounds of the choicest vegetables.

Dr. Wigmore also reports that wheatgrass therapy, along with "living foods," has helped to eliminate cancerous growths and helped many other disorders, including mental health problems. Treatment by wheatgrass rectal implants and enemas are also used.

The molecular structure of wheatgrass closely resembles hemoglobin, the oxygen-carrying protein of red blood cells, and may be the reason for the effectiveness of chlorophyll. The only difference between the two is that the metallic atom in a molecule of human blood is iron, while the metallic atom of chlorophyll is magnesium. In experiments with anemic animals, their blood count returned to normal after four to five days of receiving chlorophyll.

Yeast (Brewer's Yeast)

A yeast is a single-celled organism that can multiply at extremely rapid rates, doubling its number in two hours. It is rich in many basic nutrients such as the B vitamins (except for B_{12}), chromium, sixteen amino acids, fourteen or more minerals, seventeen vitamins (not including vitamins A, C, and E). The protein content of yeast is responsible for 52 percent of its weight. Yeast is also high in phosphorus, so be sure to add extra calcium.

There are various sources from which yeast is grown. Brewer's yeast is grown from hops (a by-product of beer), also known as nutritional yeast. Tourla yeast is grown from blackstrap molasses or wood pulp. A liquid yeast product from Switzerland, called Bio-Strath, is derived from herbs, honey, malt, etc. It is a natural product that we highly recommend.

Live baker's yeast should be avoided. Live yeast cells deplete the body of B vitamins and other nutrients. Home-baked breads are best consumed the second day because of the baker's yeast. In nutritional yeast, these live cells are destroyed.

Yeast may be consumed in juice or water, and is a good energy booster between meals. Yeast may be added to the diet to aid in certain disorders. It helps in sugar metabolism and is good for eczema, heart disorders, gout, nervousness, and fatigue. By enhancing the immune system, yeast is important during cancer therapy (radiation and chemotherapy). It also seems to increase mental and physical efficiency. Those suffering with osteoporosis should avoid yeast products. Dr. William Crook states that if a person with *Candida*-related health problems is not specifically allergic to yeast, it is all right for that person to take a food supplement containing yeast. We suggest avoiding yeast products if candidiasis is suspected.

HERBS

INTRODUCTION

The medicinal benefits of herbs have been known to man for centuries. The records of Roman, Egyptian, Persian, and Hebrew medicine show that herbs were used extensively to cure practically every known illness to man. Many herbs contain powerful ingredients that, if used correctly, can help heal the body. The early pharmaceutical industry was based upon its ability to isolate these ingredients, and make them available in a purer form. Herbalists, however, contend that nature provided other ingredients in the same herb to balance with the more powerful ingredients. These other components, though they may be relatively less potent, may help to act as a buffer, a synergist, or a counterbalance when working in harmony with the more powerful ingredient. Therefore, by using these herbs in their complete form, the body's healing process utilizes a balance of ingredients provided by nature.

All roots and bark are fungicidal and bactericidal, otherwise pathogens would destroy them in the ground. Roots, bark, and other herbs will retain their medicinal value for years when thoroughly dried and kept dry.

Many believe that the healing properties of herbs are just as effective as drugs, but without the side effects. Herbs can be very potent, so it is important to regulate their dosage. Most over-the-counter drugs are too strong. It is of interest to note that in many industrialized countries today, herbs are prescribed by physicians and prepared and sold through neighborhood drugstores. In fact, in countries where access to hospitals and doctors is limited, herbal remedies are the only form of medicine.

Herbs do perform many healing functions in the body, but they must be used appropriately, not indiscriminately. Remember, not all plant life is beneficial. There are poisonous plants and some that are deadly, especially if used for long periods of time. In fact, it is important to point out that qualified herbalists use herbs with great care. Since herbs contain active ingredients, you should be aware that some of these elements may interact negatively with prescribed medications. It is wise, therefore, to consult a health professional when there is any question about safety.

As a general guideline, most of the bitter-tasting herbs are medicinal herbs. The pleasant tasting herbs are potentially less toxic and can be used more often. Certain herbs should be used only while healing, and not for longer than six months at a time. Also, most herbal ingredients are more potent when taken from freshly picked herbs.

WHAT'S ON THE SHELVES

The fresh leaves and roots of herbs can be used in their natural form, or they can be found in tablet form, capsules, liquid beverages, bark pieces, powders, extracts, tinctures, creams, lotions, salves, and oils. The whole leaves of the herb are also dried and made available to consumers.

HOW TO USE HERBS

The many ways in which herbs can be used include:

- *Compress.* A cloth is soaked in a cool herb solution and applied directly on the injured area.
- *Decoction.* A tea is made from the bark, root, seed, or berry of a plant. These teas should not be boiled; they should only be simmered.
- *Essential oils.* All oils are derived from herbs or other plants through distilling or by cold extraction. They are usually mixed with a vegetable oil or water, and used either as a mouth, ear, or eyewash or as an inhalant, douche, or tea. These oils also can be used externally in massage or on cuts and abrasions. Essential oils readily combine with the natural fats present in the skin.
- *Extracts.* The herbs are placed in a solvent and soaked, allowing the solution to evaporate. Extracts are the most effective form of herbs to use when severely ill.

The following are some herb extracts that are very beneficial in healing. Add them to juices and take while fasting for their benefits. They can be found in health food stores.

Celery	Horsetail	Red beet crystals
Echinacea	Nettle	Red clover
Fig	Parsley	Suma
Goldenseal	Pau d'arco	Valerian root
Hawthorn	Pumpkin	

- *Herb vinegars.* Herbs are put into raw apple cider vinegar, rice, or malt and left to stand for two or more weeks.
- *Infusion.* The delicate leaf, flower, or part of the plant is used and is steeped, not boiled, for five minutes in hot water so the benefits of the herbs are not destroyed.
- *Ointment.* A powdered form of an herb is added to a salve.
- *Poultice.* A hot, soft, moist mass of herbs, flour, mustard, and other substances is spread on muslin or a cloth and applied for one to eight hours on a sore or inflamed area of the body to relieve pain and inflammation. Ground or granulated herbs are best. The cloth should be changed when cooled. *See* POULTICE in Part Three for further information on the uses of poultices.
- *Powder.* The useful part of the herb is ground into a powder and is also used in capsule or tablet form. Capsules and tablets are generally used for certain disorders and should be used for no longer than six months at a time.
- *Syrup.* Herbs are added to a form of sugar and then boiled.
- *Salves.* Salves, creams, oils, and lotions are generally used on bruises, sores, and inflammations, and for poultices.

- *Tincture.* Most tinctures contain about 50 percent alcohol; however, there are now some on the market that contain less alcohol. Powdered herbs are added to a 50-50 solution of alcohol and water. Tinctures keep for a long period of time and should only be used if severely ill.

HERB TEAS AND THEIR EFFECTS

Herb teas are good, especially when used for long periods of time. Certain beneficial herbs may be too strong, but not in the form of teas. Mild teas may be used daily as tonics and for general well-being.

If there are several herbs listed for a certain disorder, alternate the herbs to obtain the most benefits from each. To prepare herb teas, use approximately one to three teaspoons of herbs per cup of boiling water. Boil water in a kettle as you would for ordinary tea, but do not use an aluminum kettle. Pour the water into a mug or pot; leave the herbs to steep for at least five minutes, but don't leave them for longer than ten minutes or the tea may have a bitter taste. If you prefer a stronger tea, increase the amount of herbs used rather than steeping the tea for a longer period. Also, do not preserve herbs in glass.

HERBS AND THEIR USES

The following table describes which parts of each herb to use to obtain its benefits, lists its chemical and nutrient content, and explains its various uses.

Herb	Parts Used	Chemical and Nutrient Content	Actions and Uses	Comments
Alfalfa	Leaves, petals, flowers, and sprouts.	Biotin, calcium, choline, inositol, iron, magnesium, PABA, phosphorus, potassium, protein, sodium, sulfur, tryptophan (amino acid), and vitamins A, B complex, C, D, E, K, and U.	High in chlorophyll and nutrients. Alkalizes the body and detoxifies the body, especially the liver. Good for all colon disorders, anemia, hemorrhaging, diabetes, ulcers, and arthritis. Promotes pituitary gland function. Contains an antifungus agent.	
Astragalus	Roots.	Betaine, B-sitosterol, choline, dimethoxyisoflavane, glucoronic acid, kumatakenin, and sucrose.	Acts as a tonic to protect the immune system, as a diuretic to reduce edema (especially in nephritis), and as an anhydrotic. Aids adrenal gland function and digestion. Increases metabolism, promotes healing, and provides energy to combat fatigue. Effective for chronic lung weakness and produces spontaneous sweating.	

Herb	Parts Used	Chemical and Nutrient Content	Actions and Uses	Comments
Barberry	Berries, fruits, roots, and bark.	Berbamine, berberine, berberrubine, columbamine, hydrastine, jatrorrhizine, manganese, oxycanthine, palmatine, and vitamin C.	Decreases heart rate, depresses breathing, stimulates intestinal movement, reduces bronchial constriction, and kills bacteria on the skin.	
Bee pollen	Fresh pollen from bees.	Amino acids, calcium, carotene, copper, enzymes, iron, magnesium, manganese, polyunsaturated fatty acids, potassium, sodium, plant sterols, simple sugars, the B complex, and vitamin C.	Effective for combating fatigue, depression, cancer, and colon disorders. Has an antimicrobial effect. Honey is an antiseptic and salve for burns.	*Warning:* Some people (approximately .05%) may be allergic to bee pollen. Try small amounts at first and dis-continue if a rash, wheezing, discomfort, or any other symptoms occur.
Black cohosh	Rhizomes and roots.	Actaeine, cimicifungin, estrogenic substances, isoferulic acid, oleic acid, palmitic acid, phosphorus, racemosin, tannins, triterpenes, and vitamins A and B_5.	Helps relieve sinusitis and asthma. Lowers cholesterol levels and blood pressure. Relieves pain, morning sickness, hot flashes, and menstrual cramps. Helpful for poisonous bites. Reduces mucus levels.	*Warning:* Do not take if you are pregnant or have any type of chronic disease.
Black walnut	Husks, inner bark, leaves, and nuts.	Ellagic acid, juglone, and nucin.	Aids in treatment of tuberculosis, diarrhea, female disorders, sore throat, and lung disease. Aids digestion and promotes healing of sores in the mouth or throat. Cleanses the body of tapeworms and parasites.	
Bladderwrack	Various parts.	Alginic acid, bromine iodine, fucodin, and laminarin.	For obesity, goiter, and kidney function. Eliminates parasites, increases thyroid activity, and absorbs water in the intestines to produce bulk.	
Blessed thistle	Various parts.	Cincin and volatile oils.	Increases appetite and stomach secretions. Heals the liver. Improves circulation, purifies the blood, strengthens the heart, and alleviates pneumonitis (inflammation of the lung tissue). May act as brain food. Aids milk flow in the nursing mother.	*Warning:* Handle carefully to avoid toxic skin effects.
Blue cohosh	Roots.	Calcium, coulosaponin, gum, inositol, iron, leontin, magnesium, methylcystine, phosphoric acid, phosphorus, potassium, salts, silicon, starch, and vitamins B_3, B_5, B_9, and E.	A bitter, mildly toxic herb for menstrual disorders, cramps, leukorrhea, rheumatism, nervous disorders, vaginitis, colic, and diabetes. Elevates blood pressure and stimulates uterine contraction for childbirth.	

Herb	Parts Used	Chemical and Nutrient Content	Actions and Uses	Comments
Blue vervain	Roots, leaves, and stems.	Essential oil, mucilage, tannin, verbenaline, and verbenine.	Good for fever, colds, flu, pneumonia, asthma, inflammation, worms, nerves, epilepsy, delirium, headaches, skin disorders, female disorders, and stomach, bowel, and colon problems. Relieves the bladder. Also helps to expel phlegm from the throat and chest.	
Buchu	Leaves.	Barosma camphor, diasmin, l-enthone, hesperidin, mucilage, volatile and essential oils, and resin.	For inflammation of mucous membranes, sinuses, prostate, colon, vagina, and gums. Aids in controlling diabetes, ulcers, hypoglycemia, respiratory disorders, bladder and kidney problems, digestive disorders, fluid retention, gas, bloating, and pancreatic disease.	
Burdock root	Roots and seeds.	Arctiin, biotin, copper, inulin, iron, manganese, volatile oils, sulfur, tannins, vitamins B_1, B_6, B_{12}, and E, and zinc.	Helps skin disorders (i.e., boils and carbuncles) and relieves gout symptoms. Purifies the blood, restores liver and gallbladder function, and stimulates the immune system.	*Caution:* Burdock root interferes with iron absorption when taken internally.
Butcher's broom	Tops and seeds.	Alkaloids, hydroxytyramine, and ruscogenins.	For circulatory disorders, gout, leg cramps, varicose veins, hemorrhoids, phlebitis, thrombosis, and jaundice. Also good for the kidney and bladder. Relieves inflammation.	
Capsicum (cayenne)	Berries and fruits.	Apsaicine, capsacutin, capsaicin, capsanthine, capsico, PABA, and vitamins A, B_1, B_2, B_3, B_5, B_6, B_9, and C.	A catalyst for all herbs. Improves circulation, aids digestion, and stops bleeding from ulcers. Good for the kidneys, lungs, spleen, pancreas, heart, and stomach. Take for nausea, rheumatism, arthritis, and pleurisy.	Use with lobelia for nerves.
Cascara sagrada	Bark.	Anthraquinone, calcium, cascarosides, essential oils, inositol, manganese, PABA, potassium, vitamin B complex, and vitamins B_2 and B_6.	Use for liver disorders, gallstones, leukemia, colitis, parasitic infestation, and diverticulosis. Acts as a colon cleanser and as a laxative.	
Catnip	Leaves.	Acetic acid, biotin, buteric acid, choline, citral, dipentene, inositol, lifronella, limonene, manganese, nepetalic acid, volatile oils, PABA, phosphorus, sodium, sulfur, valeric acid, and vitamins A, B_1, B_2, B_3, B_5, B_6, B_9, and B_{12}.	Controls fever (catnip enemas reduce fever quickly). Also good for colic, colds, flu, inflammation, pain, and convulsions. Stimulates the appetite. Aids digestion and sleep. Relieves stress.	
Celery seed	Juice, roots, and seeds.	Iron and vitamins A, B, and C.	Reduces blood pressure. Relieves muscle spasms. Good for arthritis and liver problems. Acts as an antioxidant and as a sedative.	

49

Herb	Parts Used	Chemical and Nutrient Content	Actions and Uses	Comments
Chamomile	Various parts.	Antheme, anthemic acid, anthesterol, apigenin, calcium, chamazulene, iron, magnesium, manganese, volatile oils, potassium, tannic acid, tiglic acid, and vitamin A.	A good nerve tonic, sleep aid, appetite stimulant, and digestive aid. Relieves the bladder, colds, asthma, colitis, diverticulosis, fever, headaches, hemorrhoids, muscle cramps, and pain. Effective in the treatment of rheumatism, arthritis, worms, and jaundice.	*Warning:* Do not use for long periods of time. In the past, chamomile was planted alongside an ailing plant, but removed after a short period of time. When the ailing plant was left for a long time, it suffered a relapse. Do not use if allergic to ragweed.
Chaparral	Leaves.	Nordihydroquaiaretic acid, sodium, sulfur, and zinc.	Bitter herb that acts as a free radical scavenger. Protects from harmful effects of radiation and sun exposure. Good for skin disorders (i.e., boils), leg cramps, and arthritis. Relieves pain, purifies the blood, increases adrenal ascorbic acid levels, and protects against the formation of tumors and cancer cells. Improves kidney, lung, and liver function.	
Chickweed	Various parts.	Ascorbic acid (vitamin C), biotin, choline, copper, inositol, PABA, phosphorus, potash salts, rutin, silicon, sodium, and vitamins B_6, B_{12}, and D.	Reduces mucus build-up in the lungs. May effectively treat asthma. Use for gastrointestinal disorders, constipation, coughs, colds, rheumatism, scurvy, pleurisy, skin diseases, tumors, cancer, inflammation, and blood disorders. Use as a vitamin C supplement.	
Coltsfoot	Berries, fruits, and leaves.	Caoutchouc, volatile oils, pectin, resin, and tannins.	For various skin disorders, persistent cough, asthma, bronchitis, catarrh, inflammation, fever, diarrhea, ulcers, and burns.	*Warning:* Carcinogenic properties have been discovered.
Comfrey root	Leaves and roots.	Allantoin, consolidine, mucilage, phosphorus, potassium, pyrrolizidine, starch, tannins, and vitamins A, C, and E.	Acts as a blood cleanser. Beneficial for asthma, coughs, catarrh, ulcers, swelling, cramps, tuberculosis, pain, and burns. Also good for the stomach, kidneys, bowels, and lungs.	*Caution:* Use only under careful supervision by your physician or health care practitioner. Do not use for longer than 3 months at a time. May cause liver damage.
Cornsilk	Stylus.	Alkaloids, ascorbic acid, cryptoxanthin, fluorine, malic acid, oxalic acid, palmitic acid, pantothenic acid, resin, saponins, silicon, sitotsterol, stigmasterol, tartaric acid, and vitamin K.	A sweet herb that aids the kidneys, bladder, and small intestines. Take for hypertension, edema, urinary tract dysfunction and stones, bed-wetting, and painful urination caused by the prostrate gland. Acts as a diuretic.	

Herb	Parts Used	Chemical and Nutrient Content	Actions and Uses	Comments
Damiana	Leaves.	Arbutin, chlorophyll, damianian, volatile oils, resin, starch, sugar, and tannins.	Relieves headaches, controls bed-wetting, and stimulates muscular contractions of intestinal tract.	*Warning:* Damiana interferes with iron absorption when taken internally.
Dandelion	Leaves, roots, and tops.	Biotin, calcium, choline, fats, gluten, gum, inositol, inulin, iron, lactupicrine, linolenic acid, magnesium, niacin, PABA, phosphorus, potash, proteins, resin, sulfur, vitamins A, B_1, B_2, B_5, B_6, B_9, B_{12}, C, E, and P, and zinc.	A mildly bitter herb that cleanses the bloodstream and liver and increases the production of bile. Used as a diuretic. Improves function of the pancreas, spleen, stomach, and kidneys. Take for anemia, gout, rheumatism, jaundice, cirrhosis, hepatitis, abscesses, boils, cramps, fluid retention, constipation, and breast tumors. May aid in the prevention of breast cancer and age spots. Reduces serum cholesterol and uric acid.	
Dong quai	Roots.	Alcohols, cadinene, carotene, carvacrol, isosafrol, essential oil, safrol, sesquiterpenes, sucrose, and vitamins A, B_{12}, and E.	Used in the treatment of female problems such as hot flashes, menopause, PMS, and vaginal dryness. Increases the effect of ovarian/testicular hormones.	
Echinacea	Roots and leaves.	Arabinose, betaine, copper, echinacen, echinacin B, echinacoside, echinolone, enzymes, fructose, fatty acids, galactose, glucose, glucuronic acid, inulin, inuloid, iron, pentadecadiene, polyacetylene compounds, polysaccharides, potassium, protein, resin, rhamnose, sucrose, sulfur, tannins, vitamins A, C, and E, and xylose.	A bitter herb used for colic, colds, flu, infections, and snake bites. Has antibiotic, antiviral, and anti-inflammatory properties. Good for the immune system, lymphatic system, and glandular swelling.	Can be sold fresh, freeze-dried, dried, or as an alcohol extract, liquid, tea, capsule, or salve. (Take every 2 hours for acute inflammation and decrease dosage accordingly.) *Warning:* Alcohol tincture may destroy polysaccharides in echinacea that stimulate the immune system, although other active ingredients remain intact. Most tinctures are 20 percent in order to preserve the herb, but even 10 percent ruins the echinacea. The freeze-dried form is preferred.
Evening primrose oil	Seeds .	Gamma-linolenic acid (GLA), linoleic acid, and vitamin F (essential fatty acids).	Aids in weight loss, reduces high blood pressure, and helps to treat all skin disorders, female disorders such as cramps and heavy bleeding, hot flashes, multiple sclerosis, arthritis, alcoholism, and many other disorders.	If linoleic acid cannot convert to GLA, its desired effects cannot be achieved.

Herb	Parts Used	Chemical and Nutrient Content	Actions and Uses	Comments
Eyebright	Entire plant except the root.	Bitters, inositol, volatile oils, PABA, sulfur, tannins, and vitamins A, B_3, B_5, B_{12}, C, D, and E.	Used as an eyewash. Prevents secretion of fluids and relieves discomfort from eyestrain or minor irritation. Good for all eye disorders.	
Fennel	Berries, fruits, roots, and stems.	Anethole, calcium, camphene cymene, chlorine, dipentene, fenchone, 7-hydrozycoumarin, volatile oils, oleic acid, petroselinic acid, phellandrene, pinene, limonene, stigmasterol, sulfur, and vitamins A and C.	A sweet herb used as an appetite suppressant and as an eyewash. Promotes function of the spleen, liver, and kidneys, and also clears the lungs. Used for acid stomach. It relieves gas, gastrointestinal tract spasms, abdominal pain, and colon disorders. Effective in the treatment of gout, and good for the cancer patient after chemotherapy and radiation.	.
Fenugreek	Seeds.	Biotin, choline, inositol, iron, lecithin, mucilage, volatile oils, PABA, phosphates, protein, trigonelline, trimethylamine, and vitamins A, B_1, B_2, B_3, B_5, B_6, B_9, B_{12}, and D.	Helps asthma and sinus problems by reducing mucus. Good for lung disorders and inflammation. Acts as a bulk laxative. Reduces fever, lowers cholesterol, and lubricates the intestines. Good for the eyes.	
Feverfew	Bark, dried flowers, and leaves.	Borneol, camphor, parthenolide, pyrethrins, santamarin, and terpene.	Relieves headaches, arthritis, indigestion, colds, fever, and muscle tension. Eliminates worms. Stimulates the appetite, increases fluidity of lung and bronchial tube mucus, stimulates uterine contractions, and promotes menses.	
Flaxseed	Seeds.	Glycosides, gum, linamarin, linoleic acid, linolenic acid, mucilage, oleic acid, protein, saturated acids, tannins, and wax.	Used for female disorders, colon problems, inflammation, and tumors. Promotes strong nails, bones, and teeth and healthy skin.	
Garlic	Bulb.	Unsaturated aldehydes, allicin, allyl disulfides, calcium, copper, germanium, iron, magnesium, manganese, volatile oils, phosphorus, phytoncides, potassium, selenium, sulfur, vitamins A, B_1, B_2, and C, and zinc.	A natural antibiotic. Protects from infection, detoxifies the body, strengthens blood vessels, and lowers blood pressure. Aids in the treatment of arteriosclerosis, asthma, arthritis, cancer, circulatory problems, colds, flu, digestive problems, heart disorders, insomnia, liver disease, sinusitis, ulcers, and yeast infections. Good for all diseases, infections, fungus, and bacteria.	Odorless garlic (Kyolic) is available.
Gentian	Roots and leaves.	Gentiamarin, gentiin, gentisin, mesogentioigenin, protogentiogenin, sugar, and xanthone pigment.	Stimulates gastric secretions, aids digestion, stimulates appetite, increases circulation, and kills plasmodia (organisms that cause malaria) and worms. Good for liver and spleen function, fever, colds, and gout.	

Herb	Parts Used	Chemical and Nutrient Content	Actions and Uses	Comments
Ginger	Roots and rhizomes.	Bisabolene, borneal, borneol, camphene, choline, cineole, citral, ginerol, inositol, volatile oils, PABA, phellandrene, acrid resin, sequiterpene, vitamins B_3, B_5, and B_9, zingerone, and zingiberene.	A spicy herb used for colitis, diverticulosis, nausea, gas, indigestion, paralysis of the tongue, morning sickness, nausea, vomiting, hot flashes, and menstrual cramps. Cleanses the colon, stimulates circulation, and reduces spasms and cramps.	
Ginkgo biloba	Leaves.	Ginkgolides and heterosides.	Improves memory loss, brain function, depression, cerebral and peripheral circulation, oxygenation, and blood flow. Good for tinnitis, asthma, Alzheimer's disease, heart and kidney disorders, and glucose utilization.	
Ginseng (Siberian, American, Panax)	Roots.	Arabinose, calcium, camphor, gineosides, iron, mucilage, panaxosides, resin, saponin, starch, and vitamins A, B_{12}, and E.	Used for impotence, (stimulates male sex glands), stress (strengthens the adrenal glands), cocaine withdrawal, energy, diabetes, radiation protection, colds, and chest problems. Promotes lung function, enhances immune function, stimulates the appetite, and normalizes blood pressure.	
Goldenseal	Roots and rhizomes.	Albumin, berberine, biotin, calcium, candine, chlorine, choline, chologenic acid, fats, hydrastine, inositol, iron, lignin, manganese, volatile and essential oils, PABA, phosphorus, potassium, resin, starch, sugar, the B complex, and vitamins A, C, and E.	A bitter, cure-all type of herb that strengthens the immune system, acts as an antibiotic, has anti-inflammatory and antibacterial properties, potentiates insulin, and cleanses the body. Good for colds, flu, inflammation, glandular swelling, gum disease, morning sickness, diabetes, hypoglycemia, and ulcers. Promotes functioning capacity of the heart, the lymphatic and respiratory system, the liver, the spleen, the pancreas, and the colon. Good for stomach, prostrate, bladder, and vaginal disorders. Cleanses mucous membranes, regulates menses, improves digestion, and counters infection. Also decreases uterine bleeding, reduces blood pressure, and stimulates the central nervous system.	*Warning:* Long-term use may weaken the bacterial flora of the colon. When combined with gotu kola, goldenseal acts as a brain tonic.

Herb	Parts Used	Chemical and Nutrient Content	Actions and Uses	Comments
Gotu kola	Seeds, nuts, and roots.	Catechol, epicatechol, magnesium, theobromine, and vitamin K.	A mildly bitter herb that stimulates central nervous system, aids in the elimination of excess fluids, shrinks tissues, decreases fatigue and depression, and increases sex drive. Used for rheumatism, blood diseases, mental disorders, high blood pressure, congestive heart failure, sore throat, tonsillitis, hepatitis, urinary tract infections, veneral disease, measles, insomnia, and stress. Acts as a diuretic. May neutralize blood acids and lower body temperature. Good for liver and heart function.	May promote hair growth when combined with eclipta.
Hawthorn berries	Berries, fruits, and leaves.	Anthocyanin-type pigments, choline, citric acid, cratagolic acid, flavonoid, glavone, glycosides, inositol, PABA, purines, saponins, sugar, tartaric acid, and vitamins B_1, B_2, B_3, B_5, B_6, B_9, B_{12}, and C.	An herb used to dilate the coronary blood vessels, to restore the heart muscle wall, and to lower cholesterol levels. Used to treat heart disease, sore throats, and skin sores. Relieves abdominal distention and diarrhea.	
Hops	Berries, fruits, and leaves.	Asparagine, choline, humulene, inositol, lupulin, lupulinic acid, lupulon, manganese, essential oil, PABA, picric acids, resin, and vitamin B_6.	Good for nervousness, restlessness, pain, stress, insomnia, toothaches, earaches, gonorrhea, ulcers, circulation, muscle cramps, and shock. Decreases the desire for alcohol.	
Horehound	Flowers and leaves.	Iron, marrubiin, volatile oils, potassium, resin, tannins, the B complex, and vitamins A, C, E, and F.	Take for coughs, colds, asthma, jaundice, sore throat, intestinal gas, and worms. Decreases thickness and increases fluidity of mucus in bronchial tubes and lungs.	
Horsetail	Stems.	Aconitic acid, calcium, copper, equisitine, fatty acids, fluorine, nicotine, PABA, silica, sodium, starch, vitamin B_5, and zinc.	Used as a diuretic and in the treatment of kidney stones. Strengthens hair, nails, bone, and teeth, promotes healthy skin, and increases calcium absorption. Also used in the treatment of cystitis, intestinal disorders, rheumatism, and gout. Promotes healing of broken bones and connective tissue.	Use as a poultice to depress bleeding and to accelerate healing of wounds.
Huckleberries	Entire plant.	Fatty acids, hydroquinone, iron, loeanolic acid, neomyrtillin, sodium, tannins, and ursolic acid.	For diabetes, sinusitis, kidney and bladder problems, and ulcers. Helps to lower insulin and blood sugar levels and to ease inflammation.	*Caution:* Interferes with iron absorption when taken internally.
Irish moss	Entire plant.	Amino acids, bromine, calcium, carrageenan, chlorine, iodide, iron, manganese salts, mucins, protein, and sodium.	Use for thyroid problems (goiter), colon disorders, and obesity. Aids in the formation of bulky stools and corrects diarrhea. Used for hand lotions.	

Herb	Parts Used	Chemical and Nutrient Content	Actions and Uses	Comments
Juniper berries	Berries and fruits.	Alcohols, cadinene, camphene, flavone, volatile oils, resin, sabinal, sugar, sulfur, tannins, and terpinene.	Relieves inflammation and sinusitis. Helps in treatment of pancreas, kidney, and bladder problems, hypoglycemia, and ulcers. Regulates sugar levels. Used as a diuretic.	*Caution:* May interfere with iron absorption and other minerals when taken internally.
Kelp	Leaves.	Alginic acid, biotin, bromine, calcium, choline, copper, inositol, iodine, PABA, potassium, selenium, sodium, sulfur, vitamins A, B_1, B_3, B_5, B_6, B_9, B_{12}, C, and E, and zinc.	Reported to be very beneficial to the sensory nerves, membranes surrounding the brain, spinal cord, and brain tissue. Use for hair loss, goiter, ulcers, and obesity. Good for thyroid function, arteries, and nails. Protects from effects of radiation and softens stools. Good for those with mineral deficiency.	
Licorice root	Roots.	Asparagine, biotin, choline, fat, glycyrrhizin, gum, inositol, lecithin, manganese, PABA, pantothenic acid, pentacyclic terpenes, phosphorus, protein, sugar, vitamins B_1, B_2, B_3, B_5, B_6, B_9, and E, and yellow dye.	Beneficial for hypoglycemia, bronchitis, colitis, diverticulosis, gastritis, stress, colds, nausea, and inflammation. Cleanses the colon, promotes adrenal gland function, decreases muscle or skeletal spasms, and increases fluidity of mucus from the lungs and bronchial tubes. Has estrogen-like hormone effects; changes the voice.	Studies show licorice root stimulates the production of interferon. *Warning:* Do not use if you have high blood pressure. Deglycyrrhizinated licorice may stimulate the body's defense mechanisms that prevent the occurrence of ulcers by increasing the amount of mucous-secreting cells in the digestive tract. This improves the quality of mucous, lengthens intestinal cell life, and enhances microcirculation in the gastrointestinal lining. Licorice derivatives have been recommended as a standard nutritional support for ulcer sufferers in Europe.
Lobelia	Seeds, flowers, and leaves.	Alkaloids, chelidonic acid, isolobeline, lobelic acid, lobeline, selenium, and sulfur.	A cough suppressant and relaxant that reduces fever and cold symptoms. Beneficial in the treatment of sore throats, laryngitis, colic, asthma, bronchitis, angina pectoris, and epilepsy. Aids in hormone production.	

Herb	Parts Used	Chemical and Nutrient Content	Actions and Uses	Comments
Milk thistle (Silymarin)	Fruits (contain highest concentration), seeds, and leaves.	Active flavonoid silymarin (a unique type of flavonoid with antioxidant ability).	For all liver disorders such as jaundice and hepatitis. Contains some of the most potent liver-protecting substances known. Prevents free radical damage by acting as an antioxidant, protecting the liver. Stimulates the production of new liver cells and prevents formation of damaging leukotrienes. Also protects the kidneys and is beneficial to those with psoriasis.	
Milkweed	Roots.	Asclepiadin, asclepion, and galitoxin.	Stimulates gastrointestinal tract and increases perspiration. Aids in the treatment of gallbladder and female disorders, kidney trouble, asthma, arthritis, and bronchitis.	*Warning:* May be dangerous for children and people over 55.
Mullein	Leaves.	Aucubin, choline, hesperidin, magnesium, PABA, saponins, sulfur, verbaside, and vitamins B_2, B_5, B_{12}, and D.	For difficult breathing, asthma, glandular swelling, and hay fever. Used as a pain killer, sleep aid, and laxative. Gets rid of warts.	
Nettle	Leaves, flowers, and roots.	Chlorine, chlorophyll, formic acid, iodine, magnesium, potassium, silicon, sodium, sulfur, tannin, and vitamins A and C.	Good for colon and urinary disorders, arthritis, hemorrhoids, nephritis, cystitis, diarrhea, eczema, worms, and asthma. Improves mucous conditions of the lungs, goiter, and inflammatory conditions. A diuretic, expectorant, pain reliever, and tonic.	
Parsley	Fruits, berries, stems, and roots.	Apiin, apiol, bergapten, calcium, fatty oil, flavone glycoside apiin, furanocumarin bergapten, iodine, iron, isoimperatorin, mucilage, myristicene, volatile and essential oils, parsley camphor (apiin), petroselinic acid, phosphorus, pinene, potassium, and vitamins A and C.	A sweet plant that contains a substance in which tumor cells cannot multiply. Good for goiter, obesity, edema, bed-wetting, fluid retention, rheumatism, indigestion, gas, menstrual disorders, and worms. For thyroid, lung, stomach, bladder, liver, and kidney function. A diuretic, stimulant, carminative, and anthelmintic.	
Pau d'arco	Inner bark.	Antibacterial agent.	Bitter herb that contains a natural antibacterial agent, has a healing effect, and cleanses the blood. Good for candidiasis, smoker's cough, warts, all types of infection, diabetes, ulcers, rheumatism, allergies, tumors, AIDS, leukemia, cancer, and liver disease.	Some patients who no longer respond to pau d'arco can drink mathake herb tea. It is a good alternative. Pau d'arco needs to be boiled. Mathake is prepared as a regular tea. Resistant strains of *Candida* develop rapidly due to genetic mutation. Rotating treatment programs will be beneficial.

Herb	Parts Used	Chemical and Nutrient Content	Actions and Uses	Comments
Pennyroyal	Entire plant.	Ketone puligone and volatile oil.	For colds, phlegm, respiratory disorders, jaundice, nausea, skin disorders, ulcers, headaches, fever, menstrual disorders, and gout. Relieves gas and stomach pain. Purifies the blood, stimulates uterine contractions, and may increase perspiration. Also used as a flavoring.	*Warning:* May cause severe kidney/liver damage used in excess of two ounces. Do not use pennyroyal during pregnancy.
Peppermint	Leaves and flowering tops.	Menthol, menthone, methyl acetate, volatile oils, tannic acid, terpenes, and vitamin C.	Increases stomach acidity. Irritates mucous membranes and the gastrointestinal tract. Use for chills, colic, fever, nausea, diarrhea, heart trouble, rheumatism, convulsions, spasms, and headaches.	*Caution:* May interfere with iron absorption.
Psyllium	Seeds.	Aucubine, enzymes, fats, glycosides, mucilage, and protein.	Softens the stools, preventing constipation, colitis, and hemorrhoids. Cleans the intestines.	
Pumpkin	Seeds and husks.	Anthelmintic properties, isoprenoid compound, and vitamin F.	For prostate disorders, stomach problems, worms, and nausea (morning sickness).	
Red clover	Flowers.	Biotin, choline, copper, coumarins, glycosides, inositol, magnesium, manganese, selenium, vitamins A, B_1, B_2, B_3, B_5, B_6, B_9, B_{12}, C, and P, and zinc.	A sweet herb that is a blood purifier, an antibiotic used for tuberculosis and to fight other bacteria, a relaxant, and an appetite suppressant. Good for inflamed lungs, whooping cough, other inflammatory conditions related to gout and arthritis, skin disorders, and the AIDS virus.	Has positive effects on cancer patients when taken with chaparral.
Red Raspberry	Bark, leaves, and roots.	Citric acid, pectin, silicon, and vitamins C and D.	Good for diarrhea and female disorders such as morning sickness, hot flashes, and menstrual cramps. Strengthens the uterine wall, relaxes uterine and intestinal spasms, and decreases menstrual bleeding. Also heals canker sores and promotes healthy nails, bones, teeth, and skin.	*Caution:* May interfere with iron absorption when taken internally.
Rhubarb root	Roots.	Flavone, gallic acid, glucogallin, palmidine, pectin, phytosterol, rutin, starch, and tannins.	Helps disorders of the colon, spleen, and liver. Relieves headache, diarrhea, constipation, and hemorrhoids. Eliminates worms. Promotes healing of duodenal ulcers. Enhances gallbladder function. Antibiotic properties.	
Rose hips	Fruits.	Citric acid, flavonoids, fructose, malic acid, sucrose, tannins, vitamins A, B_3, C, D, E, and P, and zinc.	Good for all infections and bladder problems. Helps combat stress.	

Herb	Parts Used	Chemical and Nutrient Content	Actions and Uses	Comments
Sarsaparilla	Roots.	Copper, fat, glycosides, iron, manganese, essential oil, parillin, resin, saponins, sarsaponin, sitosterol stigmasterin, sodium, sugar, sulfur, vitamin A and D, and zinc.	A sweet herb used for impotence, liver problems, stress, rheumatism, gout, veneral disease (i.e., syphilis), leukorrhea, herpes, other disorders caused by blood impurities, epilepsy, and nervous system disorders. Reduces fever, clears skin disorders such as eczema and psoriasis, and controls diabetes. Also good for stomach and kidney disorders. Regulates hormones, increases energy, and protects against harmful radiation.	
Skullcap	Aerial parts.	Fat, glycoside, iron, volatile oil, sugar, tannins, and vitamin E.	Good for nervous disorders, hysteria, migraine headaches, rheumatism, epilepsy, and convulsions. Relieves pain, stress, muscle cramps, and spasms. Improves circulation, strengthens the heart muscle, and aids sleep.	
Slippery elm	Inner bark.	Calcium, mucilage, phosphorus, polysaccharides, starch, tannins, and vitamins K and P.	For inflamed mucous membranes of the stomach, bowels, and urinary tract. Good for diarrhea.	
Suma	Bark, leaves, berries, and roots.	Albumin, germanium (immune system booster that aids cancer), malic acid, volatile oils, pfaffic acid (inhibits certain cancer cells), six saponins (called pfaffosides A, B, C, D, E, and F), and tannins.	Suma has properties that combat anemia, fatigue, stress, and diabetes. An immune system booster.	In Brazil suma was reported to be more powerful than ginseng, and it is referred to as Brazilian ginseng. Research in Japan found that the suma root contains pfaffic acid, which is capable of inhibiting certain types of cancerous cells. Dr. Takemoto was the first to study suma in Japan.
Thyme	Berries, fruits, leaves, and flowers.	Borneol, cavacrol, fluorine, gum, trace minerals, essential oils, tannins, thiamine, thyme oil, thymol, triterpenic acids, and B-complex, C, and D vitamins.	For sinusitis and asthma. Eliminates gas and reduces fever, headache, and mucus. Good for chronic respiratory problems, colds, flu, and sore throat. Lowers cholesterol levels.	
Uva ursi	Leaves.	Arbutin, chlorine, ellagic acid, ericolin, gallic acid, hydroquinolone, malic acid, methyl-arbutin, myricetin, volatile oils, quercetin, tannins, ursolic acid, ursone, and a substance similar to quercetin.	A bitter herb used for kidney and bladder infections and kidney stones, diabetes, and hemorrhoids. Strengthens the heart muscle and helps disorders of the spleen, liver, pancreas, and small intestines. Used as a diuretic. Good for female disorders.	

Herb	Parts Used	Chemical and Nutrient Content	Actions and Uses	Comments
Valerian root	Roots and rhizomes.	Acetic acid, butyric acid, camphene, chatinine, formic acid, glycosides, magnesium, volatile oils, pinene, valeric acid, and valerine.	Good for nervousness, ulcers, headaches, colic, gas, pain, stress, anxiety, insomnia, convulsions, muscle cramps and spasms. Improves circulation and acts as a sedative. Reduces mucus from colds.	
Watercress	Flowers and leaves.	Calcium, chlorine, cobalt, copper, fluorine, iodine, iron, manganese, phosphorus, sulfur, vanadium, vitamins A, B_1, B_2, and C, and zinc.	Good for urinary (bladder) problems. Promotes kidney function. Helps heart disease by relieving fluid retention. Relieves indigestion and stops gas formation. Stimulates rate of metabolism.	
White oak bark	Bark.	Calcium, cobalt, iron, phosphorus, potassium, sodium, sulfur, and vitamin B_{12}.	Good for hemorrhoids, PMS, varicose veins, goiter, gallstones, kidney stones, fever, sores, and bladder problems. Also good for teeth.	Herb is used in enemas and douches.
Wood betony	Leaves.	Magnesium, manganese, phosphorus, and tannins.	Good for indigestion, stomach cramps, jaundice, Parkinson's disease, worms, headache, gout, colic, pain, colds, and tuberculosis. Stimulates the heart.	
Yarrow	Leaves, berries, and fruits.	Achilleic acid, achilleine, caledivain, volatile oils, potassium, tannins, and vitamin C.	Use for hemorrhages (i.e., bleeding from the lungs), ulcers, measles, smallpox, and chicken pox. Has healing effects on mucous membranes, eases diarrhea, and improves blood clotting.	*Caution:* Interferes with absorption of iron and other minerals.
Yellow dock	Leaves and roots.	Chrysarobin, iron, manganese, potassium oxalate, and rumicin.	A bitter herb that is good for liver and colon function, skin disorders (such as psoriasis, eczema, and urticaria), iron deficiency, anemia during pregnancy, hemorrhoids, bleeding lungs, bile congestion, and rheumatism. A blood purifier and cleanser. Tones up the entire system.	Combine with sarsaparilla as a tea for chronic skin disorders.
Yerbamate	All parts.	Chlorophyll, iron, trace minerals, and vitamins B_5, C, and E.	For arthritis, headache, hemorrhoids, fluid retention, obesity, fatigue, stress, constipation, allergies, and hay fever. Cleanses the blood, tones the nervous system, retards aging, stimulates the mind, controls the appetite, stimulates production of cortisone, and is believed to enhance the healing powers of other herbs.	To relieve constipation and allergy symptoms, use 2–3 tbsp. yerbamate in 16 oz. hot water. Consume on an empty stomach.

Herb	Parts Used	Chemical and Nutrient Content	Actions and Uses	Comments
Yucca	Roots.	Saponins.	A sweet herb used for gout. Also beneficial in treatment of urethritis and prostatitis. A blood purifier.	Routinely prescribed for arthritis (osteoarthritis and rheumatoid arthritis) in some clinics. Can cut up in water to make a natural lather as a soap substitute, can add to shampoos, or can use alone to wash hair (1 cup in 2 cups of water).

PART TWO

THE DISORDERS

INTRODUCTION

Part One explored the nutritional and dietary needs of the body. In order to be well, the parts of the body must be fueled so that a breakdown does not occur. With the growing number of stressors in the environment today, the body must obtain the proper nourishment in order to maintain a healthy immune system. If the immune system weakens, the body becomes susceptible to a number of harmful conditions.

Part Two offers an A–Z listing of the disorders that can occur if the body is overcome with stress and insuf-

ficient nutritional intake due to poor eating habits. The descriptions of the conditions may help you identify whether you have a particular illness. If your symptoms match those given for a certain illness, confirm your suspicions by visiting your physician. Once a diagnosis has been confirmed, you can refer to the dietary guidelines, recommendations, and supplementation program to help speed your recovery. Should you have any questions about the appropriateness of any suggested nutrients, speak to your physician.

Troubleshooting for Disorders

Some symptoms are indicative of a variety of illnesses. The following table lists some of the more common disorders that you may have if you are suffering from the corresponding symptom. Consult with your physician if you have any of these symptoms. Although you may experience some of the symptoms below, you may *not* have any of the illnesses

cited. Your body is simply sending a message that something may be wrong. Listening to your body can help stop a problem before it becomes serious. The illnesses listed below are in alphabetical order and do not at all reflect your chances of having any of them.

Symptom	Possible Cause
Abdominal pain	Colitis, diverticular disease, food allergies, food poisoning, hiatal hernia, irritable bowel syndrome, premenstrual syndrome
Backache	Back strain, disc disease, lack of exercise, female disorders, spinal injury
Blood in urine, stools, or vomit, or from vagina or penis	Cancer of kidneys, bladder, or uterus; hemorrhoids; infections; polyps; tumor of bowels; ulcers
Persistent cough	Food allergies, cancer, emphysema, lung disorders, pneumonia
Persistent fever	Bronchitis, colds, diabetes, chronic infection, influenza, mononucleosis, rheumatic disorders
Persistent headaches	Allergies, asthma, drugs, eyestrain, glaucoma, high blood pressure, sinusitis, stress, brain tumor, vitamin deficiency
Indigestion	Acidosis; alkalosis; allergies; poor diet; lack of enzymes or HCl; gallbladder problems; heart disease; junk foods; liver, pancreas, or adrenal disorders; stress; ulcers
Rash with blisters	Shingles, herpes zoster
Difficulty swallowing	Cancer of diverticulum of esophagus, hiatal hernia, stress
Excessive sweating	Food allergies, fever, Hodgkin's disease, infection, menopause, stress, thyroid disorder
Swelling of ankles, legs, feet, hands, abdomen	Food allergies, edema, heart disorders, kidney disorders, medications, oral contraceptives, steroids
Swollen lymph nodes	Hodgkin's disease, chronic infection, lymphoma, toxic metals, toxin build-up
Excessive thirst	Diabetes, fever, infection
Frequent urination	Bladder infection, poor emptying of bladder, diuretic effect/excessive liquid intake, cancer
Vaginal discharge	Chlamydia, genital herpes, gonorrhea, trichomoniasis, yeast infection (candidiasis)
Sudden weight gain	Edema, underactive thyroid
Unexplained loss of weight	Cancer, diabetes, hepatitis, malabsorption syndrome, mononucleosis, parasitic infection, overactive thyroid

Abscess

When pus accumulates in a particular part of the body due to infection, an abscess forms. The abscess may be located externally or internally and may result from a lowered resistance to infection that often leads to bacterial contamination or from an injury. The infected part becomes swollen, inflamed, and tender. The victim also experiences alternate bouts of fever and chills.

An abscess can form in the brain, lungs, teeth, gums, abdominal wall, gastrointestinal tract, ears, tonsils, sinuses, breasts, kidneys, prostate gland, or almost any other body part. Infections are the most common human disease and are produced by bacteria, viruses, parasites, and fungi.

Some abscesses need to be surgically treated, but most require only antibiotics, which destroy the B vitamins as well as the bacteria. Therefore, the diet must be supplemented with products containing "friendly" bacteria such as acidophilus and yogurt. The abscess may require that you get plenty of bed rest, drink plenty of fluids, and either apply ice packs or take hot baths to alleviate the pain.

NUTRIENTS

SUPPLEMENT	SUGGESTED DOSAGE	COMMENTS
Very Important		
Zinc	80 mg daily in divided doses. Use the lozenge form for effective absorption.	Powerful immune system stimulant. Necessary for T-lymphocyte function, which is needed to fight infection.
Important		
Garlic capsules (Kyolic)	2 capsules 3 times daily.	Acts as a natural antibiotic and stimulates the immune system.
Superoxide dismutase (SOD)	1 capsule taken 1 hour before meals.	Available in an antioxidant formula called Cell Guard or in SOD/CAT, both from Biotec Foods.
Vitamin A (emulsion formula)	Begin with 100,000 IU for the first 5 days; decrease to 50,000 IU for the next 5 days. Then decrease again to 25,000 IU.	By strengthening the cell walls, vitamin A protects them from invasion by bacteria. Essential to the immune system.
Vitamin E	400–600 IU	Important in circulation and tissue oxygenation. Enhances the immune system.
Vitamin C with bioflavonoids	6,000–10,000 mg in daily divided doses.	Essential in immune function and tissue repair. See ASCORBIC ACID FLUSH in Part Three.
Helpful		
Germanium	100 mg daily.	Enhances the immune system.
Multivitamin and mineral complex	As directed on label.	All nutrients are needed for healing.
Proteolytic enzymes or Intenzyme from Biotics Research or Inflazyme Forte from American Biologics	2 tablets between meals.	Aids in cleanup of the abscess. Powerful free radical scavengers.
Raw thymus extract	2 tablets before meals.	Stimulates the production of T-cells; protects against infection.

HERBS

☐ The therapeutic effects of the following herbs are beneficial for abscesses: burdock root, cayenne, chaparral, dandelion root, red clover, and yellow dock root.

RECOMMENDATIONS

☐ Perform a liquid fast using fresh juices for 24–72 hours. (See FASTING in Part Three.)

☐ Consume distilled water with fresh lemon juice and three cups daily of echinacea, goldenseal, and suma tea.

☐ Applying honey to the affected area often helps. To cleanse, apply chlorophyll liquid mixed with water to the area several times a day.

☐ Eat kelp, which is rich in vitamins and minerals.

Acidosis

Acidosis is a tendency of the body to be overacid. This occurs when the body loses its alkaline reserve. Persons who have diabetes often suffer from acidosis, and stomach ulcers are associated with this condition. The symptoms of acidosis are frequent sighing, insomnia, water retention, recessed eyes, rheumatoid arthritis, migraine headaches, abnormally low blood pressure, dry hard stools, foul-smelling stools accompanied by a burning sensation in the anus, alternating constipation and diarrhea, difficulty swallowing, burning in the mouth and/or under the tongue, sensitivity of teeth to vinegar and acid fruits, and bumps on the roof of the mouth or tongue. The causes of acidosis are kidney, liver, and adrenal disorders; improper diet; malnutrition; obesity; ketosis; anger, stress, and fear; anorexia; toxemia; fever; and excess niacin, vitamin C, and aspirin.

Although it might seem that citrus fruits would have an acid effect on the body, the citric acid they contain actually has an alkaline effect in the system, converting to carbon dioxide and water. To treat acidosis, start with small amounts of citrus fruits and gradually add larger amounts.

ACID AND ALKALINE SELF-TEST

This test will determine whether your body fluids are either too acidic or too alkaline. An imbalance can cause illnesses such as acidosis or alkalosis.

Purchase nitrazine paper, available at any drugstore, and apply saliva and/or urine to the paper. Always perform the test either before eating or at least one hour after eating. The paper will change color to indicate if your system is overly acidic or alkaline. Red litmus paper turns blue in an alkaline medium and blue litmus paper turns red in an acid medium.

Water is neutral with a pH of 7.0. Anything with a pH below 7.0 is acid, while anything with a pH above 7.0 is alkaline. The ideal pH range for saliva and urine is 6.0 to 6.8. Our body is naturally mildly acidic. Therefore, values below pH 6.3 would be considered too acidic; values above pH 6.8 are too alkaline. The pH value of milk varies from 6.2 to 7.3.

The following foods should be consumed according to the results of your test. If your test indicated one extreme or another, omit the acid- or alkaline-forming foods from your diet until another pH test shows that you have returned to normal. Alkaline-forming foods should be consumed when the body is too acidic (pH under 7). Acid-forming foods should be eaten if the pH is too alkaline. Low-level acid and low-level alkaline foods are almost neutral.

Acid-Forming Foods

alcohol	flour products
asparagus	legumes
beans	lentils
Brussels sprouts	meat
catsup	milk
chickpeas	mustard
cocoa	noodles
coffee	oatmeal
cornstarch	olives
eggs	organ meats
fish	pasta

pepper	soft drinks
poultry	sugar
sauerkraut	tea
shellfish	

Low-Level Acid-Forming Foods

butter	grains (most)
cheeses	ice cream
coconuts (dried)	ice milk (homemade)
fruits (canned/glazed)	lambsquarter
fruits (dried sulfured)	seeds and nuts (most)

Alkaline-Forming Foods

apricots	maple syrup
avocados	melons
corn	millet
dates	molasses
fruits	oranges
grapefruit	raisins
grapes	soy figs
honey	vegetables
lemons	

Low-Level Alkaline-Forming Foods

almonds	coconuts (fresh)
blackstrap molasses	dairy products, soured
Brazil nuts	lima beans
buckwheat	millet
chestnuts	

Prunes, cranberries, and plums are acid forming and remain acidic in the body. Raw fruits become acid forming when sugar is added. All foods with added sugar become acidic. Alcohol, drugs, aspirin, tobacco, and vinegar are also acid forming.

NUTRIENTS

SUPPLEMENT	SUGGESTED DOSAGE	COMMENTS
Very Important		
Tri Salts from Cardiovascular Research	As directed on label.	For acid-alkaline balance.
Helpful		
Kelp	5 tablets daily.	Reduces acid in the body. Aids in maintaining a proper balance of minerals.
Potassium	99 mg daily.	Increases metabolism. Aids in balancing the pH in the blood.

Vitamin A	50,000 IU for 1 month, then reduce to 25,000 IU.
Vitamin B complex	100 mg twice daily.

HERBS

☐ Use elder bark, hops, and willow for acidosis.

RECOMMENDATIONS

☐ Diet is important. Acidosis results from eating excess animal protein, excess processed junk foods, and cooked food. When ingested, cooked and processed foods become acid in the body. Reduce intake of beef and pork.

☐ Since excess vitamin C may lead to acidosis, reduce intake of vitamin C for a few weeks. When taking vitamin C, use the non-acid forming varieties (buffered, such as sago palm).

☐ Avoid beans, cereals, crackers, eggs, flour products, grains, oily foods, macaroni, and sugar. Reduce cooked and processed foods—cooked food often means dead food. Plums, prunes, and cranberries do not oxidize and therefore remain acid to the body. Avoid these until the situation improves.

☐ Eat 50 percent raw foods such as apples, avocados, bananas, grapefruit, grapes, lemons, pears, pineapples, and all vegetables. Fresh fruits and vegetables reduce acidosis. Phosphorus and sulfur act as buffers to maintain pH. Sulfur is now available in tablet form.

☐ Drink potato broth every day (see THERAPEUTIC FOODS in Part Three for the recipe).

☐ Externally, apply ginger compresses to the kidney area.

☐ Practice deep breathing.

☐ Check your urine pH daily using nitrazine paper (acid and alkaline self-test). See the self-testing section for a list of foods to avoid until your pH is corrected.

Acne

Acne is a skin inflammation that to some degree afflicts about 80 percent of all those between the ages of twelve and twenty-four. A sebaceous gland, located in each hair follicle or tiny pit of skin, produces oil that lubricates the skin. If some of the oil becomes trapped, bacteria multiply in the pit and the skin becomes inflamed. Several of these spots can come and go over a period of months or years. Most adolescents have acne because the sebaceous glands are stimulated by a male hormone at puberty.

No exact cause is known, but factors that contribute to acne are heredity, oily skin, and androgens (male hormones) produced in increased amounts when a boy or girl reaches puberty. Other causes include oral contraceptives, allergies, stress, and excess junk food.

Blackheads form when sebum combines with skin pigments and plugs the pores. If scales below the surface of the skin become filled with sebum, whiteheads appear. In severe cases the whiteheads build up, spread under the skin, and rupture, which eventually spreads the inflammation.

NUTRIENTS

SUPPLEMENT	SUGGESTED DOSAGE	COMMENTS
Very Important		
Chromium (GTF)	As directed.	Aids in reducing infections of the skin.
Gerovital H-3 face cream (GH-3)	As directed on label.	Relieves inflammation. Used in Europe with good results.
Lecithin	1 capsule before meals.	Needed for better absorption of the essential fatty acids.
Primrose oil	As directed on label.	Supplies the essential gamma-linoleic acids needed for healing. Used in Europe with good results. See unsaturated fatty acids below.
Unsaturated fatty acids	1 tbsp. cold-pressed sesame or flaxseed oil (linseed oil) or take in capsule form.	Needed to keep the skin smooth and soft, and to repair damaged cells.
Zinc gluconate	30–80 mg daily.	Aids in healing of tissue and helps to prevent scarring.
Important		
Vitamin A and E emulsion	100,000 IU vitamin A and 400 IU vitamin E. Use emulsion for easier assimilation.	Strengthens the protective epithelial (skin) tissue.
Helpful		
Accutane	As directed on label.	Strengthens epithelial (skin) tissue. *Caution:* Do not use if pregnant. May cause birth defects.
Chlorophyll (liquid or tablets)	As directed on label.	Aids in cleansing the blood, preventing infections.
Cod liver oil	As directed on label.	A good source of vitamins A and D, which are needed for healing of skin tissue.

Hydrochloric acid (HCl) with digestive enzymes	Take with meals.	*Caution:* Those with ulcers should not take digestive enzymes containing HCl.
Niacin	100 mg 3 times daily with meals.	Improves blood flow to the surface of the skin.
Proteolytic enzymes	2 tablets between meals.	Free radical scavengers.
Retin-A (contains retinoic acid and a vitamin A derivative)	By prescription only.	Successfully used by dermatologists to treat acne. *Caution:* Do not use if pregnant. May cause birth defects.
Vitamin B complex (high potency) with extra B$_6$ and pantothenic acid	50 mg 3 times daily.	Important for healthy skin tone.
Vitamin C with bioflavonoids	3,000–5,000 mg daily in divided doses.	Promotes immune function.

HERBS

☐ Use alfalfa, burdock root, cayenne, chaparral, dandelion root, echinacea, the herbal combinations AKN and BFC, red clover combination from Nature's Way Products, and yellow dock root. Prepare a poultice using chaparral, dandelion, and yellow dock root, and apply to the areas of skin with acne. *See* POULTICE in Part Three for directions on how to prepare and use a poultice.

☐ Use red clover, lavender, and strawberry leaves as a steam sauna on the face. Lavender kills germs and stimulates new cell growth.

RECOMMENDATIONS

☐ Keep the affected area as free from oil as possible. Wash or pat the face with lemon juice three times daily. Shampoo hair frequently.

☐ Increase your intake of raw vegetables. Avoid alcohol, butter and cream, caffeine, cheese, chocolate, eggs, fat, fish, meat, poultry, sugar, and wheat. Do not use any dairy products for one month. Acne may develop due to an allergic reaction to dairy products, and the fat content of the dairy products can worsen the condition. Add one dairy product back at a time to see if the acne returns.

CONSIDERATIONS

☐ An antibiotic cream or an oral antibiotic is sometimes prescribed for acne. If so, add some form of

acidophilus because antibiotics kill "friendly" bacteria along with "unfriendly" bacteria. Eat plenty of sour products, such as yogurt.

☐ Benzoyl peroxide, an active ingredient in many acne products, helps in mild cases. All cosmetics should be water based; do not use oil-based products.

☐ An acne treatment program called Derma-Klear from Enzymatic Therapy may help.

☐ Blackheads should be removed only with a specially designed instrument. Picking or scratching may cause scarring. Keep hands clean and avoid touching the face.

☐ Follow the fasting program. (*See* FASTING in Part Three.)

☐ *See also* SKIN PROBLEMS in Part Two.

Acquired Immune Deficiency Syndrome

See AIDS.

Adrenal Disorders

The adrenal glands are triangular-shaped organs resting on top of each kidney. Each gland normally weighs about five grams and is comprised of two parts: the cortex or outer section, which is responsible for the production of cortisone, and the medulla or central section, which secretes adrenaline.

The adrenal cortex helps to maintain salt and water balance in the body. It is also involved in the metabolism of carbohydrates and the regulation of blood sugar. The cortex produces a sex hormone similar to that secreted by the testes as well.

The medulla of the adrenal gland produces the hormone epinephrine, also called adrenaline, when the body is under stress. This hormone speeds up the rate of metabolism in order to help the body cope with stressful situations.

The functioning ability of the adrenal glands is most often impaired due to extensive use of cortisone therapy for nonendocrine diseases, such as arthritis and asthma. Long-term use of cortisone drugs causes the adrenal gland to shrink in size. Adrenocortical failure is also caused by pituitary disease and tuberculosis.

When the adrenal cortex is underactive, a rare disease called Addison's may develop. Discoloration and darkening of the skin is common in people suffering from Addison's disease; discoloration of knees, elbows, scars, skin folds, and creases in the palms are more noticeable when these body parts are exposed to the sun. The mouth, the vagina, and freckles will appear darker. This disease is also characterized by bands of pigment running the length of the nail and darkened hair. Other symptoms include a decreased amount of body hair, such as under the arms, fatigue, a loss of appetite, dizziness or fainting, an inability to cope with stress, nausea, and moodiness. The individual may also constantly complain about being cold.

Addison's disease is a lifelong condition. In order for the adrenal glands to work at their highest functioning ability, a victim of Addison's disease must take his medication as prescribed and pay strict attention to his diet; nutritional supplements are recommended.

Whereas Addison's disease results from an underactive adrenal cortex, Cushing's syndrome is a rare disorder caused by an overactive adrenal cortex. Those with this disease generally are heavy in the abdomen, face, and buttocks, but have very thin limbs. Muscular weakness and wasting of muscles are also characteristic of this syndrome. Round, red marks mimicking acne may appear on the face, and the eyelids may appear swollen. Increased growth of body hair is common, and women may grow mustaches and beards. A "Cushinoid" appearance is frequently present with prolonged cortisone use. People with Cushing's generally are more susceptible to illness and have trouble healing properly. Thinning of the skin from Cushing's syndrome often leads to stretch marks and bruising.

In order to keep the adrenal glands functioning properly, stress must be avoided. Continuous and prolonged stress from troubled marriages, bad job conditions, illness, or feelings of low esteem or loneliness can be detrimental to the adrenal glands. Because the adrenals must work harder under stressful situations, continuous stress will impair their functioning ability. Poor nutritional habits, smoking, and alcohol and drug abuse can also contribute to adrenal failure.

ADRENAL GLAND FUNCTION SELF-TEST

Reduced adrenal function may be indicated by the following: weakness, lethargy, dizziness, headaches, memory problems, food cravings, allergies, and blood sugar disorders.

The normal systolic blood pressure (the higher pressure—*120/80*) is approximately 10 mm higher when you are standing than when you are lying down.

To test adrenal function, take and compare two blood pressure readings—one while lying down and one while standing. Rest for five minutes in the recumbent position (lying down) before taking the reading. Stand up and immediately take the blood pressure again. If the blood pressure is lower after standing, suspect reduced adrenal gland function. The degree to which the blood pressure drops while standing is often proportionate to the degree of hypoadrenalism.

NUTRIENTS

SUPPLEMENT	SUGGESTED DOSAGE	COMMENTS
Essential		
Pantothenic acid (vitamin B₅)	100 mg 3 times daily.	The adrenal glands will not function adequately without pantothenic acid.
Vitamin B complex	100 mg twice daily.	All B vitamins are necessary for adrenal function.
Vitamin C plus bioflavonoids	4,000–10,000 mg daily in divided doses.	Vital for proper functioning of the adrenals.
Very Important		
L-Tyrosine	500 mg on an empty stomach.	L-Tyrosine aids adrenal gland function and relieves excess stress put on the glands.
Important		
Raw adrenal extract or freeze-dried tablets and raw adrenal cortex	As directed on label.	The protein derived from this adrenal gland substance helps to rebuild and repair the adrenal glands.
Helpful		
Chlorophyll	As directed on label.	Cleanses the bloodstream.
Coenzyme Q₁₀	60 mg daily.	Carries oxygen to all glands.
Germanium	100 mg daily.	A powerful stimulant of the immune system.
Liver	As directed on label.	Obtain from Argentine beef only, which is from livestock raised without antibiotics, pesticides, and hormones. Supplies natural B vitamins, iron, and enzymes.
Mega-multivitamin and mineral complex with beta-carotene and copper and zinc	15,000 IU daily. 3 mg daily. 50 mg daily.	Contains nutrients needed for correct functioning of all glands.
Raw spleen tissue and pituitary glandulars (freeze-dried or extract)	As directed on label.	Boosts immune function and aids healing process. Available in health food stores.

HERBS

☐ The herb astragalus improves adrenal gland function and aids in stress reduction. Using echinacea can increase white blood cell production and protect tissues from bacterial invasion. Milk thistle extract aids liver function, which in turn helps adrenal function. Siberian ginseng is an herb that helps the adrenal gland prepare the body for stressful situations.

RECOMMENDATIONS

☐ Avoid alcohol, caffeine, and tobacco; these substances are highly toxic to the adrenal gland and other glands. Stay away from fats, fried foods, ham, pork, highly processed foods, red meats, salt, sodas, sugar, and white flour. These foods put unnecessary stress on the adrenal glands.

☐ Consume plenty of fresh fruits and vegetables—particularly green, leafy ones. Brewer's yeast, brown rice, legumes, olive and safflower oils, nuts, seeds, wheat germ, and whole grains are healthy additions to the diet. Eat deep-water ocean fish, salmon, and tuna at least three times a week.

☐ Take positive action to relieve stressful situations. Moderate exercise helps to stimulate the adrenal glands. Steps must be taken to protect these glands or they can become exhausted.

CONSIDERATIONS

☐ ACTH, a hormone released by the pituitary gland when under stress, is responsible for activating substances that raise the blood pressure. The presence of this hormone leads to sodium retention and potassium excretion. As a result, the body may retain water, which can lead to hypertension.

Age Spots

"Age spots" are the flat brown spots that appear anywhere on the body as it ages. They are also called "liver spots." These brown spots are the result of a waste build-up known as "lipofuscin accumulatio," a by-product of free radical damage in skin cells (*see* RADIATION POISONING in Part Two for an inset on free radicals). These spots are thought by many to be harmless, but are actually signs that the cells are full of accumulated waste

that is slowly destroying cells in the body, including brain and liver cells. They are the surface sign of free radical intoxication of the body.

The causes of age spots include poor diet, lack of exercise, *excess sun exposure*, poor liver function, and the ingestion of rancid oils.

NUTRIENTS

SUPPLEMENT	SUGGESTED DOSAGE	COMMENTS
Very Important		
Ageless Beauty from Biotec Foods	As directed on label.	A free radical destroyer.
Vitamin B complex plus extra pantothenic acid (B₅)	100 mg 3 times daily.	Needed by the elderly for proper assimilation of all nutrients.
Vitamin C with bioflavonoids	3,000–6,000 mg daily in divided doses.	A powerful antioxidant and free radical scavenger that is necessary for tissue repair.
Important		
Lactobacillus bulgaricus (Bulgaricum I.B. from Natren)	As directed on label.	Aids in liver regeneration and digestion.
Helpful		
Bio-Strath	As directed on label.	Acts as a tonic.
Calcium and magnesium	1,500–2,000 mg daily. 750–1,000 mg daily.	The elderly need these nutrients. Asporotate or chelate form is best.
Gerovital H-3 (GH-3) cream	As directed on label.	This is a skin cream from Rumania that is excellent. Apply it externally.
Lecithin	1 capsule or 1 tbsp. with meals.	Needed for proper brain function, this emulsifier works well as an antioxidant when taken with vitamin E.
Superoxide dismutase (SOD) with selenium from Biotec Foods	Use as directed on label.	Powerful antioxidants.
Vitamin A-D-E emulsion	50,000 IU vitamin A; 400 IU vitamin D; 600 IU vitamin E (or in capsule form for 1 month).	Aids in cleaning and rebuilding the system to prevent age spots. Emulsion form is more easily assimilated.

HERBS

☐ Use ginseng, gotu kola, licorice, and sarsaparilla for age spots.

RECOMMENDATIONS

☐ A high-protein diet that includes 50 percent raw fruits and vegetables and fresh grains, seeds, and nuts is recommended. Be aware that seeds and nuts may become rancid. Avoid caffeine, fried foods, processed foods, sugar, and tobacco.

☐ Sun exposure should be limited.

☐ A fasting program may be followed for one month until spots start to disappear. (*See* FASTING in Part Three.)

☐ A liver cleanse is probably indicated. Use black radish extract or dandelion root and beet juice along with three days of fasting a month.

CONSIDERATIONS

☐ The prescription drug retinoic acid is being used with good results.

☐ *See also* AGING in Part Two.

Aging

Years can be added to life when changes are made in lifestyle. The most important changes are in the areas of diet and exercise. Diet is important because there are many nutrients that can slow the aging process. As we age, our bodies do not assimilate nutrients as they once did. As a result, higher amounts of these essential nutrients are needed. See below for a list of these nutrients.

Many of the elderly have malabsorption problems; the nutrients in food are not absorbed from the gastrointestinal tract. If you follow the suggestions below and still do not feel a positive change in your energy level, *see* COLITIS, DIVERTICULITIS, and MALABSORPTION SYNDROME, all of which are in Part Two.

NUTRIENTS

SUPPLEMENT	SUGGESTED DOSAGE	COMMENTS
Essential		
Superoxide dismutase (SOD) or SOD/CAT from Biotec Foods	Use as directed on label. Take intravenously or dissolve under the tongue under doctor's supervision.	A potent antioxidant that destroys free radicals, which damage body cells.

Very Important		
Calcium asporate or chelate and	1,500 mg daily.	Necessary to prevent bone loss and for normal heart function.
magnesium and	750 mg daily.	
vitamin D	600–1,000 mg daily.	
Coenzyme Q$_{10}$	100 mg	Aids circulation; improves cellular oxygenation.
DMG (Gluconic from DaVinci Labs)	Use as directed. Dissolve under tongue.	Improves cellular oxygenation.
L-Methionine, L-carnitine, L-cysteine, and tyrosine (amino acids)	500 mg each twice daily on an empty stomach.	*See* AMINO ACIDS in Part One on the benefits of the amino acids.
Lecithin	1 tbsp. with meals or 4–6 capsules daily.	Improves brain function and memory. Protects nervous system cells.
Mega-multivitamin with trace chelated minerals including		Each is needed for the immune system. Also important antioxidants.
vitamin A and	25,000 IU daily.	
beta-carotene and	15,000 IU daily.	
selenium or	200 mcg daily.	
Nutri-Cell and De-Oxi-Flo	As directed on label.	
Protein supplement (free form amino acids)	¼ tsp. under tongue on empty stomach, 3 times daily. A small amount of vitamins B$_6$ and C helps assimilation.	The free form amino acids are more easily assimilated. Studies have shown that most of the elderly are protein deficient.
RNA-DNA	Use as directed on label.	Do not use if you have elevated serum uric acid because you may have gout. Good for reproduction of healthy cells.
Vitamin C plus bioflavonoids	4,000–10,000 mg daily in divided doses.	A powerful antioxidant and immune system enhancer.
Vitamin E	Start with 200 IU daily and slowly increase to 800 IU daily.	Studies reveal that vitamin E slows down the aging process (*see* VITAMINS in Part One on the many benefits of vitamin E).
Helpful		
Brewer's yeast	Start with ½ tsp. and work up.	A natural source of the B vitamins.
Germanium	60 mg twice daily.	A powerful antioxidant and immune system enhancer.
Lactobacillus bulgaricus (Bulgaricum I.B. from Natren)	Use as directed on label.	Improves liver function and aids in digestion.
Multidigestive enzymes (with meals)	After meals as directed on label.	If you have ulcers, avoid those brands containing HCl. Most elderly lack sufficient amounts of HCl.
Raw thymus glandular	500 mg daily.	Stimulates the immune system.

| Unsaturated fatty acids (evening primrose oil or salmon oil) | 2 capsules with meals. | Plays an important role in cell formation. |
| Vitamin B complex with extra choline, inositol, PABA, and pantothenic acid (B₅) | 125–250 mg daily. Divide the B vitamins throughout the day in capsule form. Do *not* use hard sustained-released pills. | Injections are best. The elderly have a difficult time assimilating the B vitamins. High amounts are needed for best bodily and brain function. |

HERBS

☐ Use ginseng and ginkgo biloba extract for extra energy and improved circulation.

RECOMMENDATIONS

☐ Eat a balanced diet that includes raw vegetables, fruits, grains, seeds, and nuts. Eat quality protein. Avoid alcohol, coffee, red meat, salt, smoking, white flour, and white sugar. Decrease food consumption, but increase intake of raw foods. Include broccoli, cabbage, cauliflower, egg yolks, fish, fruits, whole grains, nuts, oats, seeds, and soybeans. A high-fiber diet is important. Take extra fiber by eating plenty of fresh vegetables, whole grains, bran, and oats. Eat only when hungry. Cut your calorie intake—experiments with rats have shown that the rats live 50 percent longer when their calorie intake is decreased.

☐ Avoid alcohol, chemicals in food, drugs, pesticides, smoking, and contaminated drinking water. These items, along with pollution, poor diet, and malnutrition, shorten life span. You can lengthen your life by changing your lifestyle and following this program.

☐ Consume steam-distilled water. Drink even when you don't feel thirsty—your body needs plenty of water.

☐ Improve your blood and oxygen with deep breathing exercise. For one month try holding your breath for thirty seconds every half hour.

☐ To keep your skin healthy, avoid prolonged exposure to the sun. Use creams and lotions to keep your skin from becoming too dry. By keeping up your appearance, exercising every day, and becoming involved in hobbies or other activities, you can keep your mind active, and this is important.

☐ Learn how to relax! Keep active and be enthusiastic about life.

AIDS
(Acquired Immune Deficiency Syndrome)

AIDS is an immune system deficiency disorder that suddenly alters the body's ability to defend itself. The AIDS virus invades the T-cells and multiplies, causing a breakdown in the body's immune system, eventually leading to overwhelming infection and/or cancer, with ultimate death. Many of those who die from AIDS have respiratory illnesses that the immune system is not able to fight (e.g., pneumocystis carinii pneumonia, a parasite found in about 60 percent of AIDS patients). At this time, there is no cure for AIDS. Eighty percent of those diagnosed with full-fledged AIDS since 1984 have already died.

The virus that causes AIDS is called HIV, which stands for human immunodeficiency virus. The origin of this virus is unknown. The earliest documented case of AIDS appeared in 1981, but doctors acknowledge that there were probably unidentified cases in the 1970s.

Many people who are carriers of the HIV virus are not even aware that they have it. They spread the virus primarily through sexual contact or through the sharing of needles during intravenous drug use. Those who abuse drugs should never share a needle. Those who engage in sexual intercourse (anal or vaginal) with persons whose sexual history is unknown or with multiple partners should consider the consequences. Adequate precautions should be taken by those who continue to practice anything but monogamy. Condoms, along with spermicide, should be used if a monogamous relationship cannot be maintained; they are about 90 percent effective against transmission of the HIV virus.

It is conservatively estimated that about 30 percent of those who are infected with HIV contract AIDS. People who are infected with this virus are more likely to contract AIDS if their immune systems are severely suppressed. When the immune system is working properly, a virus is taken into the white cells and destroyed. When a person has a full-blown case of AIDS, the AIDS virus is taken in, but the white cells can't kill it, and the virus reproduces unchecked.

The risk of developing AIDS is proportional to the degree of immune suppression and, of course, the amount and duration of exposure to the AIDS virus. With an optimal functioning immune system, AIDS can be avoided, even in high risk groups. Studies have repeatedly shown that the "immune compromised person" is at greatest risk to succumb to AIDS. Because of a weakened immune system, resistance to many viruses and bacteria results in an increased susceptibility to infections, a rare skin cancer called Kaposi's sarcoma, Epstein Barr virus (EBV), cytomegalovirus (CMV), herpes simplex virus (HSV), candidiasis, salmonella, *Mycobacterium aviumintracellulare,* tuberculosis, and toxoplasmosis.

Besides sexual contacts, AIDS is spread primarily through the sharing of needles by intravenous drug users and blood transfusions. In the United States, as well as in many other parts of the world, blood is screened for HIV and discarded if found to contain the virus. Occasionally, however, the HIV-infected blood does pass through, because the virus does not always show up in tests if it has been recently contracted. AIDS is also passed from mothers with the virus to children during birth. It is also possible for dentists and medical workers who come into close contact with bodily fluids of infected persons to become infected if they fail to use extreme caution. Many wear rubber gloves to avoid possible contact with blood products or saliva. While there are varying points of view, we believe that the virus may live for many days, even in a dried inactive state, and then become infectious again.

It takes two to five years (or longer) after infection for symptoms of the AIDS virus to appear. When the virus becomes active, some of the symptoms are nonspecific and variable. They include fever, fatigue, loss of appetite and weight, swollen lymph nodes, diarrhea, night sweats, skin disorders, and enlarged liver and/or spleen. The first sign may be a tongue that is coated with white bumps. This is oral candidiasis, or thrush. Candidiasis indicates a compromised immune system.

The immune system is the most important single factor in disease prevention. At this time, building up the immune system is the best defense for the potential AIDS victim. Correct diet, appropriate supplements, exercise, proper environment, and correct mental outlook all play significant roles in keeping the immune system working adequately at all times.

The fundamental approach in treatment is to eliminate all known causes of immune suppression and to implement the use of all therapies that stimulate immune function. (*See* WEAKENED IMMUNE SYSTEM in Part Two.)

The AIDS victim and those at risk to contract AIDS can be helped through the following program:

NUTRIENTS

SUPPLEMENT	SUGGESTED DOSAGE	COMMENTS
Very Important		
Aerobic 07 from Aerobic Life Products or Dioxychlor from American Biologics	9 drops in water 3 times daily.	For tissue oxygenation. Kills harmful bacteria.
Egg lecithin	20 g on an empty stomach, divided throughout the day.	For cellular protection.
Garlic tablets (Kyolic)	2 capsules with meals 3 times daily.	A powerful immunostimulant.
Germanium	200 mg daily.	For tissue oxygenation and interferon production.
Protein supplement (free form amino acids)	As directed on label.	Protein in this form is readily available for the body's use and more easily metabolized.
Selenium	200 mcg daily.	Free radical scavenger.
Superoxide dismutase (SOD) from Biotec Foods	As directed on label.	Free radical scavenger.
Vitamin B complex plus B₁₂ and B₆ (pyridoxine) or liver	100 mg 3 times daily in tablet form or receive injections under doctor's supervision. Injections are the most effective.	Antistress vitamins, especially important for normal brain function.
*Vitamin C plus bioflavonoids	10,000 mg in divided doses through day.	Use buffered, powdered ascorbic acid. *See* ASCORBIC ACID FLUSH in Part Three.
Important		
Acidophilus	3 times daily. Take a high-powered form.	Supplies essential "friendly" bacteria for intestinal tract.
Coenzyme Q₁₀	100 mg daily.	Supports immune system.
DMG (Gluconic from DaVinci Labs)	As directed on label.	Actively stimulates the immune system, increasing the T-cell population.
Kyo-Green	As directed on label.	Supplies nutrients needed for repair. Important in immune response.
Multimineral formula (high potency) with zinc plus copper	50 mg daily. 3 mg daily.	Hypoallergenic form is best. Omit iron supplements if fever is present. Do not exceed 100 mg zinc at any time.
Proteolytic enzymes	6 tablets between meals.	Destroys free radicals and aids digestion.
Quercetin plus bromelin	As directed on label.	Aids in preventing reactions to certain foods, pollens, and other allergens. Increases immunity.
Raw thymus plus multiglandulars including spleen from Arteria	As directed on label.	Best from lamb source. Enhances T-cell production from thymus and spleen.
Vitamin A emulsion	50,000 IU daily.	Reduce dosage if known to have liver disease, and use caution if using pill form.
Vitamin E emulsion	200 IU daily increasing to 800 IU. Emulsified form is readily and rapidly assimilated.	Both vitamins A and E destroy free radicals and enhance immune function.
Helpful		
Aloe vera	As directed on label.	Carrisyn from the aloe plant may work as the drug AZT without the side effects.

Essential fatty acids	As directed on label.	Unsaturated fatty acids are most important in the diet. Some sources are primrose oil, black currant oil, salmon oil, and linseed oil.
L-Carnitine plus L-cysteine and L-methionine and L-ornithine (amino acids)	As directed on label, taken on an empty stomach with 500 mg vitamin C and 50 mg vitamin B$_6$.	Improves immune function. Do not give children L-ornithine.
Multiple enzyme digestive formula	Take with meals.	Improves digestion.
RNA-DNA complex		

*Massive IV doses of vitamin C (100–200 grams daily) have been used safely, often with dramatic improvement, in the treatment of AIDS.

HERBS

☐ Silymarin (extract of milk thistle weed) aids in repairing the liver. Also helpful are cayenne, echinacea, Chinese ginseng, shiitake mushroom extract, and suma.

☐ An extract from a mushroom known as somastatin may bolster the immune system and improve liver function in AIDS patients.

☐ Echinacea, goldenseal, mullein, and suma are good for cleaning the blood and lymph systems, for viral and bacterial infections, and for boosting the immune system.

☐ Ginkgo biloba extract is good for the brain cells and circulation.

☐ Pau d'arco is a natural antibiotic, and potentiates immune function.

☐ Red clover is a good blood cleanser.

☐ The *AIDS Treatment News* of San Francisco, California, reported that a chemical compound called hypericin, which is found in the herb St. Johnswort, may inhibit retroviral infections, which may be useful in the treatment of AIDS patients.

☐ Black radish and dandelion help cleanse the liver.

☐ Chaparral aids in the destruction of free radicals.

☐ Garlic and rose hips aid in digestion, endurance, and strength, and reduce the risk of blood clotting. Garlic is a natural antibiotic.

☐ Siberian ginseng helps bronchial disorders and endocrine gland function, and boosts energy.

☐ Bee propolis is good for bacterial infections invading the lungs, mouth, throat, and mucous membranes.

RECOMMENDATIONS

☐ Increase your intake of fresh fruits and vegetables. Juicing is beneficial. *See* JUICING in Part Three. "Green drinks" and carrot and beet root juice should be consumed on a daily basis, with garlic and onion added. Kyo-Green is excellent three times a day, and contains chlorophyll, protein, vitamins, minerals, and enzymes.

☐ The diet should consist of 75 percent raw foods plus seeds, nuts, and grains. Obtain as much fresh air, rest, and sunshine as possible. A lack of quality protein and adequate calories in the diet is a common reason for immune deficiency.

☐ Do not smoke, and stay away from those who do. Eliminate alcohol, caffeine, colas, sugar, and sugar products, as well as red meat. (*See* CANCER in Part Two, and follow the dietary guidelines.)

CONSIDERATIONS

☐ *See* HYPOTHYROID in Part Two, and take the test to determine whether thyroid function is underactive.

☐ Determine what food sensitivities or allergies may be present. Consider a cytotoxic test and refer to ALLERGIES in Part Two for the self-test.

☐ Drink steam-distilled water only!

☐ Many drugs are being tested and developed in the search for a cure for AIDS. At the present time, there is no cure, and the best answer is prevention through enhancement of the immune system. Precautions should be taken (as mentioned above), and common sense should be used to avoid infection from this and other diseases.

☐ *See also* SEXUALLY TRANSMITTED DISEASES in Part Two.

MEDICAL UPDATES

☐ The National Cancer Institute has conducted studies on a new anti-AIDS drug, called dideoxyinosine or ddI, which appears to be more effective in controlling the AIDS virus but less toxic than AZT, the drug currently being used. Unfortunately AZT eliminates more than the AIDS virus. It also leads to anemia by destroying normal bone marrow cells. After eighteen to twenty-four months, the AIDS virus is resistant to AZT.

DDI fights the AIDS virus, inhibiting its ability to reproduce in human cells, without the side effects of AZT. The use of this important new drug could extend the life expectancy of the AIDS patient. Dr. Robert Yarchoan, a researcher at the National Cancer Institute, reported in *Newsday* that of the twenty-six patients with AIDS-related diseases using ddI for forty-two months, most experienced no serious side effects. DDI also remains active in the bloodstream twelve times as long as AZT. The availability of ddI to the AIDS patient is now under negotiation between the government and the manufacturer of ddI, Bristol-Meyers Company.

☐ A drug called N-acetylcysteine or NAC, normally prescribed for bronchitis sufferers, has shown promise in its ability to combat the AIDS virus. The drug works to prevent the weight loss common in AIDS patients. Immunologists Leonard and Leonore Herzenberg reported their findings at a conference of AIDS specialists in Geneva, Switzerland.

AIDS patients suffer from extreme weight loss, which is partially caused by the release of a chemical called tumor necrosis factor, or TNF, in those cells infected with HIV. The chemical stimulates oxidation, which promotes the reproduction of the virus and leads to cell destruction.

In a sophisticated laboratory set-up, the Herzenbergs found that NAC blocks the chemical, inhibiting the growth of the virus. NAC is an inexpensive drug, routinely prescribed in daily doses for bronchitis, and does not have the toxic side effects of AZT.

☐ A West African who came to the United States in 1987 is believed to be the first case of AIDS caused by HIV-2 reported in this country, according to doctors in Newark, New Jersey. Those with the HIV-2 virus are chiefly located in countries along the western coast of Africa. Dr. Luc Montagnier, who was one of two men to first isolate the HIV-1 virus, maintains that the HIV-2 is just as infectious and likely to result in AIDS as the HIV-1. Harvard researchers Drs. Max Essex and Phyllis Kanki disagree. They assert that the virus does not typically cause illness and seldom causes AIDS based upon their work in Western Africa, where they witnessed a high prevalence of infection with HIV-2, but a low incidence of AIDS. Although researchers have developed a screening test for HIV-2, it has not been approved for widespread use in the United States by the Food and Drug Administration. The Department of Health and Human Services has stated that screening for HIV-2 will take place when evidence that HIV-2 is spreading through the nation's blood supply warrants it.

☐ On December 7, 1989, Dr. Michael Murphy-Corb announced that his research team at the Delta Regional Primate Research Center in Covington, Louisiana, had successfully protected eight of nine monkeys from AIDS infection. The monkeys were given a vaccination of whole killed viruses, and then later injected with the live virus. Although many researchers are skeptical that a human vaccine will not be developed for at least five to ten years, the success in monkeys offers hope that AIDS can soon be prevented in human beings.

ADDITIONAL SOURCES FOR AIDS HELP

☐ The following organizations and groups provide information and help for people with AIDS:

AIDS Hot Line: 1-(800) 342-2437. This is a free national hot line for anyone with a question about AIDS. It is open twenty-four hours a day, seven days a week.

The AIDS Health Project
Box 0884, Dept. P
San Francisco, CA 94143-0884

AIDS Atlanta
1132 Peachtree Street, NW
Dept. P
Atlanta, GA 30309

AIDS Foundation Houston
3927 Essex Lane
Dept. P
Houston, TX 77027

American Foundation for AIDS Research
Box AIDS
Dept. P
New York, NY 10016

Project Inform
347 Dolores Street #301
Dept. P
San Francisco, CA 94110
1-(800) 822-7422

AIDS Action Committee
661 Boylston Street
4th Floor
Dept. P
Boston, MA 02116

National Association of People With AIDS
2025 I Street, NW
Dept. P
Washington, D.C. 20006

Alcoholism

Alcoholism is a chronic condition marked by a dependence on alcohol— either physiological or psychological. Some effects of alcohol are a loss of inhibition and damage to the brain, liver, pancreas, duodenum, and central nervous system. Alcohol is a human specific poison! It causes metabolic damage to every cell and depresses the immune defense system. If the alcoholic continues to drink, he may shorten his life span ten to fifteen years.

Alcohol is broken down in the liver. The toxic effect of alcohol on the liver is very serious. The alcoholic will first experience a fatty degeneration of cells in his liver. Next the alcoholic will develop hepatitis, a condition in which his liver cells become inflamed and die. The usually fatal final stage is cirrhosis of the liver. Prolonged consumption of alcohol inhibits the liver's production of digestive enzymes, impairing the body's ability to absorb proteins and fats. Its ability to absorb vitamins A, D, E, and K is impaired. Many essential nutrients are not retained for use by the body; they are rapidly eliminated through the alcoholic's urine.

Alcohol affects people differently. Some may become intoxicated from their first drink; others may be able to consume four or five drinks before showing any effects. Alcoholism is a progressive disease that usually starts with acceptable social drinking. Soon this leads to a drink for every mood: one to calm down, one to perk up, one to celebrate, and so on. The alcoholic soon needs no excuse to drink. One drink starts the craving for another. Now he is completely controlled by his dependence on alcohol.

Because the alcoholic lacks control, he becomes ashamed and angry at his compulsive behavior. He harbors his feelings of inadequacy inside; however, he begins taking out his pain on those closest to him. If the alcoholic wished to regain control of his life, he must avoid all alcohol. Since one sip of alcohol can renew the drinking pattern, total abstinence is the only way that the alcoholic can exercise control over this disease. He must choose *not* to drink.

It may be helpful for recovering alcoholics to avoid people, things, and places that are associated with their drinking days. New friendships should be made with people who do not drink. Taking up a hobby, becoming involved in sports, and exercising will promote self-esteem and provide a productive outlet for energy.

The alcoholic will experience severe withdrawal symptoms during the first week that he abstains from alcohol. Insomnia, visual and auditory hallucinations, convulsions, acute anxiety, rapid pulse, extreme perspiration, and fever can occur; however, with proper supervision these symptoms will pass and the alcoholic will be set free!

Women should be cautioned about drinking while pregnant. Consumption of alcohol may cause birth abnormalities in the newborn infant. Alcohol passes through the mother's placenta and into the fetus's bloodstream. This toxic substance depresses the central nervous system of the fetus, and the baby's liver must try to metabolize the alcohol. Since the fetus's liver is not fully developed, the alcohol remains in the infant's system. Women who drink during pregnancy generally give birth to babies with a lower birth weight. Growth may be retarded or stunted. The baby's brain may be small and there may be mental retardation. Limbs, joints, fingers, and face may be deformed. Heart and kidney defects may occur as well. Some of these children characteristically become hyperactive at adolescence and exhibit learning disabilities. Even moderate amounts of alcohol may be harmful to the unborn infant, especially in the first three to four months of pregnancy. Pregnant women should avoid *all* alcohol.

NUTRIENTS

SUPPLEMENT	SUGGESTED DOSAGE	COMMENTS
Essential		
Thiamine (B$_1$)	200 mg 3 times daily.	Alcoholics often are deficient in B vitamins, especially B$_1$.
Vitamin B complex and/or liver	High dosages are recommended. Injections are often necessary with extra vitamin B$_{12}$. Use only under doctor's supervision.	Liver is a rich source of vitamins and minerals, and is high in protein as well as B$_{12}$, niacin, riboflavin, and other B vitamins. Also a source of copper, iron, phosphorus, and vitamins A, C, and D.
Very Important		
Essential fatty acids (primrose oil)	2 capsules with meals.	Used successfully in Europe, this supplement is a good source of essential fatty acids.
Protein supplement (free form amino acids) with extra	500 mg each 3 times daily.	These amino acids aid in withdrawal and are needed for brain and liver function. Protein is necessary for regeneration of liver cells.
L-cysteine	Take on an empty stomach. Work up to 1 g daily.	
L-glutamine	Take 3 g with vitamin B$_6$ (pyridoxine) on an empty stomach.	Do not use glutamic acid.
L-methionine	Must be taken on an empty stomach and is best taken with small amounts of vitamins B$_6$ and C.	
Magnesium	1,000 mg daily.	Magnesium is depleted from the body with alcohol use.
Pantothenic acid (B$_5$)	100 mg 3 times daily.	

Proteolytic enzymes	2 capsules between meals plus digestive enzymes with meals.	Essential for assimilation of protein.
Vitamin C with bioflavonoids	3,000–10,000 mg daily in divided doses.	Acts as a powerful antioxidant with healing potential.
Important		
Lecithin (choline and inositol)	1 capsule or 1 tbsp. before meals.	Good for brain function. Helps correct fatty liver degeneration.
Multimineral vitamin with selenium	200 mcg daily.	Selenium is an important trace mineral that enhances immune function.
Niacin (B₃)	200–1,000 mg daily. Do not take high dose for longer than 3 months.	Can mix with niacinamide to prevent flush.
Helpful		
Calcium	2,000 mg daily.	A vital mineral that has a sedative effect.
Choline complex or acetyl complex or Oxy-Free from Nature's Plus, or phosphatidyl	As directed on label.	Effective combinations that reduce fatty liver changes, improving liver function.
DMG (Gluconic from DaVinci Labs)	100 mg 3 times daily	Carries oxygen to the cells.
Lithium (a trace mineral)	Use as directed by attending physician.	May help depression.
Maxidophilus or Megadophilus or Bulgaricum I.B. or Bifido Factor/ Life Start Two	Use as directed on label.	Needed for proper digestion. Helps the damaged liver.
Raw brain concentrate and raw duodenum concentrate (i.e., glandulars) and raw liver concentrate and raw pancreas concentrate	Available in health food stores; use as directed on label.	*See* GLANDULAR THERAPY in Part Three.
Vitamin A-D-E emulsion	25,000 IU vitamin A; 400 IU vitamin D; and 400–1,200 IU vitamin E. Do not take this dosage in pill form.	Vitamins A, D, and E are poorly absorbed when the liver is damaged. Emulsion is rapidly assimilated.

HERBS

☐ The herb valerian root, used in Germany, has a calming effect. The herb silymarin (extract of the milk thistle weed) helps to repair damage done to the liver.

RECOMMENDATIONS

☐ If you suspect someone of alcohol abuse, encourage the person to seek professional care. In the early stages of care, the alcoholic will need plenty of rest, good nutrition, and supplements to assist in the repair of bodily damage. Patience will be needed for the long, slow road to recovery.

☐ It is best to avoid tranquilizers as there is a danger of substituting one drug addiction for another. Sobriety should be drug free.

CONSIDERATIONS

☐ The latest research has found that children of alcoholics are more inclined to use drugs, including cocaine. These children are 400 times more likely to use drugs than those who do not have a family history of alcohol addiction. Studies conducted in Sweden revealed that babies of alcoholics who were adopted by nonalcoholic families eventually became alcoholics, indicating a correlation between chemical dependency and genetics.

☐ Some physicians use the drug Antabuse to help alcoholics stay sober. Those on this drug will experience nausea, vomiting, severe headaches, blurred vision, and even an impending feeling of death if they take even a small sip of alcohol. Abstention from alcohol often results with use of this drug.

☐ A ten-day cleansing fast may be beneficial. (*See* FASTING in Part Three.)

☐ *See also* CIRRHOSIS OF THE LIVER and DRUG ADDICTION, both in Part Two.

Alkalosis

Alkalosis occurs when the body is too alkaline. It is often the result of excessive intake of alkaline drugs such as sodium bicarbonate for the treatment of gastritis or peptic ulcers. It can also result from excessive vomiting, high cholesterol, endocrine imbalance, poor diet, diarrhea, and osteoarthritis. The symptoms of alkalosis include sore muscles, creaking joints, bursitis, bone spurs, drowsiness, protruding eyes, hypertension, hypothermia, seizures, edema, allergies, night cramps, asthma, chronic indigestion, night coughs, vomiting, too rapid blood clotting and thick blood, menstrual problems, hard dry stools, prostatitis, and skin thickenings with burning, itching sensations.

Alkalosis occurs less often than acidosis (*see* ACIDOSIS in Part Two). It produces overexcitability of the nervous system—the peripheral nerves are affected first. The symptoms may be manifested in a highly nervous condition, including hyperventilation. Convulsions may result.

Alkalosis may cause calcium to build up in the body, such as in bone or heel spurs.

ACID AND ALKALINE SELF-TEST

This test will determine whether your body fluids are either too acidic or too alkaline. An imbalance can cause illnesses such as acidosis or alkalosis.

Purchase nitrazine paper, available at any drugstore, and apply saliva and/or urine to the paper. Always perform the test either before eating or at least one hour after eating. The paper will change color to indicate if your system is overly acidic or alkaline. Red litmus paper turns blue in an alkaline medium and blue litmus paper turns red in an acid medium.

Water is neutral with a pH of 7.0. Anything with a pH below 7.0 is acid, while anything with a pH above 7.0 is alkaline. The ideal pH range for saliva and urine is 6.0 to 6.8. Our body is naturally mildly acidic. Therefore, values below pH 6.3 would be considered too acidic; values above pH 6.8 are too alkaline. The pH value of milk varies from 6.2 to 7.3.

The following foods should be consumed according to the results of your test. If your test indicated one extreme or another, omit the acid- or alkaline-forming foods from your diet until another pH test shows that you have returned to normal.

Acid-Forming Foods

alcohol	milk
asparagus	mustard
beans	noodles
Brussels sprouts	oatmeal
catsup	olives
chickpeas	organ meats
cocoa	pasta
coffee	pepper
cornstarch	poultry
eggs	sauerkraut
fish	shellfish
flour products	soft drinks
legumes	sugar
lentils	tea
meat	

Low-Level Acid-Forming Foods

butter	grains (most)
cheeses	ice cream
coconuts (dried)	ice milk (homemade)
fruits (canned/glazed)	lambsquarter
fruits (dried sulfured)	seeds and nuts (most)

Alkaline-Forming Foods

apricots	maple syrup
avocados	melons
corn	millet
dates	molasses
fruits	oranges
grapefruit	raisins
grapes	soy figs
honey	vegetables
lemons	

Low-Level Alkaline-Forming Foods

almonds	coconuts (fresh)
blackstrap molasses	dairy products, soured
Brazil nuts	lima beans
buckwheat	millet
chestnuts	

Prunes, cranberries, and plums are acid forming and remain acidic in the body. Raw fruits become acid forming when sugar is added. All foods with added sugar become acidic. Alcohol, drugs, aspirin, tobacco, and vinegar are also acid forming.

NUTRIENTS

SUPPLEMENT	SUGGESTED DOSAGE	COMMENTS
Helpful		
Alfalfa	As directed on label. Also use natural sources.	Has a neutralizing effect on the intestinal tract.
Ammonium chloride	As directed on label.	Found in seawater and arrowroot.
Betaine hydrochloric acid (HCl)	As directed on label.	A digestive enzyme that releases acid in the digestive tract.
L-Cysteine	500 mg twice daily.	Is necessary to produce glutathione, a major detoxifying chemical. Also aids in making the tissues more acid.
Raw kidney concentrate	500 mg daily.	Stimulates kidney function.
Selenium	200 mcg daily.	Protects against free radicals produced in alkalosis.

Sulfur (MSM from DaVinci Labs)	250 mg, 2 capsules daily.	A bioavailable source of dietary sulfur (methylsulfonyl).
Vitamin B$_6$ (pyridoxine) plus	50 mg 3 times daily.	Needed for hydrochloric acid (HCl) production. Relieves fluid retention. Vitamin B complex is essential for a stable and normal pH.
B-complex vitamins	100 mg daily.	
Vitamin C with rose hips plus citrus and bioflavonoids	3,000–6,000 mg daily in divided doses.	A potent antioxidant and free radical scavenger.

RECOMMENDATIONS

☐ Change of diet is recommended. A diet consisting of 80 percent grains should be adopted and should include beans, breads, brown rice, crackers, lentils, macaroni, nuts, soy sauce, and whole grain cereals. The other 20 percent of the diet should contain fresh fruits and vegetables and fish, chicken, eggs, and natural cheese. Sodium should be avoided.

☐ See the self-test for foods to avoid when you have this condition.

☐ Do not use antacids or mineral supplements, except those mentioned above, for two weeks.

☐ Oxygen is acidifying—the rate at which you breathe affects the alkali and acid balance of your body. Prolonged hyperventilation may cause alkalosis. Breathe into a paper bag when this occurs.

☐ Megadoses of vitamins and minerals should be cut back for two weeks.

Allergic Rhinitis

See HAY FEVER.

Allergies

An allergy is the inappropriate response by the body's immune system to a substance that is not normally harmful. The immune system is the highly complex defense mechanism that helps us to combat infection. It does this by identifying "foreign bodies" and mobilizing the body's white blood cells to fight them. In some people, the immune system wrongly identifies a nontoxic substance as an invader, and the white blood cells overreact and do more damage to the body than the invader. Thus, the allergic response becomes a disease in itself. Common responses are asthma, eczema, and hayfever.

The substances that cause allergies are called allergens. Almost any substance can cause an allergy to someone somewhere in the world, but the most common allergens are grass pollen, dust, certain metals (especially nickel), some cosmetics, lanolin, some animal hair, insect bites and stings, some common drugs (e.g., penicillin, aspirin), some foods (e.g., strawberries, eggs, shellfish), some additives (e.g., benzoic acid, sulfur dioxide), and chemicals found in soap and washing powder.

No one knows why some people are allergic to certain substances. However, allergies do run in families and it is also believed that babies that are not breastfed are more likely to develop allergies. There may be an emotional cause to the problem as well; stress and anger, especially when the immune system is suppressed, are frequently contributing factors.

MOLD ALLERGIES

Many people are allergic to mold. Molds are microscopic living organisms, neither animal nor insect, that thrive where no other life form can. Molds live throughout the house—under the sink and in the bathroom, basement, refrigerator, and any damp, dark place. They also flourish in the air, in the soil, on dead leaves, and on other organic material. They may be destructive, but they are also beneficial. They help to make cheese, fertilize gardens, and speed decaying of garbage and fallen leaves. Penicillin is made from molds.

Mold spores are carried by the wind and predominate in the summer and early fall. In warm climates they thrive year round. Cutting grass, harvesting crops, or walking through tall vegetation will provoke a reaction. Those who repair old used furniture are also at risk. Keep rooms free from dust and use a dehumidifier in the basement. Use mold-proof paint and a disinfectant on walls and furniture.

FOOD ALLERGIES

Food allergies and food intolerance are not the same. Those with an intolerance lack certain enzymes needed for digestion, and therefore do not break down the food properly. (*See* ENZYMES in Part One.) Undigested food can enter the bloodstream and cause a reaction. A food allergy occurs when a person has an antibody response to the ingested food. A few foods may provoke a reaction as soon as one starts chewing. These are easy to identify and eliminate from the diet. A delayed reaction is harder to detect. An irritating cough or tickle in the throat is most often a food sensitivity.

Research is being conducted on the ability of coenzyme Q_{10} to counter histamine for asthma and other allergy sufferers.

Food Allergy Self-Test

If you suspect that you are allergic to a specific food, a simple test can help you determine if you are correct. By recording your blood pressure after consuming the food in question, you can reveal if you are having an allergic reaction. Using a watch with a second hand, sit down and relax for a few minutes. When completely relaxed, take your pulse at the wrist. Count the number of beats in a sixty-second period. A normal pulse reading is 52–70 beats per minute. Consume the food that you are testing for an allergic reaction. Wait fifteen to twenty minutes and take your pulse again. If your pulse rate increased more than ten beats per minute, omit this food from your diet for one month, and then retest.

When taking the following nutrients, be sure to take only hypoallergenic supplements. GH-3 should not be used if sensitive to metabisulfite (sulfites).

NUTRIENTS

SUPPLEMENT	SUGGESTED DOSAGE	COMMENTS
Very Important		
Bee pollen (raw crude pollen)	2 tsp. daily, or take in capsule form, beginning with a few granules at a time.	Best when produced within a 10-mile radius of where you live.
Calcium (chelated form) with magnesium	1,500–2,000 mg daily. 750 mg daily.	Needed to help reduce stress.
Multienzymes or pancreatin	Take with meals.	Those suffering from ulcers should take a brand without hydrochloric acid (HCl).
Raw adrenal, raw spleen, and raw thymus glandulars	500 mg each twice daily.	Stimulates immune function.
Vitamin B complex (high stress) with pantothenic acid (B_5) and vitamin B_{12}	100 mg daily and up. 100 mg 3 times daily in lozenges or sublingual form.	The B complex and liver injections give fast results.
Vitamin C with bioflavonoids	2,000 mg and up, 3 times daily.	Stimulates immune function.

Important		
Beta-carotene	1,500 IU daily.	A free radical scavenger that stimulates immune response.
Quercitin-C from Cardiovascular Research with bromelin	500 mg twice daily. 100 mg twice daily.	A co-bioactive bioflavonoid that increases immunity. Needed to decrease reactions to certain foods, pollens, and other allergens.
Helpful		
Coenzyme Q_{10}	100 mg daily.	Improves cellular oxygenation and immune function.
Germanium (Dr. Asai's Ge-132 from Global Marketing)	60 mg daily.	Stimulates immune response.
L-Tyrosine and L-cysteine (amino acids) plus vitamins B_6 (pyridoxine) and C	500 mg each on empty stomach daily. 50 mg each daily.	Vitamins B_6 and C aid in assimilation.
Manganese chelate	Use for 3 months.	An important component in many of the body's enzyme systems.
Milk-free acidophilus	Follow label instructions.	Take on an empty stomach for easier access into the small intestine.
Multivitamin and mineral complex	As directed on label.	Use hypoallergenic product.
Potassium protinate or chelate form	99 mg daily.	Necessary for adrenal gland function.
Protein supplement (free form amino acids without phenylalanine) from Ecological	1-2 tsp. daily. Take sublingual form for best absorption.	This form of protein is rapidly absorbed and assimilated by the body.
Proteolytic enzymes	2 tablets between meals on an empty stomach.	Aids digestion and destroys free radicals.
Vitamin A	10,000 IU daily.	Necessary for proper immune function.
Vitamin D	600 IU daily.	Essential in calcium metabolism.
Vitamin E	600 IU daily.	Necessary for proper immune function.
Zinc	50 mg daily.	Necessary for proper immune function.

HERBS

☐ For allergies, use burdock, centaury, dandelion, fringe tree, goldenseal root, phytolacca, and St. Mary's thistle. Goldenseal root aids absorption of nutrients.

☐ If you are allergic to ragweed, take caution when using goldenseal; these herbs are from the same family.

RECOMMENDATIONS

☐ Those with allergies who smoke should stop smoking.

☐ ABC colon cleanser combined with aloe vera juice may slow absorption of food that can cause a reaction into the bloodstream. Taking fiber in the morning will work in the same way. Do not use wheat bran. Oat bran or guar gum is better. (*See* NATURAL FOOD SUPPLEMENTS in Part One for a discussion on fiber.)

☐ The *British Medical Journal* reported that aspirin allows more of the allergy-producing food to be absorbed. Avoid taking aspirin within three hours of eating.

☐ Take the temperature underarm test to determine if you have an underactive thyroid. (*See* HYPERTHYROID in Part Two for the self-test.)

☐ Follow the fasting program. (*See* FASTING in Part Three.) After a fast, you can try adding back the "foods to avoid" (listed below) in very small amounts, such as one teaspoon at a time. Record your reactions after eating. If you feel bloated or have a slight headache, an upset stomach, gas, diarrhea, a rapid pulse, or heart palpitations after eating certain foods, then you should eliminate them from your diet for sixty days and then introduce them again in small amounts.

☐ Avoid the following foods: bananas, beef products, caffeine, chocolate, citrus fruits, corn, dairy products, eggs, oats, oysters, peanuts, processed and refined foods, salmon, strawberries, tomatoes, wheat, and white rice.

☐ Avoid F, D, and C yellow #5 dyes. *The New England Journal of Medicine* reports that 100,000 Americans are allergic to these food colorings. Other additives to avoid are vanillin, benzyldehyde, eucalyptol, monosodium glutamate, BHT-BHA, benzoates, and annatto. Read labels carefully.

Sulfite Allergies

A product called Sulfitest is now available for those individuals who are sensitive to sulfites. This kit contains test strips that indicate the presence of sulfites in your foods. For more information on this product, write to:

Center Laboratories
Division of EM Industries, Inc.
Port Washington, NY 11050

FOODS AND BEVERAGES FREQUENTLY CONTAINING SULFITES

Those who are sensitive to sulfites should beware of the following foods and beverages, which often contain sulfites or sulfur dioxide:

Fresh Fruits and Beverages

- avocado (guacamole) dip
- carrots
- cole slaw
- fruit
- lettuce
- mushrooms
- peppers
- potatoes
- tomatoes

Fish and Shellfish

- dried fish
- fresh shellfish, especially shrimp
- frozen, canned, or dried shellfish
- clams
- crabs
- lobsters
- oysters
- scallops
- shrimp

Prepared Foods

- French fries (frozen)
- fruits and vegetables (frozen, canned, or dried)
- mushrooms (canned)
- pickles
- potato chips
- salad dressings (dry mix)
- sauces and gravies
- sauerkraut
- soups (dried or canned)

Miscellaneous Food Products and Beverages

- baked products (frozen doughs, cornmeal)
- beer
- cider
- cordials
- fruit juices
- gelatin
- wines

CONSIDERATIONS

☐ Allergenic persons should rotate foods. (See Rotating Foods: Daily Menus inset at the end of this section.) A different group of foods is eaten for each of four days and then the cycle is repeated. You can select as many of the foods allowed on a specific day as you like, but it is essential that no food be ingested more often than every four days. Omit the foods on the Food Sensitivity Questionnaire (see inset) for thirty days if you have consumed the foods four or more times per week.

☐ There is an abnormal immune globulin called IgE, which is an antibody that is formed in an allergic response to a food substance. When this substance is found in your lung tissue, it frequently causes a reaction such as shortness of breath or asthma. It can cause hives if found in the skin. Many intestinal problems commonly occur because IgE is most often found in the wall of the intestinal tract, often resulting in severe pain, gas, or bloating. IgE can be located anywhere in the body, causing severe problems. Even natural health foods can adversely affect the immune system.

☐ Stemming from a reaction to food pollutants, a cerebral allergy causes a swelling of the lining of the brain. Entire food families will cause allergic reactions. Schizophrenic, violent, and aggressive reactions could be an indicator. Foods such as corn, wheat, rice, milk, chocolate, and food additives may produce violent reactions in those suffering from allergies.

☐ *See also* CHEMICAL ALLERGIES in Part Two and FASTING in Part Three.

Detecting Your Hidden Food Allergies

FOOD SENSITIVITY QUESTIONNAIRE

In order to identify food allergies, it is important that you fill out the following form. Foods that are eaten daily or more often than three times a week should be omitted from the diet for thirty days, and then reintroduced one at a time after testing for a reaction to the food. See the self-test to test for specific food allergies. After you have completed this form, move on to the Rotation Diet.

For each of the following foods, note how often you consume the particular food in a given week. Record the number each week for a one-month period.

Type of Food	First Week	Second Week	Third Week	Fourth Week
Beverages				
Alcohol	_____	_____	_____	_____
Coffee	_____	_____	_____	_____
Colas	_____	_____	_____	_____
Milk (cow's)	_____	_____	_____	_____
Milk (goat's)	_____	_____	_____	_____
Milk shakes	_____	_____	_____	_____
Nut milk	_____	_____	_____	_____
Soy milk	_____	_____	_____	_____
Tea	_____	_____	_____	_____
Breads and Starches				
Pancakes	_____	_____	_____	_____
Pasta	_____	_____	_____	_____
Pastries	_____	_____	_____	_____
Pizza	_____	_____	_____	_____
Tapioca	_____	_____	_____	_____
White flour	_____	_____	_____	_____
Condiments				
Catsup	_____	_____	_____	_____
Gravy	_____	_____	_____	_____
Mustard	_____	_____	_____	_____
Pepper	_____	_____	_____	_____
Pickles	_____	_____	_____	_____
Salt	_____	_____	_____	_____

Type of Food	First Week	Second Week	Third Week	Fourth Week
Dairy Products				
Butter	_____	_____	_____	_____
Buttermilk	_____	_____	_____	_____
Cheese	_____	_____	_____	_____
Cottage cheese	_____	_____	_____	_____
Eggs	_____	_____	_____	_____
Ice cream	_____	_____	_____	_____
Margarine	_____	_____	_____	_____
Milk (cow's)	_____	_____	_____	_____
Milk (goat's)	_____	_____	_____	_____
Milk shakes	_____	_____	_____	_____
Yogurt	_____	_____	_____	_____
Fruits and Fruit Juices				
Apples	_____	_____	_____	_____
Apricots	_____	_____	_____	_____
Bananas	_____	_____	_____	_____
Blackberries	_____	_____	_____	_____
Blueberries	_____	_____	_____	_____
Cherries	_____	_____	_____	_____
Coconuts	_____	_____	_____	_____
Dates	_____	_____	_____	_____
Dried fruits	_____	_____	_____	_____
Figs	_____	_____	_____	_____
Grapefruits	_____	_____	_____	_____
Grapes	_____	_____	_____	_____
Lemons	_____	_____	_____	_____
Melons	_____	_____	_____	_____
Oranges	_____	_____	_____	_____
Nectarines	_____	_____	_____	_____
Papayas	_____	_____	_____	_____
Peaches	_____	_____	_____	_____
Pears	_____	_____	_____	_____
Pineapples	_____	_____	_____	_____
Plums	_____	_____	_____	_____
Prunes	_____	_____	_____	_____
Strawberries	_____	_____	_____	_____
Tangerines	_____	_____	_____	_____
Grains				
Buckwheat	_____	_____	_____	_____
Cereals (cold)	_____	_____	_____	_____
Millet	_____	_____	_____	_____
Oats	_____	_____	_____	_____
Rye	_____	_____	_____	_____
Wheat	_____	_____	_____	_____
Meats, Poultry, and Fish				
Bacon	_____	_____	_____	_____
Beef	_____	_____	_____	_____
Bologna	_____	_____	_____	_____
Cheeseburger	_____	_____	_____	_____
Chicken	_____	_____	_____	_____
Fish	_____	_____	_____	_____
Ham	_____	_____	_____	_____
Hamburger	_____	_____	_____	_____
Lamb	_____	_____	_____	_____
Liver	_____	_____	_____	_____
Luncheon meat	_____	_____	_____	_____

Type of Food	First Week	Second Week	Third Week	Fourth Week
Meats, Poultry, and Fish (continued)				
Pork	————	————	————	————
Sausage	————	————	————	————
Shellfish	————	————	————	————
Turkey	————	————	————	————
Veal	————	————	————	————
Nuts and Seeds				
Almonds	————	————	————	————
Cashews	————	————	————	————
Chestnuts	————	————	————	————
Hazelnuts	————	————	————	————
Peanuts	————	————	————	————
Pecans	————	————	————	————
Pistachio nuts	————	————	————	————
Sesame seeds	————	————	————	————
Walnuts	————	————	————	————
Oils				
Corn oil	————	————	————	————
Cottonseed oil	————	————	————	————
Olive oil	————	————	————	————
Peanut oil	————	————	————	————
Safflower oil	————	————	————	————
Sesame oil	————	————	————	————
Soy oil	————	————	————	————
Spreads				
Butter	————	————	————	————
Cream cheese	————	————	————	————
Jellies	————	————	————	————
Margarine	————	————	————	————
Peanut butter	————	————	————	————
Sweeteners				
Corn syrup	————	————	————	————
Fructose	————	————	————	————
Honey	————	————	————	————
NutraSweet	————	————	————	————
Saccharin	————	————	————	————
Sugar (brown)	————	————	————	————
Sugar (white)	————	————	————	————
Vegetables				
Alfalfa sprouts	————	————	————	————
Artichokes	————	————	————	————
Asparagus	————	————	————	————
Avocados	————	————	————	————
Beans (lima)	————	————	————	————
Beans (mung)	————	————	————	————
Beans (pinto)	————	————	————	————
Beans (snap)	————	————	————	————
Beans (white)	————	————	————	————
Beets	————	————	————	————
Broccoli	————	————	————	————
Brussels sprouts	————	————	————	————
Cabbage	————	————	————	————

Type of Food	First Week	Second Week	Third Week	Fourth Week
Vegetables (continued)				
Carrots	_____	_____	_____	_____
Cauliflower	_____	_____	_____	_____
Celery	_____	_____	_____	_____
Corn	_____	_____	_____	_____
Cucumbers	_____	_____	_____	_____
Eggplant	_____	_____	_____	_____
Lentils	_____	_____	_____	_____
Lettuce	_____	_____	_____	_____
Mushrooms	_____	_____	_____	_____
Okra	_____	_____	_____	_____
Olives	_____	_____	_____	_____
Onions	_____	_____	_____	_____
Parsley	_____	_____	_____	_____
Peas	_____	_____	_____	_____
Peppers	_____	_____	_____	_____
Potatoes (sweet)	_____	_____	_____	_____
Potatoes (white)	_____	_____	_____	_____
Radishes	_____	_____	_____	_____
Spinach	_____	_____	_____	_____
String beans	_____	_____	_____	_____
Squash (yellow)	_____	_____	_____	_____
Swiss chard	_____	_____	_____	_____
Tomatoes	_____	_____	_____	_____
Turnips	_____	_____	_____	_____
Zucchini	_____	_____	_____	_____
Junk Foods and Miscellaneous Foods				
Candy bars	_____	_____	_____	_____
Chocolate	_____	_____	_____	_____
Chewing gum	_____	_____	_____	_____
French fries	_____	_____	_____	_____
Fried foods	_____	_____	_____	_____
Peppermint	_____	_____	_____	_____
Potato chips	_____	_____	_____	_____
Puddings	_____	_____	_____	_____
Tofu products	_____	_____	_____	_____

Fill in the snacks that you eat weekly. _____

KEEPING A FOOD DIARY

Are you getting the proper nutrients to keep you healthy? After filling out the sensitivity questionnaire, note which foods are eaten four or more times a week. Omit these foods from your diet for a period of thirty days to give your body a rest from overconsumption of these foods. After thirty days, do the pulse self-test for these foods to identify food sensitivities. Those which cause a reaction should be omitted for an additional thirty days.

Before starting the rotation diet, you should follow the fasting program to cleanse the system of offending foods and toxins. *See* FASTING in Part Two and follow the program. After you have finished the program, consume only the following foods for the next two weeks: fresh fruits (except oranges); raw, steamed, or broiled vegetables; chicken or turkey; broiled, boiled, or baked fish; brown rice; herb teas; and unsweetened juices.

Although you may feel that these foods do not offer a variety, you can do very nicely on them. There are numerous fruits and vegetables available, in addition to a variety of fishes. You will feel good on this diet.

As you add foods back to your diet one at a time, keep a diary of your reactions to them. See the self-testing section to identify your reactions. Add only one new food a day. If you have a reaction to it, omit that food for two months. Then try to add a small amount of the food back to your diet, and record your reactions again. If you have another reaction, eliminate it from your diet. By slowly adding these foods back one at a time, you will be able to determine which foods are giving you trouble.

Sample Diary

Date	Meal	Time	Foods Consumed	Symptoms
4/12	Morning	8:38 a.m.	milk, toast	bloatedness, gas
	Noon	12:30 p.m.	pea soup, salad	no symptoms

Diary

Date	Meal	Time	Foods Consumed	Symptoms
_____	Morning			
	Noon			
	Evening			
	Bedtime			
_____	Morning			
	Noon			
	Evening			
	Bedtime			
_____	Morning			
	Noon			
	Evening			
	Bedtime			
_____	Morning			
	Noon			
	Evening			
	Bedtime			
_____	Morning			
	Noon			
	Evening			
	Bedtime			
_____	Morning			
	Noon			
	Evening			
	Bedtime			

Medications: _____

Herbs: _____

Miscellaneous: _____

Consume only one food type every four days. If you eat beans one day, don't eat beans again for the next four days. If you eat fish on a particular day, wait four days before consuming any other fish. This rotation diet will not only make you feel better, it will also stabilize your weight.

When you consume the same foods daily, your body builds up an intolerance to them. Rather than nourishing the body, these foods can cause harmful reactions.

Food sensitivity symptoms most often develop slowly, but some people will have a reaction soon after ingesting a particular food. After avoiding the allergenic foods for 60–90 days, the foods can be reintroduced without any adverse reactions in most cases.

The following symptoms are the most common that manifest from food allergies:

- Acne, especially pimples on the chin or around the mouth.
- Arthritis.
- Asthma.
- Colitis.
- Depression.
- Fatigue.
- Headaches.
- Insomnia.
- Intestinal problems.
- Overweight.
- Sinus problems.
- Ulcers.

In addition to these signs, your physician should also look for the following symptoms when trying to determine if you have an allergy:

- Anemic and exhibits a pale complexion.
- Bed-wetting.
- Cheeks exhibiting red circles (as if wearing rouge, even in children).
- Repeated colds in children.
- Conjunctivitis.
- Diarrhea.
- Dizzy spells and floating sensations.
- Excessive drooling.
- Repeated ear infections in children.
- Dark circles under the eyes or puffy eyes.
- Eye pain, tearing.
- Watery, itchy, red eyes.

- Sensitivity to light.
- Periods of blurred vision.
- Fluid retention.
- Hearing loss.
- Hyperactivity.
- Any illness that keeps recurring despite treatment.
- Learning disabilities.
- Poor memory and concentration.
- Severe menstrual cycles.
- Poor muscle coordination.
- Noises in the ear.
- Unusual body odor.
- pH balance is either too alkaline or too acid.
- Phobias.
- Stuffiness or watery nasal secretions.
- Swollen fingers and cold hands.
- Dramatic weight gains.

THE ROTATION DIET

Some people are hungry all the time, even after eating a large meal. They never feel satisfied because they are craving the foods to which they are addicted. Many recurring illnesses, such as colds, flu, and bladder and prostate infections, are indications of food allergies.

The following menus were designed to include a variety of food types in the diet. If you are sensitive to any of the foods listed, substitute that food with one that agrees with you. Try putting together daily menus for one week consisting of the foods that agree with you—you will surely see an increase in your energy level!

Sample Rotation Diet

Meal	Day 1	Day 2	Day 3	Day 4
Breakfast	_____	_____	_____	_____
Lunch	_____	_____	_____	_____
Dinner	_____	_____	_____	_____
Snacks	_____	_____	_____	_____

Rotating Foods: Daily Menus

Breakfast	Lunch	Dinner	Snacks
Day 1			
Glass of distilled water	Tomato stuffed with tuna salad or tuna burger on wheat-free bread with tomato, onion, alfalfa sprouts, and eggless mayonnaise	Broiled whitefish or salmon with dill sauce	Celery sticks
Papaya juice with vitamin C		Cole slaw or sprout salad with tomato, onion, celery, and eggless mayonnaise	Pecans
Fresh papaya or peaches		Steamed asparagus with dill sauce	Fresh papaya or peaches
Oatmeal or oat bran cereal		Herb tea or lemonade	
1 tbsp. raw honey	Fresh lemonade		
Skim milk			
1 cup rose hips tea			

Substitutions:
Cauliflower, Brussels sprouts, or sauerkraut can be substituted for asparagus.

Breakfast	Lunch	Dinner	Snacks
Day 2			
Glass of distilled water Apple juice with vitamin C Fresh apple Cream of Wheat cereal with pure maple syrup and soy milk Herb tea	Homecooked sliced turkey or chicken on whole wheat bread with lettuce and mustard Potato soup and wheat crackers (make soup with soy milk) Herb tea or apple juice *Substitutions:* Tofu soup, soy burgers, eggless egg salad, tofu mayonnaise.	Baked skinless turkey or chicken with lemon juice, garlic, and spike Baked potato with 2 tsp. sesame oil and chopped chives, dash of spike Tossed salad with radishes, zucchini, yellow squash, kale, and soy oil dressing *Substitutions:* Cornish game hens for turkey or chicken, vinaigrette dressing.	Apples Walnuts *Substitutions:* Baked apple with pure maple syrup, wheat crackers, sugar-free applesauce topped with walnuts for dessert.
Day 3			
Glass of distilled water Cranberry juice with vitamin C Sliced banana with almond milk Cream of Rice cereal or puffed rice 1 cup hot herb tea	½ avocado filled with cooked salmon, cooled rice with fresh peas, water chestnuts, dash of herb seasoning and lemon juice, topped with slivered almonds Split pea soup with rice crackers	Stir-fried vegetables with broccoli, green peppers, leeks, pea pods, sweet red peppers, bean sprouts, bamboo shoots, grated fresh ginger, served over cooked brown rice Rice cakes with almond butter 1 cup uncoffee or herb tea	Raw almonds Rice crackers with almond butter Sliced bananas
Day 4			
Glass of distilled water Grape juice with vitamin C 2 poached or soft-boiled eggs or omelette 1 slice rye toast sugar-free grape jam 1 cup herb tea	Egg salad with chopped cucumber, green onions, black olives, and low-fat cottage cheese, topped with raisins RyKrisp crackers with sugar- free grape jelly or jam Lentil soup or cool lentil salad	Spinach mushroom quiche Fresh spinach salad with hard-boiled eggs, artichoke, shredded raw beets, and raisins Olive oil and lemon dressing Iced herbed tea with grape juice for flavor	RyKrisp crackers with sesame butter and sesame seeds sprinkled on top or sugar-free grape jam Fresh grapes Raisins Hard-boiled eggs

Alopecia

See HAIR, LOSS OF.

Aluminum Toxicity

While aluminum is not a heavy metal, it has been found to be toxic. Because aluminum permeates our air, water, and soil, small amounts are present in our food. The average person consumes between three and ten milligrams of aluminum a day. Only recently has research revealed that aluminum is absorbed and accumulated in the body. Aluminum is a popular metal used to make cookware, cooking utensils, and foil. Excessive use of antacids is the most common cause of aluminum toxicity. Mylanta, Maalox, Gelusil, Amphojel, and many others have a high aluminum hydroxide content. Many over-the-counter drugs used for inflammation and pain contain aluminum, including Arthritis Pain Formula, Ascriptin, Bufferin, and Vanquish. Several douche preparations, including Massengil and Summer's Eve, contain aluminum. It is also an additive in most baking powders and is sometimes evident in drinking water.

Many symptoms of aluminum toxicity are similar to those of Alzheimer's disease and osteoporosis. Aluminum toxicity can lead to colic, rickets, gastrointestinal disturbances, poor calcium metabolism, extreme nervousness, anemia, headache, decreased liver and kidney function, forgetfulness, speech disturbances and memory loss, softening of the bones, and weak, aching muscles. Research suggests that a chronic calcium deficiency may change the way in which the body uses minerals. Bone loss and increased intestinal absorption of aluminum and silicon combine to form compounds that accumulate in the cerebral cortex of the brain. These compounds prevent impulses from being carried to or from the brain.

An accumulation of aluminum salts in the brain has been implicated in seizures and reduced mental faculties. Autopsies performed on Alzheimer's victims revealed that four times the normal amount of aluminum had accumulated in the nerve cells in the brain. This suggests that long-term accumulation of aluminum in the brain may contribute to the development of Alzheimer's disease. In addition, an unidentified protein not found in normal brain tissue has been discovered in the brain tissue of Alzheimer's victims. *See* ALZHEIMER'S DISEASE in Part Two for further information.

Because aluminum is excreted by the kidneys, toxic amounts of aluminum may impair kidney function. Working in aluminum smelting plants for long periods can lead to dizziness, impaired coordination, and losses of balance and energy. Accumulation of aluminum in the brain was cited as a possible cause for these symptoms as well.

In addition to aluminum cookware, foil, antacids, baking powders, buffered aspirin, and most city water, aluminum is also used in food processing (pickles and relishes, in particular), antiperspirants, deodorants, beer (especially when in aluminum cans), bleached flour, table salt, tobacco smoke, cream of tartar, Parmesan and grated cheeses, aluminum salts, douches, and canned goods.

Those who enjoy fast foods should be aware that processed cheese has a high aluminum content. The food product having perhaps the highest aluminum content is the cheeseburger. This mineral is added to give processed cheese its melting quality for use on hamburgers.

NUTRIENTS

SUPPLEMENT	SUGGESTED DOSAGE	COMMENTS
Helpful		
Calcium in the chelate form with magnesium	1,500 mg daily.	This chelating agent binds with aluminum and eliminates it from the body.
	750 mg daily.	
Garlic tablets (Kyolic)	2 capsules 3 times daily.	Acts as a detoxifier.
Kelp	6 tablets daily.	Has a balanced mineral content. Acts as a detoxifier of excess metals.
Lecithin	2 tbsp. 3 times daily with meals.	Aids in healing of the brain (and other cell membranes).
Multivitamin and mineral complex (high potency, hypoallergenic)	As directed on label.	Basic in stabilizing vitamin and mineral imbalance in toxic conditions.
Vitamin B complex plus	100 mg 3 times daily.	The B vitamins, especially B_6, are important in ridding the intestinal tract of excess metals and in removing them from the body.
vitamin B_6 (pyridoxine) and	50 mg 3 times daily.	
B_{12} lozenges or		
B_{12} injections	Injections under doctor's recommendation and supervision only.	

RECOMMENDATIONS

☐ Make sure that your diet is high in fiber and contains apple pectin.

☐ Use glass, iron, or stainless steel cookware. There is still much controversy as to whether aluminum collects in the neurons as a result of a dysfunction of the neurons or if it actually causes the dysfunction of the neurons. It is best to avoid aluminum as much as possible!

☐ Beware of products containing aluminum. Read the labels and avoid those that contain aluminum, bentonite, or dihydroxyaluminum.

CONSIDERATIONS

☐ If you use chelation therapy, use oral chelating agents only (*see* CHELATION THERAPY in Part Three). Aluminum cannot be chelated out of the body, but it can be displaced or moved.

☐ *See also* ALZHEIMER'S DISEASE in Part Two.

Alzheimer's Disease

The incidence of Alzheimer's disease in the United States today is more than 2.5 million, afflicting 15 percent of Americans over sixty-five. Previously classified as senile dementia, this disorder is characterized by tangled nerve fibers surrounding the hippocampus. The hippocampus is the brain's memory center. When the nerves surrounding the hippocampus become tangled, nerve impulses can no longer carry information to or from the brain. Because the brain's circuits are now disconnected, information cannot be retrieved. This entanglement does not destroy the information stored in the hippocampus, rather it prevents the information from being transferred.

Originally identified by a German neurologist in 1907, this degenerative disease is characterized by mental deterioration to the degree that it interferes with the person's ability to function socially and at work. Memory and abstract thought processes are impaired. Some characteristics of this disorder are memory loss, severe mood swings, personality changes, disoriented perceptions of space and time, and an inability to concentrate or communicate. The individual's health progressively deteriorates until he is totally incapacitated. Death will usually occur within five years if the victim is not treated.

Many people worry that their forgetfulness is a sign of Alzheimer's disease. Many of us forget where we have put our keys or glasses at one time or another; this is not an indication of Alzheimer's disease. However, when an individual forgets that he wears glasses, then he is showing signs of dementia.

Alzheimer's disease is not limited to the elderly. Presenile dementia may strike when an individual is in his forties. Because dementia is a symptom of many disorders, a diagnosis of Alzheimer's disease is usually made when all of the others have been eliminated. Currently there are no laboratory procedures or biochemical markers that can confirm Alzheimer's disease. Dementia may result from arteriosclerosis (hardening of the arteries) when the supply of blood to the brain is slowly cut off. Loss of brain tissue from a series of minor strokes or from an increased amount of fluid accumulation in the brain might cause dementia. Toxic reactions to drugs or small clots to the brain, advanced syphilis, brain tumors, and hypothyroidism often exhibit the same symptoms as Alzheimer's.

A recent study of seventy-eight patients with dementia revealed that 68 percent also had Alzheimer's disease, 5 percent had a vitamin deficiency (particularly B_{12}), 8 percent had a mild form of depression, and 5 percent had dementia from repeated strokes.

Research has revealed a strong correlation between Alzheimer's disease and excessive amounts of aluminum concentrated in the brain. Autopsies of victims of Alzheimer's disease reveal excessive amounts of aluminum and silicon in the brain. The hippocampus area and cerebral cortex of Alzheimer's patients contained not only excess amounts of aluminum, but also of bromine, calcium, silicon, and sulfur. In addition, a deficiency of boron, potassium, selenium, vitamin B_{12}, and zinc was found. These results may suggest that excessive amounts of aluminum in the diet, combined with a lack of several essential minerals, directly or indirectly predispose one to Alzheimer's disease. Although this information offers hope that Alzheimer's disease might some day be prevented, science does not yet know what can be done to allay the mental deterioration. A hair analysis may be needed to determine whether the body contains toxic metals.

In addition to the discovery of mineral imbalances in Alzheimer's patients, research indicates that estrogen levels may be upset as well. Dr. Bruce McEwen of Rockefeller University found that women with Alzheimer's disease had lower estrogen levels than their healthy counterparts (*Saturday Evening Post* 258:9).

NUTRIENTS

SUPPLEMENT	SUGGESTED DOSAGE	COMMENTS
Important		
Superoxide dismutase (SOD): AOX/PLX from Biotec Foods	Use as directed on label.	This high potency antioxidant not only improves utilization of oxygen but also contains glutathione peroxidase, a selenium enzyme.
Helpful		
Coenzyme Q$_{10}$	100 mg daily.	This natural substance carries oxygen to cells and is responsible for generating cellular energy.
Germanium	200 mg daily.	Enhances immune function.
Kelp	5 tablets daily.	Supplies minerals.
Lecithin	1 tbsp. with meals.	Needed for brain function.
Potassium from a high potency multivitamin	99 mg daily.	A necessary nutrient.
Protein supplement (free form amino acids)	Twice daily on an empty stomach.	Needed for improved brain function and tissue repair.
RNA-DNA	1 tablet contains 200 mg RNA and 100 mg DNA. Use as directed on label.	These are the brain's cellular building blocks, and are available in supplements in health food stores.
Selenium with	200 mcg daily.	
zinc and	50 mcg daily.	
vanadium and	5 mg daily.	
boron	3 mg daily.	
Vitamin B complex with	2 cc 3 times weekly.	Needed for brain function. Aids in the digestion of food.
vitamin B$_6$ (pyridoxine) and	½ cc 3 times weekly.	
vitamin B$_{12}$	1 cc 3 times weekly.	
Vitamin C with bioflavonoids	6,000–10,000 mg daily in divided doses.	Enhances immune function and increases energy levels.
Vitamin E	Start at 400 IU daily and increase to 800 IU daily.	Helps transport oxygen to the brain cells.

HERBS

☐ Use butcher's broom and ginkgo biloba.

RECOMMENDATIONS

☐ Consume steam–distilled water only.

CONSIDERATIONS

☐ The drugs sandostatin and tetrahydroaminoacridine (THA) may reduce some of the symptoms of Alzheimer's disease.

☐ The signs of alcoholism are much the same as Alzheimer's. Rita Hayworth, who was afflicted with Alzheimer's disease, was at first thought to be an alcoholic.

☐ Acid rain leeches aluminum out of the soil and into our drinking water.

☐ In his book *Beating Alzheimer's*, Tom Warren cites that diet and chemical allergies may play an important role in Alzheimer's. Include plenty of fiber in your diet. Try oat bran or Aerobic Bulk Cleanse (ABC).

☐ *See also* ALUMINUM TOXICITY in Part Two.

The Alzheimer's/Aluminum Connection

Early in 1989, Britain's highly respected medical journal, *The Lancet*, reported conclusions of a study by the British government: the risk of contracting Alzheimer's disease had risen by 50 percent in areas of Great Britain where drinking water contained elevated levels of aluminum.

While our British cousins must contend with the threat of Alzheimer's disease from aluminum-tainted water, Americans can accumulate aluminum through a wide variety of popular, nationally advertised products. Why not check the following guide, and then prune your pantry or medicine cabinet of items that are rife with potentially hazardous aluminum derivatives?

FOOD ADDITIVES

Manufacturers add aluminum to many of the food products Americans eat every day. Cake mixes, frozen doughs, self-rising flour, and sliced processed cheese food all contain from 5 to 50 milligrams of sodium aluminum phosphate per average serving. Baking powder contains from 5 to 70 milligrams of sodium aluminum sulfate per teaspoonful. Varying amounts of other aluminum compounds are contained in food starch modifiers and anti-caking agents. Pickling salts can contain one of two aluminum compounds: aluminum ammonium sulfate or aluminum potassium sulfate. Either of these will cause your pickles or maraschino cherries to taste metallic.

DOUCHES

Many popular douche preparations contain aluminum salts. These include products manufactured by Calgon and Norcliff-Thayer as well as such nationally advertised products as Massengil and Summer's Eve. Research has not yet shown how much of these solutions the body absorbs. In the meantime, it might be wise to be cautious in using them. A homemade, weak solution of vinegar and water could substitute for over-the-counter concoctions.

ANTACIDS

Several dozen antacids contain aluminum hydroxide, an aluminum salt. Depending on the product, concentrations can range from 29 milligrams (Trisogel capsules) to 265 milligrams (Estomul-M liquid) per dose. Included in this list are the nationally advertised products Di-Gel, Gelusil, Maalox, Mylanta, Riopan, and Rolaids. Because the aluminum-Alzheimer's link is so strong, the use of antacids as calcium supplements is not recommended. More than twenty aluminum-free antacid compounds are available. These can be found by reading the label before you make your purchase. Antacids that contain aluminum must state so in their list of ingredients.

BUFFERED ASPIRIN

With concentrations of 14.4 milligrams to 88 milligrams per dose, several major brands of buffered aspirin can be considered dietary sources of aluminum. One of two compounds, aluminum hydroxide or aluminum glycinate, is found in brands such as Arthritis Pain Formula, Arthritis Strength Bufferin, Ascriptin, Bufferin, Cope, and Vanquish.

ANTIDIARRHEAL PREPARATIONS

More than a dozen nonprescription antidiarrheal drugs contain aluminum salts, including kaolin, aluminum magnesium silicate, and attapulgite, in doses of 100 mg/ml to 600 milligrams per tablet. Familiar preparations include Donnagel, Kaopectate, and Rheaban.

OTHER PRODUCTS

Containers

Aluminum-coated waxed containers, used especially for orange and pineapple juices, cause juices inside to absorb aluminum. Beer stored in aluminum cans absorbs small quantities of the metal as well. Bottled beverages are a better choice because they pose less of an aluminum risk than beverages packaged in aluminum cans.

Shampoos

Selsun-Blue, and other antidandruff preparations, contain magnesium ammonium silicate. Aluminum lauryl sulfate is a common ingredient in many nationally advertised shampoos.

Aluminum Cookware

Aluminum cookware contributes significantly to the amounts of aluminum in our diet. According to a study by the University of Cincinnati Medical Center, using aluminum pots to cook tomatoes increased the aluminum content of those tomatoes by 2 milligrams to 4 milligrams per serving.

Anemia

Millions of Americans suffer from anemia, which involves a reduction in the amount of oxygen that the blood is able to carry. This reduced red blood cell count results in weakness; fatigue; dizziness; pale-appearing nails, lips, and eyelids; irritability or depression; drowsiness; soreness in the mouth; and in the female, cessation of menstruation. The first signs of slowly developing anemia are loss of appetite, headaches, constipation, irritability, and difficulty in concentrating.

Iron is an important factor in anemia because this mineral makes hemoglobin, the component of the blood that carries oxygen. The formation of red blood cells will be impaired in those lacking sufficient amounts of iron.

Of those suffering from anemia, 20 percent are women and 50 percent are children. It is a hidden disease because symptoms are not easily recognized.

Possible causes of anemia include drug use, hormonal disorders, surgery, infections, peptic ulcers, hemorrhoids, diverticular disease, heavy menstrual bleeding, repeated pregnancies, liver damage, thyroid disorders, rheumatoid arthritis, bone marrow disease, irradiation, and dietary deficiencies. Excessive aspirin usage in the elderly may cause internal bleeding.

NUTRIENTS

SUPPLEMENT	SUGGESTED DOSAGE	COMMENTS
Essential		
Raw liver extract (from Argentina)	500 mg twice daily or 2cc in injectable form biweekly. Consider injections (under doctor supervision only).	Contains all the elements needed for red blood cell production.
Very Important		
Blackstrap molasses	1 tbsp. twice daily for adults; for children and babies add 1 tsp. to milk.	Contains iron and essential B vitamins.
Iron (ferrous gluconate) or	As prescribed by doctor.	*Caution:* An excess of iron can be toxic to the immune system.
Floradix formula from Germany	2 tsp. twice daily.	A readily absorbable form of iron.
Folic acid and	800 mcg twice daily.	For red blood cell formation.
biotin	300 mcg twice daily.	
Vitamin B₁₂	2,000 mcg 3 times daily. Injections are the most effective, or take in sublingual form.	Essential in red blood cell production.

Important		
Vitamin B complex with extra pantothenic acid (B₅) and	50 mg of each 3 times daily. 100 mg daily.	Pantothenic acid and pyridoxine are important in red blood cell production.
vitamin B₆ (pyridoxine)	50 mg 3 times daily.	
Vitamin C	3,000–10,000 mg daily.	Important in iron absorption.
Helpful		
Brewer's yeast	As directed on label.	Rich in basic nutrients.
Copper plus	2 mg daily.	Copper is needed in red blood cell production. Too much zinc upsets copper metabolism.
zinc	30 mg daily.	
Raw spleen concentrate	Use as directed on label.	Available in health food stores (*see* GLANDULAR THERAPY in Part Three).
Vitamin A plus	10,000 IU daily.	Important antioxidants.
beta-carotene	15,000 IU daily.	
Vitamin E emulsion	600 IU daily or take in capsule form. Take emulsion for easier assimilation.	Important antioxidant.

HERBS

☐ Alfalfa, comfrey, dandelion, mullen, nettle, and red raspberry are good for anemia.

RECOMMENDATIONS

☐ *Calcium, zinc, and antacids interfere with iron absorption and should be taken separately.* Excess serum iron has been linked to cancer. Use iron with caution, and only under a doctor's supervision.

☐ The diet should include blackstrap molasses, broccoli, egg yolks, kelp, leafy greens, legumes (peas, but not beans), parsley, prunes, raisins, rice bran, turnip greens, and whole grains. Fish eaten at the same time as vegetables containing iron increases iron absorption. Include foods with a high vitamin C content to aid iron absorption. Avoid bran as a fiber.

☐ Foods that contain oxalic acid, which interferes with iron absorption, should be eaten in moderation or omitted. These include almonds, asparagus, beets, cashews, chocolate, kale, rhubarb, soda, sorrel, spinach, Swiss chard, and most nuts and beans. Additives found in beer, candy bars, dairy products, ice cream, and soft drinks interfere with iron absorption, as do tannins in tea, polyphenols in coffee, lead found in various products, and cadmium from smoking.

☐ Have a complete blood test to determine if you have

an iron deficiency before taking iron supplements. Excess iron can damage the liver, heart, pancreas, and lymphocyte (B- and T-cell) activity.

Anorexia Nervosa

Individuals suffering from this condition, 95 percent of which are females, have an intense fear of becoming obese. They either refuse to eat to the point of starvation or they eat and make themselves vomit immediately afterward. This disorder typically appears during adolescence, afflicting 1 to 2 percent of the female population between the ages of twelve and eighteen. Initially, anorexia nervosa was thought to be primarily of psychological origin; however, in the last few years, there are indications from medical scientists and nutritionists that some cases of anorexia nervosa may be caused by a severe zinc deficiency.

Even though they become emaciated, sufferers are obsessed with the idea that they are fat. This can result from excessive teasing by their peers or parents. Anorexics often display great fear at the prospect of growing up, and with female anorexics there is frequently a very difficult mother/daughter relationship. All forms of treatment are normally rejected, and no amount of common sense or persuasion will force them to change their mental image of how they look.

Signs of anorexia are a swollen neck, erosion of enamel on back teeth from excessive vomiting, broken blood vessels in the face, underweight, extreme weakness, dizziness, cessation of menstruation, and low pulse rate and blood pressure.

Symptoms include self-starvation, vomiting deliberately, and/or taking huge doses of laxatives. Some anorexics just quit eating, some vomit, some take laxatives, and some do all three. A major problem with laxatives is that they deplete the body of potassium. This causes irregular heartbeat, which can lead to heart failure. About 30 percent of all anorexics struggle with the disorder all their lives, while 40 percent outgrow it and 30 percent have at least one life-threatening bout with it. Nearly all victims of anorexia die prematurely. Although anorexia has been perceived as a serious and widespread problem for some time, the tragic death of singer Karen Carpenter in 1983 due to complications from this disorder brought it to the forefront. Many cases of anorexia require hospitalization in which intravenous nutrient feedings of potassium and multivitamins are given to the anorexic.

NUTRIENTS

SUPPLEMENT	SUGGESTED DOSAGE	COMMENTS
Very Important		
Multivitamins and minerals containing	Megadoses	Must be taken in extremely high doses because they are passed through the gastrointestinal tract rapidly and are poorly assimilated.
potassium and	99 mg daily.	
selenium and	200 mcg daily.	
zinc	50 mg daily.	
Important		
Acidophilus or Megadophilus	Follow directions on label. Take on an empty stomach so that it passes quickly to the small intestine.	Needed to replace the "friendly" bacteria lost from use of laxatives and/or from vomiting.
Minerals (essential) including zinc	50–100 mg daily. Do not exceed 100 mg zinc.	Needed to replace lost minerals.
Protein supplement (free form amino acids)	As directed on label.	Needed to repair all tissues.
Vitamin B complex with B₁₂ injections plus liver injections	100 mg 3 times daily. 1cc 3 times weekly. 2cc 3 times weekly.	Helps to prevent anemia. Replaces lost B vitamins.
Vitamin C	5,000 mg daily in divided doses.	Needed for the impaired immune system and to alleviate the stress that is on the adrenal glands.
Helpful		
Bio-Strath or	3 times daily.	Acts as a tonic.
Floradix formula, both from West Germany	3 times daily.	A natural source of iron.
Brewer's yeast	Start with a small amount and work up.	Contains balanced amounts of the B vitamins.
Kelp	6 tablets daily.	Needed for mineral replacement.
Proteolytic enzymes	Take between meals and with meals.	To aid in digestion and in rebuilding of tissue.
Vitamin A	15,000 IU daily.	Needed for repair of all tissues and to aid the immune system.
Vitamin D	600 IU daily.	Prevents bone loss.
Vitamin E	600 IU daily.	Increases oxygen uptake in the body for healing.

HERBS

☐ The following herbs are appetite stimulants: ginger root, ginseng, gotu kola, and peppermint.

RECOMMENDATIONS

☐ When a regular eating pattern is being established, a high-fiber, well-balanced diet is essential for maintaining good health. Consume no sugar in any form and avoid white flour products. Be aware that there might be withdrawal symptoms.

ADDITIONAL SOURCES OF INFORMATION

To learn more about eating disorders and treatments, contact any of the following:

American Anorexia/Bulimia Association
133 Cedar Lane
Teaneck, NJ 07666
(201) 836-1800

ANAD
P.O. Box 7
Highland Park, IL 60035
(312) 831-3438

ANRED
P.O. Box 5102
Eugene, OR 97405
(503) 344-1144

Center for the Study of Anorexia and Bulimia
1 West 91st Street
New York, NY 10024
(212) 595-3449

National Anorexic Aid Society
5796 Karl Road
Columbus, OH 43229
(614) 436-1112

Appetite, Poor

Emotional factors such as stress, depression, and trauma may lead to a poor appetite. Controllable factors such as alcohol, cigarette, and drug use can also result in poor appetite, as can an undetected illness, heavy metal poisoning, and nutritional deficiencies. To stimulate a poor appetite, the diet must be individualized to the patient's tolerances. Undernourished people may lose their appetite at the sight of large amounts of food. Therefore, frequent small meals may be better tolerated with a gradual increase in the volume of food. When trying to stimulate a poor appetite, consider whether the appearance and aroma of the foods are appealing, in addition to whether the environment is conducive to eating.

NUTRIENTS

SUPPLEMENT	SUGGESTED DOSAGE	COMMENTS
Very Important		
Bio-Strath	As directed on label.	Yeast and herb formula from Germany. Aids in gaining back strength and energy.
Floradix formula from West Germany	As directed on label.	Helps digestion and stimulates appetite.
Multivitamin/ mineral high potency complex with		All nutrients are needed in large amounts.
vitamin A	25,000 IU daily.	
and calcium	1,500 mg daily.	
and magnesium	750 mg daily.	
Vitamin B complex	100 mg or more daily. Vitamin B or liver injections may be necessary.	A high stress vitamin that increases the appetite.
Zinc	80 mg daily.	Zinc enhances the taste of foods. Copper is needed to balance with zinc.
and copper	3 mg daily.	
Helpful		
Brewer's yeast	Start with ½ tsp. and work up.	Rich in nutrients—especially B-complex vitamins. Improves the appetite.
Protein supplement (Spiru-Tein from Nature's Plus)	Take between meals.	Needed to build and repair tissue. Acts as an appetite stimulant.

HERBS

☐ To stimulate a poor appetite, try using catnip, fennel seed, ginger root, ginseng, gotu kola, papaya leaves, peppermint leaves, and saw palmetto berries.

RECOMMENDATIONS

☐ Do not drink liquids before or during meals.

☐ Between meals, eat any of the following: avocados, banana soy pudding, buttermilk, cheese, chicken or tuna, custard, fruit shakes, nuts and nut butters, turkey, and yogurt. In addition to promoting weight gain, these snacks are easy to digest, are high in protein and essential fatty acids, and contain "friendly" bacteria.

☐ Drink three or more cups a day of skim, soy, or almond milk. Use a soy carob drink and yogurt fruit shakes. Eat only whole grain breads, rolls, macaroni, crackers, and hot and cold cereals. Use cream (soy) soups as desired. They are usually higher in protein than broth soups. Use the kinds that your system can tolerate.

☐ Although undernourished people need their strenth to get well, it is important that they become active as soon as possible. Walking and/or moderate exercise can trigger the appetite. Exercise if possible, but avoid strenuous exercise. Some exercise helps to assimilate nutrients better and to increase appetite.

☐ Check the sections, ANOREXIA NERVOSA and BULIMIA, in Part Two to rule out these disorders. *Also see* HYPOTHYROID in Part Two for the self-test. See a doctor to rule out a disorder.

CONSIDERATIONS

☐ Try eating from red plates. This color stimulates the taste buds.

Arsenic Poisoning

Arsenic is a highly poisonous metallic element that can be found in water, pesticides, laundry aids, beer, table salt, seafood, tobacco smoke, smog, bone meal, dolomite, and kelp. Inorganic arsenic deposits in the hair, skin, and nails. Once it is in the hair follicles, it will stay in the shaft for years.

Workers involved in pesticide production, copper smelters, makers and sprayers of insecticides, miners, sheep dip workers, and those in the metallurgical industries are at a high risk for skin cancer, scrotal cancer, hemangiosarcoma of the liver, cancer of the lymphatic system, and lung cancer due to toxic levels of arsenic in their bodies.

Arsenic poisoning will primarily affect the lungs, skin, and liver. Headaches, confusion, drowsiness, convulsions, and changes in fingernail pigmentation may occur with chronic arsenic poisoning. If you have any of the following symptoms, you may have a toxic level of arsenic: vomiting, diarrhea, bloody urine, muscle cramps, gastrointestinal upsets, and convulsions. If you have any of these symptoms, have a hair analysis done to determine the level of toxic metals in your body. Toxic levels of arsenic can even result in coma and death.

NUTRIENTS

SUPPLEMENT	SUGGESTED DOSAGE	COMMENTS
Very Important		
Garlic tablets (Kyolic)	2 tablets with meals.	Kyolic acts as a potent detoxifier.
Kelp	6 tablets daily.	High in minerals and aids in detoxification.
Superoxide dismutase (SOD) from Biotec Foods	Use as directed on label.	This product is a powerful detoxifying agent.
Vitamin C (buffered form)	8,000–10,000 mg daily in divided doses.	A potent detoxifier. *See* ASCORBIC ACID FLUSH in Part Three and follow instructions.
Helpful		
L-Cysteine and L-methionine (amino acids)	500 mg each, taken daily on an empty stomach.	Potent detoxifiers of the liver. L-Cysteine contains sulfur, which eliminates arsenic.
L-Cystine (amino acid)	Take on an empty stomach as directed on label. If taken with vitamins B_6 and C, amino acids will be better assimilated.	Aids in detoxification. Contains sulfur, which eliminates arsenic.
Pectin plus antioxidant formula	Use as directed on product label.	Aids in removing arsenic from the body.
Selenium	200 mcg daily.	This element helps rid the body of arsenic.

RECOMMENDATIONS

☐ Supplement your diet with plenty of fiber on a daily basis. If you are a victim of arsenic toxicity, eat eggs, onions, beans, legumes, and garlic to obtain sulfur. You can also obtain sulfur from garlic in tablet form. Sulfur helps eliminate arsenic from the body. L-Cysteine will also provide sulfur. Sulfur can now be purchased in tablet form from DaVinci Laboratories. This source of dietary sulfur is called methylsulfonylmethane (MSM).

☐ In case of accidental arsenic ingestion, you should *immediately* take five charcoal tablets every fifteen minutes until you reach your doctor or hospital. Charcoal tablets should be kept on hand in every household in case of accidental overdose of drugs. These tablets are available in health food stores. They can be used for extreme gas, bloating, and allergies. Be careful about taking them *too* often—they also absorb good nutrients.

☐ *See also* CHEMICAL POISONING and ENVIRONMENTAL TOXICITY, both in Part Two.

Arteriosclerosis

Arteriosclerosis involves the build-up of calcium deposits on the inside of the artery walls, which causes thickening and hardening of the arteries. If the deposits are fatty substances, the condition is referred to as atherosclerosis. Both conditions have about the same effect on circulation. The condition causes strokes, coronary disease (angina), and high blood pressure. High blood pressure can also *cause* arteriosclerosis. The calcium or fatty deposits typically form in areas of the arteries that have been weakened by high blood pressure or strain. Narrowing of the arteries forces blood pressure that is already high to become even higher. As the arteries become less pliable and less permeable, cell starvation (ischemia) results due to insufficient circulation in the cells. An individual will suffer a heart attack, also referred to as a myocardial infarction (MI) or coronary occlusion (a coronary), when one of the coronary arteries becomes completely obstructed by accumulated deposits or by a blood clot that has either formed or been snagged on the deposit. Older people are at a greater risk for this kind of heart trouble. When arteriosclerosis occludes the arterial supply of blood to the brain, a cerebrovascular accident, or stroke, occurs.

Arteriosclerosis obliterans occurs when the lower limbs are affected. In the early stages the major arteries that carry blood to the legs and the feet become narrowed by fatty deposits. Early signs are aching muscles, fatigue, and cramp-like pains in the ankles and legs. Depending on which arteries are blocked, the pain may also be in the hips and thighs.

Leg pain brought on by walking that is promptly relieved by sitting is called *claudication*. Additional symptoms include numbness, weakness, and a heavy feeling in the legs. These symptoms occur when the arteries are clogged with cholesterol plaque. Pain is experienced if the amount of oxygenated blood is insufficient to meet the needs of the exercising leg muscles.

ARTERY FUNCTION SELF-TEST

A simple test can determine how well the blood is flowing through the arteries of the legs. There are three places on the lower leg where a pulsating artery can be felt by lightly touching the skin covering the artery. One spot is the top of the foot; the second spot is the inner aspect of the ankle; and the third spot is behind the knee.

Apply pressure lightly to the skin on these spots where the pulsating artery can be felt. If you cannot find a pulse, it is an indication that the artery supplying the leg is narrowed. Special studies may be needed. Consult your doctor.

Foods rich in vitamin E will help the problem. Vitamin E and vitamin C will enhance the oxygen supply in the bloodstream and in the red blood cells. It would be wise to add these supplements to your diet.

NUTRIENTS

SUPPLEMENT	SUGGESTED DOSAGE	COMMENTS
Very Important		
Dr. Rinse's Formula or	1 tbsp. in juice before meals.	Specially formulated for hardening of the arteries.
lecithin	1 tbsp. or 2 capsules with meals.	
Garlic tablets (Kyolic)	As directed on label.	Kyolic has a lipid (fat) regulating effect.
Multidigestive enzymes	Take with meals.	Important for proper digestion.
Proteolytic enzymes	Take between meals.	Aids in destroying free radicals and in digestive function.
Selenium	200 mcg daily.	Selenium promotes action of vitamin E.
Vitamin A and E emulsion or multivitamin and mineral	25,000 IU vitamin A; 400–1,000 IU vitamin E. Increase slowly.	Antioxidants that act as free radical scavengers.
Vitamin C (buffered)	6,000–10,000 mg in daily divided doses.	Antioxidant that acts as a free radical scavenger. *See* ASCORBIC ACID FLUSH in Part Three.
Important		
Coenzyme Q_{10}	100 mg daily.	Improves tissue oxygenation.
DMG (Gluconic from DaVinci Labs)	1 tablet 3 times daily.	Improves tissue oxygenation.
Germanium	200 mg daily.	Lowers cholesterol and improves cellular oxygenation.
Lipotropic factors	Use as directed on label.	Reduces lipid (fat) content of blood. Phosphatidyl choline is best because it is strongest.
Helpful		
Calcium plus	1,500 mg daily.	Use chelate or asporotate.
magnesium	750 mg daily.	
L-Methionine plus	500 mg daily.	Must be taken on an empty stomach. Take with vitamin C or with vitamin B_6 for easier assimilation.
L-cysteine	500 mg daily.	
Unsaturated fatty acids (salmon oil or MaxEPA)	As directed on label.	Salmon oil or MaxEPA are good sources of the fatty acids.
Vitamin B complex plus extra niacinamide	100 mg 3 times daily.	The B vitamins work together as a complex. Niacin (B_3) dilates the small arteries (arterioles).
Zinc chelate and copper chelate	50 mg daily. 3 mg daily.	Aids in cleansing and in the healing process. *See also* CHELATION THERAPY in Part Three.

HERBS

☐ The following herbs are helpful if you suffer from arteriosclerosis: cayenne, chickweed herb, ginkgo biloba extract, and hawthorn berries.

RECOMMENDATIONS

☐ Anticoagulants such as aspirin are given to thin the blood and prevent clotting. For effective anticoagulation, the supplement vitamin K and foods rich in vitamin K must be avoided. (*See* the dietary recommendations in CARDIOVASCULAR DISEASE, Part Two, for a list of foods to avoid.)

☐ The diet should not contain any red meat. Avoid white flour, white sugar, and salt. Do not use stimulants such as coffee, colas, and tobacco; also eliminate alcohol and highly spiced foods. Increase the amount of fiber in the diet.

☐ Drink steam-distilled water and use pure olive oil to aid in lowering cholesterol.

☐ Impotence can result from this disease. *See* IMPOTENCE in Part Two.

☐ *See also* CHELATION THERAPY in Part Three.

Arthritis

Arthritis is characterized by an inflammation and/or pain in a joint or joints. Joints of the body are found at the knees, wrists, elbows, fingers, toes, hips, and shoulders. The neck and back also have joints between the bones of the spine. Symptoms of chronic arthritis are pain, swelling, stiffness, and deformity of one or more joints. It may appear suddenly or come on gradually. Some people feel a sharp burning or grinding pain. Others compare the pain to a toothache. Moving the joint usually hurts, although sometimes there is only stiffness.

There are many different forms arthritis can take. However, here we will be discussing the most common forms: osteoarthritis and rheumatoid arthritis. A degenerative joint disease, osteoarthritis is related to the wear and tear of aging and involves deterioration of the cartilage at the ends of the bones. The once smooth surface of cartilage becomes rough, resulting in friction. The tendons, ligaments, and muscles holding the joint together become weaker, and the joint itself becomes deformed, painful, and stiff. There is usually some pain, but little or no swelling. Any disablement is usually minor. Osteoarthritis rarely develops before the age of forty. It afflicts 15.8 million Americans. It typically runs in families, but afflicts almost three times as many women as men.

Rheumatoid and juvenile rheumatoid arthritis are types of inflammatory arthritis that attack the synovial membranes surrounding the lubricating fluid in the joints. The cartilage and tissues in and around the joints and often the bone surfaces are destroyed. The body replaces this damaged tissue with scar tissue, causing the spaces between the joints to become narrow, to develop folds, and to fuse together. The entire body is affected instead of just one joint as in osteoarthritis. Rheumatoid arthritis creates stiffness, swelling, fatigue, anemia, weight loss, fever, and often crippling pain. It often occurs in people under forty years of age, including young children. Currently, 2.1 million Americans are afflicted with rheumatoid arthritis; twice as many women as men suffer from rheumatoid arthritis. Juvenile rheumatoid arthritis affects 71,000 young Americans (aged eighteen and under); six times as many girls are afflicted with juvenile rheumatoid arthritis as boys.

The onset of rheumatoid arthritis is often associated with physical or emotional stress; however, poor nutrition or bacterial infection may also be the cause.

Other forms of arthritis include gout, ankylosing spondylitis (AS), and systemic lupus erythematosus (SLE). Gout occurs more often in overweight people and those who indulge regularly in rich foods and alcohol. It typically attacks the smaller joints of the feet and hands, generally affecting the big toe. Deposits of crystallized uric acid salt in the joint cause swelling, redness, and a sensation of heat and extreme pain. Currently 1 million Americans are affected, with four times as many men suffering from gout as women.

Ankylosing spondylitis (AS) affects certain joints of the spine, which become inflamed, stiffen, become rigid, and then fuse together. If confined to the lower back, AS will cause virtually no limitation of movement. In some cases, however, the entire spine may become rigid and bent. If the joints between the ribs and spine are affected, it will cause severe breathing problems due to limited expansion of the chest wall. Postural deformities are common. Currently 318,000 Americans are afflicted; two and a half times as many men as women have AS.

Systemic lupus erythematosus (SLE) is a malfunction of the body's immune system. For reasons unknown, the body produces antibodies that act against itself. Although it mimics rheumatoid arthritis and results in painful and inflamed joints, SLE is not a crippling disease. Currently 131,000 Americans are afflicted; eight times as many women as men have this disorder.

NUTRIENTS

SUPPLEMENT	SUGGESTED DOSAGE	COMMENTS
Essential		
Primrose or salmon oil	2 capsules twice daily.	Controls arthritis pain and inflammation.

Superoxide dismutase (SOD)	As directed on label.	A free radical destroyer. Injections have given excellent results. The sublingual form is also good, or try Cell Guard from Biotec Foods.

Very Important		
Calcium plus magnesium	2,000 mg daily. 1,000 mg daily.	Chelate form is the most effective. Needed to prevent bone loss.
Coenzyme Q_{10}	60 mg daily.	Increases tissue oxygenation, which is needed to aid in repairing connective tissues.
Garlic tablets (Kyolic)	2 capsules 3 times daily with meals. Use this odorless garlic or 1 tsp. of oil.	Inhibits the formation of free radicals, which can damage the joints.
Kelp	8 tablets daily.	A rich source of minerals.
Multienzymes	Take with meals.	Avoid brands containing hydrochloric acid (HCl) if ulcers are present.
Niacin (B_3, niacinamide) plus vitamin B_6 (pyridoxine)	100 mg 3 times daily.	Increases blood flow by dilating small arteries.
Vitamin B complex with extra niacin (B_3) plus B_6 (pyridoxine) and PABA and pantothenic acid (B_5)	100 mg 3 times daily.	Use hypoallergenic variety. PABA is good for swelling.
Vitamin B_{12} and folic acid	Take lozenges daily.	Needed for proper digestion, the formation of cells, and the production of myelin, the protective coating surrounding the nerves. Prevents nerve damage.
Vitamin C plus bioflavonoids	3,000–10,000 mg daily in divided doses. 500 mg daily.	A powerful free radical destroyer.

Important		
Germanium	200 mg daily.	A powerful antioxidant that also relieves pain.
Multienzymes	Take with meals.	Bromelin enzymes help to stimulate production of prostaglandin. Also helps digestion of protein. Proteolytic enzymes protect the joints from free radical damage.
Proteolytic enzymes	Take between meals.	

Helpful		
DL-Phenylalanine (DLPA)	Take daily every other week.	Good for pain relief. *Caution:* Not for use if pregnant, have high blood pressure, or diabetic.
Gerovital H-3 (GH-3)	As directed on label.	Drug from Rumania that has given good results.
Iron (Floradix formula)	As directed on label.	Floradix is a good source of iron. Omit if anemia is not present.
L-Cysteine	500 mg twice daily on an empty stomach.	A detoxifier essential for immune function. A sulfur source.

Multivitamin complex plus vitamin A and beta-carotene	10,000 IU daily.	All nutrients are needed to protect from free radical damage and to repair tissues and cartilage.
Silicon extract (horsetail)	As directed on label.	Needed for calcium absorption and the connective tissues.
Vitamin E	400 IU daily.	A powerful antioxidant. Aids in mobilizing the joints.

HERBS

☐ If you have arthritis, the use of the following herbs can be beneficial: alfalfa leaves, black cohosh, brigham tea, cayenne, celery seed, chaparral leaves, comfrey, devil's claw tea, feverfew, parsley tea, valerian root, and yucca extract. Feverfew is good for pain and soreness. Yucca extract has been used successfully at the Desert Arthritis Clinic.

RECOMMENDATIONS

☐ Check for possible allergies.

☐ Avoid milk; vitamin D causes sore joints. Also avoid red meat, sugar products, citrus fruits, green peppers, eggplant, tomatoes, potatoes, paprika, cayenne pepper, tobacco, and salt.

☐ Exercise is essential for reducing pain and retarding joint deterioration. Hot tubs and baths provide relief. Raw lemon rubs and hot castor oil packs are also extremely beneficial.

☐ A free form amino acid complex should be part of the program to help repair tissue. Some form of fiber, such as oat bran or rice bran, should be eaten daily, and the diet should be low in fats. Foods that should be consumed include eggs; onions; garlic or asparagus whose sulfur content helps to remove metals; the amino acid histidine, which is also good for removing metals; green leafy vegetables, which are needed for vitamin K; fresh vegetables; nonacidic fresh fruits; whole grains; oatmeal; brown rice; and fish.

☐ It is important to drink steam-distilled water only.

☐ The nightshade vegetables (green peppers, eggplant, tomatoes, white potatoes) contain a toxin called sotanine that some people, particularly those suffering from arthritis, are highly sensitive to it. Sotanine interferes with enzymes in the muscles, and may cause pain and discomfort.

☐ Do not take iron. It is suspected to be involved in pain, swelling, and joint destruction. Do not take a multivitamin containing iron. Consume iron naturally in blackstrap molasses, broccoli, Brussels sprouts, cauliflower, fish, lima beans, and peas.

CONSIDERATIONS

☐ The drugs piroxicam and indomethacin relieve pain more efficiently than aspirin. In some forms of arthritis, stronger types of drugs are used: hydroxychloroquine and gold compound.

☐ The bacteria responsible for chlamydia nonspecific urethritis has been linked as a cause of one form of arthritis in young women. In nearly half of the women with unexplained arthritis who were tested, chlamydia was found in the joints. Seventy-five percent had raised antibody levels in the blood.

☐ Rheumatologist Thomas Brown, M.D., implicates the mycoplasma organism as the causative agent in rheumatoid arthritis. His apparent remarkable results using the antibiotic tetracycline, however, are questionable and need further investigation.

ARTHRITIS COMMENTS

☐ A joint afflicted with rheumatoid arthritis sounds more like crinkling cellophane, while an osteoarthritic joint makes popping, clicking, and banging noises.

☐ Over 250,000 people have used supplements in arthritis treatment; they correct 80 to 90 percent of all arthritis cases according to Robert Bingham, M.D., in the journal of the Academy of Rheumatoid Diseases.

☐ Latest research has linked rheumatoid arthritis to diet. Victims had lower blood levels of folic acid, protein, and zinc. Researchers concluded that drugs brought about new biochemical changes, creating a need for certain nutrients.

☐ Researchers report that the ulcer drug, Carafate, can give the same relief as aspirin and other anti-inflammatory drugs without damaging the stomach lining. The drug Suprol (also known as suprofen) can harm the kidneys. There have been 100 reported cases of kidney damage from this drug. If side effects occur, stop the use of the drug and notify your doctor.

Asthma

Asthma is caused by spasms in the muscles surrounding the bronchi (small airways in the lungs), which con-strict the outward passage of stale air. Typical symptoms are coughing, wheezing, a tight chest, and difficult breathing. When changes in air passages occur so that air cannot pass freely to and from the tiny air sacs in the lungs, bronchial asthma results. Cardiac asthma is the result of a malfunctioning heart.

The muscular spasms, together with increased mucus, are brought on by histamine produced by the body's immune system during an allergic response. Therefore, any kind of allergen can precipitate an asthma attack.

Researchers believe that lower magnesium uptake or a magnesium deficiency may play a role in certain types of asthma.

NUTRIENTS

SUPPLEMENT	SUGGESTED DOSAGE	COMMENTS
Essential		
Vitamin A plus	15,000 IU daily.	Needed for tissue repair and immunity.
beta-carotene	10,000 IU daily.	
Pantothenic acid (B$_5$)	50 mg 3 times daily.	B$_5$ is the antistress vitamin.
Vitamin B complex including	50 mg 4 times daily.	Stimulates the immune system, especially B$_6$. Injections are the most effective.
vitamin B$_6$ (pyridoxine) and	50 mg 3 times daily or ½ cc.	
vitamin B$_{12}$ tablets or lozenges	100 mg twice daily between meals. Dissolve lozenges in mouth slowly.	
Vitamin E	600 IU and up daily.	A potent antioxidant.
Very Important		
Magnesium	750 mg daily.	Magnesium chelate or asporotate may stop the severe asthmatic episode.
Multivitamin/ mineral complex (high potency) with		Necessary for enhanced immune function.
selenium and	200 mcg daily.	
beta-carotene	15,000 IU daily.	
Important		
Bromelin with	100 mg 3 times daily.	Powerful immunostimulants. Quercetin C has an antihistamine effect. Take together for best results.
Quercetin C	500 mg 3 times daily.	
Vitamin C plus bioflavonoids	1,500 mg 3 times daily.	
Helpful		
Bee pollen	Start with a few granules; increase slowly to 1 tsp. daily.	Best to use pollen produced within a 10-mile radius of your home.
Calcium	1,500 mg daily.	Chelated form is the most effective.
Coenzyme Q$_{10}$	100 mg daily.	Has ability to counter histamine.
DMG (Gluconic from DaVinci Labs)	As directed on label.	Improves oxygenation in lung tissue.

InspirEase from Key Pharmaceuticals	Use as directed on label.	An inhaler.
Kelp tablets	10 daily for 21 days, then reduce to 3 a day.	For minerals in balanced amounts.
L-Methionine (amino acid) plus	500 mg twice daily.	L-Methionine is an important antioxidant.
vitamin B$_6$ (pyridoxide) and	50 mg daily.	
vitamin C	500 mg daily. Take these supplements together on an empty stomach for better absorption.	
Vitamin D	600 IU daily.	

HERBS

☐ Use echinacea, horsetail, juniper berries, licorice root, Ma Huang, pau d'arco, propolis, and slippery elm bark tablets. Drink three cups daily of pau d'arco tea. It acts as a natural antibiotic. Lobelia herbal extract is helpful during an asthma attack; it is a bronchial smooth muscle relaxant. Ginkgo, an herb containing the active ingredient ginkgolide B, has also shown good results in many studies.

RECOMMENDATIONS

☐ The diet should consist primarily of fresh fruits and vegetables, nuts and seeds, oatmeal, brown rice, and whole grains. A hypoglycemic diet should be followed—one that contains no sugar, is high in protein, and is low in carbohydrates.

☐ Use beta-blocking drugs, nonsteroidal anti-inflammatory drugs, and aspirin with caution.

☐ A green drink is important. Kyo-Green from Wakunaga of America Company is excellent. Use three times a day, one half hour before meals. A juice fast, a fast using distilled water and lemon juice, or a combination of both for three days each month can help rid the body of toxins and mucus.

CONSIDERATIONS

☐ Foods to avoid include alfalfa, beets, carrots, colas, cold beverages (which may cause bronchial spasm), dairy products (including milk and ice cream), fish, red meat (especially pork), processed foods, salt, spinach, chicken and turkey, white flour, and white sugar.

☐ Also avoid furry animals; aspirin; BHA and BHT food additives; F, D, and C yellow #5 dyes; smoke and tobacco; and tryptophan.

☐ Use Dr. Christopher's Air Breathe Ease two to three times daily. Also apply castor oil packs on the back and around the lung and kidney areas. Place castor oil in a pan and heat, but do not boil. Dip a piece of cheesecloth or other white cotton material into the oil until the cloth is saturated. Apply the cloth to the affected area and cover with a piece of plastic that is larger in size than the cotton cloth. Place a heating pad over the plastic. Retain for one-half to two hours as needed.

☐ An article in volume 81 of the *Journal of Allergy and Clinical Immunology* suggested taking two salmon oil capsules before meals and eating fish three times weekly for asthma.

☐ Most restaurants use sulfites to preserve the salads, avocado dip, cut or sliced fruit, cole slaw, canned or frozen shellfish, canned mushrooms, sauces and gravies, soups, pickles, frozen French fries, potato chips, wine vinegar, cider, potatoes, baked goods, sausages, beer, and wines. Sulfites can be found in any type of food. Some people have had severe attacks after consuming foods containing sulfites; even death can result.

☐ Sulfitic agents include sodium bisulfite, potassium metabisulfite, potassium bisulfite, and sulfur dioxide. These are commonly used to prevent discoloration and bacterial growth in foods.

☐ Test strips are now available to help detect the presence of sulfites in foods. For information write to: Sulfitest, Center Laboratories, 35 Channel Drive, Port Washington, NY 11050, or call (800) 645-6335 or (516) 767-1800 if in New York. This chemically treated paper strip turns red in the presence of sulfites or green in the absence of sulfites. The strips were developed by Barbara Markley of Kansas State University.

☐ The drug Theo-Dur Sprinkle, which is sprinkled on children's foods to help prevent asthma symptoms, has been used in Canada with good results.

☐ *See also* ALLERGIES in Part Two.

Atherosclerosis

See ARTERIOSCLEROSIS.

Athlete's Foot

Athlete's foot (tinea pedis) is a fungal infection that thrives in an environment of warmth and dampness. It lives off the dead skin cells and calluses of the feet, especially the skin between the toes. Symptoms include inflammation, burning, itching, scaling, and blisters.

The fungus spreads rapidly when beneficial bacteria are destroyed by antibiotics, drugs, or radiation. It is especially prevalent and highly contagious in warm, damp places such as gyms and pool locker rooms. Care should be taken to protect the feet from direct contact with floors in these places. Athlete's foot sufferers should eat a balanced diet that includes plenty of raw fruits, vegetables, whole grains, yogurt and other acidophilus-containing foods, and megadoses of vitamins A, B, and C. Refer to CANDIDIASIS in Part Two and follow the recommended diet.

NUTRIENTS

SUPPLEMENT	SUGGESTED DOSAGE	COMMENTS
Essential		
Maxidophilus or Megadophilus	1 tsp. in water, taken on an empty stomach twice daily.	Replenishes the "friendly" bacteria that inhibit pathogenic organisms. Prevents potential systemic fungus infection, such as candidiasis.
Very Important		
Garlic tablets (Kyolic)	2 tablets three times daily.	Odorless garlic; aids in destroying fungus.
Important		
Vitamin B complex (high potency)	Use as directed on label.	Use a yeast-free product.
Vitamin C (buffered)	3,000–10,000 mg 3 times daily in divided doses.	Reduces stress. Promotes immune function.
Zinc	50 mg daily.	Inhibits fungus and stimulates the immune system.
Helpful		
Aerobic 07 from Aerobic Life Products	9 drops in a glass of water twice daily. Also apply drops directly on affected areas and let dry.	Its supply of oxygen to the cells kills germs and harmful bacteria.
Germanium	100 mg daily.	A potent antioxidant and pain reliever.
Orifresh from Amni	Use as directed on label.	Kills harmful bacteria.
Unsaturated fatty acids	As directed on label.	Supplies the essential fatty acids. Omega-3 fish oils are good sources. Try Fortified Flax from Omega-Life.
Vitamin A	50,000 IU daily for 1 month, then reduce to 25,000 IU.	Needed for healing of tissues and to stimulate the immune system.
Vitamin E	400 IU daily up to 1,000 IU, increasing slowly.	

HERBS

☐ Prepare a tea using pau d'arco; drink three cups daily. Also prepare a strong tea solution using pau d'arco and twenty drops of Aerobic 07; soak feet for fifteen minutes for fast results.

RECOMMENDATIONS

☐ Avoid cola drinks, grains, processed foods, and sugar. Eat plenty of fruits and vegetables, broiled fish, and broiled skinless chicken. Do not eat fried, greasy foods. Cut raw garlic into tiny pieces and wear in shoes for a few days. The garlic will be absorbed into the skin. Dust feet with garlic powder. Wear absorbent socks made of cotton. Air your shoes out and change socks daily. Though you can purchase nonprescription drugs that are antifungal, we believe garlic works better.

CONSIDERATIONS

☐ Keep feet dry. After a shower or bath, dry carefully between each toe. Make sure the towel is used only once and by no one else. Wear shoes or slippers in public locker rooms where the fungus flourishes.

☐ Those with recurrent fungal infections of the feet often have a fungal infection in the groin area. Both areas must be treated simultaneously. To prevent transmission of the foot fungus to the groin area, put clean socks on before putting on your underwear when dressing.

Autism

Autism is an illness that involves children who do not react to their environment. Speech development is delayed and often absent or limited to nonsense rhyming or babbling. They exhibit marked unresponsiveness to love and affection. Behavior ranges from total silence to periods of hyperactivity that include biting and pounding of their body. These children are withdrawn, have learning disabilities, and are often mentally disabled. Some children seem to have a low IQ, while others seem to fall into the normal range.

The cause of autism is unknown; however, it is not caused by parental neglect or actions as once believed. Some children seem to proceed along well only to inexplicably regress. Many become marginally self-sufficient and independent. However, most will need lifelong care. Scientific studies have conclusively shown that the combination of vitamin B$_6$ and magnesium produces good results in autistic children and adults. In addition, there has also been dramatic improvement after chemical additives and allergenic foods are eliminated from the diet.

A hair analysis should be done to rule out heavy metal poisoning. It is also advisable to test for food allergies.

Please note that the following recommended dosages are for adults who weigh 100 pounds or more. Adjust the following dosages according to age and weight for children.

NUTRIENTS

SUPPLEMENT	SUGGESTED DOSAGE	COMMENTS
Very Important		
Choline	500–2,000 mg daily.	Improves brain function and circulation to the brain. Use under supervision.
DMG (Gluconic from DaVinci Labs)	100 mg daily.	An oxygen carrier to the brain. Important for normal brain and nervous system function.
Magnesium plus	1,000 mg daily.	Essential for normal brain and nervous system function.
calcium	1,500 mg daily.	
Vitamin B complex plus		Essential for normal brain and nervous system function.
niacinamide and	300 mg daily.	
niacin (both B$_3$) and	50 mg 3 times daily.	
pantothenic acid (B$_5$)	500 mg daily.	
Vitamin B$_6$ (pyridoxine)	50 mg 3 times daily.	A vitamin B$_6$ deficiency has been linked to autism. Take in higher amounts only if under professional care.
Vitamin C	3,000–10,000 mg 3 times daily in divided doses.	A powerful free radical scavenger. See ASCORBIC ACID FLUSH in Part Three.
Helpful		
Brewer's yeast	Start with ½ tsp. and work up slowly.	Needed to effect a proper balance of the B vitamins.
L-Glutamine	Take on an empty stomach.	Needed for normal brain function.
L-Phenylalanine and L-tyrosine	Take together on an empty stomach with vitamins B$_6$ and C.	Needed for normal brain function.
RNA and	200 mg daily.	To aid in repairing and building of new brain tissues.
DNA	100 mg daily.	
Vitamin E	200–600 IU daily.	Improves circulation and brain function.

HERBS

☐ Use ginkgo biloba extract as directed on label. This herb improves circulation to the brain.

RECOMMENDATIONS

☐ Try to improve blood oxygen supply to the brain with deep breathing exercises. Hold your breath for thirty seconds every half hour for a thirty-day period. This will stimulate deeper breathing and increase oxygen levels in the tissues of the brain.

☐ Diet is very important for the autistic individual. The diet should be comprised of 50 to 75 percent raw foods. Do not consume junk foods, sugar, or white flour products. Use steam-distilled water.

☐ Exercise is important.

☐ See HYPOGLYCEMIA and HYPERACTIVITY, both in Part Two. Follow the diet programs.

CONSIDERATIONS

☐ Infants born with a protein imbalance may suffer mental disability. If detected early, a proper diet can correct the imbalance.

☐ Research cited in the October 1983 issue of *Pediatric Research* has found that low-level lead exposure in young children may be associated with impaired intellectual development and behavior problems.

☐ Processed baby foods on the market today do not supply enough vitamins and minerals. Therefore, infants and small children need their diets supplemented with vitamins and minerals. Use liquid or powdered preparations.

☐ An article in the May 1988 issue of *The New England Journal of Medicine* disclosed evidence that suggests autistic persons have a shortage of a type of nerve cell that normally transmits messages from the cerebellum to the cerebral cortex, the part of the brain that controls thinking and judgment.

Backache

Aches and pain in the lower back can be a chronic problem. Doctors believe that many cases are psychological in origin. These cases may be from deep-seated emotional or stress-related problems. Other causes are poor posture, improper footwear and walking habits, improper lifting, slouching when sitting, and sleeping on a mattress that is too soft.

Kidney and bladder problems or female pelvic disorders may also produce backache. Common causes of backache are arthritis, rheumatism, bone disease, a slipped disc, or an abnormal curvature of the spine.

Fractures are rarely the cause of back ailments. Most back problems are associated with long-term habits that eventually result in an acute attack.

If the pain is persistent after three days or radiates into the legs, seek medical advice.

NUTRIENTS

SUPPLEMENT	SUGGESTED DOSAGE	COMMENTS
Very Important		
Bone complex: calcium and magnesium (chelated form)	1,500–2,000 mg daily. 700-1,000 mg daily.	To assure assimilation use 3 different forms of calcium: carbonate, chelate, and asporotate.
DL-Phenylalanine (DLPA)	Take daily every other week; follow label instructions.	To alleviate pain. Do not use if pregnant, diabetic, or have high blood pressure.
Multimineral complex with vitamin A and vitamin E and zinc	25,000 IU daily. 400–800 IU daily. 50 mg daily.	Important in muscle and bone metabolism.
Silicon	3 times daily.	Improves calcium uptake. Horsetail extract is a good source of silicon.
Vitamin B₁₂	2,000 mg daily. Take sublingual form.	Aids in calcium absorption.
Important		
Boron	3 mg daily.	Improves calcium uptake, which is needed for bone and muscle repair. When healed, discontinue unless over age 50.
Manganese gluconate (trace mineral)	2–5 mg daily.	Aids in healing cartilage and tissue in the neck and back.
Protein supplement (free form amino acids)	As directed on label.	Essential in bone and tissue repair.
Vitamin D	400–600 IU daily.	Necessary for calcium uptake.
Helpful		
Cod liver oil	1 tbsp. 3 times daily.	Contains vitamins A and D, which aid in healing.
Enzymes with bromelin	2 tablets with meals.	Aids digestion and relieves muscle tension.
Superoxide dismutase (SOD)	Take on an empty stomach as directed.	A powerful free radical scavenger.
Vitamin B complex (high stress formula) with extra B₆ (pyridoxine) and B₁₂	Take 3 times daily as directed.	Needed for repair and to relieve stress in the back muscles.
Vitamin C with bioflavonoids	3,000–10,000 mg daily.	Needed for repair of tissues. Relieves tension in the back area.

HERBS

☐ The following herbs are recommended for backache: burdock, horsetail, slippery elm, and white willow bark. Also recommended is Arth-X, a formula containing herbs, sea minerals, calcium, and other nutrients for the bones and joints.

RECOMMENDATIONS

☐ Avoid all meats or animal protein products until healed because of their uric acid content.

☐ The following sports should be avoided:

- *Baseball, basketball, and football.* The quick responses needed for these sports, involving twisting, bending, and jumping motions, are potentially very dangerous to the back.
- *Bowling.* Lifting a heavy weight while bending and twisting puts strain on the back.
- *Golf.* A survey found that 25 percent of golf pros suffer from lower back problems caused by the twisting motion involved in the swing and the body's tendency to bend forward at the waist.
- *Tennis.* Playing tennis puts strain on the back due to the quick "stop and go" action of the game.
- *Weightlifting.* This sport is potentially the most damaging because it places great strain on the lower portion of the spine and back.

☐ See a doctor for a supervised exercise program. A lack of exercise may be the cause of the back pain. Exercises that are good for the back include swimming, cycling, walking, and rowing.

☐ Never lean forward without bending the knees. Lift with the legs, arms, and abdomen—not with the small muscles of the back. Avoid lifting anything heavier than twenty pounds. Squat down to work at low levels so that you avoid bending at the waist.

☐ Don't sleep on your stomach. Sleep on a firm mattress with your knees bent and your head supported on a pillow.

☐ Sit with your knees a little higher than your hips and your feet flat on the floor.

CONSIDERATIONS

☐ Heavy shoulder bags may produce neck, back, and shoulder pain.

☐ Follow fasting program. (*See* FASTING in Part Three.)

Baldness

See HAIR, LOSS OF.

Bedsores

Bedsores are deep ulcers that form when pressure is exerted over bony areas of the body, restricting circulation and leading to the death of cells in the overlying tissue. They are most commonly found on the heels, buttocks, hips, sacrum, and shoulder blades. They always occur during periods of prolonged bed rest. The comatose patient, paraplegic, and bedridden elderly are the most susceptible.

Proper light in the bedridden person's room and fresh air are beneficial. Use loose-fitting clothing made from an appropriate material; cotton is best because it allows air to penetrate to the skin. The patient must avoid staying in one position for too long, and should be moved to alternate positions often.

Keep the bed clean and dry. Massaging the affected area once daily is very helpful. If the patient can sit up, have him do so three to four times daily, or use pillows as a prop. Give a sponge bath daily using warm water and a mild herbal soap or one containing vitamin E. Do not use harsh soaps.

NUTRIENTS

SUPPLEMENT	SUGGESTED DOSAGE	COMMENTS
Very Important		
Vitamin E	400 IU daily and up.	Improves circulation.
Zinc plus copper	50–80 mg daily. 3 mg daily.	Important in healing.
Important		
Beta-carotene	15,000 IU daily.	Protects the lungs, improving breathing. Repairs bedsores by improving skin tissue.
Protein supplement (free form amino acids)	As directed on label.	Free form amino acids are more readily available for use by the body.
Vitamin B complex	100 mg twice daily.	Needed to reduce stress and for healing.
Vitamin C	3,000–10,000 mg daily in divided doses.	Aids in healing and improves circulation.
Vitamin D	400–1,000 IU daily.	Vitamin D is essential for healing. (A lack of sunshine inhibits healing ability.)
Helpful		
All-Purpose Bacteriaside Spray from Aerobic Life Products	As directed on label.	Use on irritated body parts. Destroys harmful bacteria.
Calcium plus magnesium	2,000 mg daily. 1,000 mg daily.	Needed for the central nervous system and to keep bones from softening through nonuse.
Garlic capsules (Kyolic)	2 capsules 3 times daily.	Has a natural antibiotic effect; protects against infection.
Kelp	6 tablets daily.	Provides necessary minerals.
Vitamin A emulsion	50,000 IU for 1 month, then decrease to 15,000 IU, or take in capsule form.	Emulsion is assimilated easier for skin healing.

HERBS

☐ Goldenseal, myrrh gum, pau d'arco, and suma are beneficial for bedsores. Marigold Ointment by Nature-Works and comfrey ointment can be used externally. Buckwheat tea and lime flower tea are also helpful.

RECOMMENDATIONS

☐ It is very important to consume liquids around the clock, even if you are not thirsty. Use steam-distilled water, herbal teas, and sugar-free juices.

☐ Fiber is important. Use oat bran, guar gum, or Aerobic Bulk Cleanse (ABC). The bowels must move every day. Use an enema for days when the bowels do not move. (*See* ENEMAS in Part Three.) Liquids and fiber are important in keeping the colon clean and the bladder functioning properly.

☐ Mix goldenseal powder, vitamin E oil, and a small amount of honey into a paste, and apply to sores often. This mixture gives fast relief and helps the healing process. Alternate with raw honey or enzyme cream, vitamin E cream, and aloe vera gel.

CONSIDERATIONS

☐ Frequent alcohol rubs stimulate circulation and prevent blood vessels from closing up. Use rubbing alcohol and cotton wool.

☐ A well-balanced diet with 70 percent raw fruits and vegetables is very important. Eliminate animal fats, fried foods, junk foods, processed foods, and sugar from the diet.

☐ There is a mattress designed for the bedridden patient. It has pockets of air connected by small tubes. When placed between the sheet and the standard mattress, it relieves the pressure points when a patient has to lay in one position for long periods of time.

Bed-Wetting

The cause of bed-wetting is often unknown. The most common theories speculate on the roles of heredity, stress, behavioral disturbances, small or weak bladders that cannot hold much urine, underlying illnesses such as urinary tract infections, psychological problems, nutritional deficiencies, too much liquid consumption before bedtime, dreaming about using the rest room, being a sound sleeper, and food allergies. Bed-wetting usually stops spontaneously by the teenage years.

The following dosages should be adjusted according to age and weight.

NUTRIENTS

SUPPLEMENT	SUGGESTED DOSAGE	COMMENTS
Very Important		
Protein supplement from a vegetable source	Follow label directions.	Helps to strengthen bladder muscle.
Important		
Calcium plus magnesium	500 mg daily. 250 mg daily.	Dosage is for children 6 to 12 years old. Dosage must be adjusted for others.
Helpful		
Multivitamin/ mineral complex plus B complex	As directed on label.	Aids in relieving stress and supplies all needed nutrients.
Potassium	As directed on label (99 mg for children 12 and older).	Aids in balancing sodium and potassium in the body.
Vitamin A or cod liver oil	As directed on label.	Vitamins A and E aid in normalizing bladder muscle function.
Vitamin E	100 IU daily for 6- to 12-year-olds; 600 IU daily for adults.	
Zinc	10 mg daily for children; 80 mg daily for adults.	For improved bladder function. Also enhances the immune system.

HERBS

☐ Use buchu, corn silk, oat straw, parsley, and plantain.

RECOMMENDATIONS

☐ Do not drink liquids around bedtime.

☐ Do not spank or scold a child for bed-wetting. This only complicates the problem. Instead, give rewards for *not* bed-wetting.

☐ Bed-wetting is often caused by an allergy. See a doctor for food sensitivity testing. Omit cow's milk, which is highly allergenic, from your diet. Eliminate carbonated beverages, chocolate, refined carbohydrates (including junk food), and products containing food coloring from your diet.

Bee Sting

There are only a few stinging insects in the United States that may cause an allergic reaction: honeybees, hornets, yellow jackets, bumblebees, wasps, spiders, and ants. The yellow jacket and honeybee are the cause of most allergic reactions to insects.

Some people are allergic to bee venom, and if they are stung, a very severe reaction can occur. Symptoms include difficulty in swallowing, hoarseness, labored breathing, weakness, confusion, severe swelling, and a feeling of impending disaster. A more severe reaction results in closing of the airway and/or shock (cyanosis and a drop in blood pressure), producing unconsciousness.

Using tweezers, immediately and carefully remove any stinger left in the skin. Reactions can occur within minutes or hours. If treatment is not sought immediately, death can result. If you have a known allergy to a particular venom, have a doctor prescribe an emergency treatment kit. *See also* INSECT ALLERGY in Part Two.

NUTRIENTS

SUPPLEMENT	SUGGESTED DOSAGE	COMMENTS
Helpful		
Calcium gluconate	1,500 mg daily.	Helps relieve pain.
Pantothenic acid (B₅)	500 mg daily.	Acts as an antiallergenic.
Vitamin C	5,000–15,000 mg daily. (Take 10,000 mg in first hour.)	*See* ASCORBIC ACID FLUSH in Part Three.
Vitamin E (capsule or oil)	Cut open capsule or use vitamin E oil and apply to sting site.	Aids in healing.

HERBS

☐ Take echinacea as a tea or in capsule form. Drink as much yellow dock tea as you can, or take two capsules every hour until symptoms are relieved. Apply poultices made from white oak bark and leaves, comfrey, and slippery elm. Also good are a lobelia poultice and a plantain poultice or salve.

RECOMMENDATIONS

☐ For a wasp or bee sting, open or crush a charcoal tablet and place on a cotton ball. Place the cotton ball on the affected area and cover with an adhesive bandage. This will reduce pain and swelling. Honeybees leave their stinger in their victim, and this should be removed immediately. A cold pack will relieve the pain.

☐ To avoid bee stings, wear plain, light-colored clothing; avoid wearing anything that is flowered or dark. Don't wear perfume, suntan lotion, hair spray, or shiny jewelry. Avoid wearing sandals or loose-fitting clothes.

☐ Researchers in Gainesville, Florida, have found that squashing a yellow jacket releases a chemical that causes other yellow jackets in the area to attack. Instead of swatting at the insect, it is best to run from it.

CONSIDERATIONS

☐ A venom extractor called "Lil Sucker" is available. It fits inside your pocket or purse. If you get stung, it produces a vacuum that sucks the venom out within two minutes. The end of the extractor can also be used to remove a honeybee stinger. For more information on this, call 1-(800) ITCHING.

☐ *See also* INSECT ALLERGY and INSECT BITE in Part Two.

Beriberi

Beriberi is a disease caused by a deficiency of the B vitamins, particularly thiamine. This disease occurs mainly in the Far East, where the principal diet consists mainly of polished rice, which does not supply sufficient thiamine. Subclinical beriberi cases that do occur in the United States are associated with alcoholism, infections, pregnancy, hypothyroidism, and stress.

Symptoms of beriberi in children include impaired growth, the wasting of tissue, mental confusion, convulsions, gastrointestinal problems, nausea, vomiting, constipation, and diarrhea. In adults the symptoms are fatigue, diarrhea, weight loss, edema, heart failure, and nerve malfunction causing paralysis.

NUTRIENTS

SUPPLEMENT	SUGGESTED DOSAGE	COMMENTS
Important		
Multivitamin and mineral complex	As directed on label.	For essential balanced vitamins and minerals.
Thiamine (B₁)	50 mg 3 times daily.	Take in addition to B complex.
Vitamin B complex	100 mg each daily, taken orally.	Injections of B vitamins may be necessary. Use intravenous treatment only under the supervision of your physician.
Helpful		
Brewer's yeast	Start with a small amount and increase to 1 tbsp. twice weekly.	Supplies the B vitamins.
Vitamin C	2,000–5,000 mg daily in divided doses.	Important for immune function, improved circulation, and healing. Needed for proper uptake of the B vitamins.

RECOMMENDATIONS

☐ Do not drink liquids with meals. Liquids wash out most of the B vitamins.

☐ Include brown rice, legumes, raw fruits and vegetables, seeds and nuts, whole grains, and yogurt in your daily diet. These foods are rich in B vitamins, particularly B₁ (thiamine).

Bite

See BEE STING; DOG BITE; INSECT ALLERGY; SNAKE BITE; SPIDER BITE.

Bitot's Spots

See EYE PROBLEMS.

Bladder Infection (Cystitis)

Bladder infections are usually caused by some type of bacteria resulting in cystitis, an inflammation of the bladder. Kidney infections are more serious and often result from cystitis. Bladder inflammations are much more frequent in women than in men due to the closeness of the bladder and urethra to the vagina. The bacteria gain access to the bladder by traveling up the urethra in females. The closeness of the anus to the vagina and urethra allows the transmission of bacteria to the bladder in women. Nearly 85 percent of urinary tract infections are caused by *Escherichia coli*, a bacterium found in the intestines. Chlamydia may also cause bladder problems in sexually active women.

Bladder infections are characterized by an urgent desire to empty the bladder. Urination is typically frequent and painful; even after the bladder has been emptied, however, there may be a desire to urinate again. The urine often has a strong, unpleasant odor and may appear cloudy. Children suffering from bladder infections may have lower abdominal pain and experience a painful burning sensation while urinating. Blood in the urine could indicate a more serious problem and warrants medical attention.

Antibiotics and analgesics may be necessary treatment. If your physician prescribes these drugs, make sure you take some form of acidophilus to replace the "friendly" bacteria that are destroyed by these drugs.

URINARY TRACT INFECTION SELF-TEST

In order to determine whether you have a urinary tract infection, a simple home kit can answer your questions. You can purchase a product called Dipstick from your local drugstore. It contains a thin strip of plastic that has been chemically treated. If the tip of this strip changes color when dipped in urine, it indicates the presence of a bacterial infection. If you are susceptible to infections, check yourself weekly. Make sure that your urine sample is collected cleanly. Begin urinating, and then collect specimen while in midstream.

The following supplement program is recommended for those suffering from bladder infections.

NUTRIENTS

SUPPLEMENT	SUGGESTED DOSAGE	COMMENTS
Very Important		
Acidophilus or Maxidophilus or Megadophilus	2 capsules 3 times daily.	Also use 1 tbsp. in 1 quart warm water as a douche; if associated with vaginitis, alternate with apple cider vinegar. Supplies the necessary "friendly" bacteria.
Vitamin C	4,000–5,000 mg daily in divided doses.	Produces antibacterial effect through acidification of urine. Also important in immune function.
Important		
Garlic capsules (Kyolic)	2 capsules 3 times daily.	Kyolic is odorless garlic and a natural antibiotic.
L-Cysteine (amino acid)	500 mg twice daily on an empty stomach.	A potent detoxifier.
SP-6 Cornsilk Blend from Solaray Products or KB from Nature's Way Products	2 capsules twice daily.	These herb formulas have a diuretic effect and reduce bladder spasm.
Thymus and pituitary raw glandulars	50 mg twice daily.	Used by many professionals and available in health food stores. Important for immune function. *See* GLANDULAR THERAPY in Part Three.
Vitamin B complex	50–100 mg twice daily with meals.	High doses are necessary when antibiotics are used.
Helpful		
Calcium and magnesium	1,500 mg daily. 750–1,000 mg daily.	Calcium reduces bladder irritability. Magnesium aids in the stress response and works best when balanced with calcium. Chelate formula is the most effective.
Vitamin and mineral complex (high potency)	As directed on label.	Needed for essential balanced vitamins and minerals. Use hypoallergenic form.
Vitamin A plus beta-carotene	10,000 IU daily. 15,000 IU daily.	Promotes the healing process and immune function.
Vitamin E	600 IU daily.	Combats infecting bacteria.
Zinc	50 mg daily.	Important in tissue repair and immunity.

HERBS

☐ Beneficial herbs include burdock root, juniper berries, marshmallow root, and rose hips. Marshmallow root increases the acid content in the urine, inhibiting bacterial growth. Juniper berries will help to restore kidney function. Goldenseal is good for bladder infections when there is bleeding; however, pregnant women should not use large amounts of this herb.

☐ Diuretics can help cleanse the system. Dandelion tea or dandelion extract acts as a diuretic and liver cleanser; it aids in relieving bladder discomfort. You might wish to try uva ursi. Use only small amounts and dilute with other herb teas. Bearberry acts as a mild diuretic and antiseptic. Birch leaves are a natural diuretic and reduce some of the pain associated with bladder infections.

RECOMMENDATIONS

☐ Do not delay emptying the bladder! Making sure that you urinate every two to three hours will help. Research shows that retaining the urine in the bladder for long periods increases a woman's risk of urinary tract infection. An Israeli study suggests that habitual holding of urine may increase the risk of bladder cancer. In addition, empty your bladder before and after exercising to avoid undue strain.

☐ Keep the genital and anal areas clean and dry. Wipe from front to back after emptying the bladder or bowels. Women should empty the bladder before and after intercourse. Avoid hygiene sprays, douches, and bubble baths; these may cause further irritation. Women should wear white cotton underwear; nylon underwear should be avoided. They should not use tampons if they frequently suffer from urinary tract infections.

☐ When bacteria cannot be cultured by the laboratory and urination is painful, discontinue use of all types of soaps and use only water to clean the vaginal area. Some women are sensitive to soap; an all-natural soap from a health food store is recommended.

☐ Take hot baths (sitz baths) twice daily for twenty minutes. Hot sitz baths will help relieve pain associated with cystitis. Batherapy, which can be found in a health food store, is excellent. In addition, you can add one cup vinegar to a sitz bath daily or to shallow bath water, positioning the knees up and apart so that the water can enter the vagina. Alternate with two cloves of crushed garlic or with garlic juice.

☐ Drink plenty of liquids, especially cranberry juice. A quality cranberry juice produces hippuric acid in the urine, a substance that acidifies the urine, inhibiting bacterial growth. Avoid Ocean Spray's cranberry juice product, as it contains less than 30 percent cranberry juice and has high fructose corn syrup added. Purchase pure juice from a natural foods store.

☐ Steam-distilled water is preferred over tap water. A six- to eight-ounce glass of quality water every hour is extremely beneficial for urinary tract infections.

☐ Avoid citrus fruits; these produce alkaline urine that encourages bacterial growth. Increase acid content in urine to inhibit bacterial growth.

☐ Stay away from caffeine, carbonated beverages, coffee, chocolate, and alcohol as well.

☐ Include celery, parsley, and watermelon in your diet. These foods act as natural diuretics. Celery and parsley juice or extract can be purchased at a health food store.

☐ Take either two teaspoonfuls of whey powder with each meal or acidophilus tablets or capsules. This is especially important during antibiotic therapy.

CONSIDERATIONS

☐ Because use of diuretics causes increased urinary excretion of magnesium, it can cause hypomagnesemia in elderly people. Magnesium is needed in conjunction with calcium to prevent bone deterioration. Potassium is also lost when using diuretics. Consult your physician before using diuretics.

☐ After menopause a reduction of the female hormone, estrogen, can prompt shrinkage of urethral and vaginal membranes, thus promoting incontinence. Because the bladder is satiated, there is a continuous dribbling of urine. Urethral dilation helps stretch the contracted urethra.

☐ Look for allergies, especially to certain foods. Allergies often cause symptoms that mimic bladder infections. Cytotoxic testing can determine which foods are causing the allergic reaction.

☐ Avoid aluminum cookware. It may cause cystitis symptoms.

☐ Bladder infections in men may signal a more serious problem, such as prostatitis. *See* PROSTATITIS in Part Two. Cystitis in men may indicate a serious underlying disease.

☐ A one-to-three-day cleansing fast can be beneficial. *See* FASTING in Part Three.

☐ Avoid taking zinc and iron supplements until healed. Bacteria require iron for growth. The body will store iron in compartments in the liver, spleen, and bone marrow when a bacterial infection is present in order to prevent further growth of the bacteria.

☐ *See also* KIDNEY AND BLADDER PROBLEMS in Part Two.

Bladder Problems

See KIDNEY AND BLADDER PROBLEMS.

Boil

A boil, referred to as a furuncle by medical professionals, is a round, tender, pus-filled raised area of skin. It may be caused by a bacterial infection, an airborne or food allergy, stress, poor hygiene, an illness, a lowered resistance, certain drugs, excessive consumption of junk foods, an infected wound, a toxic bowel and bloodstream, or thyroid disorders. It may also be caused when the deepest portion of the hair follicle becomes infected and the inflammation spreads, often with staphylococcus bacteria (spherical-shaped bacteria, usually found in clusters). A carbuncle occurs when the infection spreads and other boils are formed. The formation of a carbuncle may be an indication of immune depression.

Symptoms of boil formation include itching, mild pain, and localized swelling. Boils appear suddenly. Within twenty-four hours they become red and filled with pus. Swelling of the nearest lymph glands occur. A boil will normally heal in ten to twenty-five days. If the boils are very large, a doctor should drain them. They most often appear on the scalp, buttocks, face, and underarms.

NUTRIENTS

SUPPLEMENT	SUGGESTED DOSAGE	COMMENTS
Essential		
Chlorophyll	1 tbsp. 3 times daily in liquid form.	Wheatgrass and alfalfa are good sources. Needed to clean the bloodstream.
Garlic capsules (Kyolic)	2 capsules 3 times daily.	Kyolic is a natural antibiotic and potentiates immune function.
Germanium	200 mg daily.	Needed for the immune system. Aids in cleansing the bloodstream.
Very Important		
Proteolytic enzymes	Twice daily on an empty stomach.	Speeds up cleansing process at infection sites.
Vitamin A and E emulsion	75,000 IU vitamin A; 600 IU vitamin E daily for 1 month. Then 25,000 IU vitamin A and 600 IU vitamin E.	Necessary for proper immune system function.
Vitamin C	3,000–8,000 mg daily in divided doses.	Powerful anti-inflammatory substance and immune system stimulant.
Helpful		
Coenzyme Q$_{10}$	60 mg daily.	Important for oxygen utilization and immune function.
Kelp and high potency multimineral complex	6 tablets daily. As directed on label.	Needed for balanced minerals.
Raw thymus glandular	500 mg daily.	Stimulates the immune system. See GLANDULAR THERAPY in Part Three.
Silicon tablets or oat straw tea	Use as directed on label.	Reduces inflammatory reaction.

HERBS

☐ Use burdock root, comfrey, dandelion, echinacea, goldenseal, pau d'arco, red clover, and suma. Pau d'arco, like burdock root, is a natural antibiotic that helps rid the body of infections and toxins. Echinacea and goldenseal help to cleanse the lymph glands. Dandelion and black radish are liver cleansers.

RECOMMENDATIONS

☐ The infected area should be washed several times a day and swabbed with antiseptic. Also apply honey directly on the boil. Vitamin A and E emulsion directly on boils is effective. Use clay packs and/or chlorophyll.

☐ Warm Epsom salt baths are good. Apply moist heat three or four times a day. Prevent spreading of boils by using clean towels.

☐ A cleansing fast is important to help cleanse the system and rid the body of toxins that may cause boils. (See FASTING in Part Three.)

☐ An onion poultice may be beneficial for sores. Use between a piece of cloth—not applied directly to the area. See POULTICE in Part Three.

Bone Spur

See HEEL SPUR.

Breast Cancer

Breast cancer is the leading cause of death from malignant tumors for women in the United States. It is important to detect breast cancer in its earliest and most curable stage. Women need to reduce their risk of breast cancer by regular self-examination (see self-test), regular mammography, and changes in diet and lifestyle. A high-fat diet has been associated with breast cancer.

The breast is actually a gland and contains milk ducts, lobes, fatty tissue, and a network of lymph vessels. If you are not pregnant and have a yellow, bloody, or clear discharge from the nipple, this should be checked by a doctor. Any breast lumps should be checked by a doctor, although the majority are not cancerous. Cancerous lumps are firm, never go away, and are usually pain free.

Women accustomed to the feel of their breasts are better able to notice subtle changes. Women who detect a lump should seek medical advice without delay. A lump that does not move around may be cancerous, or may simply be caused by normal fibrocystic changes during the menstrual cycle. A biopsy will detect which kind of lump it is.

Paget's disease, which affects the nipple, cannot be detected by an examination. This form of cancer occurs when cancer cells migrate to the nipple. The symptoms are itching, redness, and soreness. Paget's disease always signals the presence of primary ductal carcinoma elsewhere in the breast tissue. Not all rashes and itching of the nipple are cancerous.

Eighty percent of all breast cancer is *infiltrating ductal carcinoma*. Ductal carcinomas invade (infiltrate) the surrounding breast tissue. They are discovered when a lump is found, or in a mammogram.

Inflammatory carcinoma is another type of ductal cancer in which the lymphatic and blood vessels become plugged with a tumor. The skin thickens and turns red. The breast becomes extremely tender and looks infected. This type of cancer spreads very quickly due to a rich blood and lymph vessel supply associated with the inflammatory reaction. Biopsy proof of malignancy is required because a benign breast condition may mimic an inflammatory carcinoma.

Intraductal carcinoma is characterized by growth of cancer cells within the ducts. Sometimes this cancer does not invade other tissues. This disease is called intraductal carcinoma in-situ (meaning "in place" or localized).

Lobular carcinoma occurs in about 9 percent of breast cancers. Lobular carcinomas occasionally occur in both breasts simultaneously.

Rare forms of breast cancer include: *tubular carcinoma, malignant cystosarcoma phylliodes, medullary carcinoma, adenoid cystic carcinoma,* and several others which are less common. These forms of cancer tend to be less aggressive. They are diagnosed and treated in a way that is similar to the more common forms of breast cancer.

BREAST SELF-EXAMINATION

It is important to examine your breasts each month at the same time. Changes naturally occur in the breast during the menstrual cycle, so do not examine them during this period. Familiarize yourself with the normal feel of your breasts so that you can detect any changes or enlargement of a lump. Any changes in your breasts should be reported to your doctor and you should be rechecked by your physician if you have any doubt concerning your examination.

1. While standing and looking in the mirror, raise your hands over your head and press them together. Notice the shape of your breast. Place your hands on your hips, apply pressure, and look for dimpling of the skin, nipples that seem to be out of position, one breast different from the other, or red scaling or thickening of the skin and nipples.
2. Raise one arm above your head. With the other hand, firmly explore your breast beginning at the outer edge. Using a circular motion, gradually work toward the nipple. Take your time when examining the area between the nipple and the armpit, and feel the armpit as well. You have lymph nodes in the armpit; they move freely and feel soft, and are not painful to the touch. Look for lumps that are hard and not mobile. Cancers are often attached to underlying muscle or the skin. Repeat on both sides.
3. Repeat step 2 while lying on your back. In this position lumps are more easily detected. Also, squeeze each nipple gently to check for blood or a watery yellow or pink discharge.

Men can get breast cancer also and should follow the above procedure as well.

NUTRIENTS

SUPPLEMENT	SUGGESTED DOSAGE	COMMENTS
Essential		
Beta-carotene	10,000 units	Powerful antioxidant that destroys free radicals.
Coenzyme Q₁₀	100 mg daily.	Improves cellular oxygenation.
DMG (Gluconic from DaVinci Labs)	As directed on label.	Improves cellular oxygenation.

Garlic capsules (Kyolic)	2 capsules 3 times daily.	Enhances immune function.
Germanium	200 mg daily.	Improves cellular oxygenation, deterring cancer growth. A potent immunostimulant.
Proteolytic enzymes or Wobe-Mugos-N-Dragees	2–6 tablets with meals. 2–6 tablets between meals.	Powerful free radical scavengers.
Selenium	200 mcg daily.	Powerful free radical scavenger.
Superoxide dismutase (SOD)	As directed on label. Consider injections.	Destroys free radicals.
Vitamin A emulsion and vitamin E	50,000–100,000 IU vitamin A daily for 10 days or for as long as on program. Start with 400 IU vitamin E daily. Increase slowly to 1,000 IU. The emulsion form is absorbed rapidly, easily assimilated, and safe at high doses (bypassing the liver).	Vitamin A is vital to immunity. A vitamin E deficiency has been linked to breast cancer. Vitamin E also aids in normal hormonal production and in immune function.
Vitamin B complex and brewer's yeast and choline	100 mg 3 times daily. 100 mg 3 times daily.	B vitamins are necessary for normal cell division and function. Choline aids in reducing estrogen production.
Vitamin C plus bioflavonoids	5,000–10,000 mg daily in divided doses.	Powerful anticancer agent. *See* ASCORBIC ACID FLUSH in Part Three.

Helpful		
Aerobic 07 from Aerobic Life Products or Dioxychlor from American Biologics	As directed on label.	Antimicrobial agents.
Comprehensive mineral and trace element supplement, rich in potassium and calcium and magnesium	2,000 mg daily. 1,000 mg daily.	Essential for normal cell division and function.
Carnitine derived from fish liver (squalene)	As directed on label.	Protects the skin in postmastectomy and the x-ray treated patient.
L-Cysteine and L-methionine (amino acids)	As directed on label.	Detoxifies harmful substances.
L-Taurine (amino acid)	As directed on label.	Functions as foundation for tissue and organ repair.
Megadophilus or Maxidophilus or Primadophilus DDS	As directed on label.	Has an antibacterial effect on the body. A milk-free brand is available.

Multiple enzyme digestive formula	Take with meals as directed.	Aids digestion.
Multivitamin	Take with meals as directed on label.	Should not be sustained release. Take formula that is iron free.
Niacin (B$_3$) and folic acid and choline	100 mg daily. 500–1,000 mg daily.	B vitamins that improve circulation, build red blood cells, and aid liver function.
Raw glandular complex with extra raw thymus	As directed on label.	Stimulates glandular function, especially the thymus (site of T-lymphacyte production).
Seaweed or kelp	5 tablets daily.	For mineral balance.
Vitamin B$_{12}$	Injections or sublingual form are recommended.	Prevents anemia.

RECOMMENDATIONS

☐ *See* CANCER in Part Two for dietary guidelines.

CONSIDERATIONS

☐ Being physically "fit" appears to help protect against breast cancer. Follow the diet and suggested supplements in CANCER in Part Two. Diet is most important in the treatment and prevention of breast cancer.

☐ When a lump turns out to be malignant (cancerous), there are different treatment options to choose from:

1. *Lumpectomy*. Only the tumor and a small amount of surrounding tissue are removed.
2. *Quandrantectomy* (partial mastectomy). Only the quadrant of the breast in which the tumor was found is removed.
3. *Simple mastectomy*. The removal of the entire breast, but only a sample of the underarm lymph nodes.
4. *Modified radical mastectomy*. The removal of the entire breast and all underarm lymph nodes.
5. *Radical mastectomy*. The entire breast, lymph nodes, and chest muscle are removed (less than 5 percent of patients still receive this type of surgery).

☐ If the cancer has spread to the nodes after surgery, part of the postoperative therapy may include radiation, chemotherapy, or hormonal therapy. Radiation is always required after a lumpectomy or quandrantectomy to assure that no more cancer cells remain. If tumors are estrogen-dependent, an alternative to conventional chemotherapy may be the drug tamoxifen (Nolvadex). This drug blocks estrogen from binding with receptors on breast cancer cells in the early stages, "starving" the cancer cells.

☐ A few women may have a problem with swelling of the arm on the side surgery was performed when the lymph nodes have been removed. This is not unusual. After surgery, avoid moving or carrying heavy objects. Wear loose-fitting clothes and gloves and avoid overexposure to the sun. Contact your physician promptly if there is any unusual swelling, redness, or pain in the hand or arm. The doctor will recommend certain arm exercises to keep the arm from becoming stiff and to assist in healing. The doctor will want to follow the patient's progress for at least five years. There is also the option of having breast reconstruction later.

☐ Family support is necessary for the breast cancer patient. Depression, anxiety, and fear are not uncommon after surgery. Usually when medications are stopped, the patient starts to feel better and look at everything in a different light. Many celebrities have had breast cancer and have gone on to have fulfilling careers. Thousands of women who have had breast cancer are living happy, normal lives today.

☐ See also CANCER in Part Two.

MEDICAL UPDATES

☐ Dr. Carlton Fredericks believes that high estrogen contributes to breast cancer. Also, a poor diet makes it difficult for the liver to rid the body of excess estrogen. Normally, estrogen produced by the ovaries is detoxified by the liver and then replaced by the ovaries throughout a women's reproductive years. The problem begins when too much estrogen is produced and the liver is unable to function normally. Estrogen is also implicated in fibrocystic disease, premenstrual disorders, endometrial cancer, and fibroid tumors of the uterus. Estrogen is needed, but only in moderation.

☐ Researchers have found that women over forty are more likely to develop breast cancer than younger women. Evidence is strong for a link between breast cancer and lifestyle. *The New England Journal of Medicine* stated that consuming as few as three drinks a week increases the potential of breast cancer by 50 percent. The National Women's Health Network is urging all women to cut their fat intake to 20 percent of total calories. Two kinds of fat, however, are good: omega-3 fatty acids from cold-water fish and olive oil.

☐ Research has shown that patients with cancer of the lung, bladder, breast, colon, and skin have levels of vitamin A that are lower than normal.

☐ The recognized risk factors for breast cancer are early start of menstruation, late menopause, giving birth late in life, a family history of breast cancer, obesity after menopause, alcoholism, and a high-fat diet.

☐ Research conducted by Dr. Clifford R. Kay at the research unit in Manchester, England, indicates that breast cancer may be linked to use of oral contraceptives. Dr. Kay evaluated more than 40,000 women and concluded that women using oral contraceptives were more than three times as likely to develop breast cancer.

☐ Silicon, which is used in breast implants, causes malignant tumors in test animals (130,000 breast implants are performed annually).

Breastfeeding-Related Problems

Breastfeeding, or lactation, is the natural way in which the mother of a newborn can feed her child instead of relying on cow's milk or artificial formula preparations. The female breasts are ideally suited for the task of nourishing the baby, and provide many benefits to the baby that bottles and formulas do not. For example, mother's breast milk is much easier to digest, prevents constipation, lowers the incidence of food allergies, and protects the baby from many infectious diseases. It also promotes healthy oral development, satisfies sucking needs, and enhances bonding and skin-to-skin contact between mother and child. In addition, breastfeeding is also beneficial to the mother in that it reduces the chance of hemorrhaging from the placental site, gives the mother an opportunity to rest, and encourages the uterus to contract, returning it to its prepregnant size.

In breastfeeding, as with anything else that is new and unfamiliar, problems will occur. This section offers explanations and solutions to the most common breastfeeding problems in order to help the new breastfeeding mother have a good experience.

ENGORGEMENT

This temporary problem can occur between two to five days after childbirth. It is caused by a combination of the increased blood supply to the breast and the pressure of the newly produced milk, resulting in the swelling of the tissues in the breast. A low-grade fever may be present, the breasts will feel full, hard, tender, and tight, and the skin on the breasts will be hot, shiny, and distended. This condition does not have to be present in order to allow nursing.

Engorgement prevention relies mainly on frequent

feedings without delay and the nonrestriction of sucking time. Feedings should not be skipped or delayed during the day or night. Do not give the baby any formula or sugar water, and allow the baby to empty each breast completely at each feeding. This should take about seven minutes on each side.

Treatment includes short, frequent feedings, using milk cups between feedings to relieve pressure, and breast massage. A feeding schedule of every one and a half to two hours day and night should be maintained while suffering from engorgement. Application of moist heat for thirty minutes preceding each feeding and massaging the breast during feedings will help to get the milk flowing. Do not use nipple shields, as they can confuse the baby's sucking pattern, damage nipples, reduce stimulation of the breast, and decrease the milk supply.

SORE NIPPLES

This problem can occur even when the nipples have been prepared in advance. It is typically caused by improper nursing positions and improper nursing schedules.

To prevent sore nipples while nursing, the following tips are recommended:

- Do not wash nipples with soap, alcohol, or petroleum-based products. This washes away their natural protection. Keep nipples dry between feedings. Expose them to sunlight and air. Feed the baby frequently to avoid a baby who is overly hungry from biting down roughly on the nipple. Change nursing positions often to rotate the pressure of the baby's mouth on the breast. Learn to break suction correctly.
- Treatment for sore nipples includes the following suggestions. Nurse on the least sore side first. However, if both breasts are sore, hand express (i.e., massage the breast) until letdown occurs and milk is readily available to the baby. Make sure that the baby's jaws exert pressure on the least tender spots. Use dry heat such as a low-wattage electric bulb placed twelve to eighteen inches from the breast for ten to fifteen minutes following each feeding. Do not pull away when the baby is about to begin feeding. Learn to relax.
- If cracked nipples accompany soreness, applying aloe vera to the nipples will alleviate pain and promote healing.

PLUGGED DUCT

Incomplete emptying of the milk ducts by the baby or the wearing of a tight bra can cause a plugged duct.

Soreness and a lump in one area of a breast is an indication of this problem. Check the nipple very carefully for a tiny dot of dried milk. When this is removed by gentle cleansing along with frequent nursing on the affected breast, the duct will clear itself within twenty-four hours. Massaging the breasts with firm pressure, from the chest wall toward the nipple, also stimulates milk flow.

Alter the position of the baby on the nipple so all the ducts are drained. Make sure you offer the affected breast first, when the baby's sucking is strongest.

MASTITIS (BREAST INFECTION)

If a plugged duct is not taken care of, mastitis can result. Soreness and redness in the breast, fever, and flu-like symptoms are indicators of this problem. In fact, in a nursing mother all flu symptoms should be considered a breast infection until proven otherwise.

Treat mastitis by drinking plenty of fluids, getting plenty of rest, and applying heat to the area with a hot water bottle or heating pad. Do not stop nursing the baby, otherwise the ducts will remain full and could worsen the problem by allowing the ducts to overfill. In addition, your health care provider may prescribe antibiotics that can be taken while nursing.

In rare cases, a breast infection results in a breast abscess in which the sore breast fills with pus. This abscess may need to be incised to allow drainage. This procedure is performed in a doctor's office. During this time, milk should be hand expressed (massaged) from the infected breast and discarded. Breastfeeding should continue on the noninfected breast until the abscess is healed.

The following supplements should be taken by the nursing mother.

NUTRIENTS

SUPPLEMENT	SUGGESTED DOSAGE	COMMENTS
Essential		
Protein supplement (free form amino acids or soy protein)		Soy protein or free form amino acids are better than animal protein.
Helpful		
Bifidobacteria (Life Start from Natren)	Dosage for mother: ½ tsp. between meals. Dosage for infant: ¼ tsp. daily added to water or juice.	Use only unchilled water in preparation. Boosts immune system and provides necessary "friendly" bacteria.
Calcium chelate and magnesium	1,000–1,500 mg daily. 500–750 mg daily.	Avoid bone meal because of the lead content.

Multivitamin and mineral complex (high potency) containing the B complex with extra folic acid plus vitamins C and D and iron and manganese	As directed on label.	This high potency preparation is needed by both mother and baby.
Vitamin B complex or brewer's yeast	50 mg twice daily. Start with a small amount of brewer's yeast and work up to 1 tbsp. in juice, 3 times daily.	Needed for production of milk and to relieve stress.

HERBS

☐ While breastfeeding, use of any of the following herbs can be beneficial: alfalfa, blessed thistle, dandelion, fennel, horsetail, nettle leaf, and raspberry. Nettle leaf has a tonic effect and contains iron in addition to many other nutrients.

☐ The following herbs decrease milk supply: bark, black walnut, sage, and yarrow.

RECOMMENDATIONS

☐ Eat plenty of brewer's yeast, eggs, nuts and seeds, and whole grains. Raw foods should be plentiful in the diet.

☐ Mother's milk is nearly a perfect food. However, it is low in vitamins C and D and iron. Therefore, after discussing the ramifications of this with your health care provider, you may decide to supplement your diet with these vitamins and minerals.

CONSIDERATIONS

☐ The UCLA Medical School reported that mother's milk kills a tiny parasite (*Giardia lamblia*), which can cause intestinal disease in children.

☐ If you need to supplement mother's milk, try almond milk or soy milk formulas and a small amount of papaya (put through a blender). This will resemble mother's milk. You can add a small amount of blackstrap molasses and brewer's yeast after the baby is a few months old. Always consult your doctor before making any changes in your baby's diet.

☐ Almost all drugs have been found to enter the mother's milk, including the following: alcohol, amphetamines, antihistamines, aspirin, barbiturates, caffeine, cocaine, cough syrups with iodine, decongestants, ergotamine, Librium, marijuana, nicotine antibiotics, opiates (morphine, codeine, Demerol), Tagamet, Tylenol, and Valium. Some of the effects of these drugs on the infant include diarrhea, rapid heart rate, restlessness, irritability, crying and poor sleeping, vomiting, and convulsions. In addition, some of these drugs may accumulate in the infant and cause addiction.

Bright's Disease

See KIDNEY AND BLADDER PROBLEMS.

Bronchitis

Bronchitis is the inflammation or obstruction of the bronchi or breathing tubes that lead to the lungs. The inflammation is followed by incessant coughing due to the irritation present, a build-up of mucus, fever, back and chest pain, sore throat, and difficulty breathing. Acute bronchitis typically follows upper respiratory tract infections such as influenza and often leads to pneumonia. Chronic bronchitis results from frequent irritation of the lungs, but it is not an infection. Allergies may be the cause of chronic bronchitis. In addition, as the space in the lung available for the exchange of oxygen and carbon dioxide diminishes, the heart has to work harder to keep an adequate volume of blood. This can lead to heart disease.

Smoking and acute upper respiratory infections are often associated with bronchial infections. If bacteria are the cause, antibiotics should be prescribed; however, cough suppressants should not be used in the treatment. A chest x-ray should be taken to rule out lung cancer.

A new type of bronchitis, probably viral in origin, has targeted many women. It is very difficult to treat, often lasting three weeks to five months. Antibiotics may help, especially Doryx.

NUTRIENTS

SUPPLEMENT	SUGGESTED DOSAGE	COMMENTS
Essential		
Vitamin C plus bioflavonoids	3,000–10,000 mg daily in divided doses.	A buffered powdered form is best. Combine with vitamin E.
Very Important		
Beta-carotene	15,000 IU daily.	Needed to protect the lung tissue.

DMG (Gluconic from DaVinci Labs)	1 tablet under the tongue twice daily.	A powerful oxygen carrier.
Proteolytic enzymes	Take between meals.	Helps reduce inflammation.
Vitamin A capsules	20,000 IU twice daily for 1 month, dropping to 15,000 IU.	For healing of tissue and protection of all tissues.
Vitamin E	400 IU and up twice daily, combined with vitamin C.	Powerful free radical scavenger. Needed for healing of tissues and improved breathing.
Important		
Chlorophyll tablets (wheatgrass) or liquid or fresh green juice	3 times daily as directed on label.	Kyo-Green is good.
Garlic tablets (Kyolic)	2 tablets with meals.	Kyolic is odorless. A natural antibiotic that reduces infection and detoxifies the body.
Multimineral formula plus zinc	50 mg daily.	All nutrients are needed for healing, especially zinc.
Helpful		
Calcium chelate or asporotate plus magnesium	1,000 mg daily. 500 mg daily.	Necessary for healing.
Coenzyme Q$_{10}$	60 mg daily.	For increased circulation and improved breathing.
L-Arginine (amino acid)	Take 2 g at bedtime with a small amount of L-lysine.	To prevent an imbalance. Aids in liver detoxification. Needed for protein synthesis to aid in healing. Depresses elevated ammonia.
L-Cysteine (amino acid)	500 mg twice daily.	Protects and preserves the cells and contains needed sulfur.
L-Ornithine (amino acid)	500 mg twice daily on an empty stomach for adults only. Take amino acids in juice—not with milk or a protein drink— because amino acids compete for entry through the gastrointestinal tract.	*Warning:* Not for children. Promotes and detoxifies ammonia.
Superoxide dismutase (SOD) from Biotec Foods	Follow label directions.	Improves healing and is an excellant antioxidant.
Vitamin B complex	100 mg 3 times daily.	Activates many enzymes needed for healing.

Note: Take all amino acids on an empty stomach with a small amount of vitamins C and B$_6$ for better assimilation.

HERBS

☐ **Bronc-Ease** from Nature's Herbs is an excellent herbal formula. It relieves congestion, coughing, and irritation. Also use black radish extract or dry herbs, chickweed, coltsfoot, echinacea tea (daily), eucalyptus, fenugreek, ginger, Iceland moss, mullein, myrrh, pau d'arco tea (daily), slippery elm bark, and wheatgrass capsules from New Moon Extracts. Inhaling the vapors of the eucalyptus leaves helps to relieve respiratory problems. Iceland moss is good for mucous congestion.

RECOMMENDATIONS

☐ Add moisture to the air. Drink plenty of fluids.

☐ For those who have chronic bronchitis, cigarette smoke—even as a passive smoker—is very harmful. Little can be done unless the irritating substances that cause the mucus to clog the air passages are eliminated. Cigarette smoke is a common irritant.

Bruising

The skin is not broken when bruised, but the underlying tissues are injured, resulting in pain, swelling, and black and blue marks due to blood that has collected under the skin. Although body parts often become bruised after banging into hard objects, there are several factors that predispose one to bruising. Anemia, overweight, malnutrition, leukemia, and excessive use of anticlotting drugs can lead to vessel rupture, clotting, and thrombosis, each of which can result in bruising. Bruising is also an early warning sign of cancer. Treat the bruise by placing an ice pack on the area for thirty minutes.

NUTRIENTS

SUPPLEMENT	SUGGESTED DOSAGE	COMMENTS
Very Important		
Vitamin C plus bioflavonoids	3,000–10,000 mg daily in divided doses.	Helps to prevent bruising.
Important		
Alfalfa tablets	5 tablets daily.	To supply vitamin K. Good food sources of vitamin K are kale, alfalfa, and fish meal.
Helpful		
Coenzyme Q$_{10}$	60 mg daily.	Essential for construction and reconstruction of body cells.

DMG (Gluconic from DaVinci Labs)	100 mg daily.	Improves oxygen metabolism in the cells and tissues.
Enzyme compound or proteolytic enzymes	Take between meals.	
Germanium	100 mg daily.	Improves circulation and boosts the immune system.
Iron (Floradix formula)	As recommended by your doctor.	Floradix formula from Germany is a good iron supplement.
Vitamin B complex plus extra folic acid	100 mg twice daily.	Aids in protecting the tissues.
Vitamin D plus calcium and magnesium	400–800 IU daily. 1,500 mg daily. 750 mg daily.	Helps protect the skin. Needed for blood cell formation.
Vitamin E	Start at 400 IU daily and increase slowly to 800 IU.	Do not exceed 400 IU if on blood thinning medication.

HERBS

☐ For bruising try alfalfa, garlic, and rose hips.

RECOMMENDATIONS

☐ The diet should include an abundance of dark green leafy vegetables, buckwheat, and fresh fruits. These foods are high in vitamin C and bioflavonoids, which help to prevent bruising. Studies show that those with a vitamin C deficiency bruise more easily than others because their blood vessels are generally weaker.

☐ Stay away from aspirin.

☐ If bruising is frequent, see your doctor.

Bruxism

Bruxism or tooth grinding usually occurs without awareness during sleep and results in loosened teeth and gum recession. Loss of teeth can occur if the disorder is not caught in time. Bruxism can develop if the teeth become sensitive to heat and cold. Sometimes the teeth are out of line and the bite needs adjusting. Most often, calcium and pantothenic acid are needed to prevent bruxism. Calcium is effective for treating involuntary movement of muscles. Pantothenic acid is important for maintaining proper motor coordination.

NUTRIENTS

SUPPLEMENT	SUGGESTED DOSAGE	COMMENTS
Essential		
Calcium and magnesium	1,500–2,000 mg daily. 750 mg daily.	A deficiency has been linked to tooth grinding.
Pantothenic acid (B₅)	500 mg twice daily.	Reduces stress.
Very Important		
Vitamin C	3,000–5,000 mg daily.	Potentiates adrenal function, acting as an antistress vitamin.
Helpful		
Multivitamin and mineral complex plus raw adrenal glandular	As directed on label.	Needed to reduce stress. *See* GLANDULAR THERAPY in Part Three.
Vitamin B complex	100 mg twice daily.	High stress formula.
Zinc	50 mg daily.	Needed to reduce stress.

RECOMMENDATIONS

☐ Do not eat any type of sugar six hours before going to bed; sometimes a light protein snack helps. Cut back on processed foods and colas.

☐ Avoid stress.

CONSIDERATIONS

☐ Hypoglycemia, related to low adrenal function, is often the cause of bruxism. Refer to HYPOGLYCEMIA in Part Two, and follow the dietary guidelines.

☐ Have a hair analysis done to determine if you have any mineral imbalances, such as abnormal levels of sodium and potassium.

Bulimia

Unlike the starvation tactics employed by the anorexic, the bulimic characteristically has abnormal increases in hunger, binges several times a day, and then induces vomiting. Long-term treatment is needed to improve self-esteem. Psychiatric consultation may be necessary, as the cause is most often psychological.

Signs of bulimia are a swollen neck and erosion of enamel on back teeth from excessive vomiting, broken blood vessels in the face, over- or underweight, extreme weakness, dizziness, cessation of menstruation, and low pulse rate and blood pressure.

Bulimics need their serotonin levels elevated to reduce their cravings for simple carbohydrates (rich binge foods). Overexercising is a problem for bulimics. They binge on foods and then try to burn up the calories through exercise. Anyone who is obsessed with exercise in order to control weight needs help.

NUTRIENTS

SUPPLEMENT	SUGGESTED DOSAGE	COMMENTS
Very Important		
Multivitamins and minerals	Take in extremely high doses because they pass rapidly through the gastrointestinal system and are poorly assimilated. See physician for amount needed.	The bulimic syndrome results in extreme vitamin and mineral deficiency.
Important		
Acidophilus or Megadophilus	Follow directions on label. Take on an empty stomach so it can pass quickly to the small intestine.	Stabilizes intestinal bacteria. Protects the liver.
Protein supplement (free form amino acids)	Follow directions on label.	Free form amino acids are more readily available for use by the body than other protein forms. Protein deficiency is a serious problem.
Vitamin B complex with	100 mg 3 times daily.	Essential for all cellular function. Needed for the digestion of foods and the assimilation of all nutrients including iron.
B$_{12}$ injections plus	1cc 3 times weekly.	
liver injections	2cc 3 times weekly.	
Vitamin C	5,000 mg daily in divided doses.	For all cellular and glandular function.
Zinc	50–100 mg daily. Do not exceed 100 mg zinc.	Necessary in protein metabolism.
Helpful		
Bio-Strath from West Germany or	3 times daily.	For increased strength and energy. Aids in repair and increases the appetite.
brewer's yeast	Start with a small amount and work up.	Contains the B vitamins and other necessary nutrients.
Iron (Floradix formula from West Germany)	3 times daily.	Source of iron that is easily assimilated.
Kelp	6 tablets daily.	Supplies essential minerals, especially iodine.
Proteolytic enzymes	Take between and with meals.	Important for proper digestion.
Vitamin A	15,000 IU daily.	Vitamins A, D, and E are necessary fat-soluble vitamins.
Vitamin D	600 IU daily.	
Vitamin E	600 IU daily.	

RECOMMENDATIONS

☐ When a regular eating pattern is being established, a high-fiber, well-balanced diet is essential for maintaining good health. Consume no sugar in any form and avoid white flour products. Be aware that there might be withdrawal symptoms when eliminating sugar from the diet.

ADDITIONAL SOURCES OF INFORMATION

☐ To obtain more information about eating disorders and treatments, contact any of the following:

American Anorexia/Bulimia Association
133 Cedar Lane
Teaneck, NJ 07666
(201) 836-1800

ANAD
P.O. Box 7
Highland Park, IL 60035
(312) 831-3438

ANRED
P.O. Box 5102
Eugene, OR 97405
(503) 344-1144

Center for the Study
of Anorexia/Bulimia
1 West 91st Street
New York, NY 10024
(212) 595-3449

National Anorexic Aid Society
5796 Karl Road
Columbus, OH 43229
(614) 436-1112

Burns

There are three degrees of burns: first degree, indicated by redness; second degree, indicated by redness and blisters; and third degree, in which the entire thickness of skin and underlying muscle is destroyed. For third-degree burns see your doctor immediately or go to a hospital emergency room.

NUTRIENTS

SUPPLEMENT	SUGGESTED DOSAGE	COMMENTS
Very Important		
Potassium	99 mg daily.	Needed to replace potassium lost from burns.

Protein supplement (free form amino acids)	As directed on label.	Important in the healng of tissues. Free form amino acids are easily absorbed and assimilated by the body.
Vitamin C plus bioflavoniods	10,000 mg daily and up.	*See* ASCORBIC ACID FLUSH in Part Three.
Vitamin E	600–1,600 IU, increasing slowly.	Needed for healing and to prevent scarring.
Zinc	30 mg 3 times daily.	Zinc gluconate is fast acting. Needed for quicker healing of tissues.
Important		
Selenium	200 mcg daily.	Needed for tissue elasticity. Provides protection at the cellular level.
Unsaturated fatty acids (linseed and/or primrose oil)	As directed on label.	Linseed oil and primrose oil are good sources.
Vitamin A	100,000 IU daily for 1 month, then drop to 50,000 IU. End with 25,000 IU.	Use emulsion for easier assimilation. Needed for tissue repair.
Helpful		
All-Purpose Bacteriaside Spray from Aerobic Life Products	As directed on label.	Kills bacteria and prevents infection.
Calcium with magnesium and vitamin D	1,500 mg daily. 750 mg daily. 400 IU daily.	Calcium is important in protein structuring. Loss of body fluids increases the need for magnesium. Vitamin D is needed for calcium uptake.
Coenzyme Q$_{10}$	100 mg daily.	Helps circulation and healing of tissue.
DMG (Gluconic from DaVinci Labs)	100 mg daily.	Enhances circulation and healing of tissue.
Germanium	200 mg daily.	Enhances circulation and healing of tissue.

RECOMMENDATIONS

☐ Put cold applications on the burn at once to reduce pain and swelling. Cover to minimize bacterial infection. Baking soda mixed with olive oil and applied to the area promotes healing and prevents scarring.

☐ Do not put ointments, salves, or butter on burns. Do not break blisters.

☐ Elevate burn injuries to prevent swelling. Watch for signs of infection, odor, pus, or extreme redness. Protect from exposure to sun.

☐ To remove hot tar, wax, or melted plastic from the skin, use ice water to harden the heated object.

☐ Tannic acid has been used in clinics for surface burns that have begun to heal. It is found in many herbs including sumac leaves, sweet gum, white oak bark, beriberi leaves, and blackberry leaves. These herbs can be used as a tea and as a wet compress.

☐ Aloe vera is good on first-degree burns when applied immediately, and on second- and third-degree burns after healing begins. Try Burn Gel from Aerobic Life Products for burns. It contains aloe vera.

☐ For third-degree burns, obtain Silvadene Cream by prescription and apply. A rare reaction to the silver sulfadiazine may occur. If so, discontinue use. Antibiotics, debridement to remove dead tissues, and hydrotherapy to loosen dead skin and keep muscles flexible should be part of a medically supervised program.

☐ Diet for second- and third-degree burns is very important. High protein is needed for tissue repair, and 5,000 to 6,000 calories per day is needed for healing. Fluid intake must be increased.

☐ Cold clay poultices are helpful. *See* POULTICE in Part Three.

☐ *See also* SUNBURN in Part Two.

Bursitis

Bursitis is an inflammation of the bursae, small fluid-filled sacs found in the joints, muscles, tendons, and bones that help to promote muscular movement by cushioning the bones against friction. It can be caused by injury, food, airborne allergies, or calcium deposits. This disorder typically afflicts the hip or shoulder joints and is also known as tennis elbow, bunions, or frozen shoulder. Tenderness of the affected body part accompanies bursitis, and acute pain that usually limits motion often follows as well. Treatment involves removing the cause of the injury, clearing up any underlying infection, and perhaps surgically removing calcium deposits.

NUTRIENTS

SUPPLEMENT	SUGGESTED DOSAGE	COMMENTS
Very Important		
Calcium plus magnesium	1,500 mg daily. 750 mg daily.	Chelate form is the most effective.
Inflazyme Forte from American Biologics or proteolytic enzymes	2 tablets between meals.	A powerful anti-inflammatory substance.

Important		
Multienzymes	Take with meals.	Avoid preparations that contain hydrochloric acid (HCl), particularly if you have ulcers.
Protein supplement (free form amino acids)	Take on an empty stomach.	Free form amino acids are more readily available for use by the body.
Vitamin A emulsion	100,000 IU daily for 1 month, then decrease to 50,000 IU daily for 2 weeks, and end with 25,000 IU daily.	Needed for tissue repair and the immune system.
Vitamin C plus bioflavonoids	3,000–8,000 mg daily in divided doses.	Reduces inflammation and potentiates immune function.
Vitamin E emulsion	Start with 400 IU and increase slowly to 1,000 IU in capsule form.	An anti-inflammatory free radical scavenger.
Helpful		
Coenzyme Q_{10}	60 mg daily.	Good for circulation.
DMG (Gluconic from DaVinci Labs)	100 mg daily.	Good for circulation and repair of free radical damage.
Germanium	100 mg daily.	Enhances the immune system and reduces inflammation and pain.
Multivitamin and mineral complex	As directed on label.	Needed for tissue repair.
Vitamin B complex	100 mg twice daily.	B vitamins are important in cellular repair.
Vitamin B_{12}	By injection or 1,000 mcg in lozenge form dissolved under tongue.	Needed for proper digestion and absorption of foods and for the repair of nerve damage.

RECOMMENDATIONS

☐ Splint and rest the affected area. Apply hot castor oil packs on sore joints. Some doctors recommend ice packs.

☐ Complete a seven-day raw food diet, followed by a three-day cleansing fast. (*See* FASTING in Part Three.)

Cadmium Toxicity

A toxic trace metal, cadmium can be detrimental to your health. Like lead, cadmium accumulates in the body and has varying degrees of toxicity. Cadmium replaces the body's stores of the essential mineral zinc in the liver and kidneys. Cadmium levels will rise in those suffering from a zinc deficiency.

Elevated levels of cadmium may result in hypertension (high blood pressure), a dulled sense of smell, anemia, joint soreness, hair loss, dry, scaly skin, and loss of appetite. Cadmium toxicity threatens the health of the body by weakening the immune system. It causes a decreased production of T-cells, which protect the body by destroying foreign cells and cancer cells. Because cadmium is retained in the kidney and liver, excessive exposure can lead to kidney disease and serious liver damage; other detrimental effects of intense cadmium exposure include emphysema, cancer, and a shortened life span.

Several recent studies have revealed that cigarette smokers have abnormally high levels of cadmium in their bodies. You can also accumulate cadmium from secondhand smoke. Cigar and pipe smoke contain cadmium as well. Cadmium is used in plastics and in the production of nickel-cadmium batteries. In addition to cigarette smoke, it can be found in drinking water, fertilizer, fungicides, pesticides, soil, industrial air pollution, refined grains, rice, coffee, tea, and soft drinks.

NUTRIENTS

SUPPLEMENT	SUGGESTED DOSAGE	COMMENTS
Important		
Alfalfa tablets	6–8 tablets daily.	Containing vitamin K and chlorophyll, alfalfa helps to remove cadmium from the body.
Calcium and magnesium	2,000 mg daily. 1,000 mg daily.	Trace metals that help rid the body of cadmium.
Garlic capsules (Kyolic)	2 capsules 3 times daily.	Odorless garlic that helps to rid the body of cadmium. A potent detoxifier.
L-Methionine and L-cysteine and L-lysine (amino acids)	Take on an empty stomach in juice, not milk. Add vitamins B_6 and C for better assimilation.	These amino acids act as antioxidants; they protect the organs, especially the liver.
Lecithin	2 tbsp. or 2 capsules with meals. Take with vitamin E for better assimilation.	Protects all cells.
Rutin	200 mg 3 times daily with a small amount of vitamin C.	Aids in removing high amounts of metals from the body.
Vitamin E emulsion	600–1,000 IU daily.	Vitamin E is assimilated easier in emulsion formula; however, you can take in capsule form as well.
Zinc	50–80 mg daily.	Needed to replace zinc that was depleted due to cadmium deposits and to prevent cadmium levels from rising.
Helpful		
Copper	3 mg daily.	Works with zinc to remove calcium deposits.

Iron from Floradix formula or ferrous fumarate from Freeda Vitamins	As directed on label.	This formula is easily assimilated into the body.

RECOMMENDATIONS

☐ Make sure that you include plenty of fiber and apple pectin in your diet. Eat pumpkin seeds, as well as other foods that are high in zinc.

☐ If you have any of the symptoms described above and suspect cadmium toxicity, you may wish to have a hair analysis done to determine the level of toxic metals in your system.

CONSIDERATIONS

☐ See also CHELATION THERAPY in Part Three for further suggestions.

☐ See also ENVIRONMENTAL TOXICITY in Part Two.

Cancer

When your body is injured—for example, if you have a cut—the cells surrounding the cut reproduce to replace the ones that have been harmed. These cells *know* to stop reproducing once they have "filled in" the cut.

With cancer, one cell gets the idea to reproduce and begins doing so for no obvious reason. The cells that it reproduces form a hard lump. This is cancer. Often, a cell from this lump, or tumor, will spread to another part of the body and begin reproduction there. These cells are not receptive to the normal signal to stop.

No one knows *exactly* why a cell will do this. We do know, however, some of the agents that cause cancer, such as cigarette smoke. Persons who are exposed to this and other irritants have higher rates of cancer. Free radicals damage the cell, often resulting in uncontrolled growth (*see* the section on free radicals in RADIATION POISONING in Part Two.

There are four main categories of cancer. *Carcinomas* affect the skin, mucous membranes, glands, and other organs; *leukemias* are blood cancers; *sarcomas* affect muscles, connective tissue, and bones; and *lymphomas* affect the lymphatic system.

One person dies every minute from cancer. Another 3 million have cancer, and one out of three will die from

it. There are more than one hundred different varieties of cancer. They all have different causes and vary in aggression (how fast they spread).

Two of what are believed to be the major causes of cancer (known as carcinogens) are environmental factors and diet, with resultant loss of immune defense. Many experts link cancer to stress and diet.

Some types of cancer are treated with chemotherapy and have apparently been cured with this treatment. The side effects of chemotherapy are hair loss, extreme nausea, vomiting, fatigue, weakness, sterility, and damage to the kidneys and heart. Vitamin B_6 and coenzyme Q_{10} help the body avoid some of the damage done by this treatment.

Vitamins and supplements should be taken daily with meals. Vitamin E should be taken before meals. Use only *natural* vitamins. Vitamin injections should be used when possible. Do not take any drugs except those prescribed by your doctor.

SELF-TESTS

Breast Cancer Self-Test

See BREAST CANCER in Part Two.

Colon Cancer Self-Test

If you suspect that you have colon cancer, a test kit can be purchased to detect whether blood is in the stool (an early sign of colon cancer). In the newest test, you simply drop a strip of chemically treated paper into the commode after a bowel movement. The paper will change to the color blue if there is blood present in the stool.

If you test positive, take a second test in three days. If the second test is also positive, see your doctor immediately. Remember that the presence of blood in the stool does not necessarily mean you have cancer. The test may prove positive after consuming red meat, or if you have diverticulitis, hemorrhoids, polyps, ulcers, or an inflamed colon. About 10 percent of those who test positive have cancer.

Testicular Cancer Self-Test

Because there is presently no cure for cancer, early detection is extremely important. Cancer can appear anywhere in the body, so self-examination should be conducted regularly. You will be better able to feel for lumps if you check for them after a warm bath or shower when the scrotal skin is relaxed. With the fingers of both hands, examine each testicle, gently rolling each between the thumb and the fingers, checking for hard lumps or nodules. If you find a suspicious lump, see your doctor.

NUTRIENTS

SUPPLEMENT	SUGGESTED DOSAGE	COMMENTS
Essential		
Beta-carotene	10,000 units	Powerful antioxidant that destroys free radicals.
Coenzyme Q$_{10}$	100 mg daily.	Improves cellular oxygenation.
DMG (Gluconic from DaVinci Labs)	As directed on label.	Enhances oxygen utilization.
Garlic capsules (Kyolic)	2 capsules 3 times daily.	Enhances immune function.
Germanium	200 mg daily.	Improves cellular oxygenation, deterring cancer growth. A potent immunostimulant. Aids in relieving pain and discomfort.
Proteolytic enzymes or	2–6 tablets with meals.	Powerful free radical scavengers.
Wobe-Mugos-N-Dragees	2–6 tablets between meals.	
Selenium	200 mcg daily.	Powerful free radical scavenger. Aids in protein digestion.
Superoxide dismutase (SOD)	As directed on label. Consider injections.	Destroys free radicals.
Vitamin A and E emulsion or capsules	50,000–100,000 IU vitamin A daily for 10 days or for as long as on program. Up to 1,000 IU vitamin E daily. (Same amount of vitamin E in capsule form.)	Emulsion is absorbed rapidly and easily assimilated, is safe at high doses, and puts less stress on the liver.
Vitamin B complex and	100 mg daily.	B vitamins are necessary for normal cell division and function.
brewer's yeast	3 times daily.	
Vitamin C plus bioflavonoids	5,000–10,000 mg daily in divided doses.	Powerful anticancer agent. *See* ASCORBIC ACID FLUSH in Part Three.
Helpful		
Aerobic 07 from Aerobic Life Products or Dioxychlor from American Biologics	As directed on label.	Antimicrobial agents.
Comprehensive mineral and trace element supplement, rich in potassium and		Essential for normal cell division and function.
calcium and	2,000 mg daily.	
magnesium	1,000 mg daily.	
Carnitine derived from fish liver (squalene)	As directed on label.	Protects against oxygen radical damage and other toxins.
L-Cysteine and L-methionine (amino acids)	As directed on label.	Detoxifies harmful substances. Protects the liver and other organs.
L-Taurine (amino acid)	As directed on label.	Functions as foundation for tissue and organ repair.
Maxidophilus or Megadophilus or Primadophilus DDS	As directed on label.	Has an antibacterial effect on the body. A milk-free brand is available.
Multiple enzyme digestive formula	Take with meals as directed.	Aids digestion.
Multivitamin	Take with meals as directed on label.	Should not be sustained release. Take formula that is iron free.
Niacin and folic acid and	100 mg daily.	B vitamins that improve circulation, build red blood cells, and aid liver function.
choline	500–1,000 mg daily.	
PABA	Less than 400 IU daily.	Protects against skin cancer.
Raw glandular complex with extra raw thymus	As directed on label.	Stimulates glandular function, especially the thymus (site of T-lymphacyte production). *See* GLANDULAR THERAPY in Part Three.
Seaweed or kelp	5 tablets daily.	For mineral balance.
Vitamin B$_{12}$	A sublingual form or injections (under doctor's supervision only) are recommended.	Prevents anemia.

HERBS

☐ Include some of the following in your cancer prevention or cancer therapy program: black radish, dandelion, echinacea, Jason Winters tea, pau d'arco, red clover, and suma. Dr. Hans Neiper, a German cancer specialist, uses carnivora, a South American plant.

☐ Many with external cancers responded well to poultices made from comfrey, pau d'arco, ragwort, and wood sage. *See* POULTICE in Part Three.

RECOMMENDATIONS

☐ Do not take supplemental iron tablets. The body withholds iron from cancer cells. Studies reported in Volume 319 of *The New England Journal of Medicine* reveal that people with excess iron levels in the blood tend to have an increased risk of developing cancer. Excess iron may suppress the cancer-killing function of the macrophages (an important type of cell that helps repair tissue) and interfere with T- and B-cell activity. The diet outline will supply the necessary amount of iron.

☐ Drink beet juice (from roots and tops), carrot juice (beta-carotene), and asparagus juice often. Dr. Hans Nieper, cancer researcher, is using fresh raw cabbage and carrot juice with excellent results. Grape, black cherry, and all dark-colored juices are good, as are black currants. Also beneficial is apple juice, if it is fresh. Fruit juices are best taken in the morning, and vegetable juices are best taken in the afternoon.

☐ Drink spring or steam-distilled water only!

☐ Eat onions and garlic. Kyolic is an odorless form of specially prepared garlic.

☐ Eat ten raw almonds every day. They are high in laetrile, which acts as an anti-cancer agent.

☐ All anti-cancer diets should include grains, nuts, seeds, and brown unpolished rice. Millet cereal is a good source of protein. Eat wheat, oat, and bran. Eat plenty of cruciferous vegetables such as broccoli, Brussels sprouts, cabbage, and cauliflower. Also consume yellow and deep orange vegetables such as cantaloupe, carrots, pumpkin, squash, and yams. Fresh cabbage and carrot juice are used in clinics around the globe. Apples, berries, Brazil nuts, cherries, grapes, legumes (including chickpeas, lentils, and red beans), and plums all help to fight cancer. The berries will protect DNA from damage.

☐ Do *not* consume the following: junk foods, processed refined foods, saturated fats, salt, sugar, or white flour. Instead of salt, use a kelp or potassium substitute. A small amount of blackstrap molasses or pure maple syrup acts as a natural sweetener in place of sugar. Use whole wheat or rye instead of white flour. Eliminate alcohol, coffee, and all teas except for herbal teas.

☐ Do not eat any animal protein—*never* eat luncheon meat, hot dogs, or smoked or cured meats. As your condition improves, eat broiled fish three times a week. Restrict consumption of dairy products; a little yogurt, kefir milk, or raw cheese occasionally is enough. Do not eat any peanuts. Limit, but don't eliminate altogether, your intake of soybean products; they contain enzyme inhibitors.

☐ Many cancer patients have good results with the macrobiotic diet.

☐ Cook all sprouts slightly, except alfalfa sprouts.

☐ *See* FASTING in Part Three, and follow the program. Take coffee enemas daily. Use cleansing enemas with lemon and water or garlic and water two or three times weekly.

☐ Because of potential low-level radiation leakage, avoid microwave ovens. Use only stainless steel or glassware for cooking. Do not sit close to television sets—sit at least eight feet away. Also avoid x-rays.

☐ Exercise is important.

☐ Avoid chemicals such as hair sprays, cleaning compounds, waxes, fresh paints, and garden pesticides. Chemicals promote the formation of free radicals in the body, which may lead to cancer. Cancer victims will further weaken their immune system by using chemicals. The body expends energy trying to protect itself from the damaging chemicals instead of fighting the cancer. Do not use aerosol products.

☐ Avoid stress!

CONSIDERATIONS

☐ Surveys indicate that 40 percent of the U.S. population rarely eats a single fruit, including that contained in fruit juices, and 20 percent never eat vegetables. In addition, 80 percent of Americans do not consume quality high-fiber cereals or whole grain bread. The American diet *must* be changed to avoid cancer and heart disease. Cancer is less prevalent in physically active people, so exercise is important.

☐ Obesity is another factor linked to cancer, especially in women. Overweight women are more likely to develop cancer of the uterine lining than other women and tend to do poorly once they have breast cancer. Fat seems to affect female hormones—the greater the amount of fat present, the greater the amount of estrogen converted from androgen-like hormones and made into a much more potent form of the female hormone. Estrogen stimulates cells to divide in the breast and reproductive system. Obesity in men may cause colon and rectal cancer; in women it can cause gallbladder, cervical, uterine, and breast cancer.

☐ *The New England Journal of Medicine* reported that calcium may prevent precancerous cells from becoming cancerous.

☐ A lack of the nutrients beta-carotene, vitamin E, and the B vitamins in lung tissue may be related to lung cancer. Researchers have found that the presence of calcium allows bile to bond with fatty acids that may irritate the colon lining and cause rapid growth in destructive cells.

☐ Two hundred scientists from around the world have discovered that niacin plays a major role in the prevention and treatment of cancer.

☐ The Cancer Control Convention in Japan reported that germanium may be one of the important factors in the prevention and cure of cancer.

☐ Japan and Iceland both have low rates of goiter and breast cancer. This may be because their soils are rich in both iodine and selenium. Breast cancer has been linked to an iodine deficiency. Breast cancer is almost nonexistent in Japanese women, who consume large amounts of fish. Colon cancer rates in Japan are also low.

☐ Studies reveal that a high-fat diet dramatically increases the incidences of colon and breast cancer, as compared to a low-fat diet. High dietary fat is a promoter of cancer.

☐ It is now thought that intestinal cancer takes about twenty years to develop.

☐ A group of seventy-five Environmental Protection Agency (EPA) experts ranked pesticide residues among the top three environmental cancer risks.

☐ Those people whose mother's smoked during pregnancy are 50 percent more likely to develop cancer later in life. These findings confirm the harmful effects smoking has on the unborn fetus. Smoking is extremely dangerous and leads to cancer no matter what age group is involved.

☐ Dr. Virginia Livingston at the Livingston-Wheeler Clinic in San Diego has prepared a vaccine against the organism that "causes" cancer (*Progenitor cryptocides*). She states that if the immune system is weakened through poor diet, "infected" foods, or old age, the microbe gains a foothold and initiates the growth of cancer cells into tumors. She has over fifteen years of experience in treating cancer patients with this PC vaccine, which is made from the patient's own body fluids. Dr. Livingston reports remarkable results. Dietary and vitamin therapy, plus the vaccine, boost immune response. She says that nine out of ten patients improved.

☐ According to the August 1989 issue of the *Medical Tribune*, the risk of prostate cancer for males who have undergone a vasectomy is three times greater than that of males who have not had a vasectomy.

☐ *See also* BREAST CANCER and SKIN CANCER in Part Two.

The Warning Signs and Possible Causes of Certain Cancers

You can save your life by knowing the warning signs of cancer. The American Cancer Society estimates that 170,000 or more Americans will die annually of preventable cancers. The table below indicates the risks and signs that have been associated with various types of cancer.

Type of Cancer	Risks	Symptoms
Bladder and Kidney	Exposure to certain chemicals such as benzidines, aniline dyes, naphthalenes; excessive smoking; excessive consumption of caffeine and/or artificial sweeteners; a history of schistosomiasis (a tropical disease); frequent urinary tract infections.	Blood in the urine and increased frequency of urination. Although it is infrequently the case, blood in the urine can signify cancer. Seek medical attention to rule out this possibility.
Breast	Women who give childbirth after age 35; women who have never had children; a family history of cancer; a high alcohol and/or caffeine intake; a high-fat diet; diabetes. There is a link between sugar intake in older women and breast cancer. Estrogens and oral contraceptives have also been linked to breast and uterine cancer.	Lump(s); thickening; any physical changes in the breast.
Cervical and Uterine	More than 5 complete pregnancies; intercourse at an early age (i.e., before 18); a history of gonorrhea; multiple sex partners; infertility.	Bleeding between menstrual periods; unusual discharge; painful menstrual periods; heavy periods.
Colon	Lack of fiber and calcium; polyps; a family history of cancer of the colon; continued constipation and/or diarrhea; a "toxic" colon; a high-fat diet.	Rectal bleeding; blood in the stool; changes in bowel habits (i.e., diarrhea and/or constipation).
Endometrium	Women who have never been pregnant; women past menopause; a family history of cancer; diabetes; obesity; hypertension.	Bleeding between menstrual periods; unusual discharge; painful menstrual periods; heavy periods.

Type of Cancer	Risks	Symptoms
Larynx	Heavy smoking; alcohol consumption.	Persistent cough; hoarse throat.
Leukemia	Hereditary factors; radiation exposure; chronic viral infections.	Signs in children include paleness, fatigue, weight loss, repeated infections, easy bruising, and nosebleeds.
Lung	Smoking; exposure to asbestos, nickel, chromates, and radio-active materials; chronic bronchitis; a history of tuberculosis; exposure to certain chemicals such as pesticides and herbicides.	A persistent cough; sputum with blood; chest pain.
Mouth and Throat	Irritants inside the mouth such as a broken tooth and ill-fitting or broken dentures; excessive alcohol intake; smoking. Chewing tobacco leads to cancer of the mouth. Smoking may lead to cancer of the mouth.	A chronic ulcer of the mouth, tongue, or throat that does not heal.
Ovarian	Women who have not had children; women on a high-fat diet.	Often no obvious symptoms until it is in its later stages of development.
Prostate	Recurrence of prostate infections; history of venereal disease; a diet high in animal fat; high intake of milk, meat, and/or coffee; use of male hormone testosterone in treatment of impotence. Risk increases after age 50.	Weak or interrupted urine flow; continuous pain in the lower back, pelvis, and/or upper thighs.
Skin	Prolonged exposure to the sun, especially for those who have fair skin; a history of moles (malignant or otherwise), moles on the feet, or in areas irritated by clothing; scars from severe burns and scars or sores that won't heal; a family history of skin cancer.	Tumor or lump under the skin, resembling a wart or an ulceration that never heals; moles that change color or size; flat sores; lesions that look like moles.
Stomach	Pernicious anemia; lack of hydrochloric acid and fiber; a high-fat diet; chronic gastritis; stomach polyps.	Indigestion and pain after consuming foods.
Testicular	Undescended testicle.	Lump(s); enlargement of a testicle; thickening of the scrotum; sudden collection of fluid in the scrotum; pain or discomfort in a testicle or in the scrotum; mild ache in the lower abdomen or groin; enlargement or tenderness of the breasts.

U.S. Cancer Rating by State

Information regarding the incidence of cancer in each state was provided by the Cancer Research Foundation of America. The states below are listed from highest to lowest cancer rate.

1. District of Columbia	16. Alabama	31. California
2. Rhode Island	Nebraska	32. Oregon
3. Florida	17. Kentucky	33. Mississippi
4. Pennsylvania	18. South Dakota	34. South Carolina
5. Massachusetts	19. Oklahoma	35. Montana
6. New Jersey	20. Wisconsin	Georgia
7. New York	21. Indiana	36. Washington
8. Missouri	22. Tennessee	37. Arizona
9. Delaware	23. Vermont	38. Nevada
10. Connecticut	Kansas	39. Texas
11. Ohio	24. North Dakota	40. New Mexico
12. Maine	25. Michigan	41. Idaho
13. West Virginia	26. Virginia	42. Hawaii
14. Arkansas	27. North Carolina	43. Colorado
15. Illinois	28. New Hampshire	44. Wyoming
Iowa	29. Minnesota	45. Utah
Maryland	30. Louisiana	46. Alaska

123

Candidiasis

Candida albicans is a type of yeast-like fungus that inhabits the intestine, genital tract, mouth, and throat. Normally this fungus lives in healthy balance with the other bacteria and yeasts in the body; however, certain conditions can cause this fungus to multiply, weakening the immune system and causing an infection known as candidiasis. Because this fungus travels through the bloodstream to many parts of the body, various symptoms may develop.

When this fungus infects the oral cavity, it is called thrush. White sores may form on the tongue, gums, and inside the cheeks. When the fungus infects the vagina, it results in vaginitis. The most common symptoms include a large amount of white, cheesey discharge and intense itching. Very often allergies to foods are present. Allergy testing is advised. Oral thrush, athlete's foot, ringworm, jock itch, and even diaper rash can develop as a result of food allergies and *Candida albicans.* (*See* ALLERGIES in Part Two for additional symptoms.)

Because candidiasis can infect various parts of the body—the most common being the ears, nose, gastrointestinal tract, and bowels—it can also be characterized by many symptoms. These include constipation; diarrhea; colitis; abdominal pain; canker sores; persistent heartburn; muscle and joint pain; sore throat; congestion; nagging cough; numb hands, legs, or face; tingling sensations; acne; vaginitis; kidney and bladder infections; arthritis; depression; hyperactivity; hypothyroidism followed by adrenal problems; and even diabetes. Some afflicted with candidiasis may develop a sensitivity to the environment. Many cannot tolerate the smell of rubber, petroleum products, tobacco, exhaust fumes, and chemical odors.

Candidiasis may affect both men and women; however, it is rarely transmitted sexually. An infected mother may pass the fungal infection known as thrush to the newborn. Most often the baby's tongue will appear red and be covered with white spots that resemble milk spots. Thrush may also infect the baby's buttocks, appearing as a rash. Because there is no simple, accurate test, this infection is difficult to detect.

Women diagnosed with a yeast infection should also be checked for diabetes. Because their vaginal environment is more conducive to the growth of yeast, diabetics are at greater risk of contracting a yeast infection such as candidiasis.

NUTRIENTS

SUPPLEMENT	SUGGESTED DOSAGE	COMMENTS
Very Important		
Capricin from Professional Specialties or	4 capsules 3 times daily with meals.	Destroys the Candida fungus.
Caprystatin from Arteria (caprylic acid)	1st week: 1 tablet twice daily. 2nd week: 2 tablets twice daily. 3rd week: 3 tablets twice daily.	
Dioxychlor from American Biologics or Aerobic 07 from Aerobic Life Products	5 drops in water twice daily.	These stabilized oxygen products destroy the fungus, while preserving the "good" bacteria.
Garlic capsules (Kyolic)	2 capsules 3 times daily.	An odorless form of garlic that inhibits the infecting organism. Kyolic vaginal suppositories also effectively treat Candida vaginitis.
Maxidophilus or Megadophilus or Non-Dairy Neo-Flora or DDS Extracts or Prime-Dophilus from Klaire Laboratories	Use as directed on label. Send for Superdophilus: Natren Inc. 10935 Camarillo St. N. Hollywood, CA 91602	Eugalan Topfer, a form of mother's milk from Germany, is the best form. A vegetarian form is also available for anyone who cannot tolerate dairy products.*
Omega 3–6 with evening primrose oil from Arteria or primrose oil or salmon oil	Use as directed on label.	A good source of essential fatty acids.
Vitamin B complex with extra biotin	100 mg 3 times daily.	Malabsorption is common in candidiasis.
Vitamin B$_{12}$ lozenges	1 lozenge (2,000 mcg) under the tongue 3 times daily, taken between meals. Vitamin B injections may be necessary.	Important for digestion. Needed for metabolism of carbohydrates, fats, and proteins. Candida prevents the absorption of nutrients from the intestinal tract.
Important		
Germanium	100–200 mg daily.	Improves tissue oxygenation.
Helpful		
Coenzyme Q$_{10}$	100 mg daily.	Improves tissue oxygenation.
L-Cysteine (amino acid)	500 mg on an empty stomach twice daily.	A potent antioxidant and free radical destroyer.
Multivitamin and mineral complex (zinc, iron, and yeast free) with	Daily as directed on label.	Nutrients are needed for proper immune function.
vitamin A and	25,000 IU	
selenium	200 mcg	

Orithrush from Cardiovascular Research	Use as a mouth rinse or as a douche.	Destroys Candida.
Protein supplement (Free Form Amino Acid Complex from Cardiovascular Research)	¼ tsp. under the tongue between meals on an empty stomach.	Rebuilds damaged tissue.

See also ENEMA in Part Three, for instructions for the *L. bifidus* retention enema to replace the "friendly" bacteria as a quick first treatment.

RECOMMENDATIONS

☐ Do not use corticosteroids or oral contraceptives until condition improves. Oral contraceptives can upset the balance of *Candida albicans*.

☐ Avoid aged cheeses, alcohol, chocolate, dried fruits, fermented foods, all grains containing gluten (wheat, oats, rye, and barley), ham, honey, nut butters, pickles, raw mushrooms, soy sauce, sprouts, sugars of all forms, vinegar, and all yeast products. Also eliminate citrus and acid fruits (e.g., oranges, grapefruit, lemons, tomatoes, pineapple, and limes) from your diet for one month; then add back only a few twice weekly. These fruits are alkaline-forming and Candida thrives on them.

☐ Your diet should be fruit free, sugar free, and yeast free. Candida thrives in a sugary environment, so your diet should be low in carbohydrates. Eat vegetables and meat instead. Eating live yogurt or applying it directly to the vagina can help inhibit the growth of the fungus. Consume also brown rice, millet, and acidophilus. Acidophilus capsules help to restore the normal balance of the bowel and vagina. This diet program has been used for years with good results. Take only hypoallergenic food supplements.

☐ Avoid chemical household products and cleaners, chlorinated water, moth balls, synthetic textiles, and damp and moldy places, such as basements.

☐ To prevent reinfection, use a new toothbrush every thirty days. This is a good preventive measure against both fungus and bacterial infections of the mouth.

CONSIDERATIONS

☐ For vaginal disorders use Yeast-Gard vaginal suppositories from Wakunaga of America Company.

☐ Candida-Forte from Nature's Plus is good for mild cases of candidiasis.

☐ All persons on long-term antibiotics or chemotherapy are at high risk for severe cases of candidiasis.

☐ Most doctors no longer use nystatin or antibiotics because they weaken the immune system and can damage certain organs. When prescribed, they are usually only for short-term treatment. Occasionally the antifungal drugs Nizoral and amphotericin B are also used for treatment. Stronger strains of yeast can develop, becoming resistant to the drugs. Higher dosages are then required, further weakening the immune system.

☐ High mercury levels can result in candidiasis. Mercury salts inhibit the growth of necessary "friendly" bacteria in the intestines. You may want to have a hair analysis done to determine the levels of toxic metals.

☐ You might want to try pau d'arco herb tea. This tea contains an antibacterial agent. It does have an alkaloid base and a small percentage of people may not benefit from its use. Those that do not benefit from this tea should try clove tea instead. It is a good idea to alternate between the two teas because clove tea has some benefits that pau d'arco does not have and vice versa. To make pau d'arco tea, boil one quart of distilled water with two tablespoons tea for five minutes. Store it in the refrigerator with the tea leaves in. Strain as much as you need. Drink three to six cups daily.

☐ Candidiasis may be related to hypoglycemia and allergies. Consult these sections for additional suggestions.

☐ Fiber is an important part of the diet. Oat bran is more easily digestible than wheat bran.

☐ *See also* YEAST INFECTION, Part Two.

Canker Sores
(Apthous Ulcers)

Canker sores occur in the mouth. They can appear on the tongue, on the inside cheeks, on the lips, or on the gums. Canker sores have white centers and are surrounded by a red border. The size of the sores can range from as small as a pinhead to as large as a quarter. They appear quickly and often leave quickly, usually lasting from four to twenty days.

These painful mouth ulcerations are contagious and occur most often in females. They may be triggered by poor dental hygiene, allergies to chocolate and other foods, and stress and/or fatigue. They may result from an abnormal immune response to normal bacteria in the mouth. Canker sores are occasionally associated with Crohn's disease, which affects the bowels. Deficiencies of iron, vitamin B_{12}, and folic acid have been linked to this disease in some people. Stress and allergies are usually the cause of open sores in the mouth.

To avoid getting canker sores, it is important to have a body chemistry that is balanced in minerals, acidity, and alkalinity. Have a hair analyis done, and *see* ACIDOSIS, Part Two, for the acid and alkaline self-test.

NUTRIENTS

SUPPLEMENT	SUGGESTED DOSAGE	COMMENTS
Very Important		
Acidophilus or Megadophilus or Maxidophilus	Use a high potency powdered form. Take as directed on label.	Aids in maintaining healthy balance of intestinal flora ("friendly" bacteria).
Iron (Floradix formula from Germany)	As directed on label.	A natural, nutritional tonic that supplies iron and herbs; easily absorbed.
L-Lysine (amino acid)	500 mg 3 times daily on an empty stomach.	A deficiency may cause an outbreak of sores in and around the mouth.
Vitamin B complex with extra vitamin B_{12} and folic acid in lozenge form	50 mg 3 times daily. 2,000 mcg B_{12}, taken under the tongue 3 times daily on an empty stomach.	Basic for immune function and healing. A deficiency has been linked to sores of the mouth.
Important		
Ascorbic acid	3,000–8,000 mg daily in divided doses.	Use a buffered form with bioflavonoids.
Pantothenic acid (B_5)	50–100 mg 3 times daily.	Antistress B vitamin necessary for adrenal function. The adrenal is the antistress endocrine gland.
Helpful		
Garlic capsules (Kyolic)	3 capsules 3 times daily.	Acts as a natural antibiotic and immunostimulant.
Multivitamin and mineral complex	As directed on label.	A balance of minerals is always important.
Vitamin A emulsion	50,000 IU for 2 weeks, then reduce to 25,000 IU. Also put a drop or two directly on the area.	Speeds healing, especially of the mucous membranes (i.e., the mouth). Emulsion is for easier assimilation.
Zinc gluconate lozenges	Dissolve in mouth every 3 hours for 2 days.	Enhances immune function.

HERBS

☐ For canker sores, use burdock, goldenseal, pau d'arco tea, and red clover. Red raspberry tea is very helpful.

RECOMMENDATIONS

☐ Eat plenty of salad with onions. Onions contain sulfur and have healing properties. Include yogurt and soured foods such as kefir milk, cottage cheese, and buttermilk in the diet. Avoid sugar, citrus fruits, and processed and refined foods. Do not eat fish or meat of any kind for two weeks. Animal protein produces excess body acid.

☐ Avoid chewing gum, lozenges, mouthwashes, smoking, coffee, and foods that you know trigger these sores.

☐ Some doctors prescribe mouthwashes that contain tetracycline, an antibiotic.

☐ The drug Zilactin is a gel-like ointment that is applied directly to the ulcer. It sticks to the canker sore and gives relief from irritating foods.

Cardiovascular Disease

The cardiovascular system is comprised of the heart and blood vessels; blood is pumped by the heart and circulated throughout the body through blood vessels. Cardiovascular disease is the leading health problem in the Western world. It is the number one cause of death in the United States, claiming more than 1 million lives annually. An estimated 50 million Americans are afflicted with heart and blood vessel disease, many of whom are asymptomatic.

The arteries supplying blood to the heart are called the *coronary arteries*. When the heart's blood vessels narrow, insufficient amounts of oxygen reach the heart, causing chest pain called *angina*. When the coronary arteries that carry oxygen and nutrients to the heart muscle become obstructed, a *heart attack*, or *myocardial infarction*, can occur, resulting in damage to the heart muscle. *Arteriosclerosis*, or hardening of the arteries, is the most common cause of obstruction. Arteriosclerosis is responsible for most of the deaths resulting from heart attacks. Blood clots in the coronary arteries also result in heart attacks. It is imperative that a person suffering from a heart attack receive immediate medical attention.

In addition to arteriosclerosis, high blood pressure is a precursor to heart problems. Whereas untreated coronary artery disease results in a heart attack, untreated high blood pressure (hypertension) results in a *stroke*.

Every minute someone dies of a heart attack. Angina pectoris is a common precursor of heart attacks. Angina is characterized by a heavy, tight pain in the chest area. It usually occurs after some type of exertion and is caused by inadequate blood flow to the heart muscle. It may feel as if someone is applying intense pressure to the chest. This pain may last for several minutes, often extending to the shoulder, arm, neck, or jaw. Other signs of heart attack include sweating, nausea, vomiting, shortness of breath, dizziness, fainting, feelings of anxiety, difficulty swallowing, sudden ringing in the ears, and loss of speech. Contact your doctor immediately if you have any of these symptoms, even if they last only a few minutes.

Unfortunately, despite remarkable new technology in both the diagnosis and treatment of heart conditions, the first sign of cardiovascular disease may be a life-threatening calamity. Disorders of the cardiovascular system are often far advanced before they become symptomatic. Unfortunately about 25 percent of heart attack victims have had no previous symptoms. Many people mistake signs of a heart attack for an upset stomach. Chest pain varies from one person to another. Some suffering from a heart attack have intense pain, while others feel only mild discomfort, as in indigestion. Some have no symptoms at all.

Cardiovascular disease is not the inevitable result of aging. Many preventive measures can be taken to avoid heart disease. Controllable factors that can contribute to heart disease include high blood pressure, cigarette smoking, elevated serum cholesterol, a type A personality, stress, obesity, a sedentary lifestyle, and diabetes. You can, therefore, alter your lifestyle to avoid a major cardiac catastrophe.

HEART FUNCTION SELF-TEST

Your heart is the most important muscle in your body. A simple pulse test can help you determine how well your heart is functioning. The best time to check the pulse is first thing in the morning. If your pulse is under 60, your heart is functioning at a good pace. If your pulse is above 80, you may need to change your diet and lifestyle. If your pulse remains rapid, consult your doctor to rule out any problems. Taken daily, this pulse test can forewarn you of oncoming illness.

NUTRIENTS

SUPPLEMENT	SUGGESTED DOSAGE	COMMENTS
Essential		
Coenzyme Q$_{10}$	50–100 mg 3 times daily.	Prevents additional heart damage caused by lack of oxygen.
Germanium	200 mg daily.	Improves oxygenation in tissues and organs.

Very Important		
Bio-Cardiozyme from Biotics Research	1 tablet 3 times daily on an empty stomach.	A complex that strengthens the heart muscle.
Calcium chelate plus magnesium	1,500–2,000 mg calcium chelate daily, divided up after meals and at bedtime; 750–1,000 mg magnesium daily, divided up after meals and at bedtime.	Important in the proper functioning of the cardiac muscle.
Garlic capsules (Kyolic) and	2 capsules 3 times daily.	Kyolic is a form of odorless garlic.
Kyo-Green	As directed on label.	Kyo-Green is concentrated barley and wheatgrass juice; it contains all the nutrients needed for the healing process.
L-Carnitine (amino acid)	500 mg twice daily on an empty stomach. Take with 50 mg vitamin B$_6$ and 100 mg vitamin C.	Reduces fat and triglyceride levels in the blood. Increases oxygen uptake and stress tolerance.
Lecithin	2 capsules or 1 tbsp. with meals. Take with vitamin E.	Acts as a fat emulsifier. Vitamin E speeds assimilation of lecithin into the body.
Phosphatidyl (choline) or lipotropic factors	As directed on label.	Reduces fat and triglyceride levels in the blood.

Important		
DMG (Gluconic from DaVinci Labs)	50 mg dissolved under the tongue 4 times daily.	Promotes the utilization of oxygen.
L-Taurine (amino acid)	Take with vitamins B$_6$ and C in juice; do not take with milk, which competes with absorption.	Helps stabilize the heartbeat by correcting cardiac arrhythmias.
MAXIMUM EPA PURE/700 from Nature's Products or MaxEPA or primrose oil or black currant oil or olive oil	As directed on label.	Sources of essential fatty acids. Prevents hardening of the arteries.
Potassium	99 mg daily.	A supplement of potassium is often needed if taking cortisone, diuretics, or high blood pressure medication.
Superoxide dismutase: AOX/PLX from Biotec Foods with selenium	As directed on label. 200 mcg daily.	Superoxide dismutase is a powerful antioxidant. Selenium deficiency has been linked with heart disease.
Vitamin E	Start at 100–200 IU daily. Increase slowly, adding 100 IU weekly until dosage is 800–1,000 IU. Use under doctor's supervision only.	Strengthens the immune system and heart muscle, improves circulation, and destroys free radicals.

Helpful		
Aslavitol or Gerovital H-3 (GH-3), both from Rumania	As directed on label.	Has shown good results, improving cardiovascular health. If you have an allergy to sulfites, do not use GH-3.
Copper	As directed by doctor.	A copper deficiency may be linked to some heart problems.
Kelp	3 tablets with meals.	A rich source of important vitamins, minerals, and trace elements.
Multienzymes plus bromelin	Between meals as directed on label. 300 mg	Inflazyme Forte from American Biologics is a good formula for proteolytic enzymes.
Octacosanol and/or wheat germ	As directed on label.	Improves endurance; relieves muscle pain.
Vitamin B complex with extra thiamine (B$_1$) and niacin (B$_3$) and B$_6$ (pyridoxine)	50 mg with meals.	B vitamins work best together. Vitamin B$_6$ is a safe diuretic. *Warning*: Do not take high amounts of niacin if you have a history of rheumatic heart disease (valvular heart problems).
Vitamin C plus bioflavonoids	1,000 mg 3 times daily.	Extremely important in treating cardiovascular disease.

HERBS

☐ Use barberry, black cohosh root, butcher's broom, cayenne pepper, dandelion, ginseng, hawthorn berries, red grape vine leaves, Solaray #8 Formula, and valerian root. The Circu herbal formula from Switzerland has given good results.

☐ Some heart patients may benefit from suma herb tea. Take three cups of this herb tea daily with ginkgo biloba extract.

RECOMMENDATIONS

☐ Eliminate stimulants such as coffee and tea, which contain caffeine. Also avoid tobacco, alcohol, sugar, butter, red meat, fats (particularly animal fats), fried foods, processed and refined foods, soft drinks, spicy foods, and white flour products, such as white bread. Avoid the herb licorice.

☐ Make sure your diet is well-balanced and contains plenty of fiber. Eat plenty of raw foods, broiled fish, turkey, and chicken. Garlic, onions, and lecithin are good additions to your diet. They effectively reduce serum cholesterol levels. Add almonds and nuts (no peanuts), olive oil, pink salmon, trout, tuna, Atlantic herring, and mackerel to your diet. These foods contain the essential fatty acids, are low in fat, and contain nutrients needed for normal heart function.

☐ Absolutely *no* salt should be included in the diet! Read all labels and avoid those food products that have "soda," "sodium," or the symbol "Na" on the label. These indicate that the product contains salt. Some foods and food additives that should be avoided on a low-salt diet include:

- Accent flavor-enhancer (monosodium glutamate or MSG).
- Baking soda.
- Canned vegetables.
- Commercially prepared foods.
- Diet soft drinks.
- Foods with mold inhibitors.
- Foods with preservatives.
- Foods with certain sugar substitutes.
- Meat tenderizers.
- Some medicines and dentifrices.
- Softened water.

☐ Keep your weight down. Obesity is a risk factor in heart attacks and high blood pressure. Moderate exercise is recommended.

☐ Avoid stress. Excessive noise for more than thirty minutes can increase blood pressure and can affect the heart for up to thirty minutes *after* the noise subsides.

☐ Learn all about the drugs that have been prescribed for you. Know what to do in case of an emergency. If you have a heart condition, someone close to you should know what to do if cardiac arrest occurs. Make sure your loved one knows how to do cardiac massage and mouth-to-mouth breathing. Emergency and ambulance numbers should be easily accessible.

CONSIDERATIONS

☐ Those people whose therapy includes anticoagulants (blood thinners) such as aspirin should limit their intake of foods high in vitamin K. Foods containing vitamin K increase blood clotting and should be eaten only in small quantities. Foods that are rich in vitamin K include alfalfa, broccoli, cauliflower, egg yolks, liver, spinach, and all dark green vegetables. To enhance the effect of the anticoagulants, add to the diet more of the following: wheat germ, vitamin E, soybeans, and sunflower seeds.

☐ Drink steam-distilled water only.

☐ *See also* ARTERIOSCLEROSIS, CIRCULATORY PROBLEMS, and HIGH BLOOD PRESSURE, all in Part Two, and CHELATION THERAPY in Part Three.

128

MEDICAL UPDATES

☐ Prevention is the key to maintaining a healthy heart. A new test may help to detect heart disease more quickly. When cardiokymography (CKG) is used with electrocardiograms (ECGs), doctors may be able to detect "silent" heart disease. A recent comparison revealed that electrocardiograms alone missed 39 percent of heart disease cases. When CKG was used with ECGs, only 8 percent of the cases were undetected.

☐ The Food and Drug Administration (FDA) recently approved nitroglycerin in spray form. It can be used on or under the tongue for the control of angina attacks. This drug is commonly prescribed to relieve chest pain and to improve the oxygen supply to the heart. Nitroglycerin is primarily used in sublingual tablets. These tablets are placed under the tongue at the first sign of chest pain. If the nitroglycerin tablets cannot be dissolved due to dry mouth, try the spray form. Nitroglycerin has some side effects including headache, weakness, and dizziness; these will usually disappear with continued use of the drug.

☐ A new substance used by cardiologists known as TPA (Tissue Plasminogen Activator) has the ability to break up clots. When injected intravenously, the drug circulates through the arteries, locating and disintegrating blood clots. This treatment may be contraindicated in patients with a history of stroke or peptic ulcers.

☐ The FDA asserts that one aspirin a day can reduce the risk for heart attack; however, a Harvard Medical School newsletter states that there is insufficient evidence to support this. If you do use aspirin, keep in mind that it can cause internal bleeding and stomach ulceration.

☐ Recent evidence suggests that allergies may be linked to some heart attacks. When a reaction in the walls of the arteries triggers a spasm in the coronary arteries, a heart attack may result. Allergy tests are recommended to determine food sensitivities. *See* ALLERGIES, Part Two, for further information.

☐ After years of research, cardiologist Dr. Kurt Oster is convinced that the enzyme xanthine oxidase, which is present in homogenized milk, can damage the heart and clog the arteries. He has asked either that the dairy industry affix a warning label on homogenized milk or that the homogenization process be changed.

☐ Certain viruses may infect blood vessels, causing changes that eventually lead to heart disease. According to *Circulation Magazine*, researchers have discovered traces of the herpes virus in blood vessels from patients during coronary by-pass surgery. Researchers theorize that viruses may injure blood vessels.

Indications of Heart Trouble

If either you or a loved one has heart trouble, you can better understand the changes in the body if you familiarize yourself with the following medical terms, which may be used by the physician:

- *Angina Pectoris.* Angina refers to pain or heavy pressure in the chest that is a warning sign of impending heart attack. This chest pain may be severe or mild and is usually associated with physical exertion.
- *Arrhythmias.* Cardiac arrhythmias are electrical disorders that disrupt the natural rhythm of the heart. Heart palpitations occur when the heart beats out of sequence. The victim will feel as if his heart is skipping beats. A recent report indicates that magnesium can correct irregular heartbeats and save the lives of many cardiac patients.
- *Cardiac arrest.* Cardiac arrest occurs when the heart stops beating. As a result, the blood supply to the brain is cut off and the victim loses consciousness. Someone in good health suffering from cardiac arrest generally has unsuspected coronary artery disease. Victims of cardiac arrest will experience brief dizziness followed by unconsciousness.

- *Congestive heart failure.* When a damaged heart becomes fatigued and is unable to pump effectively, the victim suffers from congestive heart failure. This heart exhaustion results in fluid accumulation in the lungs, labored breathing after mild exertion, and swelling in the ankles and feet. See EDEMA in Part Two for swelling.
- *Fibrillation.* When someone experiences atrial fibrillation and flutter, he has heart palpitations or an enhanced awareness of the beating of the heart. Dizziness and fainting spells often accompany atrial fibrillation.
- *Ischemic heart disease.* Ischemic heart disease is caused by arteriosclerosis, in which fatty deposits along the walls of the coronary arteries obstruct blood flow to the heart. Sections of the heart muscle may die in those suffering from chronic ischemia. Ischemia can lead to angina, myocardial infarction (a coronary), cardiac arrhythmias, or congestive heart failure.
- *Myocardial infarction (MI).* When a blood clot occludes a narrowed coronary artery, cutting off nutrients and oxygen to the heart for a period of time, the victim suffers a myocardial infarction or heart attack. Irreparable damage to the heart is involved.

Cataracts

See EYE PROBLEMS.

Celiac Disease

Celiac disease is a rare disorder caused by an intolerance to gluten. Gluten belongs to the class of proteins called prolamines, which are found in wheat, barley, rye, and oats. Symptoms of celiac disease include nausea, diarrhea, abdominal swelling, large and frequently foul-smelling stools that float, weight loss, anemia, skin rash, and joint and/or bone pain. It is often misdiagnosed as irritable bowel syndrome or spastic colon.

The intestinal lining becomes damaged and defective in this disorder, and its ability to absorb vital nutrients is impaired. Malabsorption becomes a serious problem. This results in loss of vitamins, minerals, and calories. Diarrhea compounds this problem, and these lost nutrients must be replaced. *See* MALABSORPTION SYNDROME in Part Two for poor absorption of nutrients.

Anyone suffering from celiac disease should read labels carefully and eat nothing that contains gluten. Since gluten is also found in vitamins, consume only hypoallergenic vitamins.

NUTRIENTS

SUPPLEMENT	SUGGESTED DOSAGE	COMMENTS
Very Important		
Multivitamins and minerals with	Daily as directed on label.	Use yeast-free products only.
vitamin A and	25,000 IU daily.	
vitamin E	400 IU daily.	
Protein supplement (free form amino acids)	As directed on label.	A form of protein that is more readily available for use by the body.
Vitamin B complex	Take injections if recommended and supervised by your physician: 2 cc B complex. 1 cc B$_6$. In tablet form: 100 mg 3 times daily.	Use yeast-free product only. Vitamin B$_6$ acts with many enzymes.
Important		
Alfalfa tablets	6 tablets daily.	A vitamin K source.
Copper	3 mg daily.	All minerals are needed due to malabsorption by the intestinal tract.
Zinc lozenges	50 mg daily in divided doses, dissolved in the mouth.	

Helpful		
Calcium and magnesium	1,500 mg daily. 750 mg daily.	Magnesium helps maintain the normal pH balance. A deficiency is common in celiac disease.
Glucomannan or Aerobic Bulk Cleanse (ABC)	As directed on label.	A fiber product not absorbed by the intestines. Drink large amounts of water when taking glucomannan because the fiber expands to several times its dry volume. Do not take with any other pills.
Proteolytic enzymes	3 tablets on an empty stomach between meals for adults.	Additional digestive enzymes may be needed.
Unsaturated fatty acids (primrose oil capsules or salmon oil)	As directed on label.	Primrose oil contains essential fatty acids.
Vitamin B$_{12}$ with folic acid	As directed on label. Injections or sublingual form.	Malabsorption of B$_{12}$ results from celiac disease.
Vitamin C	2,000–5,000 mg daily in divided doses.	Involved in interferon production.

RECOMMENDATIONS

☐ B vitamins are important because celiac disease causes malabsorption of the B vitamins.

☐ Avoid any food that contains gluten. Do not eat any products that contain barley, oats, rye, or wheat. Rice and corn can be eaten. Read all labels.

☐ Do not eat sugar products or processed foods. Avoid all dairy products.

☐ People with celiac disease need fiber and should eat fresh vegetables, including legumes (lentils such as beans and peas), rice bran, nuts, sunflower seeds, raisins, figs, and all "seedy" fruits such as strawberries, raspberries, and blackberries.

CONSIDERATIONS

☐ If a child gets blisters and sores all over his body, he should be checked for celiac disease. Omit all gluten-containing foods and see if the problem clears up. Milk should also be eliminated from the diet because of a possible lactose intolerance. Celiac disease can begin as early as six months to one and a half years of age.

☐ Schizophrenia occurs more often in persons with celiac disease.

☐ For free information on this disorder, write to Midwestern Celiac-Sprue Association, P.O. Box 3554, Des Moines, IA 50322. Send a large self-addressed, stamped envelope.

Chemical Allergies

When the body is exposed to certain foreign chemicals or other environmental contaminants, it usually responds by producing antibodies to defend itself against the foreign invaders. Metals such as nickel, mercury, chrome, and beryllium may cause such chemical allergies, manifesting in skin reactions. Some people may break out in a rash immediately. In others the rash may not appear for twenty-four hours after coming in contact with the irritant. Mercury and silver in dental fillings, for example, can cause heavy metal poisoning.

Common allergic responses to foreign chemicals are watery eyes, ringing in the ears, stuffy nose, diarrhea, nausea, and upset stomach. Other symptoms of chemical allergies include asthma, bronchitis, arthritis, fatigue, eczema, depression, and headache. Any of these reactions can be your body's response to air pollution; contaminants such as gas, oil, or coal fumes; formaldehyde; chlorine; phenol; carbolic acid; insecticides; disinfectants; paint; hair sprays; and household cleaning products.

In order to effectively manage chemical allergies, you must first determine which chemicals are producing the allergic reaction. Once this has been determined, you can avoid coming in contact with these chemicals.

The following supplement program is designed to protect you from chemical allergies.

NUTRIENTS

SUPPLEMENT	SUGGESTED DOSAGE	COMMENTS
Very Important		
SOD/CAT from Biotec Foods	As directed on label.	A potent free radical scavenger.
Vitamin A and vitamin E	Start with 100,000 IU vitamin A and 400–800 IU vitamin E orally. After 1 month, decrease the dose of A to 50,000 IU and then to 25,000 IU.	Powerful free radical scavengers and immune enhancers.
Vitamin B$_6$ (pyridoxine) with extra niacinamide (B$_3$)	100 mg 3 times daily. 500 mg 3 times daily.	Vitamin B$_6$ acts as a natural antihistamine. It also aids in detoxifying foreign substances through the kidneys.
Vitamin C plus bioflavonoids	3,000–15,000 mg daily in divided doses.	A powerful, natural antihistamine. *See* ASCORBIC ACID FLUSH in Part Three.
Important		
Coenzyme Q$_{10}$	60 mg daily.	Research is being conducted on coenzyme Q$_{10}$'s ability to counter histamines.
Selenium	200 mcg daily.	Essential in immune function and protection of cells.
Vitamin B complex	100–200 mg daily.	Many doctors use liver injections because absorption of the B vitamins is hindered in those with allergies.
Zinc and copper	50 mg daily. 3 mg daily.	Important in heavy metal detoxification; copper is needed to replace levels that were reduced due to high doses of vitamin C.
Helpful		
Dioxychlor from American Biologics	5 drops in water twice daily.	A potent detoxifier.
Garlic tablets (Kyolic)	2 tablets 3 times daily.	A powerful immunostimulant.
L-Methionine and L-cysteine plus L-glutamic acid (amino acids)	Take on an empty stomach with juice. Do *not* take with milk.	Excellent detoxifiers, expecially of the liver.
Manganese chelate	As directed.	Interacts with zinc and copper.
Pancreatic enzymes	3–6 tablets with meals.	Both pancreatic and proteolytic enzymes are needed for proper digestion and assimilation of necessary nutrients.
Proteolytic enzymes	6 tablets between meals.	
Thymus glandular	As directed on label.	Important for immune function.

RECOMMENDATIONS

☐ If you experience any of the symptoms described above, see an allergy specialist.

☐ Avoid foods that have been sprayed or that contain either artificial colorings (found in some apples and oranges), ripening agents, or protective waxes (found on some cucumbers).

☐ Supplement your diet with plenty of fiber. Oat bran is a good source of fiber. Pectin (found in apples) can also be a useful addition to your diet. Supplements containing pectin are available. It removes unwanted metals and toxins.

☐ Read food labels carefully. Avoid F, D, and C yellow #5 dyes.

CONSIDERATIONS

☐ Avoid antihistamines if you have glaucoma or prostate problems.

☐ Drink only steam-distilled water.

☐ *See also* ALLERGIES in Part Two.

Chemical Poisoning

Excessive exposure to toxic chemicals and radiation can lead to chemical poisoning. Like toxic metals, poisonous chemicals entering the body will decrease the functioning capacity of its organs. The body's immune system is threatened by these chemicals and will try to cleanse itself of these poisons. Damage to the liver can occur if your body cannot rid itself of these toxins.

Chemical poisoning occurs most often in people who use chemicals or are exposed to them in an industrial environment or who use excess amounts of chemical sprays. Those working in greenhouses and using insecticides may develop boils or lesions about the face and neck. This is the body's attempt to rid itself of these poisons.

NUTRIENTS

SUPPLEMENT	SUGGESTED DOSAGE	COMMENTS
Very Important		
Protein supplement (free form amino acids)	¼ tsp. under the tongue on an empty stomach twice daily.	Helps liver function. Free form amino acids allow rapid assimilation.
Raw liver extract (crude)	For severe chemical poisoning, injections are best.	Used by many physicians.
Superoxide dismutase (SOD) from Biotec Foods	As directed on label.	A powerful free radical destroyer.
Vitamin B complex (high potency) with extra choline and inositol	For severe chemical poisoning, injections are best. Use only under the recommendation and supervision of your physician.	Protects the liver and bodily functions.
Vitamin C plus bioflavonoids	5,000–10,000 mg daily in divided doses.	Aids in the elimination of the toxic substance. *See* ASCORBIC ACID FLUSH in Part Three.

SUPPLEMENT	SUGGESTED DOSAGE	COMMENTS
Important		
L-Cysteine and L-methionine (amino acids)	Take on an empty stomach with juice. Do *not* take with milk.	Removes toxins and rebuilds the body.
Selenium	200 mcg daily.	Works with vitamins C and E to detoxify the body.
Vitamin E	400–800 IU daily.	A powerful antioxidant.
Helpful		
Coenzyme Q₁₀	30–60 mg daily.	Aids in rebuilding the immune system and in providing oxygen to the tissues.
Dioxychlor from American Biologics	5 drops in water twice daily.	Delivers oxygen to the tissues.
Garlic capsules (Kyolic)	2 capsules 3 times daily.	Odorless garlic. Helps to detoxify and cleanse the bloodstream.
Multivitamin and mineral complex	As directed on label.	All nutrients are needed to aid in strengthening the immune system and lessening toxicity.

RECOMMENDATIONS

☐ A well-balanced, high-fiber diet is important. Fiber will help cleanse the system. Avoid chemicals whenever possible. Try to use all organic foods.

☐ Recommended foods include almonds, apricots, bananas, barley, beans, beets, brown rice, carrots, dates, oatmeal, fish, garlic, grapes, hazel and Brazil nuts, lemons, lentils, onions, spinach, and yogurt.

☐ A cleansing fast is recommended for three days each month to help the body get rid of toxins. *See* FASTING in Part Three, and follow the instructions.

☐ Drink distilled water only.

CONSIDERATIONS

☐ Before being tested for allergies, ask the physician about procedure. As many as 40 percent of physicians switch needles, but use the same syringe according to Jerald Koepke, M.D., of the University of Colorado. Allergy testing with reused syringes can transmit Hepatitis or even AIDS.

☐ *See also* CHEMICAL ALLERGIES in Part Two.

Is NutraSweet a Poisonous Sugar Substitute?

Due to America's obsession with dieting, the popularity of NutraSweet has soared. Because it is about 200 times sweeter than sugar, much smaller amounts of NutraSweet are needed to sweeten the taste of foods. This brand-name artificial sweetener pervades supermarket shelves. It is especially prevalent in diet products and can be found in the following products:

- instant breakfasts.
- breath mints.
- cereals.
- sugar-free chewing gum.
- cocoa mixes.
- coffee beverages.
- frozen desserts.
- gelatin desserts.
- juice beverages.
- laxatives.
- multivitamins.
- milk drinks.
- nonprescription pharmaceuticals.
- shake mixes.
- soft drinks.
- tabletop sweeteners.
- tea beverages.
- instant teas and coffees.
- topping mixes.
- wine coolers.
- yogurt.

Aspartame, the chemical name for NutraSweet, consists of three components: phenylalanine, aspartic acid, and methanol. Because NutraSweet contains methanol, a human specific and highly toxic poison, its safety should be examined.

Methanol is converted to formaldehyde and formic acid—two substances that have a toxic effect on the thymus gland. The cumulative effects of high doses of aspartame, however, are unknown. Many skeptics are concerned about its cumulative effects in people who are drinking up to one or two liters of drinks sweetened with aspartame a day.

A significant number of complaints from people allegedly suffering ill-effects from aspartame have been received by the Food and Drug Administration. Common complaints voiced by people using NutraSweet are that it causes malaise, nausea, recurrent headaches, dizziness, and visual disturbances. The FDA agrees that a small segment of the population may be sensitive to aspartame, however the same holds true for many other food substances such as strawberries and pineapples. Those individuals who have a reaction to it should refrain from using foods containing aspartame.

Aspartame is a highly toxic substance for those individuals who have inherited the disease phenylketonuria. In these individuals, amino acids accumulate in toxic amounts in the body and the phenylalanine in aspartame can be very dangerous for them.

The effects of increased consumption of the two amino acids in NutraSweet has also been raised. Although concern about the effects of NutraSweet on the fetus and children have been raised, no adverse effects have been documented.

Because NutraSweet has been on the market for a relatively short period, pregnant women should avoid NutraSweet until more extensive testing has been done on the effects of aspartame. Instead of choosing artificially sweetened beverages, drink fresh juices that are naturally sweet. These are nutritious, and do not contain artificial coloring or preservatives. Freshly squeezed juices also offer the benefits of raw foods. You can purchase a juicer from a department store, a health food store, or a mail order company.

Chicken Pox

This childhood disease is caused by a virus and first manifests as a fever and headache. About twenty-four to thirty-six hours later, small round "pimples" appear on the torso, face, and body. They are filled with fluid and look like water blisters. The fluid dislodges from the swollen areas of skin, forming a crust. These eruptions will continue in cycles, lasting from three days to one week. The blisters and crusts are infectious and very itchy. Care must be taken so that the child does not scratch them, as this could lead to infection and scarring. Keep the child's nails short and clean, and bathe the child often.

The virus that causes chicken pox in children, *Varicella zoster*, also causes shingles in adults. It is most important to keep infected children away from the elderly. Once the scabs are gone, the child is no longer infectious. Gratefully, one siege of chicken pox accords a lifetime immunity against the illness.

The dosages in the following table are for adults. Adjust the dosage for children.

NUTRIENTS

SUPPLEMENT	SUGGESTED DOSAGE	COMMENTS
Essential		
Beta-carotene	15,000 IU daily.	Heals tissues and stimulates the immune system.

Vitamin A capsules or emulsion	20,000 IU capsules daily for 1 month, dropping to 15,000 IU daily or 100,000 IU emulsion for 1 week, dropping to 75,000 IU for 1 week.	An immunostimulant that aids healing of tissues.
Vitamin C		Powerful immune stimulant that aids in keeping down fever. See ASCORBIC ACID FLUSH, Part Three.
Very Important		
Vitamin E	400–600 IU daily.	A powerful free radical scavenger that carries oxygen and promotes healing.
Potassium plus	99 mg daily.	Needed for fever and quicker healing.
zinc	80 mg daily.	
Helpful		
Raw thymus glandular	As directed on label.	Stimulates the production of T-lymphocytes by the thymus gland. Needed for immune function.

HERBS

☐ The following herbs are recommended for chicken pox: ginger, goldenseal, pau d'arco, and red clover.

RECOMMENDATIONS

☐ Take hot baths using tea prepared with some of the recommended herbs. Sponge the affected area with the tea. Wet compresses help to control the itching; use these often. Avoid scratching the spots. Give infants and older people catnip tea (sweetened with molasses) to drink.

☐ Do not give any cow's milk or formula to infants while feverish. Instead, use pure, freshly made juices that have been diluted with a combination of steam-distilled water and 100 to 1,000 milligrams of vitamin C. Give the infant lots of water. You can purchase almond or soy milk from health food stores for infants who are six months or older. If your pediatrician deems it appropriate, use catnip tea enemas to reduce fever in children over two (*see* ENEMAS in Part Three) and use a quarter teaspoon of lobelia herb extract every two hours. Increase or decrease according to the age of the child. If the child vomits, cut dose to 2–3 times a day.

☐ Give ginger baths using cool water. When the fever drops and the appetite returns, give only mashed bananas; avocados; raw, fresh applesauce; or yogurt. Do not give them cooked or processed foods.

CONSIDERATIONS

☐ If the sores become infected, an antibiotic ointment is usually prescribed.

☐ Drink juice, including protein powder and brewer's yeast. Use as much freshly made juice as possible and also pure vegetable broth.

☐ If taking adrenal cortical steroids such as cortisone, swelling can result around the larynx and cause serious problems. See your doctor.

☐ *See* FASTING in Part Three, and follow the instructions.

Chlamydia

Chlamydia is a sexually transmitted disease. It is believed to be twice as common as gonorrhea, and ten times as widespread as herpes simplex. It is estimated that between 3 to 10 million sexually active teenagers have contracted this disease. It is not known how many adult Americans have chlamydia.

No symptoms are found in 10 percent of the men and 70 percent of the women who have chlamydia. When symptoms do occur, they include genital inflammation, vaginal or urethral discharge, difficulty in urinating, painful intercourse, and itching around the inflamed area (these symptoms affect both men and women). If untreated, inflammatory disease and irreparable damage to the reproductive system can occur. Infertility may result, and hysterectomy may be required. Complications grow as time passes, so treatment for this disorder should not be delayed.

In males, prostatitis and inflammation of the seminal vesicles may be caused by chlamydia. Symptoms for men include pain when urinating and a watery mucous urethral discharge. Early treatment is important, because chronic prostatitis or infertility can result if treatment is delayed. Both sexes have similar discharges, and it is through this discharge that the disease is sexually transmitted.

Both partners must be treated for this disorder so that the disease is not transmitted back and forth. Antibiotics such as tetracycline will heal chlamydia. Persons under thirty-five who have more than one sexual partner should be tested yearly.

A new diagnostic technique called "antigen detection testing" is an inexpensive and simple test for chlamydia, and can be easily done in most laboratories. There is an inexpensive test by Syna called Micro-Trak

134

that can detect chlamydia within thirty minutes in a laboratory. Another test that is not quite as accurate is called Chlamydiazyme. This test gives results in about four hours. A simple urine test that detects chlamydia is also available.

Chlamydia has also been linked to one form of arthritis in young women. This parasite was found in the joints of nearly half of the women with unexplained arthritis who were tested.

NUTRIENTS

SUPPLEMENT	SUGGESTED DOSAGE	COMMENTS
Important		
Garlic capsules (Kyolic)	2 capsules 3 times daily.	Odorless garlic that acts as a natural antibiotic and aids in healing.
Vitamin C (buffered form)	1,500 mg 4 times daily.	Immunostimulant that aids healing.
Vitamin E	600 IU daily.	Can also be used directly on the inflamed site. Cut the capsule open and apply.
Helpful		
Coenzyme Q10	60 mg daily.	Aids in healing and is a powerful antioxidant and immune stimulant.
Germanium	200 mg daily.	Carries oxygen to the cells and benefits the immune system.
Kelp	6 tablets daily.	A rich source of minerals.
High potency multivitamin complex with beta-carotene	As directed on label.	Necessary for healing.
Proteolytic enzymes	3 tablets between meals and at bedtime.	Acts as an anti-inflammatory.
Superoxide dismutase (SOD) from Biotec Foods	As directed on label.	Important for immune function.
Zinc	50 mg daily.	Important for immune function and healing.

HERBS

☐ Echinacea, goldenseal, pau d'arco, and red clover aid in healing.

RECOMMENDATIONS

☐ Acidophilus is needed to replenish the "friendly" bacteria destroyed by the antibiotics.

☐ Diet is an important aid in healing. Avoid highly processed foods and junk foods. Diet should consist mainly of fresh vegetables, fruits, brown rice, whole grains, seeds and nuts, white fish, and turkey. Avoid fried foods and chicken. Approximately one-third of all chickens in this country contain pathogenic bacteria such as salmonella. This type of bacteria is not found in turkey. Drink steam-distilled water, sugar-free juices, and herb teas.

☐ *See also* SEXUALLY TRANSMITTED DISEASES in Part Two.

Cholesterol Problems

See HIGH CHOLESTEROL.

Chronic Fatigue Syndrome

The Epstein Barr virus (EBV) is what causes chronic fatigue syndrome, a condition that has become widespread in the United States. The virus is also the cause of mononucleosis. EBV is a member of the herpes family and is related to the viruses that cause genital herpes and shingles.

The symptoms of chronic fatigue syndrome, also called the "yuppie disease," are fever, sore throat, swollen glands (lymph nodes), extreme fatigue, appetite loss, recurrent upper respiratory tract infections, intestinal problems, jaundice, anxiety, depression, irritability and mood swings, sleep disturbances, sensitivity to light and heat, temporary memory loss, difficulty in concentrating, headache, spasms, and aching muscles and joints. The symptoms of this syndrome resemble flu and other viral symptoms, so it is not always diagnosed correctly. It is often misdiagnosed as hypochondria, psychosomatic illness, or depression, because the tests that are routinely ordered by doctors give negative results. A cure or vaccine for this virus has not yet been developed. It is difficult for doctors to identify, and the symptoms vary widely. This syndrome is three times more prevalent in women than in men.

The Center for Disease Control in Atlanta estimates that tens of thousands of people are infected with this virus. Many are only carriers of the virus and are unaware that they have it because they have no symptoms. Once EBV is contracted, it remains in the body, but most people develop antibodies to EBV.

Epstein Barr virus is highly contagious. It can be passed from one person to another by close contact, kissing, sharing food, and coughing, and it can be sexually transmitted. A person cannot become immune to

EBV, and antibiotics will not help, because it is a viral disease. The virus causes "overreaction" of the immune system, which results in a type of immunity "burnout."

Chronic fatigue syndrome may also be caused by the fungus *Candida albicans*, chronic mercury poisoning from dental amalgam fillings, anemia, hypoglycemia, hypothyroidism, and sleep problems.

If a person has elevated antibodies and if several of the symptoms mentioned above persist for two to three months, EBV is suspected, especially if all other symptom-producing illnesses have been ruled out. Sixteen experts have said that a diagnosis of EBV can be made only when the physician notes persistent fatigue over six months with at least eleven other symptoms that persist or recur over six months. The physician must rule out endocrine diseases, AIDS, infections, anemia, parasites, and the other diseases that cause similar symptoms.

Even though EBV is not life threatening, it is still incurable and can do serious damage to the immune system. It is important that family members fully understand this disorder and realize that the person suffering from this virus is not exaggerating or faking the symptoms.

NUTRIENTS

SUPPLEMENT	SUGGESTED DOSAGE	COMMENTS
Very Important		
Ascorbic acid (buffered) with bioflavonoids	5,000–10,000 mg daily.	Has a powerful antiviral effect.
Coenzyme Q$_{10}$	75 mg daily.	Enhances the effectiveness of the immune system.
Egg lecithin	As directed on label. Must be taken with meals.	Promotes energy and enhances immunity.
Maxidophilus or Megadophilus or Bifido Factor/ Life Start Two	As directed on label.	EBV and candidiasis are commonly found together. Candida destroy the necessary "friendly" bacteria.
Proteolytic enzymes	2–3 tablets between meals and at bedtime on an empty stomach.	Removes undigested food from the bloodstream and reduces inflammation.
Vitamin A and E emulsion	50,000 IU vitamin A for 1 month. 400–800 IU vitamin E for 1 month. Slowly drop to 25,000 IU vitamin A and 400 IU vitamin E.	Powerful free radical scavengers. Use caution when taking vitamin A in pill form because liver disorders are related to this disease. Powerful free radical destroyers. Emulsion is assimilated quickly.
Important		
DMG (Gluconic from DaVinci Labs)	50 mg 3 times daily.	Enhances oxygen utilization and destroys free radicals.
Garlic capsules (Kyolic) plus Kyo-Green	2 capsules with meals.	Promotes immune function and increases energy.
Germanium	200 mg and up.	Improves tissue oxygenation and immune function.
Protein supplement (Free form amino acids from Ecological Formulas)	Take daily as directed on label.	For tissue and organ repair.
Vitamin B complex (stress formula) or	100 mg 3 times daily.	Essential for increased energy levels and normal brain function. Use hypoallergenic brand.
vitamin B complex (injectable form) and	2 cc under doctor's supervision only.	
liver and	2 cc	
vitamin B$_{12}$	1 cc	
Helpful		
Black currant oil capsules	2 capsules with meals.	Used successfully in Europe. Contains GLA (gamma-linoleic acid) and all of the essential fatty acids.
Multivitamin and mineral complex (high potency and hypoallergenic) with	100 mg 3 times daily.	
beta-carotene and	15,000 IU daily.	
calcium and	1,500 mg daily.	
magnesium and	1,000 mg daily.	
potassium and	99 mg daily.	
selenium and	200 mcg daily.	
zinc	50 mg daily.	
Raw thymus and spleen plus raw glandular complex	As directed on label.	Potentiates immune system. *See* GLANDULAR THERAPY in Part Three.

HERBS

☐ Teas brewed from the herbs burdock root, dandelion, echinacea, goldenseal, and pau d'arco will promote healing. Combine or alternate the teas, and drink four to six cups daily.

RECOMMENDATIONS

☐ Sixty percent of the people infected with EBV also have Candida, and should add some form of acidophilus to their diet. Eat soured products such as yogurt. Consume plenty of water—eight glasses a day—and juices. Make sure that the bowels move daily, and add fiber to the diet. Occasionally, cleansing enemas should be used. *See* ENEMAS in Part Three. Eliminate each of the following from the diet: fried foods; junk foods; processed foods; stimulants including coffee, tea, and soft drinks; sugar; and white flour products such as bread and spaghetti.

☐ A well-balanced diet of 50 percent raw foods and fresh "live" juices is beneficial. The diet should consist mostly of vegetables, fruits, whole grains, seeds, raw nuts, skinless turkey, and deep-water fish. These quality foods supply nutrients that ultimately renew energy and build immunity. Do not eat shellfish.

☐ Take chlorophyll in tablet form or obtain from the liquid of vegetables, such as a "green drink" from leafy vegetables, wheatgrass, or Kyo-Green from Wakunaga of America Company. Plenty of rest and a proper diet are very important. Take a protein supplement from a vegetable source—Spiru-Tein from Nature's Plus is a good protein drink for between meals.

☐ No aspirin should be taken because Reye's syndrome may result. Make sure that you do not overexert yourself with heavy exercising.

☐ For more information on EBV, contact the National Institute of Allergies and Infectious Diseases, 9000 Rockville Pike, NIAID-OC, Building 31, Room 7A-32, Bethesda, MD 20892, or call this service at (301)496-5717.

☐ *See also* MONONUCLEOSIS in Part Two.

Circulatory Problems

There are many disorders associated with circulatory problems. High blood pressure or hypertension results when cholesterol plaque deposits along the walls of the arteries, and causes them to harden and constrict. Because the arteries are constricted, the blood exerts a greater force against the walls of the blood vessels, causing the blood pressure to rise. Arteriosclerosis or "hardening of the arteries" is associated with lack of circulation due to narrowing of the arteries from fatty deposits as well. In addition, circulatory problems can lead to stroke and angina pectoris (chest pain). *See* CARDIOVASCULAR DISEASE, ARTERIOSCLEROSIS, and HIGH BLOOD PRESSURE in Part Two for additional information.

Another circulatory disease brought on by chronic inflammation of the veins and arteries in the lower parts of the body is Buerger's disease. This disease is most prevalent among people who smoke. Early signs of Buerger's disease are a tingling sensation (commonly referred to as "pins and needles") and a burning sensation in the fingers and toes.

Another serious circulatory condition called Raynaud's disease is characterized by constriction and spasm of the blood vessels in the extremities, such as in the fingers, toes, and tip of the nose. Cold, stress, smoking, and other factors may cause fingers and toes to numb; extremities may appear colorless due to lack of circulation and arterial spasm. This disease most commonly affects women and occasionally leads to gangrene. *See* RAYNAUD'S DISEASE in Part Two for further information. In addition, poor circulation can result from varicose veins that have developed due to a loss of elasticity in the walls of the veins (*see* VARICOSE VEINS in Part Two).

Because sluggish circulation can be caused by several things, you should see your doctor if it is persistent.

NUTRIENTS

SUPPLEMENT	SUGGESTED DOSAGE	COMMENTS
Essential		
L-Carnitine (amino acid)	500 mg twice daily.	Helps to strengthen the heart muscle and to promote circulation by transporting long fatty acid chains.
Very Important		
Chlorophyll	Liquid or pill form as directed on label.	Enhances circulation and helps build healthy cells. Also prepare as fresh "green drink" made from green leafy vegetables.
Coenzyme Q$_{10}$	100 mg daily.	Improves tissue oxygenation.
Garlic capsules (Kyolic)	2 capsules with meals.	This odorless garlic helps to strengthen the heart muscle and lowers blood pressure.
Lecithin	2 capsules 3 times daily or 1 tbsp. in dry form before meals.	Dr. Rinse's Formula is sometimes used instead of lecithin. Lecithin emulsifies (breaks up) fats.
Multidigestive enzymes	Take with meals as directed on label.	Aids digestion and circulation and enhances oxygen use in all body tissues.
Vitamin B complex with extra folic acid, B$_6$, B$_{12}$, thiamine (B$_1$), and PABA	Injections may be helpful.	Improves circulation by metabolizing fat and cholesterol.
Vitamin C plus bioflavonoids	5,000–10,000 mg daily in divided doses.	Helps prevent blood clotting.
Important		
Calcium and magnesium	1,500–2,000 mg calcium and 750–1,000 mg magnesium, divided up after meals and at bedtime.	Calcium is essential in normal blood viscosity and also strengthens the heartbeat.
DMG (Gluconic from DaVinci Labs)	50 mg twice daily.	Enhances tissue oxygenation.
Germanium	200 mg daily.	Enhances tissue oxygenation.

| Multivitamin and mineral complex | As directed on label. | Basic to good circulatory function. |
| Vitamin A and E emulsion | 50,000 IU vitamin A daily. Use this form for safe assimilation, or start at 200 IU vitamin E and increase slowly to 1,000 IU. | Vitamin A aids in storage of fat and acts as an antioxidant. Vitamin E also inhibits the formation of free radicals. |

Helpful		
Choline with inositol and niacin (B₃)	100 mg each 3 times daily with meals.	Choline helps to remove fat deposits and improve circulation. Inositol and niacin help to lower cholesterol.
Copper	3 mg daily.	Needed for mineral balance with zinc.
L-Methionine and L-cysteine (amino acids)	Take with vitamins B₆ and C on an empty stomach with juice. Do *not* take with milk.	Protects and preserves cells by detoxifying harmful toxins. Prevents accumulation of fat both in the liver and in the arteries (which may obstruct blood flow).
Proteolytic enzymes	2 tablets between meals.	Acts upon undigested food in the colon and bloodstream.
Selenium	200 mcg daily.	Selenium deficiency has been linked to heart disorders.
Zinc chelate	50 mg daily.	Needed for immune function.

HERBS

☐ Use black cohosh, butcher's broom, cayenne, chickweed, Circu formula (an herbal combination from Switzerland), gentian root, ginkgo biloba extract, goldenseal, hawthorn berries, horseradish, horsetail, hyssop, licorice root, pleurisy root, rose hips, and wormwood. Cayenne increases the pulse rate, while black cohosh slows it. Ginkgo is being used for circulation disorders in many clinics.

RECOMMENDATIONS

☐ Make sure that your diet is high in fiber. Oat bran can help lower your cholesterol levels. Include the following in your diet: bananas, broccoli, brown rice, endive, garlic, lima beans, onions, pears, peas, and spinach. Eliminate animal protein and fatty foods (such as red meat), white flour, and sugar from your diet. Do not use stimulants such as coffee, colas, and tobacco, or foods with a lot of spices.

☐ Give yourself a dry massage over your entire body using a loofah sponge or natural bath brush. Also dip a towel in cold water and rub it briskly over parts of the body.

☐ Regular exercise is important to help blood flow and keep arteries soft and unclogged.

☐ Keep your weight down.

CONSIDERATIONS

☐ Use steam-distilled water only.

☐ *See also* CARDIOVASCULAR DISEASE, HIGH BLOOD PRESSURE, HIGH CHOLESTEROL, HYPOTHYROID, RAYNAUD'S DISEASE, and VARICOSE VEINS, all in Part Two.

☐ *See also* CHELATION THERAPY in Part Three.

Cirrhosis of the Liver

Cirrhosis of the liver is a degenerative, inflammatory disease in which damage and hardening of the liver cells occur. The liver is unable to function properly due to its scarred tissue, which can eventually prevent the passage of blood through the liver.

Whereas the most common cause of cirrhosis of the liver is excessive alcohol consumption, a less frequent cause is viral hepatitis. Malnutrition and chronic inflammation can also lead to liver malfunction.

In its early stages cirrhosis of the liver is characterized by constipation or diarrhea, fever, upset stomach, and jaundice. Those in the later stages of the disease may also exhibit the following: anemia, bruising due to bleeding under the skin, and edema.

NUTRIENTS

SUPPLEMENT	SUGGESTED DOSAGE	COMMENTS
Essential		
Phosphatidyl and choline and inositol	As directed on label.	Take for fatty liver.
Vitamin B complex (high potency) with extra vitamin B₁₂ and folic acid plus niacin (B₃)	Megadoses daily. / 100 mg niacin (do not exceed this dosage). Injections may be necessary. Intravenous treatment should be used only under the supervision of your physician.	Necessary for absorption of nutrients and formation of red blood cells. Allows proper digestion in the liver.
Very Important		
Garlic capsules (Kyolic)	2 capsules or tablets with meals.	Detoxifies the liver and bloodstream.

L-Methionine and L-carnitine and L-cysteine and L-glutathionine (amino acids)	As directed on label.	L-Methionine and L-carnitine help prevent accumulation of fat in the liver. L-Cysteine helps detoxify harmful toxins. L-Glutathionine is a powerful antioxidant.
Lecithin liquid or capsules	1 tbsp. or 2 capsules with meals.	A powerful fat emulsifier.
Liver extract (liquid) from Argentine beef only	As directed on label.	Prevents anemia and aids in building the liver.
Multidigestive enzymes with betaine hydrochloric acid (HCl) and ox bile extract		Needed for digestion to lessen the strain on the liver. Ox bile extract replaces the digestive enzymes produced by the gallbladder.
Important		
Alfalfa tablets or liquid	As directed on label.	Helps to build a healthy digestive tract and prevent bleeding common in those suffering from cirrhosis caused by vitamin K deficiency. Good sources of vitamin K are alfalfa sprouts and green leafy vegetables.
Calcium and magnesium chelate	1,500 mg daily divided up after meals and at bedtime. 750 mg daily magnesium chelate.	Promotes healing of tissue. Beneficial for the nervous system.
DMG (Gluconic from DaVinci Labs)	As directed on label.	Supplies oxygen for healing.
L-Arginine (amino acid)	As directed on label.	Helps to detoxify the high amounts of ammonia that can accumulate when the liver isn't functioning properly. Found in fish, legumes (kidney beans, peas, and soybeans), and seeds.
Life Start by Natren	As directed on label.	Repairs liver cells and aids in healing.
Vitamin C	3,000–8,000 mg daily in divided doses.	Buffered form is best.
Helpful		
Aerobic 07 from Aerobic Life Products	As directed on label.	Supplies oxygen in a molecular form.
Aloe vera	¼ cup in the morning and evening.	A bowel cleanser and healer. George's is a good source.
Coenzyme Q$_{10}$	100 mg daily.	Promotes oxygenation.
Germanium	200 mg daily.	Aids the immune system and relieves discomfort.
Protein supplement (free form amino acids)	As directed on label.	For a good source of protein that is easy on the liver.
Selenium	200 mcg daily.	A good detoxifier.
Spiru-Tein from Nature's Plus	Take between meals.	A vegetable protein drink that supplies essential amino acids and stabilizes the blood sugar.

Vitamin A, D, and E emulsion	As directed on label.	This form assimilates quickly, relieving stress on the liver. Avoid vitamin A in pill form.
Zinc	50 mg daily.	Needed for the immune system and the healing process.

HERBS

☐ The following herbs can be beneficial: barberry, black radish, burdock, celandine, cheonanthus, dandelion, echinacea, fennel, goldenseal, hops, horsetail, Irish moss, milk thistle extract, red clover, rose hips, suma, thyme, and wild Oregon grape. Milk thistle is beneficial because it protects the liver. Studies have shown that milk thistle extract (silymarin) repairs and rejuvenates the liver. Take two capsules of silymarin three times daily. Herbal formulas that aid in liver function include Organ Toner and Clear Stream from New Moon Extracts. Liv-R-Actin from Nature's Plus is an excellent herbal combination.

RECOMMENDATIONS

☐ A high-protein diet is beneficial, particularly if obtained from vegetable sources; do not eat foods containing animal protein. Drinking fresh vegetable juices, such as beet, carrot, dandelion extract, and "green drink," is healthful. Raw foods should comprise 75 percent of your diet. If cirrhosis is severe, consume only fresh vegetables and fruits and their juices for two weeks.

☐ Some foods to include in your diet are almonds, brewer's yeast, grains and seeds, raw goat's milk, and products derived from goat's milk.

☐ Do *not* eat raw or undercooked seafood. Limit your intake of fish—haddock, blue fish, salmon, and sardines—to two a week. The liver cannot handle the vitamin A contained in these foods. Avoid cod liver oil; never take cod liver oil with alcohol.

☐ Eliminate the following from your diet: alcohol, animal fats, candies, milk, pasteries, pepper, salt, spices, stimulants of any kind including caffeine and colas, white rice, and products containing either sugar or white flour. All prepared foods contain some of the above.

☐ Read all food labels carefully. Avoid the following products: all margarines and butters and any other hardened fats, fried and fatty foods, potato chips, melted and hard cheeses, rancid nuts and oils, and all refined and processed foods. These overwork and damage the liver. Use only nitrogen-packed nuts and cold-pressed oils.

☐ A clean colon is important. Toxins accumulate in the colon and must be excreted by the liver and kidneys. Do not use harsh laxatives to cleanse the system. Lemon enemas are preferred; take these twice weekly. Taking aloe vera juice daily will help to keep the colon clean. A product from New Moon Extracts called Mainstream is also beneficial. It contains wheatgrass. You can alternate wheatgrass enemas with coffee enemas for two weeks. They detoxify the liver. These are retention enemas; one pint is used and retained for fifteen minutes. *See* ENEMAS, Part Three.

☐ Avoid drugs unless prescribed by your doctor.

☐ Drink steam-distilled or barley water. You can make barley water by boiling one cup of barley in six pints of water for three hours. Sip the barley water throughout the day.

CONSIDERATIONS

☐ *See also* ALCOHOLISM and HEPATITIS in Part Two.

The Liver

Weighing about four pounds, the liver is the largest gland of the body and the only organ that will regenerate itself when part of it is damaged. Up to 25 percent of the liver can be removed, and within a short period of time, it will grow back to its original shape and size.

The liver has many functions, perhaps the most important of which is its secretion of bile. This fluid is stored in the gallbladder for release when needed for digestion. Bile is necessary for the digestion of fats; it breaks fat down into small globules. Bile also assists in the absorption of fat-soluble vitamins A, D, E, F, and K, and helps to assimilate calcium. In addition, bile converts beta-carotene to vitamin A. It promotes intestinal peristalsis as well, which helps prevent constipation.

After food has been absorbed into the bloodstream through the intestinal wall, it is transported by way of the hepatic portal system to the liver. In the liver nutrients such as iron and vitamins A, B_{12}, and D are extracted from the bloodstream and stored for future use. These stored substances are utilized for everyday activities and in times of physical stress. In addition, the liver plays an important role in fat metabolism, in the synthesis of fatty acids from amino acids and sugars, in the production of lipoproteins, cholesterol, and phospholipids, and in the oxidation of fat to produce energy. Finally, excess food is converted to fat in the liver, which is then transported to the fatty tissues of the body for storage.

The liver also acts as a detoxifier. Protein metabolism and bacterial fermentation of food in the intestines produces the by-product ammonia, which is detoxified by the liver. The liver regulates protein metabolism. In addition to detoxifying ammonia, the liver also combines toxic substances including metabolic waste, insecticide residues, drugs, alcohol, and chemicals with other substances that are less toxic. These substances are then excreted from the kidneys. Thus in order to have proper liver function, you must also have proper kidney function. Physicians have found that when either the liver or kidney appears to be malfunctioning, treating both organs produces the best health results.

In addition to its many other functions, the liver is responsible for regulating blood sugar levels by converting thyroxine, a thyroid hormone, into its more active form. Inadequate conversion by the liver may lead to hypothyroidism. The liver creates GTF (Glucose Tolerance Factor) from chromium and glutathione. GTF is required for insulin to regulate blood sugar levels properly. Excess sugar will be stored in the body as glycogen, and then converted back to sugar when needed for energy. The liver also breaks down hormones like adrenalin, aldosterone, estrogen, and insulin after they have performed their needed functions.

The following nutrients can help maintain proper liver function.

NUTRIENTS

SUPPLEMENT	SUGGESTED DOSAGE	COMMENTS
Coenzyme Q_{10}	60 mg daily.	Supplies oxygen to the liver. A potent liver protector.
Free form amino acids	Take on an empty stomach, as directed on label.	Source of protein that is easy on the liver because it has already been broken down.
Lecithin	1 tbsp. before meals or take in capsule form.	Prevents fat build-up (i.e., fatty liver).
Liv-R-Actin from Nature's Plus	2 capsules before meals.	Contains milk thistle, which is important for rebuilding the liver.
L-Cysteine and L-glutathione and L-methionine (amino acids)	500 mg each of L-cysteine and L-methionine daily; 100 mg glutathione. Take before meals.	Aids in liver detoxification and protects the liver cells.
Liver injections plus vitamin B_{12} or dessicated liver from Argentine beef tablets	Use only under doctor's supervision.	Supplies needed B vitamins, iron, and other nutrients that help to rebuild the liver cells.
Multidigestive enzymes including ox bile	As directed on label.	Aids in digestion. Relieves the liver of some of its burden.
Multivitamin and mineral complex containing		Needed for repairing of all tissues.
B complex and	50 mg daily.	
selenium and	200 mcg daily.	
zinc	30 mg daily.	

Phosphatidyl choline	As directed on label.	Prevents fatty build-up and is important for energy production in the liver.
Unsaturated fatty acids	As directed on label.	Needed for cell protection.
Vitamin C	5,000 mg daily in divided doses.	An immune enhancer and powerful antioxidant. Neutralizes toxic substances.
Vitamin E	600 IU daily.	A powerful antioxidant. Protects the liver from damage.

HERBS

☐ Use silymarin extract and calandine daily to help maintain liver function.

RECOMMENDATIONS

☐ Do not use more than 10,000 IU vitamin A and avoid cod liver oil.

☐ Avoid constipating foods. The liver has to work twice as hard if you are constipated. Be sure the diet contains sufficient amounts of choline, inositol, lecithin, bulk, and fiber.

☐ A three-day juice fast once every thirty days is important in any liver detoxification program. *See* FASTING in Part Three. To help cleanse the liver while fasting, drink beet juice, carrot juice, black radish extract, and dandelion extract. Chlorophyll and distilled water with lemon are excellent blood purifiers and liver cleansers. Regular cleansing of the body, especially the liver, is vital to maintaining good health.

☐ Increase consumption of foods high in potassium, kelp, dulse, blackstrap molasses, brewer's yeast, rice and wheat bran, almonds, raisins, prunes, bananas, and seeds.

☐ Do not smoke and avoid all alcohol, coffee, fish, fowl, meat, salt, soft drinks, sugar, tea, and spicy or fried foods until the liver is functioning properly again.

☐ Drinking plenty of water, especially steam-distilled, is very important. When taking supplements, always take with a full glass of water.

CONSIDERATIONS

☐ Animal studies indicate that the American diet produces liver damage. Improper diet results in allergies, digestive disorders, a low energy level, and an inability to detoxify harmful substances. The four basic reasons for poor liver function are:

1. *The presence of cumulative poisons*. The presence of alcohol, insecticides, preservatives, and other toxins can impair the liver. Even though the particular toxin may not accumulate in the liver, liver function suffers because the functioning of the pancreas and kidneys is adversely affected by the toxin.
2. *An improper diet.* A diet that is low in protein and high in carbohydrates and fats, especially saturated rancid fats from fried foods and hydrogenated fats, does not provide the individual with sufficient protein building blocks necessary for repair. Protein from a vegetable source is beneficial.

    Poor food choices containing little nutrients harm the liver, which tries to convert the food product to a useful substance, but instead produces a substance that has been robbed of all its nutritional value. Poor food choices include refined white flour products, white sugar products, and imitation foods that appear and taste like an original product. These imitations have reduced vitamin, mineral, and enzyme content. Processed foods must be avoided for good health. Also avoid junk foods and foods with additives, preservatives, and chemicals.
3. *Overeating.* Overeating is the most common cause of liver malfunction. The liver absorbs food like a sponge. Overeating creates excess work for the liver, resulting in liver fatigue. When the liver is overworked, it may not detoxify harmful substances properly before they enter the bloodstream.
4. *Drugs.* Drugs put a great strain on the liver. All drugs are foreign and unnatural to the body. These foreign substances cause the liver to work overtime in excreting these toxins. The liver neutralizes the effects of drugs on the body. When excessive amounts of alcohol enter the liver, the liver begins to lose its functioning capacity. When organic substances are used to treat disease, this rarely occurs. In fact, using organic substances actually aids and fortifies the body.

Other factors that contribute to liver malfunction include the presence of *Candida*, the use of contraceptives, and the consumption of caffeine.

Cold

See COMMON COLD.

Cold Sores (Fever Blisters)

Cold sores or fever blisters are caused by herpes simplex virus I. They usually occur with a fever, infection, or cold, or after exposure to sun and wind, when under stress, during menstruation, or when the immune system is depressed. These sores are very contagious. They appear three to ten days after exposure and may last up to three weeks. If you are prone to allergies, you most likely have a weak immune system and may be susceptible to cold sores. (*See* ALLERGIES in Part Two.)

The first sign of a cold sore is a local tenderness with a small bump. When this bump turns into a blister, there may be more tenderness in the area. The adjacent lymph nodes may become swollen and tender. In some cases, pus oozes from the blisters, which makes eating difficult. Fortunately, there is always less discomfort with a reoccurrence of cold sores.

NUTRIENTS

SUPPLEMENT	SUGGESTED DOSAGE	COMMENTS
Essential		
L-Lysine cream	As directed on label.	Apply on sores. Eliminates the virus.
Vitamin B complex (high stress formula)	100–150 mg twice daily.	Important for healing and immune function.
Zinc gluconate lozenges	Dissolve in mouth every 3 hours for 2 days. Then reduce to 2 lozenges daily.	Lozenges are absorbed quickly and stimulate immune function in order to fight the virus.
Very Important		
Acidophilus or Megadophilus	As directed on label.	Inhibits pathogenic organisms, such as the herpes virus.
Garlic capsules (Kyolic)	2 capsules 3 times daily.	Acts as a natural antibiotic and immunity enhancer.
Vitamin C	3,000–6,000 mg daily in divided doses.	Use a nonacidic form such as calcium ascorbate or sago palm. Eliminates the virus and potentiates immune function.
Important		
Calcium and magnesium	1,500 mg daily. 750–1,000 mg daily.	Relieves stress.
L-Lysine (amino acid)	50 mg twice daily.	Don't take this antiviral amino acid for long periods—no longer than 6 months. Prolonged use causes imbalance of the essential amino acid arginine.
Unsaturated fatty acids	As directed on label.	Aids skin in healing.
Helpful		
Multivitamin and mineral complex		
Vitamin A emulsion	Emulsion as directed on label or 50,000 IU daily in capsule form.	Vitamins A and E are needed for healing of tissue in mouth and lip area.
Vitamin E	400 IU daily.	

HERBS

☐ For cold sores, use goldenseal, echinacea, pau d'arco, and red clover.

RECOMMENDATIONS

☐ Eat raw vegetables, yogurt, and soured products. If cold sore outbreaks occur often, check for low thyroid function (*see* HYPOTHYROID in Part Two).

CONSIDERATIONS

☐ The prescription drug acyclovir is being used for cold sores in oral or topical form.

☐ *See also* HERPES VIRUS in Part Two.

Colitis

Colitis refers to an inflammation of the colon. The mucous membranes of the colon become inflamed, and small, pouch-like areas are formed. This condition may be acute or chronic. It often strikes young and early middle-aged adults. Its symptoms include cramps in the abdominal area, diarrhea, and an almost continual need to eliminate. Often there is blood in the stool.

There are several types of colitis, and they range from mild to serious. Enteritis and ileitis are types of inflammation of the small intestine often associated with colitis. Severe colitis is called ulcerative colitis. With this condition, the colon is both inflamed and lined with ulcers.

Some of the causes of colitis are poor eating habits, stress, and an allergy to certain foods. A food sensitivity test is advised.

NUTRIENTS

SUPPLEMENT	SUGGESTED DOSAGE	COMMENTS
Essential		
Proteolytic enzymes and	2 tablets between meals.	Vital for proper digestion.
multidigestive enzymes (low in hydrochloric acid (HCl), high in pancreatin)	2 tablets after meals.	Anti-inflammatory enzymes.

Very Important		
Acidophilus	Twice daily on an empty stomach.	Normalizes the intestinal bacteria. If you have a milk intolerance, use a milk-free product.
Aerobic Bulk Cleanse (ABC)	1 tbsp. in juice on an empty stomach in the morning.	A colon cleanser.
Alfalfa capsules or liquid	3 times daily as directed on label.	Supplies needed vitamin K and chlorophyll for healing.
Protein supplement (free form amino acids)	Twice daily on an empty stomach.	Free form amino acids are more readily available for use by the body.
Vitamin A capsules with	25,000 IU daily.	Needed for tissue repair.
vitamin E capsules	Up to 800 IU daily.	
Vitamin B complex	50–100 mg daily in divided doses.	Essential for the breakdown of fats, protein, and carbohydrates and for proper digestion. Select a hypoallergenic brand.

Helpful		
Aerobic 07 from Aerobic Life Products or Dioxychlor from American Biologics	Twice daily as directed on label.	Provides "stabilized" oxygen to the colon and destroys unwanted bacteria.
Garlic capsules (Kyolic)	2 capsules with meals.	Use yeast-free Kyolic. Has a healing effect on the colon. A natural antibiotic.
Mineral supplement with extra calcium and chromium and magnesium and zinc	As directed on label.	Malabsorption of these essential minerals is a problem with colitis. Calcium is needed for the prevention of cancer, which may occur due to constant irritation.
Raw thymus glandular	500 mg twice daily.	Important in immune function. See GLANDULAR THERAPY in Part Three.
Unsaturated fatty acids	As directed on label.	Important in cell formation. Linseed oil and primrose oil are good sources.
Vitamin C with bioflavonoids	3,000–5,000 mg daily in divided doses.	Needed for immune function and for healing of the mucous membranes. Use a nonacid-forming brand.

HERBS

☐ Chamomile, dandelion, garlic, feverfew, papaya, red clover, and yarrow extract or tea are beneficial for colitis, as is pau d'arco tea. Also good is comfrey pepsin. Use two capsules of comfrey pepsin twice daily. Do not use for more than a two-month period during flare-ups. Aerobic Bulk Cleanse (ABC) also contains healing herbs that cleanse the colon. Mix with half fruit or vegetable juice and half aloe vera juice, and take before meals. Take ½ cup of aloe vera juice in the morning and at bedtime as well. It will aid in healing the colon, thereby easing pain.

RECOMMENDATIONS

☐ Follow these "anti-colitis" dietary suggestions. Put oat bran, steamed vegetables, or raw vegetables through a blender. Add one tablespoon of oat or rice bran daily to cereals, juice, etc. This will add the bulk needed for cleansing the colon. Or you can add one tablespoon of Aerobic Bulk Cleanse to juice and drink it on an empty stomach upon arising. Try the junior baby foods for two weeks with fiber (glucomannan). Earth's Best baby foods are organic and are available in health food stores. Glucomannan should be taken one-half to one hour before meals with a large glass of liquid. Don't take glucomannan within an hour of taking medication or other supplements. Drink carrot and cabbage juices, "green drinks," or use chlorophyll liquid in juices. Use wheatgrass (as a retention enema; see also ENEMAS in Part Three) and alfalfa or barley.

☐ Eliminate any grain, seeds, or nuts except for well-cooked brown rice. Drink plenty of liquids. Do not eat any dairy products, red meat, sugar products, fried foods, spices, or processed foods. A low-carbohydrate, high-protein diet from a vegetable source is preferred.

☐ Use cleansing enemas with two quarts lukewarm water. This will help rid the colon of undigested foods and relieve pain. For severe gas and bloating, see ENEMAS in Part Three and follow instructions on the L. bifidus enema. Lobelia tea is good to drink. Also use it as an enema for inflammation of the colon; it gives quick relief.

☐ Stretching exercises are important for improved digestion. Partially digested starches may allow food to pass through the colon too rapidly.

☐ When magnesium is given intravenously with vitamin B_6, it relaxes the muscles in the walls of the bowels and controls the attack of a spastic colon. For less severe attacks, use oral magnesium and vitamin B_6.

☐ A vitamin K deficiency has been linked to gastrointestinal disorders and ulcerative colitis. Sulfa drugs and mineral oil destroy vitamin K. Vitamin K is found in alfalfa and dark green leafy vegetables.

☐ See FASTING in Part Three, and follow the program once a month. Also see MALABSORPTION SYNDROME in Part Two.

☐ Don't wear clothing that is tight around the waist.

☐ Have a regular colonoscopy.

☐ See also DIVERTICULITIS in Part Two.

Diet for Colitis

Colitis is a particularly painful and temporarily disabling condition. Diet is probably the most significant factor in the remission of colitis. Shari Lieberman, nutritionist and author, recommends the following dietary guidelines for controlling and abating colitis.

- The most important thing to do is keep a daily record of what you have eaten. This way you can see which foods have aggravated or improved your condition. Some people are sensitive only to certain foods, such as yeast products, wheat products, or dairy products. By checking your daily record, you can see which food caused a flare-up or made you feel great.
- Eat a high-fiber diet. Oat bran, brown rice, barley and other whole grains, lentils, and related products such as rice cakes are good.
- Stay on a low-fat diet. Fats and oils exacerbate the diarrhea that comes with colitis. Keep fats and oils out of your diet, and stay away from high-fat milk and cheeses. Spicy foods and coffee will also irritate this condition.

- Eat broiled or baked foods, not foods that are fried or sautéed. Avoid sauces made from butter.
- Find nonfat dairy foods. If you have a lactose intolerance, try lactose-free milk. Many people with a lactose intolerance can tolerate low-fat yogurt.
- Try low-fat cheese or soy-based cheese. Try soy milk instead of dairy milk.
- Obtain your protein from turkey or chicken without skin. Eat baked or broiled seafood, not fried or sautéed.
- Drink spring water, club soda, or seltzer water to make up for the fluid lost with diarrhea. Aloe vera juice is very good, especially for ulcerative colitis (and regular ulcers, too). It is a natural juice made from the aloe vera plant.
- If you want to eat fruit, do not eat it on an empty stomach; eat fruit at the end of a meal. Fruit juice should be diluted with spring water or club soda and taken during or after a meal.
- Eat lots of vegetables. If you cannot tolerate raw vegetables, steam them.

Common Cold

The symptoms of the common cold include head congestion, difficult breathing, coughing, headache, fever, restlessness, sneezing, watery eyes, and aches and pains. Don't use a nasal decongestant to relieve congestion—let the mucus flow. This is the body's way of getting rid of the infection.

The common cold is hard to cure because the virus has the ability to change in size and shape and has hundreds of different forms, making it almost impossible to formulate a vaccine against the virus.

A cold is always in the upper respiratory tract; if there is congestion in the chest, it is best to consult a doctor, as chest (lung) infections can be dangerous. Also contact the doctor if your fever goes above 102°F for more than three days, or if yellow or white spots appear in the throat, the lymph nodes under the jaw and in the neck become enlarged, and/or chills and shortness of breath occur.

NUTRIENTS

SUPPLEMENT	SUGGESTED DOSAGE	COMMENTS
Essential		
Vitamin A plus	15,000 IU daily.	Helps heal inflamed mucous membranes and strengthens
beta-carotene	15,000 IU daily.	the immune system.
Vitamin C	5,000–10,000 mg daily in divided doses.	Destroys the cold virus. *See* ASCORBIC ACID FLUSH in Part Three and follow directions. For children, use buffered vitamin C or calcium ascorbate.
Zinc gluconate lozenges	Dissolve 1 under the tongue every 3 hours during the first 3 days, then drop to 1 every 4 hours for 1 week.	Keep these tablets on hand and use at the first sign of a cold. Use until symptoms cease. Follow the same guidelines for children.
Important		
Garlic capsules (Kyolic)	2 capsules 3 times daily.	A natural antibiotic and immune system enhancer.
Protein supplement (free form amino acids)	As directed on label.	Free form amino acids are more readily available for use by the body.
Helpful		
Bifido Factor/ Life Start Two from Natren	As directed on label.	For infants and children. Replaces the "friendly" bacteria.
Cold-Control Capsules (a Power Herb natural product)	2 capsules 3 times daily.	Can be purchased at a natural foods store.
Fenu-Thyme or Fenu-Comf (Nature's Way herb formulas)	2 capsules 3 times daily.	Helps rid nasal passages of mucus.
Multiminerals or kelp	5–10 tablets daily.	Kelp is a rich source of necessary minerals.
Proteolytic enzymes	2–4 tablets between meals.	Anti-inflammatory.
Vitamin B complex in a multivitamin complex	50–100 mg 3 times daily.	For healing and immunity.

HERBS

☐ Echinacea, ginger, pau d'arco, slippery elm, and yarrow tea can help the common cold. For fever, take catnip tea enemas and ¼–½ teaspoon lobelia tincture every three to four hours until fever drops. This dosage can be used for children also.

☐ Also good is one tablespoon slippery elm bark powder mixed with one part boiling water and a half cup of honey for cough and sore throat. Put this in a jar and take one teaspoonful every three to four hours.

☐ Eucalyptus oil is also helpful. Put five drops in a hot bath or six drops in a cup of boiling water, put a towel over your head, and inhale.

☐ A tincture of echinacea and goldenseal is best for children. Put eight to ten drops in liquid every three hours until all symptoms are gone. This formula can also be obtained by contacting McZand Herbal, P.O. Box 5312, Santa Monica, CA 90405. This company's product is called Zand Formula.

RECOMMENDATIONS

☐ Children who frequently have colds or flus should be checked for thyroid malfunctions. Take the child's temperature rectally or under his arm before he arises in the morning. If the temperature is low when he is not ill, see a doctor. Also, allergies can cause frequent cold or flu symptoms. In this case, an allergy test is recommended.

☐ *See* HYPOTHYROID in Part Two for the thyroid self-test.

☐ Flush tissues after they have been used. Because they harbor the virus, these tissues can pass on the virus or cause you to reinfect yourself. Wash your hands often.

☐ Sip hot liquids such as turkey or chicken broth.

☐ Be cautious about giving children aspirin (*see* REYE'S SYNDROME in Part Two).

CONSIDERATIONS

☐ We can, in a sense, catch a cold from ourselves. When our immune system weakens from factors such as stress and a poor diet, our dormant viruses take hold.

☐ Drink Potato Peeling Broth twice a day—make it fresh daily. To make it, peel the potato so that the peelings are a half inch thick, including the skin. Discard the center of the potato. Boil the half-inch peelings for about twenty to thirty minutes. Strain, cool, and drink. You can add a carrot or a stalk of celery to your drink.

Constipation

Constipation results when waste material moves too slowly through the large bowel, resulting in its infrequent passage. Many ailments arise from constipation including hemorrhoids, gas, insomnia, headaches, bad breath, varicose veins, obesity, indigestion, diverticulitis, appendicitis, piles, hernia, and bowel cancer.

In most cases, constipation arises from insufficient amounts of fiber and fluids in the diet. It may also be a side effect of some drugs such as iron tablets, pain killers, and antidepressants. Constipation also occurs during pregnancy.

It is important that the bowels move on a daily basis. The body normally excretes waste in eighteen to twenty-four hours. Harmful toxins can form after this period.

NUTRIENTS

SUPPLEMENT	SUGGESTED DOSAGE	COMMENTS
Important		
Aloe vera juice	½ cup in the morning and at night.	Has a healing and cleansing effect and aids in forming soft stools.
Glucomannan or Aerobic Bulk Cleanse (ABC) from Aerobic Life Products	Take before meals with a large glass of water. Do not take with other supplements or medication.	Particularly good for high and low blood sugar problems. Creates bulk in the stool for improved function of the colon.
Naturalax #2 from Nature's Way Products	Take 2 after meals until the bowels move regularly. Take 2 or 3 times a day—whichever works best for you.	An herbal formula that helps heal and move the bowels regularly.
Helpful		
Acidophilus or Maxidophilus or Megadophilus or milk-free acidophilus	1 tsp. twice daily.	Allows survival and rapid passage of "friendly" bacteria through the stomach into the small intestine.
Apple pectin	500 mg daily.	A source of fiber that aids in correcting constipation.
Multidigestive enzymes	2 tablets after meals.	Avoid products that contain hydrochloric acid (HCl) if you suffer from ulcers.
Multivitamin and mineral complex	As directed on label.	Constipation leads to malabsorption, resulting in vitamin and mineral deficiency.
Vitamin B complex (high potency) with extra vitamin B_{12}	50 mg before meals.	Aids in proper digestion of fats, carbohydrates, and protein.

Vitamin D plus	400 mg daily.	Aids in preventing colon cancer.
calcium and	1,500 mg daily.	
magnesium	750 mg daily.	
Vitamin E	400 IU before meals.	Aids in healing of the colon.

HERBS

☐ The following will help if you suffer from constipation: cascara sagrada, comfrey, flaxseed, goldenseal, Green Magma (barley juice from Green Foods Corporation) or wheatgrass for chlorophyll, Naturalax 2 from Nature's Way Products, pepsin, psyllium seed, and senna leaf.

RECOMMENDATIONS

☐ Exercise is important. Physical activity speeds the movement of waste through the intestines and reduces the time that potential cancer-causing waste is in contact with tissues.

☐ Prunes are still one of the best natural laxatives. Linseed oil helps to soften stools. Use two to three tablespoons daily.

☐ Avoid foods that stimulate secretions by the mucous membranes. Eat fresh fruits; raw green leafy vegetables; and brown rice daily. Do not eat dairy products, white flour, or sugar. It is important that you drink extra amounts of water since you are adding fiber to the diet.

CONSIDERATIONS

☐ Continued use of laxatives will clean out the intestinal bacteria and cause chronic constipation. If you have been a heavy laxative user, take Megadophilus, Maxidophilus, or DDS (dairy-free) acidophilus to replace the "friendly" bacteria.

☐ If constipation is persistent, take cleansing enemas (see ENEMAS in Part Three) when the bowels have not moved for a few weeks. Keep bowels clean. Foul-smelling stools and a burning feeling in the anus may be signs of acidosis (see ACIDOSIS in Part Two for the self-test).

☐ If added natural fiber and herb laxatives do not improve constipation, you may have muscle incoordination. Normally, the upper muscles in the bowel contract as the lower ones relax. Problems occur when the lower muscle tightens and goes into a spasm instead of relaxing.

☐ It is helpful to fast periodically (see FASTING in Part Three).

Copper Toxicity

Like other metals, small amounts of copper are essential while exposure to too much copper can be harmful to one's health. Because the presence of copper is necessary for absorption of iron in the body, copper is usually found in foods containing iron. If the body does not acquire a sufficient amount of copper, hemoglobin production is decreased and copper deficiency anemia can result. Various enzyme reactions require copper as well. The liver and brain contain the largest amounts of copper in the body; however, other organs will contain smaller amounts.

Because copper deficiencies can produce various symptoms, copper is classified as an essential mineral. Insufficient amounts of copper can lead to inefficient utilization of iron and protein, diarrhea, and stunted growth. Long-term use of oral contraceptives can upset the balance of copper in the body (causing either excessively high or excessively low copper levels) and cause high cholesterol levels. For the body to work properly, it must maintain the proper balance of copper and zinc; an imbalance can lead to thyroid problems. In addition, low (and high) copper levels can be found in those with mental and emotional problems.

A copper deficiency will occur in babies who are fed soy milk; development of nerve, bone, and lung tissue of the baby will be impaired and the structure of these body parts may be altered. Adults suffering from a copper deficiency will lose protein. Those suffering from sprue and kidney disease characteristically have a copper deficiency. Megadoses of zinc can also lead to a copper deficiency.

Copper levels can be determined through blood serum, urine samples, and hair analysis. Hair analysis gives a very reliable reading. Normal urine levels collected over a 24-hour period will contain 15 to 40 micrograms of copper. Those suffering from a copper deficiency should increase their intake of foods rich in copper such as legumes (especially soybeans), nuts, seafood, raisins, molasses, avocados, whole grains, and cauliflower.

Although small amounts of copper are essential, *excess* amounts of copper in the body can be toxic. Too much copper in the system can lead to hemolytic anemia, emotional problems, behavioral disorders, mood swings, depression, nephritis, schizophrenia, eczema, sickle cell anemia, and severe damage to the central nervous system.

A popular mineral, copper is found in beer, copper cookware, copper plumbing, insecticides, pasteurized milk, and both city and well water. This metal can also be found in hair permanents, swimming pools, and various foods.

Using oral contraceptives and smoking (tobacco) can cause a rise in the amount of copper found in the blood and may cause hypertension. Excess serum copper is characteristic of cirrhosis of the liver, pregnancy, anemia, heart attack, infections, leukemia, high blood pressure, mental illness, stuttering, insomnia, hypoproteinemia, and niacin (vitamin B_3) deficiency. Wilson's disease, which can be fatal, is associated with high levels of copper and anemia.

NUTRIENTS

SUPPLEMENT	SUGGESTED DOSAGE	COMMENTS
Important		
Zinc chelate	50–80 mg daily.	A zinc deficiency predisposes one to excessive copper levels. Zinc and copper levels must be balanced.
Helpful		
Ascorbic acid plus bioflavonoids	2,000–4,000 mg daily in divided doses.	Bioflavonoids and vitamin C are copper chelators (*see* CHELATION THERAPY in Part Three). Rutin, a by-product of buckwheat and a bioflavonoid, lowers serum copper. Take 60 mg rutin daily.
Iron chelate	As directed on label.	May lower serum copper levels.
L-Methionine and L-cysteine and L-cystine (amino acids)	Take on an empty stomach.	Aids in elimination of copper from the body and protects the liver.

RECOMMENDATIONS

☐ People who have excessively high levels of copper in their bodies should increase their intake of sulfur, found in such foods as eggs, onions, and garlic. These will rid the body of copper. In addition, they should supplement their diets with pectin, which can be found in apples.

☐ If you suspect that you may have excessive or insufficient amounts of copper in your body, it can be confirmed through a hair analysis.

☐ *See also* ENVIRONMENTAL TOXICITY in Part Two.

Cramps

See MUSCLE CRAMPS; PREMENSTRUAL SYNDROME.

Crohn's Disease

Crohn's disease is characterized by a chronic and long-lasting inflammation of a section of the digestive tract. The inflammation extends through all layers of the intestinal wall and involves the adjacent lymph nodes. The inflamed parts heal and leave scar tissue that narrows the passageway. This disorder is not infectious and the cause is still uncertain. Risk increases with a history of food allergies.

Symptoms of Crohn's disease include diarrhea, periodic cramping, lower right abdominal pain, fever, malabsorption, possible anemia, and losses of energy, appetite, and weight.

The onset of Crohn's disease is typically around the age of twenty. Attacks may occur every few months to every few years. In rare cases it appears once or twice and does not return. If the disease continues for many years, bowel function gradually deteriorates. If left untreated, it can become very serious and increase the risk of cancer.

Lack of nutrients from malabsorption may weaken the immune system, prolonging healing time needed for the inflammation. Chronic bleeding may cause iron-deficiency anemia. If the inflamed intestinal wall leaks, peritonitis results. Sometimes Crohn's disease is misdiagnosed as appendicitis because pain is located in the same area.

NUTRIENTS

SUPPLEMENT	SUGGESTED DOSAGE	COMMENTS
Important		
Acidophilus (nondairy form)	1 tsp. in glass of water twice daily.	Aids in digestion.
Garlic capsules (Kyolic)	2 capsules with meals.	Odorless garlic that combats free radicals involved in Crohn's disease. Aids healing.
Protein supplement (free form amino acids from Ecological Formulas) plus	1/4 tsp. under the tongue twice daily.	Protein is essential in the healing of the intestine. Easily absorbed and bypasses the gastrointestinal tract.
magnesium	1,000 mg daily.	
Helpful		
Aloe vera juice (George's or Aerobic 07)	1/2 glass 3 times daily.	Softens stools and has a healing effect.
Essential fatty acids (primrose oil)	2 capsules 3 times daily.	Primrose oil is a good source.

147

Liver injections plus	2cc	Needed for proper digestion. Injections bypass possible malabsorption problems. Use only under doctor's supervision.
vitamin B$_{12}$ and	1cc twice weekly.	
vitamin B complex and	3 times daily.	
vitamin B$_{12}$ nasal gel	daily	
Multivitamin and mineral complex	Liquid, powder, or capsule form as directed.	A vitamin and/or mineral deficiency is common in this disorder.
Spiru-Tein from Nature's Plus	2 tablets between meals.	Supplies necessary protein. Helps stabilize the blood sugar between meals.
Vitamin A and E emulsion	50,000 IU daily.	Emulsion is readily absorbed. Aids in controlling infection.

HERBS

☐ Use echinacea, garlic, goldenseal root, pau d'arco, rose hips, and YerbaMate for Crohn's disease.

RECOMMENDATIONS

☐ Avoid stress. Resting during an attack is important. Make sure the bowels move daily. Use a heating pad to help reduce pain in the abdomen.

☐ Drink plenty of liquids such as steam-distilled water, herb teas, and fresh juices. Diet should consist mainly of nonacidic fresh vegetables such as broccoli, Brussels sprouts, cabbage, carrots, celery, kale, spinach, and turnips. During an attack, eat baby foods and vegetables. Avoid spicy foods, fried and greasy foods, pepper, tobacco, caffeine, alcohol, dairy products, margarine, all carbonated beverages, chocolate, animal products, and meat. However, white fish from clear waters is permissible. Steam, broil, boil, or bake your foods. Limit intake of grains—mainly wheat. Mucus-forming foods such as processed foods should be avoided.

☐ Check stools daily for bleeding. Avoid rectal suppositories that contain hydrogenated chemically prepared fats.

Croup

Croup is a respiratory infection that causes the larynx or trachea to narrow due to swelling. The larynx spasms and the victim experiences difficult breathing, a harsh cough, hoarseness, tightness in the lungs, and feelings of suffocation.

A trademark of croup is an abnormal noise that is made when air is breathed in through the constricted windpipe over inflamed vocal cords. This noise occurs in young children, since their airways are much narrower than adults and often become clogged with mucus when accompanied by an inflammation. Croup is usually caused by a cold, bronchitis, or an allergy, but can also occur when a foreign body is inhaled. Attacks frequently occur at night.

Children who have difficulty breathing should be admitted to a hospital for x-rays of the larynx. Antibiotics and oxygen may be needed. Take some form of acidophilis if antibiotics are taken. Most children recover in a few days.

The dosages in the following table are for children six years or older. Adjust the dosage for children under six years.

NUTRIENTS

SUPPLEMENT	SUGGESTED DOSAGE	COMMENTS
Essential		
Vitamin C	500 mg 4 times daily. Those under age 4 should take 100 mg 4 times daily.	Helps control infection and fever by boosting the immune system. See ASCORBIC ACID FLUSH in Part Three.
Zinc lozenges	5 mg 3 times daily for 3 days for those age 3 and up.	Lozenges are absorbed faster. Zinc promotes immune function, and is necessary in healing.
Very Important		
Vitamin A	2,000 IU daily.	Needed for healing of the mucous membranes. Use emulsified form.
Vitamin E	50 mg daily.	Destroys free radicals and carries oxygen to all cells. Use emulsified form.
Important		
Cod liver oil	1 tbsp. twice daily in juice.	Use for children in place of vitamin A.

HERBS

☐ The following herbs are recommended for those with croup: comfrey, echinacea tincture, fenugreek, goldenseal, thyme, and Herbal C by Green Farms (for congestion). Echinacea tincture should be taken if a fever is present. Put fifteen drops of this herb in liquid every three to four hours. Fenu-Thyme combination from Nature's Way Products is also good.

☐ Use eucalyptus oil from a health food store; use a vaporizer to steam and inhale.

☐ Take very warm ginger herb baths, wrap yourself in a heavy towel or blanket, and go directly to bed to perspire. This helps loosen mucus and rid the body of toxins.

RECOMMENDATIONS

☐ Apply hot onion packs over the chest and back three times a day. Slice onions and place between cloths, and then apply a heating pad. The onion pack has a healing effect by opening the pores and relieving congestion.

Cystic Fibrosis

Cystic fibrosis is a hereditary disease involving the endocrine and exocrine glands. It is characterized by recurrent lung infections and impaired gastrointestinal absorption. Symptoms begin early in life.

This disease affects certain glands in the body such as the pancreas, lungs, male reproductive organs, and sweat glands. The mucous membranes in the glands of the lungs produce thick mucus which blocks lung passages and promotes the growth of harmful bacteria.

Those with cystic fibrosis usually suffer from malnutrition because the body lacks the necessary digestive enzymes. The body does not absorb required nutrients. Victims of this disease also lose excessive amounts of salt through their sweat glands.

Since this disorder most often strikes children, the supplement doses recommended below must be altered accordingly. Consult your doctor!

NUTRIENTS

SUPPLEMENT	SUGGESTED DOSAGE	COMMENTS
Very Important		
Pancreatin	Take with meals.	Needed for protein digestion.
Proteolytic enzymes	2 tablets between meals on an empty stomach.	Aids in controlling infection, helps digestion, and thins the thick mucus secretions of the lungs.
Vitamin B complex with extra riboflavin (B₂)	100 mg 3 times daily with meals.	Aids in digestion, healing, and tissue repair.
Vitamin B₁₂ lozenges	200 mcg 3 times daily on an empty stomach.	Needed for proper digestion and assimilation of nutrients including iron.
Vitamin C	3,000–6,000 mg daily in divided doses.	For tissue repair and immune function.
Vitamin K	6 tablets daily.	Vitamin K deficiency is common in those with this disease. Needed by the gastrointestinal tract for proper digestion. Alfalfa is a good source.
Important		
Protein	As directed on label.	From a vegetable source or from free form amino acids, which are easily digested. Protein is needed for healing.

Unsaturated fatty acids (primrose oil)	As directed on label.	Primrose oil is good. Relieves inflammation.
Vitamin A	50,000 IU daily.	Use part beta-carotene. For tissue repair. Potentiates immune system. Emulsified form is best.
Vitamin E	400–1,000 IU daily. If using capsule or tablet form, increase dosage slowly.	Emulsion form enters system quickly, and is better assimilated.
Zinc chelate	50 mg daily.	Important in immune function and healing of tissue. Gluconate lozenges are fast acting.
Helpful		
Coenzyme Q₁₀	100 mg daily.	Acts as an immunostimulant.
Germanium	200 mg daily.	Aids tissue oxygenation and potentiates immune function.
Kyo-Green or chlorophyll or alfalfa liquid	As directed on label.	Supplies minerals and chlorophyll needed to control the infection.
L-Cysteine and L-methionine (amino acids)	500 mg each on an empty stomach twice daily.	Needed for repair of lung tissue and protection of the liver.
Raw thymus and raw spleen and raw pancreas extract or tablets (glandulars)	As directed on label.	Relieves inflammation. *See* GLANDULAR THERAPY in Part Three.
Selenium and copper	200 mcg daily.	Low levels of selenium and copper have been linked to cystic fibrosis.
Vitamin D	400 IU daily.	Aids in protecting the lungs.

HERBS

☐ Use echinacea, ginger, goldenseal, and yarrow tea for cystic fibrosis.

RECOMMENDATIONS

☐ If using antibiotics, take acidophilus to replace "friendly" bacteria.

☐ During hot weather, drink plenty of fluids and increase salt intake.

☐ Do not eat foods that stimulate secretions by the mucous membranes. Cooked and processed foods cause excess mucus build-up and drain the body of energy. These types of foods are harder to digest. Do not eat processed foods, dairy products, animal products, sugar, or white flour products. The diet should consist of 75 percent raw fruits and vegetables and raw nuts and seeds.

CONSIDERATIONS

☐ Low levels of selenium and vitamin E have been linked to cystic fibrosis and cancer.

☐ Researchers have recently identified the gene responsible for one of the mutations associated with cystic fibrosis. Now that this gene has been identified, a test that can identify a carrier can be developed for the general population. Researchers can now closely study the gene to try to discover what has gone wrong with it in those with cystic fibrosis, and are thus closer to developing a comprehensive treatment program.

☐ For more information on cystic fibrosis, call the Cystic Fibrosis Foundation: 1-(800) FIGHT-CF.

Cystitis

See BLADDER INFECTION.

Dandruff

Dandruff is caused by dysfunctional sebaceous glands in the scalp. When these glands secrete abnormally, the scalp forms scales that may itch and burn.

Consult your doctor for dandruff treatment. It is best not to use over-the-counter ointments. They can often do more harm than good. A dermatologist usually prescribes cleansing lotions containing a drying agent with sulfur and resorcin or Deprosone cream.

NUTRIENTS

SUPPLEMENT	SUGGESTED DOSAGE	COMMENTS
Very Important		
Kelp tablets	5 tablets daily.	Supplies needed minerals, especially iodine, for better hair growth and healing of the scalp.
Unsaturated fatty acids	As directed on label.	Primrose oil and salmon oil help to relieve pain and inflammation.
Vitamin B complex plus extra vitamin B$_6$ (pyridoxine)	100 mg twice daily with meals.	Use high stress formula.
Vitamin E	400 IU and up.	For improved circulation.
Zinc lozenges	5 tablets dissolved in mouth daily for 1 week.	Protein metabolism depends on zinc. The scalp is primarily protein.

Important		
Vitamin A and beta-carotene	Up to 20,000 IU daily. 15,000 IU daily.	Helps prevent dry skin. Aids in healing of tissue.
Helpful		
Lecithin	3 times daily.	Protects the scalp and strengthens cell membranes of the scalp and hair.

HERBS

☐ Those with dandruff can benefit from the use of dandelion, goldenseal, and red clover. Chaparral may be used as a hair rinse.

RECOMMENDATIONS

☐ Avoid fried foods, dairy products, sugar, flour, chocolate, nuts, and seafood. The diet should consist of 50 to 75 percent raw foods. Eat soured products such as yogurt. *See* FASTING in Part Three, and follow the program once a month.

☐ Don't pick or scratch the scalp. Avoid irritating soaps and greasy ointments and creams. Make sure you wash your hair frequently, and use a nonoily shampoo. Try using a hair product that does not contain chemicals. Some people have found that the sun helps clear up dandruff, but others state that the problem becomes worse after sun exposure.

☐ If antibiotics are prescribed, don't fail to take extra B-complex vitamins. You should also take acidophilus or Megadophilus supplements to replace the "friendly" bacteria that are destroyed by antibiotics.

☐ *See also* SEBORRHEA in Part Two.

DDT Poisoning

When DDT was first introduced as an insecticide in 1939, it was hoped that it would protect the farmer's crops from invading insects. Although the Environmental Protection Agency (EPA) banned its use in December of 1972, the toxic insecticide DDT remains a threat due to its long-lasting effects on the environment. Studies revealed that a high concentration of DDT is found in the fatty tissues of some species, particularly in those that are further along in the food chain. For example, birds will have a higher concentration of DDT than fish because they will acquire DDT not only from the fish they have consumed, but also from the microorganisms and algae eaten by the fish, and so on. DDT was thus shown to be a cumulative poison that is stored primarily in the fatty tissues of the body.

Although the United States has outlawed the use of DDT by American farmers on crops produced in this country, there are no such controls on foreign imports or exports. Many of the crops grown in Israel, including those sprayed with DDT, cannot be consumed by the Jewish population because the chemicals used on the produce prevent it from being certified as kosher. Although the Israeli Jews cannot eat these foods, Israel does sell such produce to the United States.

Even though DDT was banned over ten years ago, it has found its way back into our foods. It has been a by-product in pesticides used mainly on citrus fruits and cotton. A DDT by-product called dicofol has been used in pesticides, including the name brands Kelthane, Mitigan, and Acarin. In October 1984 the EPA proposed a total ban on the substance.

Because fat supplies will be used by the body when a person is dieting, a crash diet can be harmful if toxic amounts of DDT are released from the fat stores into the bloodstream too quickly. Because the body is unable to rid itself of this poison, severe damage could result. If you choose to fast, do so only on fresh juices. Never fast on water alone. (See FASTING in Part Three.)

NUTRIENTS

SUPPLEMENT	SUGGESTED DOSAGE	COMMENTS
Very Important		
AOX/SOD from Biotec Foods	As directed on label with a large glass of water in the morning.	A powerful free radical scavenger.
Garlic capsules (Kyolic)	2 capsules 3 times daily.	A potent immunostimulant and detoxifier.
Kelp tablets	6 tablets daily.	Provides necessary vitamins, minerals, and trace elements. Aids in removing toxic metals.
Selenium	200 mcg daily.	An especially important antioxidant.
Vitamin C	2,000–10,000 mg daily in divided doses.	A powerful detoxifier and immune system stimulator.
Helpful		
Lecithin	1 tbsp. or 2 capsules with meals.	A fat emulsifier that releases DDT from fat deposits.
Maxidophilus or Megadophilus	Take on an empty stomach as directed on label.	DDT damages the important "friendly" bacteria.
Multivitamin and mineral complex	As directed on label.	Necessary for healing and protection.
Vitamin A and E	100,000 IU vitamin A daily; 800–1,200 IU vitamin E daily.	Emulsified form is best. *Warning:* Do not start with high amounts of vitamin E if you have high blood pressure. Work up slowly. Vitamins A and E are powerful free radical scavengers.

RECOMMENDATIONS

☐ Supplement your diet with pectin and plenty of fiber. Oat bran is a good source of fiber. Yogurt and all forms of soured milk can protect against DDT poisoning.

CONSIDERATIONS

☐ Drink only steam-distilled water.

☐ *See also* CHEMICAL POISONING and ENVIRONMENTAL TOXICITY, both in Part Two.

Depression

Some people do not admit sadness or guilt; instead they withdraw and hide from society. They lose all interest in things around them and become incapable of any pleasure. Things appear bleak and time passes slowly for them. They are typically angry and irritable. They often try sleeping off their depression or do nothing but sit or lay around. In most people depression is not severe. They can still function, but do so at a lower capacity and at a slower pace.

Symptoms of depression include chronic fatigue syndrome, insomnia or sleeping frequently and for excessive periods of time, loss of appetite or a ravenous appetite, headaches, backaches, colon disorders, and feelings of worthlessness and inadequacy. Many think of death and consider suicide.

Depression may be caused by tension, upset stomach, stress, headache, nutritional deficiencies, poor diet, sugar, mononucleosis, thyroid disorders, endometriosis (linked to depression in women), any serious physical disorder, or allergies. Some people become more depressed in the winter months when days are shorter and darker. The sun and bright light seem to trigger a response to a brain hormone known as melatonin (produced by the pineal gland), which is, in part, responsible for preventing the "blues." Stay in brightly lit rooms on dark days. Research reveals that two hours of morning sun is very effective in lifting depression. The evening light had comparatively little results.

Depression begins with a disturbance in the part of the brain that governs moods. Most people can handle everyday stresses; their bodies readjust to these pressures. When stress is too great for a person and his adjustment mechanism is unresponsive, depression may be triggered.

It has been discovered that foods greatly influence the brain's behavior. Diet is most often the cause of depression, related to poor eating habits and constant snacking on junk foods. The brain's neurotransmitters, which regulate our behavior, are controlled by what we eat. The neurotransmitters are dopamine, serotonin, and norepinephrine. When the brain produces serotonin, tension is eased. When it is produces dopamine or norepinephrine, we tend to think and act more quickly and are generally more alert. Eating carbohydrates alone seems to have a calming effect, while proteins increase alertness. Protein meals containing essential fatty acids and/or carbohydrates are recommended for increased alertness. Salmon and white fish are good choices. Avoid foods high in saturated fats; consumption of pork or fried foods, such as hamburgers and French fries, leads to sluggishness, slow thinking, and fatigue. Fats inhibit the synthesis of neurotransmitters by the brain in that they cause the blood cells to become sticky and to clump together, resulting in poor circulation, especially to the brain.

At the neurochemical and physiological level, neurotransmitters are extremely important. These substances carry impulses between nerve cells. The substance that processes the neurotransmitter called serotonin is the amino acid tryptophan. It increases the amount of serotonin made by the brain. Complex carbohydrates, which raise the level of tryptophan in the brain, have a calming effect; protein promotes the production of dopamine and norepinephrine, which promote alertness. A balance is achieved when the diet contains a combination of these two nutrients. A turkey sandwich on whole wheat bread is a good combination: the turkey is high in protein and tryptophan, and the whole wheat bread supplies complex carbohydrates. Consume more carbohydrates than protein if you are nervous and wish to become more relaxed or eat more protein than carbohydrates if you are tired and wish to become more alert. A depressed person who needs his spirits lifted would benefit from eating foods like turkey and salmon, which are high in tryptophan and protein.

Beware: The body will react more quickly to the presence of sugar than it does to the presence of complex carbohydrates. The increase in energy supplied by the simple carbohydrates is quickly accompanied by fatigue and depression.

Tyrosine is also needed for brain function. This amino acid may be good for those who have prolonged and intense stress. Uncontrollable stress may thereby be prevented or reversed if this essential amino acid is obtained in the diet.

Heredity is a significant factor in depression. In up to 50 percent of people suffering from recurrent episodes of depression, one or both of the parents were depressive.

NUTRIENTS

SUPPLEMENT	SUGGESTED DOSAGE	COMMENTS
Essential		
Vitamin B complex or	100 mg 3 times daily.	Necessary for normal brain function.
B complex with	2cc	Use injections only under a doctor's supervision if depression is severe.
vitamin B₆ and	½cc	
vitamin B₁₂ or	1cc	
liver injections plus	2cc	
vitamin B₁₂	1cc	
Important		
Choline and inositol or lecithin	100 mg twice daily.	Important in brain function and nerve transmission. Not for manic depressives.
Gerovital H-3 (GH-3) from Rumania	As directed on label for those 35 years or older.	Inhibits production of monoamine oxidase (MAO) in the brain, which builds up in those over 45. Directly linked to depression.
L-Tyrosine (amino acid)	Up to 100 mg per kg of body weight daily taken on an empty stomach with 1,000 mg vitamin C and 50 mg vitamin B₆.	Tyrosine alleviates stress by boosting production of adrenaline and raises dopamine levels, which influence moods. Lack of tyrosine results in a norepinephrine deficiency at a specific brain location, resulting in mood disorders such as depression.
Niacin (B₃) plus niacinamide	100 mg 3 times daily. 200 mg daily.	Improves cerebral circulation.
Helpful		
Aslavitol or Megavital HP Forte with RNA from Futurebiotics	As directed on label.	Especially good for the elderly.
Calcium and magnesium	1,500 mg daily. 1,000 mg daily.	Has a calming effect. Needed for the nervous system. Asporotate and chelate forms are the most effective.
Chromium (GTF)	300 mcg daily.	Aids in mobilizing fats for energy.
GABA (gamma-amino butyric acid)	750 mg daily.	Has a tranquilizing effect.
Lithium	By prescription only.	For manic depressives.

Multivitamin and mineral complex plus zinc chelate and GTF	As directed on label.	Vitamin and mineral deficiencies are associated with depression.
Primrose oil or black currant oil	2 capsules twice daily.	Essential fatty acids are needed by every cell.
Spirulina and raw crude bee pollen	5 tablets between meals.	Improves energy. Spiru-Tein from Nature's Plus is good.
Vitamin B₆ (pyridoxine) plus pantothenic acid (B₅)	50 mg 3 times daily. 500 mg daily.	B₆ is needed for normal brain function. B₅ is an "antistress" vitamin that may help depression.
Vitamin C plus rutin, a by-product of buckwheat	2,000–5,000 mg daily in divided doses.	Needed for immune function. Aids in preventing depression.

RECOMMENDATIONS

☐ A raw fruit and vegetable diet, with soybeans and their by-products, is important. Diets too low in complex carbohydrates can cause serotonin depletion and depression.

☐ Avoid phenylalanine. It contains the chemical phenol, which is highly allergenic. Most depressed people are "allergic" to certain substances. However, there is a brand of amino acids available that does not contain phenylalanine; it is produced by Ecological Formulas.

☐ Those suffering from manic depression should avoid choline, ornithine, and arginine. These substances may make the disorder worse.

☐ *See* HYPOTHYROID in Part Two and take the underarm test to detect an underactive thyroid. If the temperature is low, take a thyroid extract product. We recommend Armour Thyroid Extract.

☐ If taking MAO inhibitor drugs, avoid tyrosine. It can raise the blood pressure. Also consume the following foods in moderation: avocados, cheese, chocolate, herring, meat tenderizer, raisins, sour cream, soy sauce, yeast extracts, yogurt, and wine and beer.

☐ Beware of hypoglycemia, allergies, hypothyroid, and malabsorption. In these conditions vitamin B₁₂ and folic acid are blocked from entering the system, thus leading to depression.

☐ Keep your mind active and get plenty of rest. Avoid stressful situations as much as possible.

CONSIDERATIONS

☐ Steroid drugs and oral contraceptives may cause serotonin levels in the brain to drop.

Dermatitis

Dermatitis is an allergy that produces scaling, flaking, thickening, color change, and itching upon contact with the skin. It may be caused from contact with metal alloys such as gold, silver, and nickel, perfumes, cosmetics, rubber, medicated creams and ointments, and plants such as poison ivy. If the irritant remains in constant contact with the skin, the dermatitis will spread and become extremely severe.

NUTRIENTS

SUPPLEMENT	SUGGESTED DOSAGE	COMMENTS
Essential		
Vitamin B complex (high stress formula) with extra vitamin B₆ (pyridoxine) and niacin (B₃)	50 mg 3 times daily. 100 mg 3 times daily.	The B complex is needed for healthy skin and for proper circulation. Aids in reproduction of all cells.
Important		
Kelp tablets	5 tablets daily.	Minerals and iodine are needed for healing of tissues.
Unsaturated fatty acids (vitamin F) or MaxEPA	As directed on label.	Vitamin F promotes lubrication of the skin. Use any one of the following: black currant oil, linseed oil, primrose oil, or salmon oil.
Vitamin E	400 IU daily and up.	Relieves itching and dryness.
Zinc	100 mg daily (do not exceed 100 mg).	Aids healing.
Helpful		
Protein supplement (free form amino acids)	As directed on label on an empty stomach.	Protein is important in the construction and repair of all tissues. Free form amino acids are more readily available for use by the body.
Vitamin A emulsion	100,000 IU for 1 month, then decrease to 50,000 IU for 2 weeks. Maintain with 25,000 IU or tablets.	Needed for smooth skin. Aids in preventing dryness.
Vitamin D	400–1,000 IU daily.	Aids in healing of tissues.

HERBS

☐ For dermatitis, use comfrey, dandelion, myrrh gum, pau d'arco, and red clover.

RECOMMENDATIONS

☐ To relieve itching and promote healing, try mixing goldenseal root powder with vitamin E oil. Add a little honey until it is the consistency of a loose paste, then apply to the infected area.

☐ A gluten-free diet is of therapeutic benefit in controlling dermatitis. Omit wheat, rye, oats, and barley from the diet for six weeks. Add one back to the diet at a time, and see if the dermatitis changes.

CONSIDERATIONS

☐ Avoid dairy products, sugar, white flour, fats, fried foods, and processed foods. Remember that food allergies could be the cause of the dermatitis.

☐ Primrose oil and vitamin B_6 (pyridoxine) have helped infants with dermatitis.

☐ See also SKIN PROBLEMS in Part Two and the section on food allergies in ALLERGIES, Part Two.

Diabetes

There are two types of diabetes: *diabetes insipidus* and *diabetes mellitus*. *Diabetes insipidus* is a rare metabolic disorder caused by a deficiency of the pituitary hormone, which is usually the result of damage to the pituitary gland. *Diabetes insipidus* is characterized by enormous amounts of urine that are produced by the body regardless of how much liquid is consumed.

Diabetes mellitus results from the production of insufficient amounts of insulin by the pancreas. Without insulin the body cannot utilize glucose, thus creating a high level of glucose in the blood and a low level of glucose absorption by the tissues. *Diabetes mellitus* is generally divided into two categories: type I, called insulin-dependent or juvenile diabetes, and type II in which the onset of the diabetes occurs during adulthood.

The symptoms of the type I diabetic include irritability, frequent urination, abnormal thirst, nausea or vomiting, weakness, fatigue, and unusual hunger. This type of diabetes occurs mostly in children or young adults. The type I diabetic may have an insulin reaction in an instant, seeming perfectly normal one second and becoming unconscious the next. The early warning signs of this type of reaction are hunger, dizziness, sweating, confusion, palpitation, and numbness or tingling of the lips. If left untreated, the insulin-dependent diabetic may also experience double vision, trembling, and disorientation, may perform strange actions, and may eventually lose consciousness. While experiencing any one of these symptoms, quick consumption of a piece of candy, some soda pop, or anything else that contains sugar will bring blood sugar levels back to normal.

Recovery is more difficult for the diabetic whose insulin reaction is left untreated for a long period of time. An insulin reaction producing low blood sugar can be life threatening. Therefore, it is safer to "spill" small amounts of urine sugar when taking insulin.

The second type of diabetes, often referred to as maturity-onset diabetes, is likely to occur in those with a family history of diabetes and is characterized by blurred vision, itching, unusual thirst, drowsiness, obesity, fatigue, skin infections, slow healing, and tingling or numbness in the feet. Onset of symptoms is usually later in life.

Diet often controls this type and insulin is not usually required. Obesity is a major factor in type II diabetes.

An estimated 5.5 million Americans are being treated for diabetes. Studies indicate that there are 5 million adults with undetected type II diabetes, and another 20 million have impaired glucose tolerance that may lead to full-blown diabetes. The National Institutes of Health report that undiagnosed diabetes is the reason behind millions losing their vision. Those who are overweight face the greatest risk of developing diabetes. It is the third leading cause of death in the United States.

Other signs of diabetes include lingering flu-like symptoms, loss of hair on legs, increased facial hair, small yellow bumps anywhere on the body (known as xanthomas-cholesterol), and inflammation of the penile skin. Diabetes is associated with arteriosclerosis.

DIABETES SELF-TESTS

Type I Diabetes
(Insulin-Dependent or Juvenile Diabetes)

To test for type I diabetes:

1. Purchase chemically treated plastic strips at the drugstore.

2. Prick your finger and apply a drop of blood to the tip of the strip.

3. Wait one minute and compare the color on the strip to a color chart, which lists various glucose levels. (There are various electronic devices available that can analyze the test strip for you and give you a numerical read-out of the glucose level.)

There is a new device called Glucometer 2 (Miles Laboratories, Elkhart, Indiana) that can be used at home at your convenience. You simply prick your finger with the spring-loaded needle, apply a drop of your blood to the test strip, and place it into the machine for analysis. This test will give you immediate feedback on your condition.

Type II Diabetes (Maturity-Onset Diabetes)

Those who do not have an onset of diabetes until adulthood (type II diabetics) are not able to perceive sweet tastes. While addressing the American Diabetic Association, Dr. J. Shan said, "This abnormality may play an important role in how food is perceived by patients and their compliance with diet therapy."

Obesity is common among type II diabetics (those who became diabetic during adulthood). A weight reduction program is usually all that is required to control this type of diabetes without the use of drugs. However, the inability of these patients to perceive sweet tastes makes it more difficult for them to lose weight. Because they do not recognize the sweet taste of substances, they often consume sugary products that they do not appreciate as sweet. If the type II diabetic attains a better understanding of his food and exercises greater care in his food choices and carefully reads food labels, he will be able to control the problem and avoid drugs or insulin.

The following test can detect this impaired ability to taste sweets.

1. Do not consume stimulants (coffee, tea, soda) or sweets for one hour before the test.

2. Label seven identical glasses as having no sugar, 1/4 teaspoon sugar, ½ teaspoon sugar, 1 teaspoon sugar, 1½ teaspoons sugar, 2 teaspoons sugar, or 3 teaspoons sugar. Fill each glass with eight ounces of water and add the appropriate amount of sugar. Have someone place the glasses out of order and hide the labels.

3. Take a straw and sip from each glass, marking which amount you think it is. Between each test rinse your mouth with water.

According to Dr. Shan, "Most normal people perceive a sweet taste with only one teaspoon or less of sugar in the eight ounces of water. Those with adult-onset diabetes will not perceive sweetness until they have tasted the equivalent of 1½ to 2 teaspoons of the sugar water."

NUTRIENTS

SUPPLEMENT	SUGGESTED DOSAGE	COMMENTS
Essential		
Chromium (GTF)	200 mcg daily.	Helps to stabilize blood sugar and increases energy.
L-Carnitine and L-glutamine	500 mg twice daily on an empty stomach.	Fat mobilizers. Avoid L-cysteine—it interferes with absorption of insulin by the cells.
Very Important		
Glucomannan or guar gum	Take with a large glass of water and drink down quickly before it thickens.	Good fiber source and fat mobilizer.
Magnesium	750 mg daily.	Important for the enzyme system and pH balance.
Raw pancreas concentrate	As directed on label.	*See* GLANDULAR THERAPY in Part Three.
Important		
Vitamin A (emulsion or capsule form)	15,000 IU daily.	Avoid beta-carotene; diabetics cannot convert it to vitamin A.
Vitamin B complex plus biotin and inositol	50 mg 3 times daily.	Avoid large amounts of vitamin B. It interferes with the absorption of insulin by the cells.
Helpful		
Calcium	1,500 mg daily.	Important for pH balance.
Copper complex (Athrinol from American Biologics)	As directed on label.	Aids in protein metabolism and in many enzyme systems.
Enzyme compound plus proteolytic enzymes	Take with meals. / Take between meals.	Proper digestion is essential in management of diabetes.

HERBS

☐ If you suffer from diabetes, you may wish to try the following herbs: buchu leaves, dandelion root, goldenseal, and uva ursi. In addition, huckleberry helps to promote insulin production and a tea made of ginseng is believed to lower the blood sugar level.

RECOMMENDATIONS

☐ A high-carbohydrate, high-fiber diet reduces the need for insulin and also lowers the fat levels in the blood. Olive oil may help adult-onset diabetes. Fiber will reduce blood sugar surges. Eat crackers with nut butters or cheese. Use oat and rice bran crackers. High fat levels are linked to heart disease.

☐ Spirulina helps produce a stable blood sugar level. Go on a spirulina diet consisting of raw fruits and vegetables as well as fresh juices. This diet will help to reduce sugar in the urine. Foods that help normalize blood sugar include berries, brewer's yeast, dairy products (especially cheese), egg yolks, fish, garlic, sauerkraut, soybeans, and vegetables. A low-protein diet consisting of less than 40 grams of protein each day is recommended for diabetic nephropathy (kidney disease).

☐ Avoid fish oil capsules, large amounts of PABA, white flour products, and salt. Consumption of these products results in an elevation of blood sugar. It is important to get protein from a vegetable source.

CONSIDERATIONS

☐ Do not take large doses of cysteine. It has the ability to break down the bonds of the hormone insulin. Be careful not to take extremely large doses of vitamins B_1 and C. Excessive amounts may inactivate insulin. They may, however, be taken in normal amounts.

☐ Type II diabetics should avoid large amounts of niacin, but niacinamide for type I diabetics slows down destruction of beta cells in the pancreas and enhances their regeneration, extending the remission time.

ADDITIONAL SOURCES OF INFORMATION

For more information on diabetes, contact the following organizations:

American Diabetes Association
1660 Duke Street
Alexandria, VA 22314
(703) 549-1500

International Diabetes Center
5000 W. 39th Street
Minneapolis, MI 55416
(612) 927-3393

Joslin Diabetes Foundation
One Joslin Place
Boston, MA 02215
(617) 732-2415

Juvenile Diabetes Foundation
60 Madison Avenue
New York, NY 10010-1550
(212) 889-7575

Diarrhea

Diarrhea is characterized by frequent and loose watery stools, and is sometimes accompanied by severe vomiting. Symptoms include runny stools, cramping, frequent bowel movements, thirst, and abdominal pain. Some people run a fever as well. Diarrhea may be caused by incomplete digestion of food, food poisoning, stress, certain foods such as beans, infection, disease of the pancreas, cancer, drugs, laxatives, antacids, caffeine, parasites, colitis, viruses, bacteria or other microorganisms, consumption of water in foreign countries, foods or chemicals the body cannot tolerate (allergens), green fruits that have not ripened on the vine, and rancid foods.

Loss of fluids can lead to dehydration and loss of minerals. Drink plenty of liquids such as hot carob drink, carrot juice, and "green drinks." If the condition persists or if there is blood in the stools, see your doctor. Have an allergy test to determine if you have any food allergies.

NUTRIENTS

SUPPLEMENT	SUGGESTED DOSAGE	COMMENTS
Very Important		
Charcoal tablets	4 tablets every hour with water until the diarrhea subsides. Take in the evening.	Never take with other vitamins or drugs.
Kelp tablets	5 tablets daily.	Replaces lost minerals.
Potassium	99 mg daily.	Needed to replace potassium lost in watery stools.
Important		
Garlic capsules (Kyolic)	2 capsules 3 times daily.	Kills bacteria and parasites.
Maxidophilus or Megadophilus	1 tsp. in distilled water, taken on an empty stomach twice daily.	Replaces "friendly" bacteria.
Helpful		
Calcium	1,500 mg daily.	To replace calcium depleted from the body. Also aids in forming stools.
Digestive enzymes	Take with meals.	High in pancreatin. Needed in normal digestive process.
Magnesium	1,000 mg daily.	Needed for calcium uptake. Promotes pH balance.
Psyllium seed or guar gum or oat bran	4 capsules at bedtime.	Aids in forming stools.
Unsaturated fatty acids	As directed on label.	Aids in forming stools.

Vitamin B complex plus vitamin B₁ and niacin and folic acid	200 mg daily for 2 weeks. 50 mg daily.	Because of malabsorption, injections of vitamin B by your physician may be necessary.
Vitamin C	500 mg 3 times daily.	Use a nonacid type.
Vitamin D	400 IU daily.	Needed for calcium uptake.
Vitamin E	400 IU daily up to 1,000 IU.	Protects the cell membranes that line the colon wall.

HERBS

☐ If you suffer from occasional bouts of diarrhea, you may wish to use blackberry root, chamomile tea, and raspberry leaves. Herbs can be added to applesauce, bananas, pineapple, or papaya juice. Take cayenne capsules two to three times daily. Ginger tea is good for cramps and abdominal pain. Slippery elm bark is also beneficial. Take six capsules or take three teaspoonfuls per eight ounces of water.

RECOMMENDATIONS

☐ A high-fiber diet is important. Eat oat bran, rice bran, raw foods, yogurt, and soured products daily. Increase liquids, adding sea water concentrate to steam-distilled water.

☐ Do not take any medication to stop diarrhea for at least two days. It is the body's way of throwing off toxins. You should contact your doctor, however, if any of these conditions occur: the diarrhea lasts for more than two days, there is blood in the stool, the stool appears as black tar, you have a fever above 101°F, you have severe pain in the abdomen or rectum, you suffer from dehydration evident by dry mouth or wrinkled skin, or urination is reduced or stopped.

☐ Do not consume milk products—they are highly allergenic. Also limit fats, wheat, and foods containing gluten.

CONSIDERATIONS

☐ A treatment consisting of rice water can be beneficial for diarrhea. Boil half a cup of brown rice in three cups of water for forty-five minutes, strain, and drink three cups daily of the rice water. Eat the rice as well. The rice helps to form stools and supplies the needed B vitamins.

☐ Chronic diarrhea in children is evident if the child has five or more watery stools a day.

Diverticulitis

In those with diverticulitis, the colon's mucous membranes become inflamed, resulting in the formation of small, pouch-like areas (diverticula) in the large intestine. These pouches typically form when an individual is constipated. Greatly increased pressure is required to force small portions of hard, dry stool through the bowel when constipated. This rise in pressure can cause pouches to form at weak points in the wall of the colon. The diverticula themselves cause no symptoms, but if waste matter becomes trapped in them, they can become infected and inflamed.

Symptoms of diverticulitis include cramping, tenderness on the left side of the abdomen that is relieved by passing gas or a bowel movement, constipation or diarrhea, and nausea. Some people have no symptoms at all. Poor eating habits and stress compound the problem. If an allergy is suspected, a food sensitivity test is advised. Partially digested starch may cause food to pass through the colon too rapidly. A poor diet, a family history of the disease, gallbladder disease, obesity, and coronary artery disease increase the possibility of developing diverticulitis.

NUTRIENTS

SUPPLEMENT	SUGGESTED DOSAGE	COMMENTS
Essential		
Fiber (oat bran, glucomannan, or Aerobic Bulk Cleanse (ABC))	Take 1 hour before meals with a large glass of liquid. Do not take within 1 hour of medication or supplement.	Helps prevent constipation. Prevents infection by preventing accumulation in "pouches" of the colon.
Vitamin B complex	100 mg 3 times daily.	Use a hypoallergenic brand.
Very Important		
Multidigestive enzymes	Take with meals.	High in pancreatin. Needed to break down proteins.
Proteolytic enzymes	Take between meals.	Aids in digestion and reduces inflammation of the colon.
Important		
Acidophilus	3 times daily on an empty stomach.	Use nondairy form if allergic to milk.
Garlic capsules (Kyolic)	2 capsules with meals.	Odorless garlic. Use yeast-free type.
Vitamin K tablets or alfalfa	100 mcg daily in pure tablet form.	A deficiency has been linked to intestinal disorders. Alfalfa is a good source of vitamin K. Take 1 tbsp. liquid 3 times daily or 3 tablets daily.

157

Helpful		
Aloe vera juice	As directed on label.	Helps prevent constipation and colon problems. George's tastes like spring water and needs no refrigeration.
Essential fatty acids	As directed on label before meals.	Important for correct bowel function.
Protein supplement (free form amino acids)	½ tsp. 3 times daily taken under the tongue on an empty stomach.	Free form amino acids are more readily absorbed and assimilated.
Raw thymus glandular	As directed on label.	See GLANDULAR THERAPY in Part Three for its benefits.
Vitamin A capsules	25,000 IU daily.	Protects and heals the lining of the colon.
Vitamin C (buffered)	3,000–8,000 mg daily in divided doses.	Use nonacid-forming brand. Needed to reduce inflammation and potentiates immune response.
Vitamin E capsules	Up to 800 IU daily.	A powerful antioxidant that protects the mucous membranes.

HERBS

☐ Use cayenne, chamomile, garlic, papaya, psyllium, red clover, and yarrow extract or tea for diverticulitis. Psyllium seed cleans the intestines and softens the stools. Drink two cups daily of pau d'arco tea. Clay tablets are also beneficial and should be taken on an empty stomach upon arising.

RECOMMENDATIONS

☐ Check stools daily for blood. If the stool is black, take a portion of it to your doctor for an analysis. Try to have a bowel movement the same time each day. Take fiber and acidophilus first thing in the morning before breakfast to help bowels move at this time.

☐ In severe cases, use liquid vitamins. Put all vegetables and fruits through a blender. Baby foods are good until healing is complete. Earth's Best baby foods are organically grown and can be found in a health food store. Add fiber to the baby food. Make steamed vegetables only. Gradually add raw fruits and vegetables. Drink carrot juice, cabbage juice, "green drink," or use chlorophyll liquid in juices (alfalfa).

☐ Do not eat grains, seeds, or nuts, except for well-cooked rice. Dairy products should also be eliminated, as should red meat, sugar products, fried foods, spices, and processed foods. A low-carbohydrate, high-protein diet from vegetable and fish sources is recommended.

☐ Take cleansing enemas (see ENEMAS in Part Three), using two quarts of lukewarm water. These enemas help to rid the colon of undigested and entrapped foods and to relieve pain. Four charcoal tablets or capsules will absorb trapped gas. Do not take with other vitamins or drugs. Take with a large glass of water.

CONSIDERATIONS

☐ To relieve pain massage the left side of the abdomen. Stand up and do stretching exercises.

☐ If the diverticula are infected, the doctor may prescribe antibiotics. Be sure to consume plenty of soured products and some form of nondairy acidophilus if on antibiotics.

☐ Fasting is beneficial. (See FASTING in Part Three.)

☐ See also COLITIS in Part Two.

Dog Bite

The first thing a dog bite victim should do is remove the animal saliva from the wound. Wash it thoroughly with warm water, then add soap and wash for at least five minutes. Rinse for a few more minutes with plain water. Cover with a gauze dressing. See your doctor to make sure that you don't need stitches. The doctor may prescribe antibiotics to prevent infection. If so, make sure that you take acidophilus to replace the "friendly" bacteria that antibiotics destroy.

There is always danger of infection from a dog bite, especially if it is deep. Any bite also carries the risk of rabies. In most states, you are required to report the incident to your local health department. The dog must be kept under observation for any signs of rabies—viciousness, paralysis, growling, foaming at the mouth, or agitation. If the animal can't be located, you must consider rabies shots. Most household pets have been immunized against rabies, but the possibility of infection still exists.

It is also possible to contract a tetanus infection from a dog bite. You should have a tetanus booster shot if you haven't had one in six years or more.

NUTRIENTS

SUPPLEMENT	SUGGESTED DOSAGE	COMMENTS
Very Important		
Vitamin C	4,000–10,000 mg for 1 week, then reduce to 3,000 mg daily.	Reduces infection. Important for repair of collagen and connective tissue.

Important		
Proteolytic enzymes	2 tablets between meals.	Acts as an anti-inflammatory.
Helpful		
Garlic capsules (Kyolic)	2 capsules 3 times daily.	Odorless garlic that acts as a natural antibiotic.
L-Cysteine and L-methionine (amino acids)	500 mg each daily on an empty stomach for 2 weeks.	Powerful detoxifying agents.
Vira-Plex 135 from Enzymatic Therapy	As directed on label.	Can be used alone if bite is not severe. Aids in healing and reduces infection.
Vitamin A and vitamin E	25,000 IU daily. 400 IU daily.	Powerful antioxidants that aid the immune system and assist healing of skin.
Vitamin B complex	50 mg each 3 times daily.	Aids in tissue oxidation and antibody production.

HERBS

☐ Pau d'arco and echinacea tea are good for dog bites, as are red clover and goldenseal.

Drug Addiction (Substance Abuse)

In our drug-oriented society, there is a pill available to solve any minor discomfort. If you have a headache, you can reach into your medicine cabinet and take some aspirin or acetaminophen to relieve the pain. If you are upset by work or marital problems, you can drown your sorrows in a stiff drink. If you have trouble sleeping, you can take a couple of tranquilizers. It is not surprising, therefore, that many adolescents and adults have drug problems.

Although perceptions of alcohol and cigarette use have dramatically changed due to publicized health reports, they are still two of the most accessible drugs. Most young people generally start with these, and then later try the illegal drug marijuana. Many of these young drug users mistakenly believe that alcohol and marijuana are harmless. They also believe that they will never become dependent on drugs and that they can quit at any time. Unfortunately, many later turn to stronger drugs, including heroin (smack) and cocaine (coke). The new potent form of cocaine, popularly referred to as crack, has become a recent problem. It is less expensive than cocaine, easy to conceal, and offers a quick "high." Newspaper reports have cited cases in which the use of this drug has even filtered down to the elementary school level.

Most people are aware that an overdose of cocaine kills; however, many do not realize that this poison kills in other ways. Recent studies show that angina, heart attack, coronary artery spasm, and life-threatening damage to the heart muscle occur with the use of cocaine and heroin.

Cocaine and heroin are not the only drugs with these deadly effects. All drugs weaken the immune system in one way or another. Studies have shown that marijuana use weakens the immune response by as much as 40 percent by damaging and destroying our protective white blood cells (Harvard Medical School letter, Volume 4, Number 5). Without a strong immune system, the body is vulnerable to degenerative disease and AIDS.

Prolonged drug use can lead to other problems. The body may build up a tolerance to the drug, so that the user must keep increasing the dosage to experience the same pleasant effect and to prevent withdrawal symptoms. In order to maintain the desired effect, some users increase the dosage to the point that they nearly die or do die from overdose.

Drug addiction is marked by a decreased desire to work, extreme drowsiness, inattentiveness, frequent mood swings, restlessness, and a loss of appetite. Those addicted to drugs typically want to be alone, lose their temper easily, experience crying spells, and have slow, slurred speech. The pupils of the eye may also change.

An individual can be addicted to substances other than illegal drugs. Many are addicted to nicotine, caffeine, colas, alcohol, sugar, and even certain foods. Although these addictions may not pose as great a health risk, withdrawal may still be painful and difficult. Those who use these substances may be more susceptible to illness and disease because these addictive substances deplete the body of needed nutrients.

An individual addicted to a drug will experience withdrawal symptoms when deprived of the drug. Drug withdrawal symptoms include headache, insomnia, sensitivity to light and noise, diarrhea, hot and cold flashes, sweating, deep depression, irritability, irrational thinking, and disorientation. To minimize withdrawal symptoms, withdrawal from any drug should be done slowly. The dose should be decreased gradually over a period of four weeks or longer. This task cannot be accomplished alone; most often it will require hospitalization and/or professional help.

Substances That Rob the Body of Nutrients

Different substances deplete the body of different nutrients. Use the list below to determine which supplements should be added to the diet when on prescription or over-the- counter medication. Some products like alcohol, caffeine, and fluoride are also listed. These rob the body of vitamins and minerals as well.

Substance	Depleted Nutrients
Alcohol	Magnesium, vitamin B complex, vitamins C, D, E, and K
Allopurinol	Iron
Antacids	Calcium, phosphate, vitamins A, B complex, and D
Antibiotics	Vitamins B and K (Antibiotics also deplete the body of "friendly" bacteria.)
Antihistamines	Vitamin C
Aspirin	Calcium, folic acid, iron, potassium, vitamins A, B complex, and C
Barbiturates	Vitamin C
Caffeine	Biotin, inositol, potassium, thiamine (vitamin B_1), zinc
Carbamazepine	(Dilutes) blood sodium
Chlorothiazide	Magnesium, potassium
Cimetidine	Iron
Clonidine (alpha-adrenergic blocker)	Calcium, vitamin B complex
Corticosteroids	Calcium; vitamins A, B_6, C, and D; potassium; zinc
Digitalis preparations	Thiamine (B_1), vitamin B_6 (pyridoxine), zinc
Diphenylhydantoin (Dilantin)	Vitamin D
Diuretics	Calcium, iodine, magnesium, potassium, riboflavin (B_2), vitamin C, zinc
Estrogen	Folic acid, vitamin B_6 (pyridoxine)
Fluoride	Vitamin C
Glutethimide	Folic acid, vitamin B_6
Guanethidine (and false neurotransmitters)	Magnesium, potassium, riboflavin (B_2), vitamin B_6 (pyridoxine)
Hydralazine	Vitamin B_6 (pyridoxine)
Indomethacin	Iron
Isoniazid	Niacin, vitamin B_6 (pyridoxine)
Laxatives (excluding herbs)	Potassium, vitamins A and K
Lidocaine	Calcium, potassium
Nadolol	Choline, chromium, pantothenic acid (B_5)
Nitrates and nitrites (coronary vasodilators)	Niacin, selenium, pangamic acid (B_{15}), vitamins C and E
Oral contraceptives	Vitamin B complex, vitamins C, D, and E
Penicillin	Niacin (B_3), niacinamide, vitamin B_6 (pyridoxine)
Phenobarbital	Folic acid, vitamin B_6 (pyridoxine), vitamin B_{12}, vitamins D and K
Phenylbutazone	Folate, folic acid, iodine

Substance	Depleted Nutrients
Phenytoin	Calcium, folic acid, vitamins B_{12}, C, D, and K
Prednisone	Potassium, vitamins B_6 (pyridoxine) and C, zinc
Propranolol	Choline, chromium, pantothenic acid (B_5)
Quinidine	Choline, pantothenic acid (B_5), potassium, vitamin K
Reserpine (sympathetic inhibitor)	Phenylalanine, potassium, riboflavin (B_2), vitamin B_6 (pyridoxine)
Spironolactone	Calcium, folic acid
Sulfa drugs	PABA (Sulfa drugs also destroy "friendly" bacteria.)
Thiazides	Magnesium, potassium, riboflavin (B_2), zinc
Triamterene	Calcium, folic acid
Trimethoprim	Folic acid

Marijuana Use

The main active ingredient in marijuana, THC (delta-9-tetrahydrocannabinol), is the most active ingredient of the sixty related chemicals found in the resin that covers the flowers and leaves of the cannabis plant. These leaves and flowers are ground up and are most often smoked in a cigarette or pipe. The pure resin, called hashish, can also be smoked, eaten, or even drunk. New cultivation and propagation techniques have resulted in an increased THC content in marijuana. The amount of THC has risen by at least 200 percent.

The intoxicated state that accompanies marijuana use varies; however, it is usually characterized by a calm, mildly euphoric state. Time may seem to pass more slowly, and the senses—sight, sound, and touch—are enhanced. The marijuana user may feel exhilarated and experience a rapid flow of ideas, accompanied by a reduction in short-term memory. In addition, the user may have an increased appetite and slightly bloodshot eyes. His heart rate may speed up as well. The effects of smoking marijuana last approximately four hours, while the effects of marijuana ingested orally can last up to twelve hours.

Since the user's reaction time and coordination are dramatically impaired when under the influence of marijuana, operating complex equipment such as automobiles is extremely dangerous. Even though the user may no longer be intoxicated, his functioning ability will still be impaired for several hours.

Some individuals may have disturbing reactions to marijuana. They may experience acute anxiety, followed by paranoia. Often the marijuana user is in a state of delirium marked by agitation, confusion, disorientation, incoordination, and hallucinations. These reactions are analogous to those experienced by an LSD user on a "bad trip," except that they are milder with marijuana. Long-term use of the drug can result in psychotic reactions, including hallucinations, inappropriate emotions, and disordered thinking. Studies indicate that marijuana smoking may increase the chance of relapse in the schizophrenic patient (Harvard Medical School letter, Volume 4, Number 5).

Marijuana impairs the functioning of the brain, immune system, reproductive system, and lungs. Marijuana smoke contains the same carcinogenic agents as those found in tobacco smoke, but in a much higher concentration. Since marijuana smoke is inhaled deeply and held in the lungs longer than tobacco smoke, it causes severe damage to the lungs. Marijuana use can lead to bronchitis, emphysema, and lung cancer. By impairing the immune system, marijuana also contributes to cancer, AIDS, and other diseases (Harvard Medical School letter, Volume 4, Number 5).

Addiction to marijuana is a serious problem. Those dependent on this drug are either constantly thinking about marijuana, intoxicated from the drug, or recovering from its effects. Because mental and physical health is impaired with marijuana use, the user's work habits, family life, and friendships suffer. Evidence indicates that long-term use causes significant mental and emotional deterioration. The individual usually lacks ambition and direction, and is typically passive, apathetic, and uncommunicative. Withdrawal from this drug can result in anxiety, insomnia, tremors, and chills. These symptoms can last for many days.

NUTRIENTS

SUPPLEMENT	SUGGESTED DOSAGE	COMMENTS
Very Important		
Vitamin B complex plus	2 cc B complex daily.	Take when under stress and to rebuild the liver.
B$_{12}$ injections	1 cc vitamin B$_{12}$ daily.	
Important		
Calcium and	1,500 mg at bedtime.	Nourishes the central nervous system and helps control
magnesium (chelate form)	1,000 mg at bedtime.	tremors by calming the body.
GABA (gamma-amino butyric acid)	As directed on label.	Acts as a relaxant and lessens cravings.
L-Glutathione	As directed on label.	Aids in detoxifying drugs. Reduces their harmful effects.
L-Lithium carbonate	As directed on label.	This relaxant aids in relieving depression.
L-Phenylalanine	1,500 mg in the morning.	Necessary as a brain fuel. Use for withdrawal symptoms. Caution: Pregnant women and those with high blood pressure should not use this supplement.
Pantothenic acid (B$_5$)	500 mg 3 times daily.	Essential for the adrenal glands and for stress.
Protein supplement (free form amino acids) plus	Take on an empty stomach as directed on label.	L-Tyrosine and valerian root taken every 4 hours have given good results for cocaine withdrawal.
L-glutamine and	500 mg 3 times daily on an empty stomach.	
L-tyrosine	500 mg twice daily on an empty stomach.	
Sodium ascorbate (buffered vitamin C)	2,000 mg every 3 hours. Intravenous form may be necessary under a doctor's supervision.	Detoxifies the system and lessens the craving for the drug.
Helpful		
Multivitamin and mineral complex (high potency)	As directed on label.	All nutrients are needed in high amounts.
Niacinamide	500 mg 3 times daily.	Important for brain function.

HERBS

☐ Siberian ginseng helps cocaine withdrawal.

RECOMMENDATIONS

☐ Many drug users suffer from malnutrition. Because drugs rob the body of necessary nutrients, those addicted to drugs need higher amounts of supplements. See FASTING in Part Three, and follow the instructions. High-protein drinks should be added to the diet. Heavily processed foods and all forms of sugar and junk food should be avoided; these foods are a quick source of energy, but are accompanied by a low feeling that may make some people turn to drugs.

CONSIDERATIONS

☐ The latest research has found that children of alcoholics are more inclined to use drugs, including cocaine. These children are 400 times more likely to use drugs than those who do not have a family history of alcohol addiction. Studies conducted in Sweden revealed that babies of alcoholics who were adopted by nonalcoholic families eventually became alcoholics, indicating a correlation between chemical dependency and genetics. Evidence also suggests that those who become addicted to cocaine carry a gene that predisposes them to chemical dependency.

☐ See also ALCOHOLISM and SMOKING DEPENDENCY, both in Part Two.

Dyspepsia

See INDIGESTION.

Ear Infection

Up to 95 percent of children have had ear infections by the age of six. If the ear infections are persistent, they may lead to eardrum damage and eventual loss of hearing. Infection of the outer or middle ear causes pressure to build up in restricted spaces, and this pressure on sensitive nerve endings causes pain.

A leading cause of ear infection in children may not be recognized by doctors. A bacterium called Branhamell catarrahalis (B-cat) that used to be harmless has since learned to resist standard antibiotics. Fortunately, there is a new antibiotic called Augmentin that can destroy the B-cat bacterium.

There are several types of ear infections, but the most common type is otitis exterma or outer ear infection (swimmer's ear). The ear canal extending from the eardrum to the outside becomes inflamed and swollen. Symptoms include slight fever, discharge from the ear, pain that worsens when the earlobe is touched or pulled, and temporary loss of hearing in the inflamed ear.

If there are symptoms of dizziness, ringing in the ears, bleeding or a bloody discharge, sudden pain, and hearing loss in one or both ears, see your doctor immediately. These symptoms could indicate a ruptured eardrum. Don't blow your nose while you have an ear infection, and keep the ear canal dry. Put cotton in the ear canal when showering or bathing. Don't swim or go out in the rain.

Causes of a ruptured eardrum are sudden inward pressure to the ear from swimming, diving, a slap, a nearby explosion, or a sudden high pressured kiss over the ear. A ruptured eardrum is most often caused by a severe middle ear infection.

Middle ear infections (*otitis media*) are very common in infants and children. The site of the infection is behind the eardrum where the small bones of the ear are located. Symptoms include earache, fullness and pressure in the ear, and a fever as high as 103°F or higher. Children often pull at their ears in an attempt to relieve the pressure. High altitudes and cold climates increase the risk of this infection. Decompression in air travel commonly triggers the infection.

Avoid unsanitary conditions. This type of ear infection may be caused from a lowered resistance due to a recent illness. Nonprescription ear drops may relieve the pain. A nasal spray may help open up the Eustachian tube and relieve the pressure. However, antibiotics may still be needed. See your doctor.

The dosages in the following table are for adults. Reduce the doses for children.

NUTRIENTS

SUPPLEMENT	SUGGESTED DOSAGE	COMMENTS
Very Important		
Manganese	10 mg daily.	A deficiency has been linked to ear disorders.
Vitamin A and E emulsion	50,000 IU vitamin A. 600 IU vitamin E.	Aids in controlling the infection. Use 1 tsp. cod liver oil for children.
Vitamin C	3,000–7,000 mg daily in divided doses.	Use buffered C (calcium or zinc ascorbate).
Zinc lozenges	10 mg 3 times daily for 5 days. Then take in pill form once daily.	Quickens immune response. Aids in reducing infection.
Important		
Vitamin B complex plus extra vitamin B₆ (pyridoxine)	50 mg 3 times daily. 50 mg daily.	Essential for healing and immune function. Relieves ear pressure.
Vitamin E	400–800 IU (increase dosage gradually).	Enhances immune function.
Helpful		
Immuno-Plex #402A from Enzymatic Therapy	As directed on label.	Use if problem persists. Helps the immune system.

RECOMMENDATIONS

☐ Surgical draining of the affected area and antibiotics may be necessary. See your doctor.

☐ Take garlic enemas if toxins accumulate to dangerous levels and cause the body to react. Toxic levels manifest in fever, chills, and general aches and pains. (*See* ENEMAS in Part Three.)

☐ For ringing in the ears, mix one teaspoonful of salt and one teaspoonful of glycerine (from the drugstore) in one pint of warm water. Use a nasal spray bottle to spray each nostril with the solution until it begins to drain in the back of the throat. Also spray the throat. Do this several times a day.

☐ To alleviate pain, use a little warm olive oil or garlic oil in the ear, then a drop or two of lobelia tincture. You can also make a paste using onion powder or clay packs and apply to the outside of the ear to relieve pain.

CONSIDERATIONS

☐ Ear problems are more prevalent in the homes of smokers.

☐ Children who have frequent ear infections should have a food allergy test. *See also* ALLERGIES in Part Two for the food allergy test.

Eating Disorders

See ANOREXIA NERVOSA; APPETITE, POOR; BULIMIA; OBESITY; UNDERWEIGHT.

Eczema

See SKIN PROBLEMS.

Edema

Edema, sometimes called dropsy, is fluid accumulation in the body. It often occurs in the feet and ankles, but any part of the body may have edema. Persistent edema may be caused by kidney, bladder, heart, or liver problems.

The bloating and swelling of edema causes muscle aches and pains. Persistent edema in which little "pits" appear in the feet and ankles after being pressed with the finger indicates a serious problem, and your doctor should be consulted.

Fluid retention is often caused by allergies. Food allergy testing is recommended. *See* ALLERGIES in Part Two for the food allergy test.

NUTRIENTS

SUPPLEMENT	SUGGESTED DOSAGE	COMMENTS
Very Important		
Protein supplement (free form amino acids)	As directed on label.	Sometimes edema is caused by inadequate protein assimilation. Protein deficiency has been linked to water retention.
SP6 Cornsilk Blend herbal combination from Solaray Products	2 capsules 3 times daily.	A safe and natural diuretic.
Vitamin B$_6$ (pyridoxine) plus B complex	50 mg 3 times daily.	Vitamin B$_6$ reduces water retention.
Important		
Alfalfa	3 tablets 3 times daily.	Supplies necessary minerals and chlorophyll. A potent detoxifier.
Calcium and magnesium	1,500 mg daily. 1,000 mg daily.	With correction of edema (i.e., diuresis), lost minerals must be replaced.
Silicon	2–3 tablets daily.	A natural diuretic.
Helpful		
Bromelin	6–8 tablets daily.	A pineapple enzyme that helps digestion and allergies.
Garlic tablets (Kyolic)	2 tablets with meals.	A detoxifier.
Kelp	5 tablets daily.	Supplies needed minerals.
L-Taurine	As directed on label.	Aids heart function.
Potassium	99 mg daily.	Very important if taking diuretics.
Raw Kidney Complex #406 from Enzymatic Therapy	As directed on label.	Improves kidney function.
Superoxide dismutase (SOD)	As directed on label.	Helpful in heart and liver disorders.
Vitamin C	3,000–5,000 mg daily in divided doses.	Essential for adrenal function and production of its hormones. These hormones are vital to fluid balance and control of edema.
Vitamin E	400 IU and up daily.	Aids circulation.

HERBS

☐ The following herbs can be beneficial if you are suffering from edema: alfalfa, butcher leaves, cornsilk, dandelion root, garlic, horsetail, juniper berries, kelp, lobelia, marshmallow, pau d'arco tea, and parsley.

RECOMMENDATIONS

☐ Exercise daily and take hot baths or saunas twice a week. Avoid stress!

☐ Increase your intake of raw food. Eat plenty of onions, apples, beets, and grapes. A high-fiber diet is important. Eat eggs, broiled white fish, and broiled skinless chicken or turkey. Eat small amounts of cottage cheese, yogurt, buttermilk, and kefir.

☐ Avoid salt and caffeine, animal protein, fried foods, soy sauce, pickles, olives, beef, dairy products, dried shellfish, gravies, white sugar, white flour, chocolate, coffee, tea, alcohol, and tobacco.

Emphysema

Emphysema is characterized by a shortness of breath that mainly occurs upon exertion. This difficulty is caused by loss of elasticity and dilatation of the lung tissue. The patient cannot exhale without great effort. Stale air remains trapped in the lungs, preventing the needed exchange of oxygen and carbon dioxide. The most common symptoms of emphysema are breathlessness followed by coughing, no matter how slight the exertion. Emphysema patients are usually elderly, but the condition may begin during youth or middle age depending on previous respiratory problems. Some people suffer from this disease due to a deficiency in serum protein; however, the majority of cases are related to smoking. If you have emphysema and smoke, you must quit. Smoking increases the chances of developing this progressive and eventually fatal disease.

There is no known cure for emphysema, which is classified along with asthma as a form of chronic obstructive pulmonary disease (COPD).

NUTRIENTS

SUPPLEMENT	SUGGESTED DOSAGE	COMMENTS
Essential		
Chlorophyll (Kyo-Green from Wakunaga of America Company)	3 times daily.	Supplies live enzymes. Vitamins, minerals, and chlorophyll aid in clear breathing.
Very Important		
Coenzyme Q$_{10}$	60 mg daily.	A powerful antioxidant.
Garlic capsules (Kyolic)	2 capsules with meals.	Odorless garlic that acts as a natural antibiotic to help prevent infection.
Germanium	200 mg daily.	Improves tissue oxygenation.
L-Cysteine and L-methionine (amino acids)	500 mg twice daily on an empty stomach.	Aids in repairing damaged lung tissue.
Protein supplement (free form amino acids)	As directed on label.	Important for repair of lung tissue.
Vitamin A emulsion	100,000 IU for 1 month, then drop to 50,000 IU. End with 25,000 IU (or same amount in capsule form, adding 10,000 IU of beta-carotene).	Needed for tissue repair and the immune system.
Vitamin C	5,000–10,000 mg daily in divided doses.	Strengthens immune response and aids healing of inflamed tissue.
Important		
Raw thymus and raw lung complex from Enzymatic Therapy	Use as directed.	*See* GLANDULAR THERAPY in Part Three for its benefits.
Vitamin E emulsion	1,000 IU (or in capsule form, start at 400 IU and increase slowly to 1,600 IU).	An oxygen carrier and potent antioxidant. A deficiency can lead to destruction of the cell membrane.
Helpful		
Aerobic 07 by Aerobic Life Products	9 drops in water once daily.	Supplies oxygen and kills bacteria.
Calcium chelate and magnesium	2,000 mg daily. 1,000 mg daily.	Acts as a nerve tonic, protects nerve endings, and promotes a sound sleep.
Kelp	5 tablets daily.	
Multienzymes and proteolytic enzymes	Take with meals. Take between meals.	Keeps infection in check by cleansing the lungs.
Protein supplement from a vegetable source		Repairs damaged lung tissue.

HERBS

☐ If you have emphysema, use the following herbs and herb products: comfrey with fenugreek, fresh horseradish, mullein tea, rosemary, and thyme. Life Extension has a CX1 combination, which helps in detoxification. Thyme is also very helpful.

RECOMMENDATIONS

☐ Upon arising, take one teaspoonful of pure, cold-pressed olive oil. This will supply essential fatty acids while aiding in the elimination of toxic waste in the gallbladder and large intestine.

☐ The diet should consist of 50 percent raw foods. Include onion and garlic daily. Avoid salt. Avoid foods that cause excess mucus to be formed in the gastrointestinal tract, lungs, sinuses, and nasal cavity. Foods that lead to the formation of mucus are meats, eggs, dairy products, processed foods, tobacco, junk foods, and white flour products.

☐ Consume foods that require less chewing. Those with chronic lung disease have difficulty breathing while chewing. Avoid gas-forming foods such as lentils (beans) and cabbage. These foods cause abdominal distention and interfere with breathing. Do not eat a typical American breakfast. Instead sip hot, clear liquids (such as herb teas) to help clear the mucus. ABC colon cleanser is helpful after consuming the liquids. Mix ABC with a glass of juice and drink quickly. This will help rid the colon of excess mucus and reduce gas and distention.

☐ Use castor oil packs on the chest and back.

☐ Avoid air pollution. Change jobs if necessary because your present environment may be dirty, dusty, and toxic to inhale. Do not use aerosol products.

☐ Rest and avoid stress. Get plenty of fresh air.

☐ Go on a cleansing fast using carrot, celery, spinach, and "green drink" fresh juices. (*See* FASTING in Part Three.)

CONSIDERATIONS

☐ *See also* ASCORBIC ACID FLUSH in Part Three and ENVIRONMENTAL TOXICITY in Part Two.

Endometriosis

Endometriosis is a condition in which the cells lining the inside of the uterus, or the endometrium, also grow elsewhere. No proof exists as to what causes endometrial cells to grow outside the uterine body. Nonetheless, doctors continue to expand their knowledge about the course, treatment, and effects of endometriosis.

During the normal menstrual cycle, the endometrium is stimulated by a continually changing cycle of hormones. In the absence of conception, these hormones cause it to "die," slough off, and pass through the vagina during the menses. However, during the menstrual cycles of women who suffer from endometriosis, both the cells of the endometrium and the cells of endometrial origin that have grown outside the uterus respond to these cyclic hormonal messages.

The growth of endometrial tissue outside of the endometrium occurs most often in or on the ovaries, the fallopian tubes, the urinary bladder, the bowel, the pelvic floor, the peritoneum, and within the uterine musculature. According to a recent Stanford University study, the most common site of endometriosis is the deep pelvic peritoneal cavity, or the cul-de-sac. The presence of endometriosis outside the pelvic area is uncommon.

Endometriosis produces a host of symptoms. These include incapacitating pain in the uterus, lower back, and organs in the pelvic cavity prior to and during the menses; intermittent pain throughout the menstrual cycle; painful intercourse; excessive bleeding including the passing of large clots and shreds of tissue during the menses; nausea, vomiting, and constipation during the menses; and infertility. Because menstruation is heavy, iron deficiency anemia is common.

Endometriosis produces adhesions, which are formed when endometrial tissue is not fully discharged. Adhesions attach to various pelvic organs, causing them to bind together. This produces the characteristic severe abdominal pain. Endometrial or "chocolate" cysts are common on the ovaries. These are usually found to contain moderate amounts of oxidized blood having an appearance of chocolate syrup.

Several theories have been proposed to explain the cause of endometriosis, including the reflux menstruation theory developed by John Sampson, M.D., in 1920. Reflux menstruation occurs when menstrual fluid backs up into the fallopian tubes and drips into the peritoneal cavity. While this theory appears to answer the question of what causes endometriosis, it has not been scientifically proven. Another popular theory states that endometriosis is caused when endometrial cells are spread through blood and lymph channels.

Despite disagreement over the cause, more is known today about this perplexing condition than ever before. Once labeled the "working woman's disease," endometriosis is now known to affect 12 million American women—approximately 10 percent of the female adult population—from all walks of life.

Most sufferers of endometriosis have never been pregnant. The exact relationship between infertility and endometriosis remains somewhat unclear. There is debate in the medical mainstream over whether endometriosis causes infertility itself, or whether delaying childbearing results in the gradual breakdown of the female reproductive organs, of which endometriosis is a symptom.

Treatment is varied according to how far the condition has progressed. Doctors commonly prescribe Danazol and birth control pills in an attempt to control the blood flow and pain and with the hope of keeping the abnormal tissue from spreading. They may also use a synthetic male hormone to stop the menstrual period completely. This type of hormone causes excess facial hair growth and a deepening of the voice. If drug therapy fails, radical excision via hysterectomy may be recommended. A less traumatic excision option used to treat milder cases is laser surgery via laparoscopy to identify and vaporize adhesions and cysts.

NEW THEORIES AND TREATMENTS

An alternative theory of the origin of, and new surgical treatment for, endometriosis was developed in the United States by David Redwine, M.D., of St. Charles Medical Center, Bend, Oregon. It is being used by several other gynecological surgeons in the United States, among them, Dan Martin, M.D., of Baptist Memorial Hospital, Memphis, Tennessee; and Russ Malanack, M.D., and Jim Wheeler, M.D., both of Baylor College of Medicine, Houston, Texas.

Rejecting the mainstream prognosis, Dr. Redwine claims that endometriosis is curable. Data collected from his follow-up studies indicate that after a procedure called "near-contact" laparoscopy, 75 percent of his patients experienced complete relief of symptoms, and 20 percent experienced an improvement in their symptoms from disabling pain to minimal pain. No relief was reported by 5 percent.

Since 1979, Redwine has performed near-contact laparoscopy on nearly 400 women. In near-contact laparoscopy, the surgeon examines the entire pelvic cavity and the entire peritoneal surface at very close range to identify any possible endometrial lesions. All suspected endometrial growths in or on the peritoneum, along with all other suspected endometrial lesions (whether typical black-colored or atypical and multicolored), are removed. (The body regenerates the removed portions of the peritoneum within several weeks.) Each biopsied tissue sample is identified, then sent to the lab for confirmation that it is endometrial in origin. This identification method has enabled Dr. Redwine to prove that excised lesions other than "black powder" lesions have been endometrial in origin.

Disagreeing with the mainstream of gynecological surgeons who accept reflux menstruation as its cause, Redwine proposes that endometriosis is actually an unrecognized congenital birth defect. He proposes that during fetal development, endometrial cells migrate toward ducts that develop into the ovaries, uterus, and vagina to form the uterine lining—and some cells are left behind. These cells become imbedded in the ectopic sites and grow. Redwine supports the theory that states that endometrial growths change color until they appear as the classic dark-colored implants primarily found in patients in their thirties.

According to Dr. Redwine, "Endometriosis actually is a disease of predominantly fertile women of any age suffering from predominantly nonmenstrual pelvic pain caused by lesions that are predominantly nonblack and easily missed and that do not spread progressively throughout the pelvis with advancing age. Infertility and dysmenorrhea are less common symptoms and frequently are not due to endometriosis. Anatomic and physiologic derangements frequently accompany, but are not necessarily the result of, endometriosis."

Though endometrial lesions vary in color (white, clear, yellow, blue, red, and black), most surgeons remove only the black "powder burn" lesions and chocolate cysts. The reason why so many women have recurring problems with endometriosis, in spite of surgery, is that only a portion of their endometrial implants have been removed in surgery, Redwine states. In fact, he claims that surgeons who excise only typical black lesions could leave from 50 to 60 percent of the disease behind. For example, the surgeon reports that only 40 percent of 143 women he treated with endometriosis had typical black powder burn lesions. The multicolored, "atypical" type was found in 60 percent of these women. Dr. Redwine attributes his success rate—measured as the lack of recurrence and lessening of symptoms—to the removal of both typical and atypical endometrial lesions not only within the pelvic cavity, but on the peritoneum, as well.

ENDOMETRIOSIS THEORIES CONTRASTED

Accepted Theories	Dr. Redwine's Theories
Caused by retrograde menstruation.	Caused by embryonic defect in cell differentiation.
Lesions bleed monthly.	Lesions do not bleed.
Frequent recurrence following removal of typical lesions.	Little recurrence following removal of both typical and atypical lesions.
Progressive disease.	Positionally static disease.

Disease primarily of women over 30.	Disease of women of all ages.
Associated with menstruation.	Independent of menstruation.
Black lesions prevalent.	Multicolored lesions prevalent.
Causes infertility.	Is not an actual cause of infertility.
Peritoneal implants not considered endometrial in origin.	Peritoneal implants proven to be endometrial in origin.
Hysterectomy recommended for severe cases. Provides undependable levels of relief.	Removal of typical and atypical lesions by near-contact laparoscopy provided complete relief for 75 percent of a sample group of 400.

The following nutrients may help keep the disorder in check if diagnosed in the early stages:

NUTRIENTS

SUPPLEMENT	SUGGESTED DOSAGE	COMMENTS
Very Important		
Vitamin E	Start at 400 IU daily. Increase slowly to 1,000 IU.	Aids hormone imbalance.
Important		
Iron (Floradix formula)	As directed on label.	Floradix formula is easily assimilated.
Unsaturated fatty acids (primrose oil)	2 capsules 3 times daily.	Provides necessary unsaturated fatty acids and gamma-linoleic acid (GLA).
Vitamin B complex and pantothenic acid (B_5) plus	100 mg 3 times daily.	Promotes blood cell productivity and hormone balance.
vitamin B_6 (pyridoxine)	50 mg 3 times daily.	B_6 assists in water balance.
Vitamin C (buffered ascorbic acid plus bioflavonoid complex)	2,000 mg 3 times daily.	Important in healing process.
Helpful		
Calcium chelate and magnesium	1,500 mg / 1,000 mg taken at bedtime.	Supplies needed minerals.
Kelp tablets	2 tablets 3 times daily.	Supplies needed minerals.

HERBS

☐ The herbs dong quai, raspberry leaves, and Siberian ginseng should be part of the program.

RECOMMENDATIONS

☐ Diet is very important. Avoid caffeine, salt, sugar, animal fats, butter, dairy products, all hardened fats, fried foods, red meats, poultry (unless farm raised and skinless), and junk foods or fast foods.

☐ The diet should include 50 percent raw vegetables and fruits. In addition, eat only whole grain products, raw nuts, seeds, and fish. Eliminate shellfish from the diet.

☐ It is important to fast for three days before the menstrual period begins. Use steam-distilled water and fresh live juices. (*See* PREMENSTRUAL SYNDROME in Part Two and FASTING in Part Three.)

☐ A "green drink" from dark green leafy vegetables should be part of the diet. Daily moderate exercise such as walking or stretching is beneficial.

CONSIDERATIONS

☐ Some natural physicians have theorized that endometriosis is related to the body's inability to absorb calcium properly.

☐ For more information contact: Endometriosis Association, P.O. Box 92187, Milwaukee, WI 53202, or call 1-(800) 992-ENDO.

☐ A videotape documenting Dr. David Redwine's studies can be obtained by writing to: Nancy Petersen, R.N., St. Charles Medical Center, 2500 N.E. Neff Road, Bend, OR 97701, or call (503) 382-4321.

Environmental Toxicity

Today there is reason to be concerned about the quality of our water and food supply and the effects of radiation and toxic metals, particularly on our immune system. The body's immune system is a complex network that protects us from particular disease agents such as viruses, bacteria and other microorganisms, allergens (substances that induce allergic reactions), and other pathogens (substances that cause disease). When foreign matter threatens the body, the body's defense mechanism responds by forming protective antibodies. Maintaining the function of the kidney and liver is particularly important, as they work to free the body from toxins. It is vital that we maintain our immune system at its highest level of function so that it can combat radiation, toxic metals, and other toxins present in our environment.

Certain minerals such as calcium and zinc are necessary to sustain life; small amounts of other minerals like copper are essential, but are toxic in larger amounts. Some, unfortunately, not only have no nutritional value but are also toxic in any amount. These toxic metals—lead, aluminum, cadmium, and mercury—pervade our environment and threaten our health, impairing the function of our organs. Pesticides, herbicides, insecticides, fungicides, fumigants, and fertilizers seep into our soil and food. Food additives, preservatives, and artificial coloring pervade our supermarkets. Fruits and vegetables are sprayed, ripening agents are used, and protective waxes are applied to make them appear more appetizing. Toxic fumes, chemicals, and radioactive waste have contaminated our air and water supply.

Products and environmental factors that can have a detrimental effect on your health include disinfectants, hair sprays, paint, bedding, animal hair, household cleaning products, dust, and mold. Some chemical products used in the home emit volatile components: styrene from plastics, benzene from solvents, and formaldehyde from manufactured wood products. Smoke from cigarettes, cigars, or pipes raises the level of toxic substances not only in the smoker, but also in passive smokers (those receiving secondhand smoke). Some people use either an air cleaner or an ion fountain to find symptomatic relief. These remove dust, animal odors, smoke, pollen, smog, and bacteria.

These various pollutants invade our bodies, causing such reactions as watery eyes, diarrhea, nausea, upset stomach, and ringing of the ears. Symptoms are so varied that they also include asthma, bronchitis, stuffy nose, arthritis, fatigue, headache, eczema, and depression.

A hair analysis is often used to identify environmental toxins producing harmful effects in the body. Exposure to environmental toxins has been linked to immune deficiency and cancer.

NUTRIENTS

SUPPLEMENT	SUGGESTED DOSAGE	COMMENTS
Essential		
Coenzyme Q₁₀	30 mg 4 times daily.	Important in immune function. Counters histamine production and benefits allergy sufferers.
Very Important		
Cell Guard from Biotec Foods with superoxide dismutase (SOD)	Use as directed on label.	A powerful antioxidant that protects against free radical formation and radiation.

Garlic capsules (Kyolic)	2 capsules 3 times daily.	Odorless garlic that is a potent immunostimulant.
L-Methionine plus L-cysteine and L-carnitine and glutathione (amino acids)	500 mg 3 times daily.	Protects the lungs, heart, and liver by destroying free radicals.
Proteolytic enzymes and pancreatic enzymes	6 tablets between meals. 3–6 tablets with meals.	Important for proper digestion and detoxification.
Important		
Vitamin A and vitamin E plus beta-carotene	100,000 IU daily. 400-800 IU daily. After 1 month decrease daily amount of vitamin A to 15,000 IU.	Both vitamins act as powerful antioxidants and detoxifiers.
Vitamin B complex (high stress) plus extra vitamin B$_6$ (pyridoxine) and niacinamide and pantothenic acid (B$_5$)	50 mg 3 times daily. Up to 500 mg daily. 100 mg 3 times daily.	Vital to cellular function and repair.
Helpful		
Calcium pantothenate plus copper and germanium and manganese chelate and zinc	50 mg daily. 3 mg daily. 200 mg daily. 50 mg daily. 80 mg daily.	These trace minerals aid the immune system. Germanium is a trace mineral that acts as a potent immunostimulant.
Thymus extract or tablets	500 mg daily.	Improves T-cell production. *See* GLANDULAR THERAPY in Part Three for its benefits.

RECOMMENDATIONS

☐ It is advisable to see an allergy specialist to have a Rast (Radio Allergo Sorbent Test) if you experience any of the symptoms listed above. You may also want to have a hair analysis to determine the level of toxic substances in your system.

☐ Fiber sources such as Aerobic Bulk Cleanse (ABC), oat bran, wheat bran, and guar gum are a very important part of the diet. Apple pectin can also be beneficial.

CONSIDERATIONS

☐ Drink only steam-distilled water.

☐ Injecting patients with liver has produced some good results.

☐ *See also* ALUMINUM TOXICITY, ARSENIC POISONING, CADMIUM TOXICITY, CHEMICAL ALLERGIES, CHEMICAL POISONING, COPPER TOXICITY, DDT POISONING, FOOD POISONING, LEAD POISONING, MERCURY TOXICITY, and NICKEL TOXICITY, all in Part Two.

Epilepsy

Epilepsy is characterized by seizures, which are caused by electrical disturbances in the nerve cells in one section of the brain. These seizures vary in their severity. Petit mal seizures are mild—the person will stare into space and may twitch slightly. Grand mal seizures are more extreme—the person will fall to the ground, become unconscious, and have convulsions. Seventy-five percent of the seizures begin in childhood and are characterized by staring spells and a few seconds of mental absence. Twenty-five percent of seizures start later in life.

Epilepsy can be caused by infection, meningitis, rickets, rabies, tetanus, malnutrition, hypoglycemia, sports injuries, head injuries, fever, or allergies. It may also result from scar tissue from an eye injury or a stroke, lack of oxygen, spasm to the blood vessels, and arteriosclerosis. It is thought that it may also be hereditary. Often its cause is unknown.

According to research done by Arizona State University's Biochemical Department, NutraSweet has been associated with seizures. Aluminum toxicity and lead poisoning may also contribute to the problem. A hair analysis should be done to rule out these metal toxicities.

TYPES OF SEIZURES

There are several types of seizures including:

- *Absence (petit mal)*. Most common in children and characterized by a blank stare. During these seizures children are unaware of their surroundings.
- *Atonic (drop attack)*. A childhood seizure in which the child loses consciousness for about ten seconds after his legs have collapsed.
- *Complex partial (temporal lobe)*. Blank stares, random activity, and a chewing motion are characteristic of this type of seizure. The person may be dazed and unaware of his surroundings, and may act oddly. There is no memory of this seizure.

- *Generalized tonic-clonic (grand mal).* Characterized by sudden cries, a fall, rigidity and muscle jerks, shallow breathing, and bluish skin. Loss of bladder control is possible. The seizure usually lasts two to five minutes, and is followed by confusion, fatigue, or memory loss.
- *Myoclonic.* Brief, massive muscle jerks occur.
- *Simple partial (Jacksonian).* Jerking begins in the fingers and toes and progresses up through the body while the person is conscious.
- *Simple partial (sensory).* The person may see, hear, or sense things that do not exist. May occur as a preliminary symptom of a generalized seizure.

Nutritional supplementation is important for those who suffer from epilepsy.

NUTRIENTS

SUPPLEMENT	SUGGESTED DOSAGE	COMMENTS
Essential		
L-Taurine and L-tyrosine (amino acids)	500 mg 3 times daily.	Important for proper brain function.
Magnesium (magnesium chloride)	700 mg taken between meals on an empty stomach with apple cider vinegar or betaine HCl.	Use magnesium chloride (an excellent source of magnesium).
Vitamin B₆ (pyridoxine)	100–600 mg daily in divided doses under supervision.	All B vitamins are extremely important in the central nervous system.
Vitamin B₁₂ lozenges	200 mcg, dissolved under the tongue twice daily, on an empty stomach.	
Very Important		
Calcium	1,500 mg daily.	Important in normal nerve transmission.
Vitamin B complex with extra vitamin B₆ and vitamin B₁₂ and folic acid and pantothenic acid and niacin	See above for dosage. See above for dosage. 50 mg daily.	Important in nerve transmission. Injections of vitamin B complex under doctor's supervision may be necessary.
Zinc	50–80 mg daily.	Valuable in RNA/DNA synthesis.
Important		
DMG (Gluconic from DaVinci Labs)	50 mg under the tongue in the morning and at night.	Stimulates immune response.
Germanium	200 mg daily.	Improves cellular oxidation.

Helpful		
Chromium (GTF)	200 mcg daily.	Important in cerebral sugar metabolism. Picolinate form is effective.
Kelp or alfalfa	5 tablets daily.	For necessary mineral balance.
Proteolytic enzymes and digestive enzymes	Take between meals. Take with meals.	
Raw thymus concentrate and thyroid extract	As directed on label.	Both the thymus and thyroid are important in proper brain function. *See* GLANDULAR THERAPY in Part Three for its benefits.
Vitamin A	25,000 IU daily.	An important antioxidant that aids in protecting brain function.
Vitamin C plus bioflavonoids	2,000–7,000 mg daily in divided doses.	Vital to functioning of the adrenal gland, which is the antistress gland.
Vitamin E	Start with 400 IU. Gradually increase to 1,600 IU.	Aids circulation and immunity.

HERBS

☐ Those with epilepsy should include black cohosh, hyssop, and lobelia in their program.

RECOMMENDATIONS

☐ If you are present when someone has a seizure, do the following:

1. Move sharp or dangerous objects away from him.
2. Place the person on a bed or the floor.
3. Loosen tight clothing.
4. Turn the person on his side, if possible.
5. Do not put anything in his mouth. Swallowing objects is more dangerous than biting the tongue.
6. Stay calm and remember that the person feels nothing during a seizure.

☐ Eat soured milk products like yogurt and kefir. Drink juices made from green vegetables, peas, green beans, seaweed, beets, carrots, and red grapes. Include raw nuts, seeds, chard, beet tops, soybeans, green leafy vegetables, eggs, raw milk, and raw cheese.

☐ Avoid alcoholic beverages, animal protein, caffeine, artifical sweeteners such as NutraSweet, and nicotine. Avoid refined foods and sugar.

☐ Eat small meals, don't drink a lot of liquids at once, and take two tablespoons of olive oil daily.

☐ If the bowels do not move each day, take a lemon enema before going to bed. (Combine the juice of two lemons and two quarts of water.)

☐ Take Epsom salt baths twice a week.

☐ Stay away from pesticides.

☐ Work toward self-care. Keep drug dosages as low as possible, and work toward becoming as free from drugs and seizures as possible. The correct diet is a key to the control of epilepsy. Improved circulation to the brain is important. Exercise is extremely beneficial! Avoidance of stress and tension is also important.

CONSIDERATIONS

☐ A manganese deficiency in pregnant women may result in the birth of epileptic children.

☐ Some good results have been reported using hyperbaric (high pressure oxygen) therapy.

☐ Tranxene, a drug used in a Japanese study of twenty-nine epileptics, helped twenty-one in the study. The only side effect was a slight impairment in memory.

☐ The side effects of antiseizure medications include liver problems, mental fatigue, mental fogginess, fatigue, leukemia-like symptoms, and, in some cases, death.

☐ Check for alkalosis (*see* ALKALOSIS in Part Two).

Epstein Barr Virus

See CHRONIC FATIGUE SYNDROME.

Eye Problems

We have all experienced eye trouble at one time or another—eyes that are bloodshot, burning, dry, infected, irritated, itchy, sensitive to light, ulcerated, or watery, to name just a few. Eye disturbances are often an early sign of disease elsewhere in the body. Watery eyes are a symptom of the common cold; eye disturbances can indicate a host of other illnesses as well. A thyroid problem may be indicated by protruding or bulging eyes and reading difficulties. Allergies are also reflected in the eyes. Dark circles under the eyes and eyes that are red, swollen, and/or watery indicate allergies. Yellowing of the eyes from jaundice can be a sign of hepatitis, gallbladder disease, or gallstone blockage. High blood pressure and diabetes often manifest themselves in periodic blurring of vision. In addition, droopy eyes are often an early sign of *myasthenia gravis*, a disorder in which the muscles of the eye weaken. Pupils that are drastically different in size could indicate a tumor somewhere in the body as well.

A deficiency of just one vitamin can lead to various eye problems. In order to avoid or correct eye trouble, you can supplement your diet with vitamins and minerals. Some of these supplements will protect against the formation of free radicals, which can damage the eye. Some eye problems that can be helped by supplementing the diet with vitamins and other nutrients are described in this section.

HERBS

☐ For various eye problems including inflammation and eyestrain, use eyebright capsules orally, prepare eyebright as a tea, and/or use it to rinse the eye. Goldenseal can be used as an alternative or in addition to eyebright; however, do not use goldenseal in large amounts if pregnant. Take two capsules of SP herb formula from Solaray three times daily. Bayberry bark, red raspberry leaves, and cayenne taken by mouth are beneficial as well.

RECOMMENDATIONS

☐ Include the following in your diet: broccoli, raw cabbage, carrots, cauliflower, green vegetables, dessicated liver, squash, sunflower seeds, and watercress. Eliminate sugar and white flour from your diet.

☐ Carrot juice can help prevent or alleviate certain eye problems. Two tablespoons of cod liver oil can also be helpful.

CONSIDERATIONS

☐ The combination of nicotine, sugar, and caffeine may temporarily affect vision.

☐ Tinted eyeglasses prevent needed light from entering the eyes. If you wear glasses, wear only clear ultraviolet spectacles. See the section on light for its influence on the master glands.

☐ Those who wear contact lenses need to take precautions against eye disease because of the associated risk of infecting the eye.

☐ Gary Price Todd, M.D., author of *Eye Talk*, states that the use of margarine and vegetable shortening is dangerous for those with certain eye disorders. Butter and

Maintaining Healthy Eyes

Like all other parts of the body, the eye needs to be rested properly. In addition to making sure that the eyes are not strained by intense close reading or inadequate light, proper eye care includes a healthy diet containing sufficient amounts of vitamins and minerals. A well-balanced diet replete with fresh fruits and vegetables can help keep your eyes healthy. In order to promote good eyesight, you must make sure your diet contains the proper amounts of vitamins A, B complex, C, and E, selenium, and zinc. Fresh fruits and vegetables are good sources of these vitamins and minerals; include plenty of these in your diet, including carrots, yams, and cantaloupe.

NUTRIENTS

SUPPLEMENT	SUGGESTED DOSAGE	COMMENTS
Protein supplement (free form amino acids)	As directed on label.	Free form amino acids are assimilated best.
Selenium in a vitamin complex	200 mcg daily.	Selenium destroys free radicals, which can damage the eye.
Vitamin A emulsion plus beta-carotene	75,000 IU emulsion or 15,000 IU in capsule form. 15,000 IU beta-carotene.	Vitamin A is absolutely necessary for proper eye function. Protects the eye from free radicals.
Vitamin B complex	100 mg twice daily.	Needed for intracellular eye metabolism.
Vitamin C	2,000 mg 3 times daily.	An antioxidant that reduces intraocular pressure.
Vitamin E	400 IU daily.	Important in healing and immunity.
Zinc	50 mg daily.	Zinc deficiency has been linked to retinal detachment.

RECOMMENDATIONS

A cold compress applied to the closed eye can be helpful.

---

vegetable oils can be used as substitutes. He also suggests taking a multivitamin and mineral supplement the evening before eye surgery, including 10,000 IU vitamin A, 1,000 milligrams of vitamin C, and 1,200 IU vitamin E. He recommends continued use of these after surgery, adding 2 milligrams of copper and 20 milligrams of zinc.

☐ Be careful when using drugs. Some may cause eye problems. Drugs that can damage the optic nerve, retina, and other vital parts of the eye include:

- ACTH.
- Allopurinol, which is used for gout.
- Anticoagulants.
- Aspirin.
- Corticosteroids.
- Diabinese.
- Diuretics, antihistamines, and digitalis preparations, all of which can cause disturbances in color distinction.
- Indomethacin.
- Marijuana, which can cause color disturbances.
- Nicotinic acid, if used for long periods.
- Streptomycin.
- Sulfa drugs.
- Tetracycline.

According to a report from *Ocular Diagnosis and Therapy*, ocular abnormalities can be hastened by anti-infection drugs, diazepam, haloperidol, psychotropic drugs, quinine, and sulfonamides.

BITOT'S SPOTS

Bitot's spots are distinct, elevated, white patches on the white part of the eye (the cornea). If you have Bitot's spots, avoid eyestrain and smoke-filled rooms.

NUTRIENTS

SUPPLEMENT	SUGGESTED DOSAGE	COMMENTS
Vitamin A emulsion	Start at 100,000 IU for 2 weeks, and then take 50,000 IU for 1 month. Decrease to 25,000 IU in capsule form.	Aids in dissolution of Bitot patches, which may be caused by vitamin A deficiency.

BLOODSHOT EYES

For this common ailment of the eyes, wash the eye with raspberry leaves to alleviate redness and irritation. Prepare as a tea, allow to cool, and then apply to the eye as a compress.

BLURRED VISION

If objects appear hazy and unclear at times, supplement your diet with vitamin A and potassium.

NUTRIENTS

SUPPLEMENT	SUGGESTED DOSAGE	COMMENTS
Potassium	99 mg daily.	Balances excess sodium.
Vitamin A	25,000–50,000 IU daily.	Necessary for proper balance of intraocular fluid.

CATARACTS

When the lens of the eye becomes clouded or opaque, it is unable to focus on close or distant objects. This eye condition is called cataracts. Some causes of cataracts are injury to the eye, the use of certain drugs such as steroids, diabetes, and heavy metal poisoning. Cataracts are the number one cause of blindness.

The most common form of cataracts is senile cataracts, which affects those over sixty-five. This form of cataracts is often caused by free radical damage. Exposure to ultraviolet rays and low-level radiation from x-rays leads to the formation of reactive chemical fragments in the eye. These free radicals attack the structural proteins, enzymes, and cell membranes of the lens.

NUTRIENTS

SUPPLEMENT	SUGGESTED DOSAGE	COMMENTS
Copper plus manganese and selenium and	3 mg copper daily.	These minerals are important for proper healing and for retarding the growth of cataracts.
zinc	50 mg zinc daily.	
L-Lysine (amino acid)	As directed on label.	Important in collagen formation in tissue, which is necessary for lens repair. Also neutralizes viruses implicated in lens damage.
Pantothenic acid (B$_5$)	500 mg daily.	An antistress vitamin.
Thiamine (B$_1$) and riboflavin (B$_2$)	50 mg each daily taken with the B complex.	Important for intracellular eye metabolism. Riboflavin deficiency has been linked to cataracts.
Vitamin A	25,000–50,000 IU daily.	Vital for normal visual function.
Vitamin C	3,000 mg daily in divided doses.	A necessary free radical destroyer. Lowers intraocular pressure.
Vitamin E	400 IU daily.	An important free radical destroyer.

Recommendations

☐ If you have cataracts, avoid antihistamines. Bilberry herbal extract contains bioflavonoids, which aid in the removal of chemicals from the retina of the eye.

COLOR BLINDNESS

For those who have a hard time distinguishing colors, take vitamin A.

NUTRIENTS

SUPPLEMENT	SUGGESTED DOSAGE	COMMENTS
Vitamin A	50,000 IU daily.	May be beneficial. (Improves night blindness.)

CONJUNCTIVITIS (PINK EYE)

Conjunctivitis is an ailment characterized by an inflammation of the membrane lining the eyelid. It is highly contagious when it is caused by a viral infection. Eyes may appear swollen and bloodshot; they are often itchy and irritated. Because the infected membrane is often filled with pus in conjunctivitis, the eyelids often stick together after being closed for an extended period. Factors that can contribute to conjunctivitis include bacterial infection, injury to the eye, allergies, and substances that are irritating to the eye such as fumes, smoke, contact lens solutions, chlorine from swimming pools, chemicals, make-up, or any other foreign substance that enters the eye. If pain or blurred vision occurs, seek medical attention immediately.

NUTRIENTS

SUPPLEMENT	SUGGESTED DOSAGE	COMMENTS
Vitamin A emulsion	100,000 IU daily for 1 month; then switch to 25,000 IU daily in capsule form.	Vitamin A, vitamin C, and zinc all help to promote immunity, which is especially important in common viral conjunctivitis.
Vitamin C	2,000–6,000 mg daily in divided doses.	Protects the eye from further inflammation. Enhances healing.
Zinc	50 mg daily.	Important in all eye disorders. Enhances immune response.

Herbs

☐ Chamomile, fennel, and red eyebright can be used to make herbal teas. Use these teas for hot compresses.

Considerations

☐ Pink eye associated with hay fever can be treated with drops containing steroids, which can be obtained from your physician.

☐ A bacterial infection is typically treated with antibiotics if the eye does not heal within four days of supplement use.

☐ If your eyelids are swollen, you might want to peel and grate a fresh potato, wrap it with gauze, and place it over your eyes. It acts as an astringent and has a healing effect.

DIMNESS OR LOSS OF VISION

A condition marked by vision loss that affects smokers is commonly referred to as tobacco amblyopia. It is seen most often in pipe smokers.

Recommendations

☐ Avoid smoking!

DRY TEAR DUCTS

Your eyes have dry tear ducts when they do not produce enough fluid to keep them moist. Dry eyes generally stem from a lack of vitamin A. See your doctor if you have dry tear ducts. This could be a symptom of rheumatoid arthritis.

NUTRIENTS

SUPPLEMENT	SUGGESTED DOSAGE	COMMENTS
Essential fatty acids (primrose oil)	2 capsules 3 times daily.	A good source of essential fatty acids.
Vitamin A ointment and/or vitamin A	As directed on label. 25,000 IU	Tears contain vitamin A. Vitamin A is beneficial for eyes that seem dry and scratchy.

Recommendations

☐ If your tear ducts are swollen, add more calcium to the diet and avoid processed foods.

☐ Avoid products that claim they can "get the red out."

FARSIGHTEDNESS

See HYPEROPIA in this section.

"FLOATERS"

Bits of debris floating within the eye are commonly referred to as "floaters." Because these "floaters" cast shadows over the retina, the individual will see small specks. Most of these specks eventually float out of view and are not considered bothersome. If you see a large number of floaters, however, you should be examined by an ophthalmologist. It is normal to see a few floaters at times, but if you see a large number of them, you should not delay seeking treatment. A detached retina requiring lengthy surgery can result from delayed treatment.

GLAUCOMA

Glaucoma is a serious eye disease marked by an increase in pressure that the fluids within the eyeball exert on the other parts of the eye. If this pressure is unrelieved, the eyeball may harden. The pressure of the fluid may harm the retina and ultimately damage the optic nerve, resulting in blindness. See also GLAUCOMA in Part Two.

NUTRIENTS

SUPPLEMENT	SUGGESTED DOSAGE	COMMENTS
Vitamin C	10,000–15,000 mg daily. You can increase this ascorbic acid flush to 30,000 mg (30 g) under a doctor's supervision.	Reduces intraocular pressure.

Recommendations

☐ Avoid the herb licorice and high amounts of niacin. Also avoid tranquilizers and antihistamines.

HYPEROPIA (FARSIGHTEDNESS)

More commonly known as farsightedness, hyperopia is characterized by burning, itchy, scaly, and tired eyes, and by red-rimmed eyelids. Because the eyeball is abnormally short, light rays fall behind the retina. Those who are farsighted can see far away objects clearly, but have trouble seeing near objects distinctly.

NUTRIENTS

SUPPLEMENT	SUGGESTED DOSAGE	COMMENTS
Vitamin B complex with extra riboflavin (B₂)	50–100 mg daily.	Improves intraocular cellular metabolism.

ITCHY EYES

If you have tired, itchy eyes, supplement your diet with vitamin B complex with extra riboflavin (B₂).

NUTRIENTS

SUPPLEMENT	SUGGESTED DOSAGE	COMMENTS
Vitamin B complex with extra riboflavin (B₂)	50–100 mg daily.	Improves intraocular cellular metabolism.

MUCUS

If your eyes are filled with mucus, wash each eye with goldenseal root. Do not use goldenseal in large amounts if pregnant.

PAIN BEHIND THE EYE

Pain behind the eye is probably due to eyestrain or an eye muscle problem.

NUTRIENTS

SUPPLEMENT	SUGGESTED DOSAGE	COMMENTS
Vitamin B complex with extra riboflavin (B₂)	50–100 mg daily.	Improves intraocular cellular metabolism.

PHOTOPHOBIA

An individual with photophobia is unable to withstand light. Light hurts the eyes.

NUTRIENTS

SUPPLEMENT	SUGGESTED DOSAGE	COMMENTS
Vitamin A	50,000 IU daily.	All eye disorders need vitamin A.

RETINAL VASCULAR LEAKAGE, MICROANEURISMS, AND RETINAL EDEMA

Other problems of the eye include leakage in the vessels that transmit the fluids of the eye, abnormally enlarged blood vessels in the eye, and accumulation of too much fluid in the eye.

NUTRIENTS

SUPPLEMENT	SUGGESTED DOSAGE	COMMENTS
Calcium and magnesium	1,000 mg daily. 500 mg daily.	A 2-to-1 ratio of calcium to magnesium helps microcirculation in the eye.
Selenium and superoxide dismutase (SOD) and vitamins A, C, and E	100–200 mcg daily. As directed on label. Megadoses.	Selenium, SOD, and vitamins A, C, and E are all potent free radical scavengers. Free radicals have been implicated in damage to the retina and microcirculation.
Vitamin B complex	100 mg daily.	Improves intraocular cellular metabolism.

SHINGLES (HERPES ZOSTER)

If painful blisters called shingles develop near the eyes, damage to the cornea can occur and may produce blindness. When shingles appear on the forehead near the eyes or on the tip of the nose, seek treatment from an ophthalmologist. If the proper supplements are taken when blisters first appear, the blisters may dry up within twenty-four hours and discomfort may be alleviated.

NUTRIENTS

SUPPLEMENT	SUGGESTED DOSAGE	COMMENTS
Vitamin and mineral complex (high potency)		
Vitamin B₁₂	2,000 mcg dissolved in mouth 3 times daily on an empty stomach.	Prevents nerve damage to the eyes.
Vitamin E	1,000 IU daily.	Do not take this amount if you have high blood pressure and have not taken vitamin E previously. Instead, start with 400 IU and work up slowly.

175

Recommendations

☐ Applying zinc oxide cream to the blisters and affected area may help. After the blisters have healed, try applying aloe gel and vitamin E to the area.

☐ If none of the above works to heal the blisters within three days, intravenous injections of 25 grams of vitamin C provides relief almost immediately.

Considerations

☐ *See also* SHINGLES in Part Two.

SCOTOMA

Those who occasionally see spots in front of the eyes have scotoma. Those with scotoma have a blind spot in their visual field, usually due to trouble in the retina.

NUTRIENTS

SUPPLEMENT	SUGGESTED DOSAGE	COMMENTS
Vitamin A emulsion	100,000 IU for 2 months. 25,000 IU in capsule form.	The emulsion formula is absorbed into the system quicker and is better assimilated.

STYES

Styes form from an infection within the oil glands of the eyelid. Because the tissues of the eye become inflamed from the infection, the styes will appear as pimples. Early treatment is necessary to avoid further complications. If a stye does not heal promptly, it may need to be drained surgically. Do not try to squeeze the lump or it may spread into the bloodstream and cause a fatal infection.

Recommendations

☐ If you suffer from styes frequently, supplement your diet with vitamin A. Those with frequent styes often suffer from a vitamin A deficiency.

☐ Hot compresses on the afflicted area may relieve discomfort.

☐ Treatment using antibiotics may be necessary.

☐ Prepare raspberry leaves as a tea and apply as an eyewash to alleviate styes.

THINNING OF EYELASHES

If you supplement your diet with B vitamins, you can help prevent thinning of eyelashes.

NUTRIENTS

SUPPLEMENT	SUGGESTED DOSAGE	COMMENTS
Vitamin B complex with extra riboflavin (B_2) plus	50–100 mg daily.	Prevents loss of eyelashes.
brewer's yeast and niacin (B_3)	2 tbsp. brewer's yeast daily.	Brewer's yeast is a good source of B vitamins.

Recommendations

Rub linseed or castor oil on eyelashes at bedtime.

ULCERATED EYE

When the normal coverings of the eye are damaged, the eye becomes inflamed. This results in an ulcerated eye. Ulcerated eyes are usually viral in origin.

NUTRIENTS

SUPPLEMENT	SUGGESTED DOSAGE	COMMENTS
Vitamin C	6,000 mg daily in divided doses.	A healing and antiviral substance.

ULCERATED EYELIDS

When the eye becomes inflamed due to ulcerated eyelids, use yellow dock. You can also use this as a poultice; steep as a tea, saturate a cloth with the tea, and apply to inflamed eyelid.

XEROPHTHALMIA

Xerophthalmia is an inflammation of the covering of the eye in which the eye is marked by dryness.

NUTRIENTS

SUPPLEMENT	SUGGESTED DOSAGE	COMMENTS
Vitamin A	25,000–50,000 IU daily.	Specifically for dry eyes.
Vitamin B_6 (pyridoxine) and	50 mg daily.	Vitamin B_6, vitamin C, and zinc work well together to heal dry eyes.
vitamin C and	2,000–4,000 mg daily in divided doses.	
zinc	50 mg daily.	

Fatigue

Chronic fatigue is usually the result of a high-fat and refined carbohydrate diet and emotional stress. Drugs, caffeine products, alcohol, smoking, stress, and incorrect eating habits are energy robbers. Chronic fatigue may also signify an undetected illness such as diabetes, candidiasis, anemia, cancer, hypoglycemia, allergies, malabsorption, hypothyroid, poor circulation, Epstein Barr virus (EBV), or mononucleosis. Fatigue is not a disorder in itself; it is a symptom.

Fatigue that is characterized by lack of energy only can also be caused by boredom. If you find no physical reason for your fatigue, then you should seriously consider changing your lifestyle!

NUTRIENTS

SUPPLEMENT	SUGGESTED DOSAGE	COMMENTS
Very Important		
Bee pollen	Start with a few granules increasing to 2 tsp.	Often dramatically increases energy.
Brewer's yeast or Bio-Strath	Start with a small amount and work up.	Bio-Strath is a good tonic that increases energy levels. From Germany with B complex and herbs.
Iron (Floradix formula or desiccated liver tablets)	As directed on label.	Supplies iron and herbs. Use liver only from Argentina.
Multivitamin and mineral (high potency) including GTF or chromium plus		Vitamin deficiencies have been associated with a lack of energy.
potassium and	99 mg daily.	
selenium and	100 mcg daily.	
vitamin A and	25,000 IU daily.	
zinc	50 mg daily.	
Octacosanol capsules	As directed on label.	Aids tissue oxygenation and increases endurance.
Protein supplement (free form amino acids)	As directed on label.	Amino acids in free form are absorbed and assimilated quickly by the body.
Vitamin B complex plus	100 mg 3 times daily.	Insufficient B complex results in fatigue.
vitamin B$_{12}$ lozenges	Place under the tongue. Consider vitamin B injections (under a doctor's supervision only) if severe fatigue exists.	
Important		
DMG (Gluconic from DaVinci Labs)	3 tablets daily.	Increases energy levels.
Vitamin C plus bioflavonoids	3,000–8,000 mg daily.	Increases energy levels.
Helpful		
Energen C from Alacer Corporation and/or vitamin C	As directed on label. 4,000–10,000 mg daily in divided doses.	Increases energy levels quickly due to rapid assimilation into the body.
Energy Now from FoodScience or PEP Formula from Vital Health Enterprises	As directed on label.	Formulated to counteract fatigue.
Gerovital H-3 (GH-3) or Aslavital, both from Rumania	As directed on label.	Dr. Aslan's formula is for those over 35. Used in clinics around the world to lift depression and to increase energy levels.
L-Aspartic acid and L-citrulline and L-phenylalanine (amino acids)	500 mg on an empty stomach twice daily.	Mood elevators.
Magnesium and calcium chelate or asporotate	750 mg daily. 1,500 mg daily.	Calcium provides energy and plays an important role in protein structuring (RNA-DNA).
Royal jelly from Montana Pollen	2 capsules 3 times daily.	Increases energy levels.
Vitamin B complex with extra choline and pantothenic acid (B$_5$) and thiamine (B$_1$)	50 mg with meals.	Needed for normal brain function, hormone production, and conversion of fats, carbohydrates, and protein to energy.

HERBS

☐ Acacia, cayenne, ginkgo biloba extract, Siberian ginseng, gotu kola, and guarana help combat fatigue.

RECOMMENDATIONS

☐ A proper diet is important. Emphasis should be on including more fresh fruits and vegetables, grains, seeds, and nuts. Avoid energy robbers like sugar, alcohol, fats, caffeine, white flour products, and highly processed foods. Eat less red meat and more white fish.

☐ Exercise is important as is adequate rest. Reducing weight to normal is necessary.

□ During exercise, the brain produces endorphins and enkephalins, pain-killing chemicals. Immunological researchers have found that exercise strengthens the immune system more than any other single factor. Exercise also releases a chemical that produces a "natural high." Most of those who exercise claim that they really feel good afterward. This may explain why exercise is the best way to get rid of depression!

□ Use spirulina, an excellent protein source. Take four spirulina tablets three times a day with bee pollen, octacosanol, 3,000 milligrams of vitamin C, and free form amino acids. This has been used for fatigue with good results.

□ See FASTING in Part Three, and follow once monthly.

□ See HYPOTHYROID in Part Two. Take the underarm temperature test as described in that section to determine if you have a low thyroid function. Also, see ALLERGIES and WEAKENED IMMUNE SYSTEM in Part Two. Allergies are often the cause of fatigue. Make sure you do not have an allergy to molds.

Fever

A fever is an elevation in body temperature often indicating an infection. Normal body temperature ranges from 98°F to 99°F. One should not have undue concern unless the body temperature rises above 102°F in adults or 103°F in children. In this case, consult your doctor immediately. This is a signal that the infection is getting worse. Fever can cause brain injury and dehydration if the temperature is too high, especially for prolonged periods.

A fever is not a disease. It is actually a symptom that indicates the presence of a disease. In fact, running a temperature is often helpful to the body. This defense mechanism of the body acts to destroy foreign microbes. If the fever does not get too high, let it run its course. In some cases, it helps to eliminate toxins.

NUTRIENTS

SUPPLEMENT	SUGGESTED DOSAGE	COMMENTS
Very Important		
Vitamin A	Use as directed on label in emulsion form. Or take 50,000 IU daily in pill form for 1 week, then lower to 25,000 IU. Children over 2 years old should take 1,000–10,000 IU daily.	Enters system quicker and is essential in immune system function. Needed to fight infection and to strengthen the immune system.
Important		
Protein supplement (free form amino acids)	3 times daily on an empty stomach.	Free form amino acids are a readily absorbed form of protein that helps repair tissue damaged during the fever.
Vitamin C		*See* ASCORBIC ACID FLUSH in Part Three, and follow the program. Children should use calcium ascorbate—it won't produce heavy diarrhea. Needed to flush out toxins and reduce fever.
Helpful		
Garlic capsules (Kyolic)	2 capsules 3 times daily.	Odorless garlic that acts as a natural antibiotic and powerful immunostimulant.
Royal jelly	3 times daily.	Has antifungal properties and improves adrenal function.
Spiru-Tein from Nature's Plus	Take between meals as directed on label.	A protein drink that contains all the amino acids, vitamins, and minerals needed for nourishment.

HERBS

□ Lobelia extract or tincture will help lower the fever if given half a teaspoon every four hours. If an upset stomach occurs, cut back to a quarter teaspoon.

□ Hyssop, licorice root, thyme, and yarrow tea combination can help a fever. Blackthorn, echinacea, fenugreek seed, feverfew, ginger, and poke root are also beneficial. You can make a poultice from echinacea root to lower fever (see POULTICE in Part Three).

RECOMMENDATIONS

□ While feverish, avoid taking a multivitamin and mineral complex that contains iron and zinc. While an infection is present, the body will throw off extra iron into the tissues in an attempt to lower the fever. Therefore, a supplement containing iron will cause undo strain on the body. In addition, zinc will not be absorbed while a fever is present.

□ Catnip tea enemas twice daily are important because constipation and congestion keep the fever up. (See ENEMAS in Part Three.) The catnip tea is also good to drink along with lobelia and dandelion teas to lower fever. Take several cool sponge baths.

□ Drink plenty of distilled water and juices, but avoid solid food until the condition has improved.

CONSIDERATIONS

If flu-like symptoms linger or are recurrent, check for diabetes (especially in children) and Epstein Barr virus (in adults and teenagers). *See* CHRONIC FATIGUE SYNDROME in Part Two.

☐ Never give children aspirin. (*See* REYE'S SYNDROME in Part Two.)

Fibrocystic Disease of the Breast

Upwards of fifty percent of adult females have fibrocystic disease of the breast. The Medical College of Pennsylvania states that an iodine deficiency is a common reason for fibrocystic disease. Other factors include hormone imbalance and abnormal breast milk production (caused by high amounts of the hormone estrogen).

In fibrocystic disease round lumps that move freely and are either firm or soft are produced. Symptoms include tenderness and lumpiness in the breasts. Pain is usually most severe before menstruation. The cysts may change in size.

In this disease, the cysts become filled with fluid and fibrous tissue surrounds the cysts and thickens like a scar. The pressure causes pain. Fluid is reabsorbed by the breast tissue when a hormone imbalance or abnormal milk production occurs. The milk-producing glands multiply and carry milk into the supporting fibrous tissue, resulting in fibrocystic disease of the breast. As a woman ages, it becomes more difficult for the lymph system to absorb this fluid completely. Fluid is trapped and results in cysts and inflammation of the breast. These cysts are benign.

A cyst is tender and moves freely—it feels like an eyeball behind the lid. A cancerous growth usually does not move freely, is most often not tender, and does not go away.

In a simple office procedure, the doctor will use a needle to diagnose fibrocystic disease. The needle is used to remove fluid from the cysts. A mammogram is usually taken to rule out cancer.

The drug Danazol (a hormone) acts through the pituitary gland, reducing the function of the ovaries. This, in turn, decreases the amount of estrogen in the breast, shrinking the lumps. Danazol is not effective in all women, but about 60 percent have shown results within a few weeks. Many patients reported less pain or tenderness. The drug may have some side effects. Use only if the following suggestions fail to give the desired results.

There have been good results using primrose oil to reduce the size of the cysts. The diet below will also help.

NUTRIENTS

SUPPLEMENT	SUGGESTED DOSAGE	COMMENTS
Essential		
Coenzyme Q$_{10}$	100 mg daily.	Similar to vitamin E in action, but more potent. A powerful antioxidant.
Germanium	100 mg daily.	A fast-acting pain killer. Also improves tissue oxygenation.
Kelp	6 tablets daily.	A rich source of iodine. Iodine deficiency has been linked to this disease.
Primrose oil capsules	2 capsules 3 times daily.	Extremely important—may work alone to reduce the size of the cysts. Used successfully in Europe.
Vitamin E emulsion	1,000 IU daily for 1 month or start at 400 IU in pill form and increase slowly to 1,000 IU.	Vitamin E supplements alone may resolve fibrocystic disease.
Very Important		
Vitamin A plus	15,000 IU daily.	Necessary for the mucous membranes of the breast's ductal system.
beta-carotene	10,000 IU daily.	
Vitamin B$_6$ (pyridoxine) and	50 mg 3 times daily.	Important in fluid retention and hormone regulation.
thiamine (B$_1$) and	50 mg 3 times daily.	
B complex	daily	
Important		
Vitamin C	3,000–7,000 mg daily in divided doses.	Necessary for hormone (especially adrenal) production and balance.
Helpful		
High-quality multimineral complex	As directed on label.	Balanced body minerals are important.
Proteolytic enzymes (Intenzyme Forte from Biotics Research or Inflazyme Forte from American Biologics)	As directed on label.	Reduces secondary inflammation and pain.

HERBS

☐ The following herbs should be included in the program: echinacea, goldenseal, herbal squaw vine, mullein, pau d'arco, poke root, and red clover.

RECOMMENDATIONS

☐ A low-fat and a high-fiber diet is important! Eat more raw foods, including seeds, nuts, and grains. Be sure nuts are not rancid. Include in your diet, three or more times a day, apples, grapes, grapefruit, bananas, unroasted nuts, seeds, yogurt, and fresh vegetables. Whole grains and beans are also an important part of the diet.

☐ Avoid alcohol, animal products, cooking oils from supermarket shelves, rancid foods, fried foods, salt, sugar, tobacco, and all white flour products. Avoid animal fats such as those found in bacon, sausage, gravies, ham, beef, and pork.

☐ The most important substances to avoid are coffee, tea (except herbal teas), cola drinks, and chocolate. These foods contain caffeine. According to research done by Dr. John Peter Minton of the Department of Surgery at Ohio State University College of Medicine, Columbus, women who eliminate caffeine-containing substances from their diets had a high rate of disappearance and elimination of cysts.

☐ Make a poultice of poke root for the breast. See POULTICE in Part Three.

☐ See HYPOTHYROID in Part Two, and take the temperature test.

Flu

See INFLUENZA.

Food Poisoning

Each year more than two million Americans report illnesses that have been traced to foods that were eaten. Food poisoning occurs when a person consumes food containing harmful bacteria. The actual number of food poisoning cases is well above the number of reported cases because most people mistake the symptoms of food poisoning for intestinal flu. In fact, up to 275 million of the cases of diarrhea reported annually are directly related to foods eaten.

Symptoms of food poisoning include nausea, vomiting, and cramps lasting from a few hours to a few days. If you suspect that you have been poisoned from a public restaurant or other eating place, contact your local health department right away so that others might be saved from possible food poisoning. Some types of food poisoning, such as botulism, are more serious, especially for elderly people and children. As many as

9,000 deaths occur annually from all types of food poisoning. In addition, many cases of food poisoning lead to chronic health disorders, such as reactive arthritis.

Pathogenic and toxigenic organisms—those that can cause disease and those that can produce toxins—are silent killers because neither the taste, odor, nor appearance of the food indicates their existence. All types of bacteria can potentially become toxigenic.

The most common cause of food poisoning is *Salmonella*. *Salmonella* bacteria are part of the natural intestinal flora of animals. They are easily transmitted to others through human food supplies, knives, table tops, cracked eggs, and the hands of food preparers. *Salmonella* thrive in livestock that has been given antibiotics. More than 50 percent of cattle, poultry, and swine are given antibiotics in their feed to make them grow faster and to prevent disease in crowded and unsanitary conditions. At least one-third of all chickens in the United States are contaminated with *Salmonella* bacteria. The Livingston-Wheeler Clinic in California forbids the consumption of chickens or eggs by their patients.

Symptoms of salmonella poisoning can range from mild abdominal pain to severe diarrhea and dehydration to typhoid-like fever. Diarrhea may be the first sign of food poisoning. Outbreaks of salmonella poisoning occur primarily in the warmer months. Salmonella poisoning can also weaken the immune system and cause kidney and cardiovascular damage and arthritis.

Most salmonella poisoning is contracted from contaminated foods—primarily chicken, eggs, beef, and pork products. People who eat raw or poorly cooked meats are at greater risk for salmonella poisoning. Cooks who first handle raw hamburger and then other foods will endanger others; in addition, those cooks who lick their hands or fingers after handling raw meat put themselves at risk for salmonella poisoning. Those taking antibiotics are also at greater risk for salmonella poisoning. Even though antibiotics can effectively treat bacterial infections, they can also promote infection by destroying good, competing bacteria and permitting the growth of bacteria that are antibiotic resistant.

In 1985 an outbreak of salmonella poisoning from contaminated milk occurred in five mid-western states. As a result, 17,000 people became ill and 2 died. Until recently eggs were thought to be free of *Salmonella* bacteria; however, there has been a dramatic increase in the number of reported cases of food poisoning from foods containing raw or only partly cooked eggs, particularly in the Northeast. Foods such as ice cream, hollandaise sauce, eggnog, and Caesar salad dressing are not cooked well enough to kill *Salmonella* bacteria. Of thirty-five outbreaks of illness that were reported from 1985 to 1987 and determined to be food poisoning, twenty-four were caused by contaminated eggs or foods containing these infected eggs. Certain strains of bacteria will not be destroyed in eggs that are poached or in eggs made over easy or sunny side up, in addition to other ways.

In addition to eggs, salmonella poisoning has been reported with raw clams, oysters, and sushi (a popular Japanese delicacy). Although this type of poisoning does not occur as often, it does exist. Sushi (raw fish) has been contaminated with a worm-like parasite called anisakis. This parasite appears as a tightly coiled, clear worm, about one-half to three-quarters of an inch in length. It commonly embeds itself in herring and other fish. A sushi chef can spot this parasite easily, so illness from sushi is a rare occurrence.

In 1988 a bacterium called *Lesteria monocytogenes* was found in packaged dairy products and a brand of chocolate dipped ice cream bars called Polar Bars. These products were recalled in twenty-five states. Fortunately they were removed in time, and no illnesses were reported.

Next to *Salmonella*, *Staphylococcus aureus* is the second most frequent cause of food-borne illnesses. Because this microorganism is commonly found in the nose and throat, sneezing and coughing on food can contaminate it. Before you eat from a salad bar, make sure that it is protected and clean. *Staphylococcus aureus* are responsible for approximately 25 percent of all food-borne illnesses. Symptoms of food contamination by this bacterium include diarrhea, nausea, and vomiting within two to six hours after eating. These responses occur because the body is trying to rid itself of the toxins produced in the presence of this bacterium. For this reason it may be wise to induce vomiting. If the symptoms are severe or prolonged, see your doctor.

Food kept at room temperature is the most likely to encourage the growth of bacteria. One of the problems with eating in some restaurants and food service companies is that they often prepare large servings of turkey, chicken, beef, and many other foods that have been left out at room temperature. Bacteria called *Clostridium botulinum*, sometimes referred to as the "cafeteria germ," and *Salmonella* often breed in food that has not been kept cold or hot.

The bacterium *Clostridium botulinum* commonly inhabits the soil in the form of harmless spores. It is easily destroyed when frozen or heated properly. Of the various types of food poisoning, botulism is the most severe and affects the central nervous system. In botulism, toxins produced by the organism block the transmission of impulses from the nerve to the muscles. Those suffering from botulism may feel extremely weak and have double vision, droopy eyelids, and trouble swallowing in the early stages. The symptoms typically appear twelve to forty-eight hours after ingestion.

Paralysis and death may result in severe cases.

Even though the Centers for Disease Control reported only thirty cases of botulism in 1982, botulism still remains a threat. Freezing, the presence of chemicals such as sodium nitrite, and drying will prevent the spores from growing. Heating foods to 176°F for twenty minutes or 194°F for ten minutes will also help to destroy the spores. Canned foods, especially those canned at home, may become contaminated with this potentially lethal organism. Beware of bulging cans, cracked jars, or loose lids on products. These can indicate botulism. In addition, beware of rusty cans and check home canning as well. This toxin has been found in asparagus, beets, corn, stuffed eggplant, smoked and salted fish, green beans, ham, lobster, luncheon meats, mushrooms, peppers, sausage, soups, spinach, and tuna. Occasionally botulism can occur even though the food containers show no signs of damage. One restaurant allowed a large batch of sautéed onions to be kept out at room temperature throughout the day instead of keeping them refrigerated and taking small amounts when needed. Several people became very ill from the botulism toxin found in the onions.

A microorganism called *Complobacter jejuni* has recently been implicated in human illness, although it has been known to cause illness in cattle for some time. Thirty-one cases of this illness have been reported, although officials believe that the actual number of cases is much higher because many people mistake it for a stomach virus. People tend not to associate their illness with food because it takes three to five days for these bacteria to produce abdominal cramps, diarrhea, and possibly blood in the stool. Because *Complobacter jejuni* are present in the intestinal tracts of healthy cattle, turkeys, chickens, and sheep, they are spread to all parts of the meat during the slaughtering process. Fortunately, heat destroys the bacteria. Hamburger and all other meats should be cooked at least until they turn brown. Rare meat that is even a little pink in color may still carry the bacteria. To insure that the bacteria have been destroyed, it is best to cook the meat until it is well done.

Four other types of food poisoning include *staphylococcal*, *campylobacteriosis*, *perfringens*, and *giardiasis*. The *Staphylococcus* produce a toxin that often contaminates meat, poultry, egg products, tuna, potato and macaroni salads, and cream-filled pastries. Symptoms such as diarrhea, nausea, vomiting, abdominal cramps, and prostration will occur thirty minutes to eight hours after eating.

Campylobacteria, which are found in poultry, cattle, and sheep, can cause similar symptoms within two to five days after eating. Those suffering from this type of food poisoning commonly have abdominal cramps, diarrhea, and fever; often they have blood in the stool as

---

Tips for Preventing Food Poisoning

Here are some fast, easy rules to help prevent food poisoning at home and while eating out.

- Keep food either hot or cold. Foods left at room temperature encourage rapid bacteria growth.
- Keep perishable products refrigerated.
- Refrigerate leftovers as soon as possible.
- Cook meat, poultry, and seafood thoroughly. Meats should be cooked at a temperature of at least 165°F.
- Wash your hands before handling food. Harmful bacteria are transmitted after diapering a baby or blowing your nose.
- Keep two cutting boards: one for cutting meat and the other for vegetables. This will prevent the transfer of bacteria from meat to vegetables. Wash your cutting boards with a bleach-water solution at least three times a week.
- Go home directly after grocery shopping, especially in warm weather. Store foods immediately according to labels.
- Clean any utensil that has come in contact with raw hamburger, poultry, or seafood. Utensils that have been used with raw meats should not be used to mix other foods until they have been disinfected. These measures will prevent the spread of harmful bacteria.
- Wash out lunch boxes and thermoses after every use.
- Throw away cans having loose lids and those that are bulging, rusted, bent, or sticky. Beware of cracks in jars and leaks in paper packaging.

- Reheat food thoroughly and bring to a rapid boil, if possible.
- Set refrigerator temperature at 40°F or below. Freezers should be set at 0°F or below.
- Wash kitchen towels and sponges with a bleach-water solution daily.
- Picnic foods, such as mayonnaise, salad dressing, and milk products, can be trouble if they are left in the sun or at room temperature.
- Avoid creamed foods, foods containing mayonnaise, and soups that are not kept at near boiling temperatures at salad bars. Do not eat at salad bars that do not look fresh and clean or have a protective glass.
- Giving honey to a newborn can produce a toxin inside the infant's immature intestine and can lead to infant botulism. Honey is safe for babies after age one.
- Mold commonly grows on spoiled food products. The following foods should be avoided if mold is growing on them: bacon, bread, cured luncheon meats, soft dairy products, flour, canned ham, hot dogs, dried nuts, peanut butter, roast poultry, soft vegetables, and whole grains. Also avoid any other cooked or raw foods covered with mold.
- Thaw all foods, especially meats and poultry, in the refrigerator.
- Do not stuff a chicken or turkey with dressing until you are ready to put it in the oven. The dressing can contaminate the poultry. Cook and/or store the dressing separately, and then place it in the poultry immediately before putting it in the oven.

---

well. These symptoms may last up to ten days.

Perfringens are bacteria that survive heat and multiply when meat and meat products cool and when they are stored. This type of food poisoning can be very serious in elderly victims. Common symptoms are mild nausea and vomiting that usually lasts the day or less.

Giardiasis is associated with consumption of contaminated water. It can also be transmitted to raw foods that have grown in contaminated water. Cool, moist environments are conducive to the growth of this type of microorganism. Symptoms generally occur within one to three weeks and include diarrhea, constipation, abdominal pain, flatulence, loss of appetite, nausea, and vomiting.

NUTRIENTS

SUPPLEMENT	SUGGESTED DOSAGE	COMMENTS
Important		
Garlic capsules (Kyolic)	2 capsules with meals.	A powerful detoxifier.
Potassium	99 mg daily.	Needed for the proper balance of sodium and potassium.
Helpful		
Acidophilus	Twice daily.	Replaces essential intestinal bacteria.
Aerobic 07 from Aerobic Life Products	Add 20 drops to a glass of water every 3 hours.	Destroys harmful bacteria such as *Salmonella*.
Antioxidant formula containing L-cysteine plus	500 mg daily.	All of these nutrients are essential in immune function.
L-methionine and	500 mg daily.	
selenium and	200 mcg daily.	
superoxide dismutase (SOD) and	5,000 mg daily.	
vitamin C plus		
bioflavonoids and	8,000 mg daily.	
vitamin E	600 IU daily.	
Fiber	Twice daily.	ABC (Aerobic Bulk Cleanse) and oat bran are recommended.
Kelp	5 tablets daily.	Contains needed minerals.

HERBS

☐ Use lobelia herb tea enemas to rid the body of the poison.

RECOMMENDATIONS

☐ Make sure that you have easy access to emergency telephone numbers. If you suspect food poisoning, call your regional poison center immediately. The poison center can be reached twenty-four hours a day, and can provide you with up-to-date information regarding treatment.

☐ If food poisoning occurs, protect your immune system by immediately taking six charcoal tablets. These are available at most health food stores and should be kept on hand for emergencies. After six hours, take six more tablets. The agents in these tablets will circulate through the bloodstream and help neutralize and eliminate the poison.

☐ If vomiting occurs, make sure that the victim does not choke. Keep enough of the vomit for analysis. If the poisoning is severe, as from a chemical or drug, call a physician to obtain an antidote, if possible.

CONSIDERATIONS

☐ For some cases of poisoning, induced vomiting may be desirable. One syrup that is available in drugstores that can induce vomiting is Ipecac. Use this syrup only if recommended by your physician.

☐ If the person suffers from severe headache and vomiting, suspect food allergies. Take the charcoal tablets as prescribed above along with a coffee retention enema to help rid the body of the poisonous toxins. *See* ENEMAS in Part Three, and refer to the section on coffee enemas.

Fractures

A fracture is a break in a bone. A fracture is called closed or simple when the skin stays intact, and open or compound when the bone breaks the skin. A fracture should be covered immediately. If possible, make a splint to immobilize the area. A doctor should be seen as soon as possible. After the doctor has set the bone, the following supplements will aid in healing.

NUTRIENTS

SUPPLEMENT	SUGGESTED DOSAGE	COMMENTS
Very Important		
Calcium	1,000–2,000 mg divided up after meals and at bedtime.	Vital for proper bone repair.
Kelp	5 tablets daily.	Rich in calcium and minerals in a natural balance.
Magnesium	1,000 mg daily.	Needed to balance with calcium.
Mineral complex and trace minerals	As directed on label.	Needed for repair of tissues.
Mixed raw bovine neonatal tissue from Biotics Research	As directed on label.	Promotes healing. *See* GLANDULAR THERAPY in Part Three for its benefits.
Proteolytic enzymes	Take on an empty stomach between meals.	Reduces associated inflammation.
Silicon	As directed on label.	Needed for calcium uptake and connective tissue repair. Springtime horsetail herb is a good source.
Vitamin C with bioflavonoids	3,000–6,000 mg daily in divided doses.	Important in bone muscle trauma.
Vitamin D	400–1,000 IU daily.	Needed for calcium absorption and repair.
Zinc	80 mg daily.	Important in tissue repair.
Helpful		
Octocosanol	3,000 mg daily.	Improves tissue oxygenation.
Pantothenic acid (B₅)	100 mg 3 times daily.	Antistress vitamin. Aids in vitamin utilization.
Potassium	99 mg daily.	Needed to keep swelling down and balance with sodium.
Protein supplement (free form amino acids)	As directed on label.	Sublingual free form amino acids speed healing.
Raw liver concentrate (from Argentine beef only)	As directed on label.	Supplies balanced B vitamins and other needed vitamins and minerals. *See* GLANDULAR THERAPY in Part Three.
Vitamin A emulsion	Start at 50,000 IU daily, then drop to 25,000 IU daily.	Emulsion enters the system more quickly. Protein is *not* utilized without vitamin A.

RECOMMENDATIONS

☐ Turmeric paste makes a good poultice. Combine it with a little hot water and apply to the site of the injury on a gauze dressing. This is also good for bruises and helps the swelling. Clay poultices and a poultice of fresh mullein leaves are also good. (*See* POULTICE in Part Three.)

☐ Avoid consumption of red meat as well as colas and any other products containing caffeine. Preserved foods should also be limited due to their phosphorus content. Phosphorus can lead to bone loss.

☐ *See also* SPRAINS, STRAINS, AND OTHER INJURIES OF THE MUSCLES AND JOINTS in Part Two.

Frigidity

Frigid women are unable to experience pleasure from sexual intercourse. Evidence has indicated that frigidity is generally of psychological origin, stemming from fear, guilt, and feelings of inferiority. Unpleasant childhood and adolescent experiences are often factors. In such cases, help from a mental health professional is advised. In other women, however, frigidity may result from physiological factors. Some women may find intercourse painful due to insufficient lubrication, inadequate stimulation, or some other physiological factor. Consult your physician to explore the various alternatives, such as surgery, which may alleviate painful intercourse. Vitamin deficiency can cause a deficiency in estrogen levels and result in improper lubrication. If this is the cause, follow the supplement program listed below.

NUTRIENTS

SUPPLEMENT	SUGGESTED DOSAGE	COMMENTS
Very Important		
Gerovital H-3 (GH-3) from Rumania	As directed on label.	This drug produces excellent results, increasing sexual vitality.
Kelp	8 tablets daily.	A good source of important minerals and iodine.
Vitamin B complex	100 mg twice daily.	
Vitamin E	Start at 200–400 IU. Increase slowly to 1,600 IU daily.	Necessary in reproductive function of the glands.
Helpful		
Fish liver oil	1 tbsp. before meals.	Supplies vitamins A and D.
Lecithin	3 tbsp. or 5 capsules daily.	Contains essential fatty acids.
L-Phenylalanine and tyrosine (amino acids)	Take with 50 mg vitamin B$_6$ and 500 mg vitamin C on an empty stomach.	*Caution:* Do not use in large amounts if you have high blood pressure or diabetes or are pregnant.
PABA (para-aminobenzoic acid)	100 mg daily.	B vitamin that stimulates vital life functions.
Vitamin C plus bioflavonoids	3,000–6,000 mg daily in divided doses.	Important in glandular function and stress response.
Zinc	50–80 mg daily.	A zinc deficiency results in impaired sexual function.

HERBS

☐ Use bee pollen, damiana, Fo Ti, sarsaparilla, saw palmetto, and Siberian ginseng or gotu kola.

RECOMMENDATIONS

☐ Make sure that you include the following in your diet: alfalfa sprouts; avocados; fresh eggs from hens (not those stored cold in the supermarket); olive oil; pumpkin seeds, as well as many other seeds and nuts; soy and sesame seed oil; and wheat.

☐ Avoid poultry, red meat, and sugar products.

☐ Avoid smog conditions. Smog is highly toxic and dangerous; it adversely affects immune function, hormone activity, as well as a host of other body functions.

CONSIDERATIONS

☐ Hypothyroidism may be the underlying problem. *See* HYPOTHYROID in Part Two and take the self-test.

Fungus

A yeast (fungus) or mold may infect the skin, mouth, or vagina, and grow under the nails, between the toes, or on internal surfaces. A fungus under the nails or between the toes may cause discoloration and swelling, and the nails may raise above the surface of the nail bed, resulting in infection.

Moist red patches anywhere on the body often indicate fungus (yeast) infections. When in the vagina, a cheesy discharge is present.

A depressed immune function is a leading cause of fungus infections, and is more likely to infect the obese or those who are ill, diabetic, or using oral contraceptives. It especially affects those taking antibiotics. Those who perspire heavily are also at risk.

NUTRIENTS

SUPPLEMENT	SUGGESTED DOSAGE	COMMENTS
Essential		
Acidophilus or Maxidophilus or Megadophilus	As directed on label.	Supplies the "friendly" bacteria that are deficient in fungus infections.
Garlic capsules (Kyolic)	2 capsules 3 times daily with meals.	Odorless garlic that neutralizes most fungi.
Important		
Aerobic 07 from Aerobic Life Products	9 drops in 8 oz. of water twice daily.	Destroys unwanted bacteria and increases tissue oxygenation needed to combat the fungus.

Pantothenic acid (B₅) plus vitamin B complex	50 mg 3 times daily.	Needed for correctly balanced bacteria in the body.
Vitamin C	3,000–10,000 mg 3 times daily.	*See* ASCORBIC ACID FLUSH in Part Three. Needed for proper immune function.
Vitamin E emulsion or capsules	400-800 IU daily.	Needed for proper immune function. Emulsion is assimilated faster.
Zinc	50 mg daily.	Needed for proper immune function.
Helpful		
Essential fatty acids	Use as directed on label.	Salmon, primrose, and black currant oils relieve pain and inflammation.
Vitamin A	25,000 IU daily.	Aids healing of skin and mucous membranes. Needed for proper immune function.

RECOMMENDATIONS

☐ If nails are affected, apply Aerobic 07 drops directly on the area. Soak infected hands or feet in a solution of Aerobic drops and pau d'arco tea daily for fifteen minutes. Keep nails dry and clean.

☐ Apply honey to the fungus, alternating with crushed garlic.

☐ Keep all body parts clean and dry.

☐ Eliminate those foods from the diet that tend to promote secretion of mucus. Exclude dairy products, grains, meat, and fish. Avoid processed foods. Eat 60–70 percent raw food.

☐ *See* FASTING in Part Three and follow the program.

☐ *See also* ATHLETE'S FOOT and CANDIDIASIS, both in Part Two.

Gallbladder Disorders

The gallbladder is a small organ located directly under the liver. It acts as a bile reservoir, concentrating the bile that the body uses to digest fats. Bile contains cholesterol, bile salts, lecithin, and other substances.

When the gallbladder becomes inflamed, the patient has severe pain in the upper right abdomen. This is accompanied by fever, nausea, and vomiting. This condition must be treated immediately. If left untreated, the inflammation of the gallbladder, called cholecystitis, can be life threatening.

Sometimes the cholesterol crystallizes and combines with bile to form gallstones. Often a patient with gallstones will have no symptoms. When a stone blocks the bile passage, nausea, vomiting, and severe pain in the upper right abdominal region occur. These symptoms often arise after the patient has eaten fried or fatty foods.

NUTRIENTS

SUPPLEMENT	SUGGESTED DOSAGE	COMMENTS
Helpful		
Alfalfa	10 tablets 3 times daily.	Take for 2 days with a glass of warm water. A liver cleanser, rich in vitamins and minerals.
Lecithin	1 tbsp. before meals or in capsule form as directed.	Aids fat (cholesterol) digestion. A fat emulsifier.
Multienzymes (containing ox bile)	Take with meals.	*Caution:* If heartburn is present, use pancreatin after meals. Do not use products containing hydrochloric acid (HCl).
Unsaturated fatty acids	As directed on label.	
Vitamin A	25,000 IU capsules daily.	Emulsified vitamin A is more easily assimilated.
Vitamin B complex (high potency) with B₁₂ and		Necessary for proper digestion.
choline and	500 mg daily.	Important in cholesterol metabolism and liver and gallbladder function.
inositol	500 mg daily.	
Vitamin C	3,000 mg daily.	A lack of vitamin C can cause gallstones.
Vitamin D	400 IU daily.	Gallbladder malfunction interferes with vitamin D absorption.
Vitamin E	600 IU daily.	Prevents fats from becoming rancid.

HERBS

☐ Use barberry root bark, catnip, cramp bark, dandelion, fennel, ginger root, horsetail, parsley, and wild yam.

☐ Peppermint oil capsules are used in Europe to cleanse the gallbladder.

RECOMMENDATIONS

☐ *For inflammation:* Eat no solid food for a few days, only distilled or spring water. Then begin to drink juices such as pear, beet root juice (Biotta brand is good), and apple juice for three more days. Then add solid foods: shredded raw beets with two tablespoons of olive oil, fresh lemon juice, and freshly made uncooked applesauce.

☐ *For gallstones:* Use three tablespoons of olive oil with the juice of a lemon before retiring and upon awakening. Many stones pass in the stool with this technique. Look for them! Grapefruit juice can be used instead of lemon juice. Try a castor oil pack on the gallbladder area.

☐ A detoxification program for the liver and colon is important for improved gallbladder function. Use a cleansing enema when there are chronic problems.

☐ Do not overeat. Obesity and gallbladder disease are related. The female who is forty and overweight and who has had children is more likely to suffer from disorders of the gallbladder.

☐ Avoid surgery if the stones show up on an x-ray but are without symptoms. A gallstone may slip into a bile duct, which drains the gallbladder and the liver. If this occurs, then extraction or surgical removal might be necessary. Sometimes the stones remaining in the gallbladder can be "fragmented" without surgery. Bile acid preparations used to dissolve stones work very slowly and can be used only on small stones.

☐ Eat 75 percent raw foods. Also include in the daily diet applesauce, eggs, yogurt, cottage cheese, broiled fish, fresh apples, and beets. Avoid sugar and products containing sugar. Avoid all animal fat and meat, fried foods, spicy foods, margarine, soft drinks, commercial oils, coffee, chocolate, and refined carbohydrates.

☐ For five days consume as much pure apple juice as possible. Add pear juice occasionally. Beet juice will also cleanse the liver.

☐ Rapid weight change may cause gallbladder problems.

☐ *See* FASTING in Part Three, follow the program, and use a coffee enema for a few days when "toxic." (You will know when you are toxic when you have pain and nausea/vomiting and fever.) The coffee enema is important. You can also use garlic in the enema. *See* ENEMAS in Part Three.

Gangrene

There are two types of gangrene, wet and dry. Dry gangrene does not involve bacterial infection. It is caused by stopped or reduced blood flow, which results in oxygen-deprived tissue. It may also be caused by hardening of the arteries, poor circulation, diabetes, or arterial embolism (a blockage in the bloodstream).

Sometimes gangrene is caused by frostbite. The oxygen-deprived area dies, but in frostbite the gangrene does not spread to any other area. As the flesh dies, it may be painful, but once the skin is dead, it becomes numb and slowly darkens.

Dry gangrene is caused by an injury or disease that cuts off the blood supply to injured tissues. It most often occurs in the feet and toes. When it involves an acute arterial obstruction, emergency surgery must be performed. If, following an injury, the area injured becomes red, swollen, and painful, or develops an odor, see a doctor without delay.

Symptoms of the most common type of dry gangrene are a dull, aching pain and coldness in the area. Pain and pallor of the injured area are early signs. Slowly developing gangrene may be reversed by revascularization (i.e., arterial surgery). Chelation is an alternative (*see* CHELATION THERAPY in Part Three).

Wet gangrene is the result of a wound or injury that becomes infected. The infection prevents adequate venous drainage, depriving the area of needed blood supply and oxygen. Careful hygiene can usually prevent this type of gangrene. Antibiotics and surgical removal of the dead tissue are usually necessary.

NUTRIENTS

SUPPLEMENT	SUGGESTED DOSAGE	COMMENTS
Essential		
DMG (Gluconic from DaVinci Labs)	100 mg 3 times daily and up.	Enhances oxygen utilization by affected tissue.
Very Important		
Chlorophyll liquid or tablets	1 tbsp. liquid 4 times daily. 2 tablets 4 times daily.	A blood cleanser.
Coenzyme Q$_{10}$	100 mg twice daily.	Improves circulation.
Germanium	200 mg daily.	Increases oxygen utilization and reduces dangerous free radical formation.
Potassium	99 mg daily.	Aids in reducing tissue swelling.
Proteolytic enzymes	2 between meals and with meals.	Aids in damaged tissue "clean up" and repair.
Vitamin A and E emulsion	50,000 IU vitamin A. 400 IU up to 1,600 IU vitamin E daily. Do not take this amount of vitamin E in pill form.	Emulsion enters the system more quickly. Vitamin A is essential for tissue repair. Vitamin E improves circulation. Both enhance immune function.
Vitamin C plus bioflavonoids	4,000–10,000 mg daily.	For tissue repair and improved circulation.
Important		
Kelp	6 tablets daily.	Rich source of chlorophyll and minerals. Good for circulation, and is a blood cleanser.

Helpful		
Aerobic 07 from Aerobic Life Products	As directed on label. Apply a few drops directly on the area.	Kills infecting bacteria. A stabilized oxygen product.
Calcium and magnesium	2,000 mg daily. 1,000 mg	For connective tissue repair.
Multivitamin and mineral complex	As directed on label.	For connective tissue repair.
Zinc	50–80 mg	Speeds healing. Necessary for tissue repair and immune function.

HERBS

☐ Butcher's broom is important for circulation. Also use bayberry, cayenne, echinacea, ginkgo biloba, goldenseal, and red seal.

RECOMMENDATIONS

☐ "Green drinks," made from vegetables such as spinach, beet tops, or any leafy greens are important! *See* JUICING in Part Three.

☐ Honey applied to the affected area is very healing.

☐ *See also* ARTERIOSCLEROSIS and CIRCULATORY PROBLEMS in Part Two.

Maintaining a Healthy Glandular System

A gland is any organ of the body that secretes fluids from its cells. There are two types of glands in the body: exocrine and endocrine. The hypothalamus is the section of the brain that regulates the activities of both the exocrine and endocrine glands. Exocrine glands are those that secrete their fluids through ducts or channels, such as the salivary glands and the mammary glands. The salivary glands excrete saliva in the mouth and the mammary glands produce milk. Other exocrine glands help digestion by secreting gastric and pancreatic juices and bile.

Unlike exocrine glands, which secrete fluids through a duct, endocrine secretions do not pass through a tube, but rather are emitted as hormones directly into the bloodstream. Endocrine glands are called ductless glands for this reason.

By secreting hormones into the bloodstream, the endocrine glands help to regulate practically all body activities. The hormones circulate through the blood, sending messages that either speed up or slow down normal body processes. Hormones help to control our rate of metabolism, circulation, pH balance, and growth. Hormones also play a role in the repair of all body tissue, protect the body from bacterial invasion, help the body deal with stress, and control reproduction.

The endocrine glands include the pituitary, the parathyroids, the thyroid, the thymus, the adrenals, the islets of Langerhans, and the gonads or sex glands; it is believed that the pineal gland, located in the brain, is also an endocrine gland. Known as the "master gland," the pituitary gland is responsible for regulating the functions of the other glands and is located in the base of the brain. The pituitary gland helps to regulate growth. The parathyroid glands are imbedded in the thyroid gland, which is an H-shaped gland located in the neck. The thyroid gland helps control the body's rate of metabolism. The parathyroid

glands help maintain the proper level of nutrients, such as calcium and phosphorus.

Although the thymus gland is found beneath the breastbone of infants, it later becomes smaller, but remains vital to the immune system due to its production of T-cells. Above each kidney is an adrenal gland that secretes adrenalin and many other hormones, such as cortisone. Adrenalin helps the body deal with stress. The pancreas, located near the stomach and duodenum, helps in the digestion of foods and also is an endocrine gland. A section of cells of the pancreas that appear as islands, called the islets of Langerhans, is responsible for the production of insulin. Insulin is necessary for the maintenance of normal blood glucose levels in the body.

The gonads are reponsible for the development of sex characteristics, including amount of body hair, range of voice, and body shape. The gonads include the ovaries, which are located in the pelvic area of females and attached to the uterus, and the testes, which are located in the scrotum of males and attached to the prostate and seminal vesicles.

Like all body parts, the glands need nutritional replenishment. When the body is under stress, it is depleted of nutrients and requires more nourishment. Glandular therapy may assist in this need. Glandulars are primarily protein substances made from individual glands that supply the body with hormones, enzymes, nucleic proteins, vitamins, trace minerals, and other active substances.

The glands work with the other organs of the body to keep it in a state of health. The liver, tonsils, lungs, heart, male and female sex organs, gallbladder, and appendix all act to maintain the healthy function of the body. When one gland is not functioning properly, it needs to be treated or all of the glands will eventually malfunction.

NUTRIENTS

SUPPLEMENT	SUGGESTED DOSAGE	COMMENTS
Very Important		
Kelp	5 tablets daily.	Rich in minerals and the element iodine, which are necessary for thyroid function.
Vitamin A plus beta-carotene	15,000 IU daily.	All organs with duct systems need vitamin A.
Vitamin B complex with extra pantothenic acid (B_5)	100 mg twice daily.	This supplement is especially important if you are under stress.
Vitamin C	3,000–5,000 mg daily in divided doses.	Important for adrenal function. *See* ASCORBIC ACID FLUSH in Part Three.
Zinc	50 mg daily.	Needed by the immune system and for tissue repair. Vital in all enzyme systems. Especially important for the sex glands.
Important		
Lecithin	1 tbsp. or 1 capsule before meals.	All cells and organs have lecithin surrounding them for protection.
Raw thymus plus multiglandular complex (sublingual)	As directed on label.	Stimulates immune function and aids glandular function. Putting this under the tongue will insure faster action and by-pass the gastrointestinal tract.
Helpful		
Germanium	200 mg daily.	A potent detoxifier and oxygen carrier.
L-Cysteine and L-methionine and L-glutathione (amino acids)	Take with a small amount of vitamins C and B_6 for better assimilation.	Aids in detoxifying glands of harmful pollutants.
Selenium	200 mcg daily.	A free radical scavenger that protects the glandular system.
Silicon (silica)	500 mg twice daily in tablet form and/ or drink as a tea.	Aids in healing the glands and tissues. High in calcium. Obtain from the herbs oat straw or springtime horsetail.
Superoxide dismutase (SOD): Cell Guard from Biotec Foods	As directed on label with a large glass of water on an empty stomach.	A potent detoxifier that also transports oxygen for healing in the glandular system.
Unsaturated fatty acids (primrose, salmon, or linseed oil)	As directed on label.	Needed to nourish the glands. You can obtain these from primrose oil, salmon oil, and linseed oil.
Vitamin E	400–800 IU daily.	Rids the body of toxic substances when combined with vitamin C and selenium.

HERBS

☐ Use black cohosh tea, dandelion, echinacea, black radish extract, goldenseal root, licorice, lobelia (no capsules), mullein, parsley, and red clover. Echinacea helps to clean the lymph glands. Burdock root and chapparal help rid the body of toxins.

RECOMMENDATIONS

☐ Alfalfa, beet, black radish, and dandelion juice are good for cleansing the liver and gallbladder. *See* JUICING in Part Three.

☐ Using olive oil and pure apple juice will stimulate the gallbladder and help excrete bile and even small gallstones. *See* GALLBLADDER in Part Two.

☐ *See* FASTING in Part Three and follow the program once monthly to allow glands time to heal and rest.

☐ *See* HYPOTHYROID in Part Two and follow the self-test instructions for temperature test to determine how well the thyroid is functioning.

☐ If toxic substances circulate through the bloodstream due to bad eating habits, drugs, and/or a nutritional deficiency, it is reflected in the lymph system. The lymph glands act as a filter, removing poisons from the body. *See* BLOOD PURIFIER in Part Three and follow the instructions.

☐ The appendix and tonsils are important in immune function. Remove only when absolutely necessary.

Light, Aging, and the Pineal and Pituitary Glands

The pineal gland, located in the center of the brain and shaped like a pine cone, has many important hormonal functions in the body. Although this small gland was considered the "seat of the soul" in ancient times, only recently have scientists uncovered the role it plays in the aging process. The pineal gland, like the pituitary gland, regulates certain endocrine functions. Through its interaction with various glands of the body, the pineal plays a role in degenerative disease and aging.

The pineal gland regulates other glandular functions through its inhibitory mechanisms. Blood pressure, body temperature, growth, motor function, the reproductive system, and sleep habits are all regulated by this important gland.

There is much that we do not know about the pineal gland. While I was in medical school, a professor of pathology informed me that this "rudimentary" organ had no role in human physiology. Today it is known that the pineal gland at least partially controls the following bodily functions:

- The passage of calcium into and out of all cells.
- Carbohydrate metabolism.
- Catecholamine production.
- Cellular respiration.
- Collagen synthesis.
- DNA synthesis.
- Enzyme activity.
- Lymphocyte production.

The pineal gland, of primary importance to the endocrine system, is hardly a rudimentary gland. Regulated by sunlight and geomagnetic fields, the pineal gland plays an integral role in body cycles, controlling metabolism, behavior, and physiological function.

In addition to its intimate relationship with the pituitary or "master" gland, the pineal gland also has a direct effect upon the adrenal glands when the body is under stress and threatened. Its effect on the parathyroid and on calcium metabolism is not yet understood. In addition, the pineal gland has an inhibitory action on the thyroid gland and is important in the hormonal functions of the thymus. This important gland also stimulates the release of prostaglandin, which affects circulation and cardiovascular disease. It plays a role in the regulation of temperature as well.

Because large toxic molecules can enter into the pineal gland, they are a potential threat. The blood barrier prevents these toxic substances from harming the other areas of the brain. Dangerous toxins, free radicals, and viruses entering through the pineal gland effect changes in the other glands that can result in abnormal growths, such as cancerous cells, or degeneration, such as in arteriosclerosis.

Eight chronic, degenerative diseases that are characteristic of aging are:

1. Alzheimer's disease.
2. Arteriosclerosis.
3. Arthritis.
4. Cancer.
5. Diabetes.
6. Menopause.
7. Osteoporosis.
8. Parkinson's disease.

Any theory concerning aging must include the pineal gland, which plays a dominant role. According to Bradford Research, administering pineal gland extract to animals can increase their life span by 25 percent.

Excessive amounts of stress and nutritional deficiency can markedly reduce the functioning capacity of the pineal gland. Vitamin A deficiency is particularly detrimental. Degenerative disease and aging will also result from the reduction of oxygen levels that occurs when viruses and toxins surround or enter the pineal and pituitary glands.

Light, working through the pineal and pituitary glands and the hypothalamus, is extremely important in the longevity of life. Part of the mystery of aging and agelessness lies in the relationship between these three body parts. According to Bradford Research, studies indicate that the hypothalamus is the primary site responsible for aging. The hypothalamus regulates autonomic responses—those that require no conscious effort, such as hormone and enzyme secretions, fluid regulation, sleep patterns, heart contractions, temperature control, and perspiration. It is the hypothalamus that coordinates the activities of the endocrine system.

The unprotected eye should be allowed to partake of environmental light on a regular basis to reap its benefits. *Make sure that you never look directly into the sun.* Reflected light upon the retina is preferred—without interposed glass. Try to stimulate the endocrine glands as often as possible by allowing reflected sunlight through the retina of the eye to reach the pineal and pituitary glands.

The use of light for therapy is currently being explored. Light treatment or photomedicine has been used in the medical community to counteract jaundice in premature babies by exposing them to blue light. In addition, ultraviolet rays are used to treat psoriasis. Other applications of light currently being explored include the adjustment of the wavelengths of laser beams to project any color of light. Lasers have successfully been used in certain types of eye, cardiac, and urologic surgery.

In addition to the use of light in surgery, phototherapy or exposure to bright light seems to reverse the effects of "seasonal affective disorder" (SAD). This disorder, often referred to as the "wintertime blues," is now recognized by the American Psychiatric Association as a psychiatric syndrome. A decrease in productivity and difficulties in interpersonal relationships are common for individuals with SAD. This disorder can be severely incapacitating in extreme cases, and is characterized by social isolation, depression, withdrawal, a craving for carbohydrates, weight gain, loss of energy, tendency to sleep longer, and a decreased sexual drive.

Glaucoma

Glaucoma is the second leading cause of blindness. There are approximately 7 million known cases of glaucoma today. This condition usually affects people over forty, and is typically more common in women than in men. It is characterized by an increase in pressure of the fluid within the eyeball and a hardening of the surface of the eyeball. Symptoms of glaucoma include eye pain or discomfort mainly in the morning, blurred vision, halos around light, inability of the pupils to adjust to a dark room, and peripheral vision loss. The disease has many causes, but most often is related to stress and nutritional problems. Whenever stress is a major factor, B-complex injections appear to have good results.

If medication cannot control the glaucoma, laser treatments may help before having other forms of surgery. Each person is unique, so be sure to have at least two opinions before making a decision.

In open angle glaucoma, new testing has shown laser treatment to be effective. The laser beam is aimed at the iris to make a small hole to relieve the pressure. If the problem is acute or angle closure glaucoma, when the cornea is clouded by edema from high pressure, the laser treatment may not be the best approach and more aggressive surgery may be needed.

GLAUCOMA SELF-TEST

See your doctor immediately if you suspect you have glaucoma or have a tendency for glaucoma. You can also take a simple test that may indicate whether or not you have glaucoma, but any diagnosis must be confirmed by your attending physician.

The self-tonometer is a self-testing device that ophthalmologists encourage their patients to use to measure intraocular pressure (the pressure inside the eyes). This device measures the light reflected from a membrane that touches the cornea of the eye.

First, desensitize the cornea using anesthetic eyedrops or by wearing a thin, plastic contact lens during the test. Next, look into the device and focus on a cross circle to position the tonometer, and then press a plastic bulb to record the pressure.

If your ophthalmologist recommends medication to control the glaucoma and it is working to your satisfaction, continue to use it faithfully. Also take vitamin C in high doses, but only under supervision.

NUTRIENTS

SUPPLEMENT	SUGGESTED DOSAGE	COMMENTS
Very Important		
Choline	1,000–2,000 mg daily.	An important B vitamin.
Pantothenic acid (B$_5$)	100 mg 3 times daily.	Antistress vitamin needed for the adrenal glands.
Rutin	50 mg 3 times daily.	Important part of the vitamin C complex that aids in reducing pressure behind the eye.
Vitamin B complex	50 mg 3 times daily with meals.	Injections may be necessary.
Vitamin C plus bioflavonoids	3,000–7,000 mg 3 times daily.	Greatly reduces intraocular pressure. *See* ASCORBIC ACID FLUSH in Part Three.
Vitamin E	400 IU daily.	Recent research indicates that vitamin E is helpful in removing particles from the lens of the eye.
Helpful		
Germanium	100 mg when having discomfort or 200 mg daily.	Increases needed oxygen supply to tissues and relieves pain.
Inositol	Use as directed on label.	An important B vitamin. Reduces stress.
Multivitamin and mineral complex containing vitamin A and beta-carotene	Use as directed on label.	All nutrients are needed to aid in healing and to relieve pressure behind the eyeball.

RECOMMENDATIONS

☐ Avoid prolonged eye stress such as watching television and reading.

☐ Avoid smokers, coffee, alcohol, nicotine, and all caffeine. Drink only small amounts of liquid at any given time.

☐ Warm fennel herb eye baths alternated with the herbs chamomile and eyebright are helpful, or use an eye dropper and apply three drops to each eye three time a day.

CONSIDERATIONS

☐ The drug Forskolin, made from the coleus plant, has been reported by Yale University to be effective for glaucoma without side effects.

☐ You may wish to contact either of the following for more information on laser surgery:

David K. Dueker, M.D.
Assistant Professor of Ophthalmology
Harvard Medical School
Massachusetts Eye and Ear Infirmary

W. Morton Grant, M.D.
Professor of Ophthalmology
Harvard Medical School
Massachusetts Eye and Ear Infirmary

Gout

Gout occurs when there is too much uric acid in the blood, tissues, and urine. The uric acid crystallizes in the joints, acting as an abrasive and causing swelling and pain. Uric acid kidney stones may be a related problem. Approximately 90 percent of gout patients are male.

Uric acid is a by-product of certain foods, so this condition is closely related to diet. It can be brought on by stress. Obesity and an improper diet increase the tendency for gout.

If you think you may have gout, be sure and be tested. The best method is for the doctor to insert a needle into the affected joint and aspirate the fluid. Then he examines the fluid under a microscope for the characteristic uric acid crystals to verify whether the serum uric acid level is elevated.

A low-purine diet is important in treatment. Purines are constituents of nucleoproteins from which uric acid is derived. See the recommendations for which purine-rich foods to avoid.

NUTRIENTS

SUPPLEMENT	SUGGESTED DOSAGE	COMMENTS
Very Important		
Vitamin B complex with extra folic acid	100 mg twice daily. As directed on label.	*Caution:* Avoid high amounts of niacin. Folic acid is an important aid in nucleoprotein metabolism.
Vitamin B$_5$ (pantothenic acid)	500 mg daily in divided doses.	The antistress vitamin.
Vitamin C	3,000–5,000 mg divided up during the day.	Lowers serum uric acid.
Important		
Germanium	100 mg twice daily.	Good for pain and swelling.
Kelp	6 tablets daily.	Contains complete protein and vital minerals to reduce serum uric acid.
Superoxide dismutase (GP/ CAT from Biotec Foods)	Once daily (morning is best) on empty stomach with full glass of water.	An antioxidant and potent free radical destroyer.
Vitamin E	Start with 100 IU daily; increase slowly to 600 IU daily.	Neutralizes free radicals and improves circulation.
Zinc	50–80 mg daily.	Important in protein metabolism and tissue repair.
Helpful		
Calcium and magnesium (chelate)	1,500 mg daily. 750 mg daily.	Works well while sleeping.
Vitamin A	25,000–50,000 IU daily; reduce to 15,000 in 1 month.	Another potent antioxidant (free radical destroyer).

HERBS

☐ Use birch, burdock, hyssop, and juniper.

RECOMMENDATIONS

☐ Eat only raw fruits and vegetables for two weeks. Juices are best. Also include grains, seeds, and nuts in your diet. Frozen or fresh cherry juice is excellent! Cherries and strawberries neutralize uric acid, so eat lots of them. Also drink celery juice diluted with distilled water—drink only distilled water.

☐ Eat no meat of any kind. Meat contains extremely high amounts of uric acid. Avoid gravies and rich foods such as cakes and pies—leave white flour and sugar products out of your diet. If you are prone to gout, limit your intake of dried beans, cauliflower, fish, lentils, oatmeal, peas, poultry, spinach, and yeast products.

☐ Avoid purine-rich foods including anchovies, asparagus, consommé, herring, meat gravies and broths, mushrooms, mussels, all organ meats, sardines, and sweetbreads. Never mix these foods with alcohol if you are prone to gout! Alcohol increases the production of uric acid and must be eliminated from the diet.

☐ Avoid restricted weight loss diets. Abruptly cutting back on foods or a fast of longer than three days may result in increased uric acid levels.

CONSIDERATIONS

☐ The drug allopurinol, prescribed for control of gout, has been linked directly to skin eruptions, vasculitis (inflammation of the vessels), and liver toxicity. If the patient has kidney problems, treatment with this drug should be carefully monitored.

☐ Note: Because of the cellular destruction associated with chemotherapy in cancer treatment, uric acid is often released in extreme amounts, resulting in gouty arthritis.

☐ *See also* ARTHRITIS in Part Two.

Growth Problems

Growth problems occur when the pituitary gland or the thyroid gland does not function as it should. The pituitary gland distributes hormones to various parts of the body, including the growth hormone *somatotropin*. This hormone stimulates the growth of muscle and bone in growing children.

An overproduction of these hormones can cause growth abnormalities, as will underproduction. Too little secretion by the pituitary will cause dwarfism, and too much causes the body to grow too large and is characterized by large hands, feet, and jaw. This malfunction of the pituitary may be caused by a tumor of the pituitary gland that can be removed surgically or treated with drugs or by other means.

In some cases, growth problems are caused by the failure of the thyroid gland to function properly. The thymus gland may also be involved. If the thymus gland of an infant is damaged, development is retarded and there is an increased susceptability to infection. Malnutrition may also play a significant role in the growth and development of a child. If not, hormone therapy and these suggestions will help.

Dosages in the following table should be adjusted according to the size and weight of the patient.

NUTRIENTS

SUPPLEMENT	SUGGESTED DOSAGE	COMMENTS
Very Important		
Cod liver oil	As directed on label.	Needed for proper growth. Contains vitamins A and D for strong tissues and bones.
Kelp liquid from World Organic Corporation	As directed on label.	An iodine deficiency may be the cause of growth problems. Kelp contains natural iodine.
L-Lysine	As directed on label.	Needed for normal growth and bone development.
Unsaturated fatty acids	As directed on label.	For normal growth.
Zinc	As directed on label.	A deficiency has been linked to growth problems.
Important		
Calcium and magnesium	As directed on label.	Needed for normal bone growth.
Protein (free form amino acids)	As directed on label.	A deficiency has been linked to growth disorders.
Raw pituitary glandular (for children)	As directed on label.	Stimulates growth.
Helpful		
Gerovital H-3 (GH-3) or Aslavital	As directed on label.	From Rumania. Use under supervision only.
L-Ornithine (amino acid)	As directed by physician.	Helps release the growth hormone. Use only under a physician's supervision.
Vitamin B$_6$ (pyridoxine) plus B complex		Needed for uptake of the amino acids and for proper growth.

CONSIDERATIONS

☐ One reason behind slow growth is "kwashiorkor," a protein deficiency disorder that causes children to grow slowly and have very little resistance to disease. If caught early, it can be corrected.

☐ High levels of lead, a toxic metal, may cause growth problems. Have a hair analysis done to rule out this metal toxicity. (*See* LEAD POISONING in Part Two and HAIR ANALYSIS in Part Three.)

Gum Disease

See PERIODONTAL DISEASE.

Hair (Loss of)

Baldness or loss of hair is referred to as alopecia. *Alopecia totalis* means loss of all the scalp hair. *Alopecia universalis* means loss of all body hair. When the hair falls out in patches, it is termed *alopecia areata*. Factors that are involved in male hair loss include heredity, hormones, and aging. Women sometimes have the same type of hair loss, but it is not as severe and usually occurs after menopause. In addition, most women lose some hair two or three months after having a baby because hormonal changes during pregnancy prevent normal hair loss.

Some factors that promote hair loss are poor circulation, acute illness, surgery, radiation, skin disease, sudden weight loss, iron deficiency, diabetes, thyroid disease, drugs such as those used in chemotherapy, stress, poor diet, vitamin deficiency, and pregnancy.

NUTRIENTS

SUPPLEMENT	SUGGESTED DOSAGE	COMMENTS
Very Important		
Biotin	As directed on label.	Use shampoo and conditioner with biotin as an ingredient.
Raw thymus glandular	500 mg daily.	Stimulates immune function and improves functioning capacity of glands.
Ultra-Hair from Nature's Plus		If condition is not severe, you may use this complex alone. It contains necessary nutrients to stimulate hair growth.
Unsaturated fatty acids (primrose oil, linseed oil, or salmon oil)	As directed on label.	Improves hair texture. Prevents dry, brittle hair.
Vitamin B complex with		The B vitamins are important for the health and growth of hair.
pantothenic acid (B$_5$) and	100 mg 3 times daily.	
vitamin B$_6$ (pyridoxine) and	50 mg 3 times daily.	
inositol and	100 mg twice daily.	
niacin (B$_3$)	50 mg 3 times daily.	
Vitamin C	3,000–10,000 mg	Aids in improving scalp circulation.
Vitamin E	Start with 400 IU and slowly increase to 800–1,000 IU.	Increases oxygen uptake, which improves circulation to the scalp. Improves health and growth of hair.
Zinc	50–100 mg daily.	Stimulates hair growth by enhancing immune function.
Important		
Coenzyme Q$_{10}$	60 mg daily.	Improves scalp circulation. Increases tissue oxygenation.
DMG (Gluconic from DaVinci Labs)	100 mg daily.	Good for circulation to the scalp.
Kelp	5 tablets daily.	Supplies needed minerals for proper hair growth.
Helpful		
Copper chelate	3 mg daily.	Works with zinc to aid in hair growth.
Dioxychlor from American Biologics	5 drops in water twice daily.	Destroys harmful bacteria.
L-Cysteine	500 mg twice daily.	Improves quality, texture, and growth of hair.
L-Methionine	Take on empty stomach with vitamins B$_6$ and C for better assimilation.	Helps prevent hair from falling out.
PABA (or para-aminobenzoic acid in GH-3)	PABA: 50 mg twice daily. GH-3: 2 tablets daily.	For graying hair.
Silica from horsetail herb	2 tablets twice daily.	Keeps hair looking shiny and sleek.

HERBS

☐ Use sage tea as a rinse to help hair grow.

RECOMMENDATIONS

☐ Apple cider, used as a rinse, may help hair grow.

☐ If large amounts of hair are lost, see a physician. Do not use a brush or fine-tooth comb.

☐ Lie head down on a slant board fifteen minutes a day to allow the blood to reach the scalp. Massage the scalp daily.

CONSIDERATIONS

☐ Taking large doses of vitamin A (100,000 IU or more daily) over long periods can trigger hair loss, but stopping the vitamin A will reverse the problem. Often the hair grows back when the cause is corrected.

☐ The drug minoxidil (used to grow hair on the scalp) may cause heart changes if used for long periods of time, report researchers at the University of Toronto. Although this drug does result in hair growth, the quality of the hair is usually poor and hair growth ceases when use of the drug is stopped. The cost of this prolonged drug program may be prohibitive.

☐ Be careful of using products that are not natural on the hair. Allergic reactions to chemicals added to these products occur frequently. Alternate all-natural hair products.

☐ Hypothyroidism is often the cause of hair loss. *See* HYPOTHYROID in Part Two and take the temperature self-test.

☐ Remember that it is normal to lose fifty to one hundred hairs a day.

☐ *See also* HYPOTHYROID and THYROID in Part Two.

Halitosis
(Bad Breath)

Halitosis is typically caused by poor dental hygiene. However, other factors can include gum or tooth decay, nose or throat infection, improper diet, constipation, excessive smoking, foreign bacteria in the mouth, liver malfunction, indigestion, and inadequate protein digestion.

Bad breath may be a sign of poor health. Have a thorough checkup if the following suggestions do not improve the condition.

NUTRIENTS

SUPPLEMENT	SUGGESTED DOSAGE	COMMENTS
Very Important		
Chlorophyll (alfalfa liquid or wheatgrass or barley juice)	1 tbsp. in juice twice daily.	Green drinks are one of the best ways to combat bad breath. Chlorophyll can also be used as a mouth rinse— 1 tbsp. to ½ glass of water.
Fiber (Aerobic Bulk Cleanse (ABC) from Aerobic Life Products or oat bran or rice bran)	1 tbsp. in juice on an empty stomach twice daily.	*Note:* Do not take fiber at the same time that you take vitamins or medications, because the fiber may absorb them.
Vitamin C	2,000–6,000 mg daily.	Important in healing mouth and gum disease and in preventing bleeding gums. Also a good detoxifier; rids the body of excess mucus and toxins that can cause bad breath.
Important		
Acidophilus	Use as directed on label.	Needed to replenish "friendly" bacteria in the colon. Insufficient "friendly" bacteria and an overabundance of harmful bacteria can cause bad breath.
Alfalfa tablets or liquid	6 tablets daily or 1 tbsp. liquid in juice or water 3 times daily.	Chlorophyll cleanses the bloodstream and colon, where bad breath often begins.
Garlic capsules (Kyolic)	2 capsules with meals and at bedtime.	Odorless garlic that acts as a natural antibiotic, destroying foreign bacteria in both the mouth and colon.
Helpful		
Bee propolis	Use as directed on label.	Aids in healing the gums, aids control of infection in the body, and has an antibacterial effect.
Vitamin A plus beta-carotene	15,000 IU daily. 10,000 IU daily.	Needed for control of infection and in healing of the mouth.
Vitamin B complex plus vitamin B$_6$ (pyridoxine) and niacin (B$_3$)	100 mg 50 mg 50 mg 3 times daily.	Vitamin B$_6$ is needed for all enzyme systems in the body. Niacin dilates tiny capillaries for improved blood flow to infection sites.

HERBS

☐ Use myrrh (to brush teeth and rinse mouth), peppermint, rosemary, and sage.

RECOMMENDATIONS

☐ Brush the teeth and *tongue* after every meal. Change toothbrushes every month to prevent bacteria build-up. Use dental floss and a chlorophyll mouthwash daily. A bacteria-destroying toothbrush sanitizer can be purchased that has been proven effective in tests conducted by the University of Oklahoma School of Dentistry. The device automatically turns on every half hour for two minutes to provide thorough sanitization of the bristles twenty-four hours a day. Call 1-(800) 543-3366 for more information.

☐ A cleansing fast with fresh lemon juice and water is important. (*See* FASTING in Part Three.)

☐ Stim-U-Dent wooden toothpicks can be purchased from the drugstore. Use after every meal by massaging between each tooth.

☐ Go on a five-day raw food diet. Eat at least 50 percent raw foods daily.

☐ *See also* PERIODONTAL DISEASE in Part Two.

Hay Fever

Hay fever (allergic rhinitis) affects the mucous membranes of the nose, eyes, and air passages. Dust, pollen (from trees, grass, and flowering plants), feathers, and animal hair are often the cause; however, allergies could also be the underlying cause. Symptoms include itchy eyes, watery discharge from the nose and eyes, sneezing, and nervous irritability.

Those who suffer from hay fever are typically atopic—they also suffer from asthma and dermatitis. Those who suffer from hay fever symptoms throughout the year are said to have perennial rhinitis.

Hay fever sufferers should take supplements designed for allergies. The Rast test is easily done and gives good results (*see* ALLERGIES in Part Two for the Rast test).

NUTRIENTS

SUPPLEMENT	SUGGESTED DOSAGE	COMMENTS
Very Important		
Coenzyme Q$_{10}$	30 mg twice daily.	Improves oxygenation and immunity.

Raw thymus glandular	500 mg twice daily.	Promotes immune function.
Vitamin A	Start with 100,000 IU; then drop to 25,000 IU after 1 month.	A powerful immunostimulant. The emulsified form is best.
Vitamin B complex plus extra vitamin B$_6$ (pyridoxine) and pantothenic acid (B$_5$)	50 mg twice daily. 100 mg 3 times daily.	Enhances immune function.
Vitamin C plus bioflavonoids	3,000–10,000 mg 3 times daily in divided doses.	A potent immunostimulant. Esterified or buffered form is best.

Important		
Germanium	100 mg twice daily.	Improves immune system function.
Proteolytic enzymes	Take with and between meals.	Necessary for digestion of essential nutrients that boost immune function.
Royal jelly capsules from Montana Pollen and Herbs	As directed on label.	Helps to reduce fever and to destroy bacteria.
Zinc	50–80 mg daily.	When feverish, zinc should be omitted.

Helpful		
Alfalfa liquid	Twice daily in juice.	Needed for chlorophyll and vitamin K.
Dioxychlor from American Biologics or Aerobic 07 from Aerobic Life Products	5 drops in water twice daily.	Stabilized oxygen.
Kelp	5 tablets daily.	A rich source of minerals.
Superoxide dismutase (SOD) from Biotec Foods	As directed on product label.	A powerful antioxidant.
Vitamin E	400–800 IU daily.	Boosts the immune system.

RECOMMENDATIONS

☐ Eat more fruits, vegetables, grains, raw seeds, and nuts. Eat yogurt or any soured products three times a week. Stay on a high-fiber diet. No dairy products, white flour products, sugar, packaged or canned foods, tobacco, coffee, chocolate, soft drinks, pies, cakes, or any other junk foods.

CONSIDERATIONS

☐ Perform a cleansing fast. (*See* FASTING in Part Three.)

☐ *See also* ALLERGIES in Part Two and ASCORBIC ACID FLUSH in Part Three.

Headache

Those who frequently suffer from headache may have reactions to wheat, chocolate, monosodium glutamate (MSG), sulfites (used in restaurants on salad bars), sugar, hot dogs, luncheon meats, citric acid, fermented foods (cheeses, sour cream, yogurt), alcohol, vinegar, or marinated foods.

There are a number of other causes including stress, tension, anxiety, constipation, diseases of the eye, nose, and throat, trauma to the head, pollution, sinusitis, drugs, tobacco, fever, perfume, after-shaves, or allergies. Other possibilities to consider are bowel problems, mold allergy, brain disorders, anemia, low blood sugar, toxic overdoses of vitamin A (can be reversed upon discontinuation), vitamin B deficiency, hypertension, grinding of teeth, and coffee consumption.

If any of the following symptoms accompany the headache, consult your doctor: blurred vision, sensitivity to light, pressure behind the eyes relieved by vomiting, food allergies, pressure in the facial sinus area, throbbing of head and temples, heart pounding, visual color changes, and feeling as though your head will explode.

Poor vertebral alignment may produce reduced blood flow to the brain. See your doctor. Chiropractic alignment is often helpful. This is often caused by flat feet or by wearing high heels.

NUTRIENTS

SUPPLEMENT	SUGGESTED DOSAGE	COMMENTS
Helpful		
Calcium and magnesium	1,500 mg daily. 1,000 mg daily.	Chelated form offers best assimilation.
Coenzyme Q$_{10}$	30 mg twice daily.	Improves oxygenation.
DMG (Gluconic from DaVinci Labs)	1 tablet twice daily, dissolved in mouth.	Improves oxygenation.
Niacin (B$_3$) and niacinamide	Combinations up to 500 mg. Start with 300 mg daily and increase dosage daily. Stop and maintain with dosage that provides relief.	Professional supervision advised.
Potassium	99 mg daily.	For the proper sodium and potassium balance, which is needed to avoid water retention. Water retention may put undue pressure on the brain.

Vitamin B$_6$ (pyridoxine) plus	50 mg 3 times daily.	Headache sufferers should avoid yeast-based products. B$_6$ removes excess water build-up in tissues. In severe cases, B-complex injections may be advisable (under doctor's supervision only).
B complex	50 mg 3 times daily.	
Vitamin C plus bioflavonoids	2,000–8,000 mg in divided doses.	Esterified or buffered form is best.
Vitamin E	Start with 400 IU and work up to 1,200 IU.	Improves circulation.

HERBS

☐ The following herbs may relieve headache pain: brigham, burdock root, feverfew, goldenseal root, lavender, lobelia, marshmallow, mint, and rosemary.

RECOMMENDATIONS

☐ Try eliminating the following foods from your diet: alcohol, bananas, caffeine, cheese and sour cream, chicken, chocolate, citrus fruits, cold cuts, smoked fish, herring, onions, peanut butter, pork, vinegar, wine, and fresh-baked yeast products. A West German publication reported that these foods contain the amino acid tyramine, a substance that causes the blood pressure to rise, resulting in a dull headache. Reintroduce one food at a time and see which ones produce the headache. Keep a food allergy diary.

☐ Charcoal tablets (from a health food store) should be used if you suspect a sensitivity to the food you are about to eat. Take five tablets within an hour before eating, and three tablets after eating. As soon as possible, take a cleansing enema and a coffee retention enema. If you have severe headaches after consuming a food, this will relieve it quickly by eliminating the toxic substances.

Do not take charcoal tablets daily as they also absorb the good nutrients.

☐ Avoid the amino acids tyramine and phenylalanine, found in market brands Equal, Accent (trade name for MSG, a common seasoning), NutraSweet, and nitrites (preservatives found in hot dogs and luncheon meats).

CONSIDERATIONS

☐ Inositol, tryptophan, and/or calcium, if taken before bedtime, will aid sleeping. A grapefruit half also helps. Do not eat sweet fruit or anything sweet after 5 p.m.

☐ Eat a well-balanced diet. Headaches are often caused by allergies. Avoid chewing gum, ice cream, iced beverages, salt, and excessive sunlight.

☐ Some doctors prescribe the drug lidocaine for headaches that occur in bunches called "cluster" headaches. Used in nose drop form, it gives relief in minutes.

☐ *See also* MIGRAINE and ALLERGIES in Part Two.

Heart Problems

See CARDIOVASCULAR DISEASE; MYOCARDIAL INFARCTION.

Heartburn

Heartburn is a burning sensation in the stomach. It often occurs when hydrochloric acid, which is used by the stomach for digestion, backs up into the esophagus. It can be caused by excessive consumption of spicy or fatty and fried foods, alcohol, coffee, citrus fruits, chocolate, and tomato-based foods, as well as by hiatal hernia, ulcers, gallbladder problems, stress, allergies, and enzyme deficiency.

"Acid stomach" may in fact be a heart problem (*see* CARDIOVASCULAR DISEASE in Part Two). If symptoms persist, see a doctor.

STOMACH ACID SELF-TEST

Hydrochloric acid (HCl) is necessary for the breakdown and digestion of many foods. You can determine if you need hydrochloric acid (HCl) with this simple test. Take a tablespoon of apple cider vinegar or lemon juice. If this makes your heartburn go away, then you need more stomach acid. If it makes your symptoms worse, you have too much HCl. Therefore, do not take enzymes that contain HCl.

NUTRIENTS

SUPPLEMENT	SUGGESTED DOSAGE	COMMENTS
Very Important		
Aloe vera from Aerobic Life Products	As directed on label.	Aids healing of the intestinal tract.
Proteolytic enzymes: pancreatin	Take with meals.	Necessary for proper digestion.

RECOMMENDATIONS

☐ Chew your food well. Eat slowly and enjoy your food!

☐ Do not consume fried foods, carbonated beverages, fats, sugar, processed foods, or spicy or highly seasoned foods. These seem to be the main cause of heartburn. Eat more raw foods.

☐ Try raw potato juice. Do not peel the potato—just wash it and put it in the juicer. Drink one-half juice and one-half water. (*See* JUICING in Part Three). Drink immediately after preparation, three times a day.

☐ At the first sign of heartburn, drink a large glass of water. This often works.

☐ Do not take digestive enzymes containing hydrochloric acid (HCl). Do not lie down immediately after eating. Avoid stress.

☐ Relief from heartburn can be obtained by sipping one tablespoon of raw apple cider vinegar, mixed with water, while eating a meal. Do not drink liquids with meals (except the vinegar and water).

☐ *See* FASTING in Part Three and follow the instructions. *Also see* the self-tests in ACIDOSIS and CARDIOVASCULAR DISEASE, both of which are in Part Two.

CONSIDERATIONS

☐ Read labels of over-the-counter antacids. Check the main ingredient of antacids. Do not take over-the-counter antacids that contain aluminum and sodium. Calcium carbonate works as an antacid and contains no aluminum. A product called Acidaid, by Nutritional Factors, has shown promising results. It may be purchased at health food stores. Acidaid is aluminum free.

Antacids often provide relief of symptoms regardless of whether the individual has an acid stomach, and therefore masks the underlying cause. Over-the-counter antacids contain excess sodium, aluminum, calcium, and magnesium. With prolonged use of these products, a dangerous mineral imbalance can occur. Excess sodium can aggravate hypertension, and excess aluminum has been implicated in Alzheimer's disease. Some of the antacids available are:

- *Aluminum Salts or Gels.* Amphojel, ALternaGEL, Aludrox, Basaljel, Phosphagel, Rolaids.
- *Aluminum/Magnesium Mixtures.* Di-Gel, Gaviscon, Gelusil, Maalox, Mylanta, Riopan.
- *Calcium Carbonate.* Alka-Mints, Chooz, Titralac, Tums.
- *Magnesium Salts or Gel.* Phillips' Milk of Magnesia.

- *Sodium Bicarbonate.* Alka-Seltzer, Bromo Seltzer, Citrocarbonate.

☐ *See also* HERNIA, HIATAL and ULCERS, both in Part Two.

Heel or Bone Spur

A bone spur is a pointed growth on the bone, most commonly located in the heel. A bone spur may be caused by calcium deposits in unwanted areas of the body. Most people who have heel disorders are middle-aged or overweight. Heel spurs are common in people who have arthritis, neuritis, alkalosis, and tendonitis.

X-rays may reveal a bony spur within the heel. The presence of a bony spur may lead to the formation of tiny tumors at the end of several nerves, and these may be very painful. It is best not to remove a heel spur surgically unless it is extremely irritating.

NUTRIENTS

SUPPLEMENT	SUGGESTED DOSAGE	COMMENTS
Very Important		
Betaine HCl (hydrochloride)	As directed on label.	Needed for calcium uptake. A deficiency of HCl is more common in the elderly. Do not use this substance if you have a history of ulcer problems or severe heartburn.
Calcium and magnesium chelate	1,500 mg daily. 750 mg daily.	A proper balance of calcium and magnesium will prevent abnormal calcium deposition.
Important		
Proteolytic enzymes (Intenzyme Forte from Biotics Research)	As directed on label.	Aids in absorption of nutrients and in control of inflammation and irritation.
Vitamin C	2,000–4,000 mg daily.	Acts as an anti-inflammatory; important for collagen and connective tissue.
Helpful		
Bioflavonoids	100 mg daily.	These vitamin C activators relieve pain.
Vitamin B complex plus additional vitamin B₆ (pyridoxine)	50–100 mg daily.	B vitamins work best when taken together; pyridoxine is necessary for production of hydrochloride.

HERBS

☐ Use arnica and chamomile to bathe the foot. You can also wrap the herbs in a cloth and apply.

RECOMMENDATIONS

☐ Select shoes with rubber heels; these will be better for the foot than leather. You should choose footwear for comfort—not for looks. Some jogging shoes can be very comfortable. Avoid hard surfaces such as concrete, wood, or hard floors without carpeting. Adding heel cushions to footwear helps to relieve pain.

☐ If you are in pain, use a linseed hot pack.

☐ Ice massages on the bottom of the feet can be helpful. Alternate hot and cold foot baths.

☐ If you walk or jog for exercise, try bicycling or swimming instead.

☐ Do not eat any citrus fruits, especially oranges. Eliminate sugar, alcohol, or coffee from your diet. These will inhibit the healing process and upset the body's mineral balance.

CONSIDERATIONS

☐ Drink distilled water only!

☐ A raw food fast for two weeks or a cleansing fast can be beneficial. *See* FASTING in Part Three.

☐ *See also* ARTHRITIS in Part Two.

Hemophilia

Hemophilia is a rare blood disease that is found only in men. The blood of hemophiliacs will not clot, and coagulation time is prolonged. Even a small cut is dangerous for the hemophiliac because he will bleed excessively.

There is no known cure for hemophilia. Often fresh whole blood is required for transfusion in emergencies. Because of the need for frequent blood transfusion and clotting factors in fresh blood serum, AIDS is a serious threat to the hemophiliac. *See* AIDS in Part Two.

NUTRIENTS

SUPPLEMENT	SUGGESTED DOSAGE	COMMENTS
Helpful		
Calcium and magnesium	1,500 mg daily. 1,000 mg daily.	Calcium is essential for blood clotting.
Liver injections or extract	1 cc once weekly.	Contains vital nutrients for blood clotting.

Multivitamin and mineral complex	As directed on label.	Provides necessary vitamins and minerals.
Niacin (B₃) plus niacinamide and B complex	As directed on label.	The B vitamins are essential in blood formation and clotting.
Vitamin C plus bioflavonoids	3,000 mg daily.	Important in normal blood coagulation.
Vitamin K and/or alfalfa tablets	300 mcg daily.	Essential in blood clotting mechanism. See below for food sources of vitamin K.

RECOMMENDATIONS

☐ Eat a diet high in vitamin K. Foods that contain a measurable amount of this vitamin are alfalfa, broccoli, cauliflower, egg yolks, kale, liver, spinach, and all green leafy vegetables.

☐ "Green drinks" made from the vegetables listed above are very healthful. Drink one of these a day for vitamin K and other essential clotting factors.

Hemorrhoids

Hemorrhoids are swollen veins around the anus that may protrude out of the rectum. They are usually related to constipation, pregnancy, improper diet, lack of exercise, prolonged periods of sitting, heavy lifting, obesity, liver damage, and allergies.

Hemorrhoids may itch, tear, and bleed, causing discomfort and pain. Severe hemorrhoids may warrant surgery. Consult your doctor.

NUTRIENTS

SUPPLEMENT	SUGGESTED DOSAGE	COMMENTS
Very Important		
Aerobic Bulk Cleanse (ABC) from Aerobic Life Products	Use with ½ fruit juice and ½ aloe vera juice. Drink down quickly before the fiber thickens.	Keeping the colon clean relieves pressure on the rectum.
Calcium chelate or asporotate plus magnesium	1,500 mg daily. 750 mg daily.	Essential for blood clotting and helps prevent cancer of the colon.
Vitamin C with bioflavonoids	3,000–5,000 mg daily. 100 mg daily.	Aids in healing and normal blood clotting.
Vitamin E	600 IU daily.	Promotes normal blood clotting and healing.

Important		
Vitamin B complex plus vitamin B$_6$ (pyridoxine) and vitamin B$_{12}$ and choline and inositol	50 mg 3 times daily with meals.	For improved digestion, resulting in reduced stress on the rectum.

Helpful		
Coenzyme Q$_{10}$	100 mg daily.	Increases cellular oxygenation and assists in healing.
DMG (Gluconic from DaVinci Labs)	1 tablet twice daily.	Improves cellular oxygenation.
Key-E suppositories from Carlson Labs	Use as directed on label.	Shrinks inflamed hemorrhoidal tissue.
Vitamin A and	15,000 IU daily.	Aids in healing of mucous membranes and tissues.
beta-carotene	15,000 IU daily.	
Vitamin D	600 IU daily.	Aids in healing of mucous membranes and tissues. Also needed for calcium uptake.

HERBS

☐ Use buckthorn bark, collinsonia root, parsley, red grape vine leaves, and stone root. An elderberry poultice can relieve the pain associated with hemorrhoids. See POULTICE in Part Three for instructions.

RECOMMENDATIONS

☐ Learn not to strain when moving the bowels. Keep bowels clean and avoid constipation.

☐ It is very important to include foods high in fiber or cellulose in the diet if you suffer from hemorrhoids. Apples, beets, Brazil nuts, broccoli, foods in the cabbage family, carrots, green beans, guar gum, oat bran, lima beans, pears, peas, psyllium seed, and whole grains are recommended.

☐ Exercise is important.

☐ Drink plenty of liquids.

☐ Linseed oil helps to soften stools. Use one or two tablespoons daily.

☐ Take a sitz (mineral) bath daily. We recommend Batherapy, a powder that is added to bath water. This can be found in a health food store.

☐ A peeled clove of garlic or a raw potato made into a suppository is beneficial for hemorrhoids. Use three times a week.

☐ Vitamin K is good for bleeding hemorrhoids. Food sources are alfalfa, kale, and all dark green leafy vegetables.

CONSIDERATIONS

☐ A new laser technology is being used to treat hemorrhoids. It was developed in Europe, and is now available in the United States. This is an improvement over conventional surgery because no hospitalization or general anesthesia is needed.

☐ A product on the market called Anurex supplies a space-age ice pack. When applied directly to the affected tissues, it reduces swelling. This stops the bleeding, relieves discomfort, and promotes healing. It can be ordered directly from Anurex Relief Labs, 2895 Biscayne Boulevard, Suite 392, Miami, FL 33137. Each ice pack is reusable for six months.

☐ Holistic Rectal Ointment and Key-E suppositories give relief from itching and pain. Cayenne and garlic enemas keep the bowels clean. A plain warm water enema will relieve pressure and pain in most cases and is fast acting. See ENEMAS in Part Three.

Hepatitis

The most common forms of hepatitis are hepatitis A and serum hepatitis B. Both forms of this disorder are caused by a virus and are contagious.

Hepatitis A is spread through person-to-person contact, eating, drinking, and other forms of contact. Beware of contaminated water or foods from polluted waters.

Hepatitis B is spread through the use of contaminated syringes, needles, bloodsucking insects, blood transfusions, and some forms of sexual activity. This disease affects 85 percent of the homosexual population. It is extremely contagious and potentially lethal.

The symptoms of hepatitis include fever, weakness, nausea, vomiting, muscle aches, drowsiness, headache, abdominal discomfort, and often jaundice. This flu-like stage may be mild or severe.

Infectious hepatitis is contagious two to three weeks before and one week after jaundice appears. The feces are contaminated with the hepatitis virus; therefore, the isolation technique should be used. Hands and all clothing should be washed often. Bathrooms should be decontaminated frequently.

Toxic hepatitis, which is not virus related, can be caused by chemicals, injection, ingestion, or absorption of toxins through the skin. Chlorinated hydrocarbons and arsenic are examples of severe hepatotoxic agents. The amount of exposure to them determines the extent of liver damage.

NUTRIENTS

SUPPLEMENT	SUGGESTED DOSAGE	COMMENTS
Essential		
Milk thistle extract (herb)	2 capsules 3 times daily.	Important for all liver disorders. Rebuilds and repairs.
Raw liver extract	As directed on label. 1–2 cc intramuscular weekly under doctor's supervision only.	Rapid improvement is noted with liver extract injections.
Very Important		
Bifido Factor/ Life Start Two or Life Start from Natren	As directed on label.	Needed for normal liver function and for healing.
Coenzyme Q$_{10}$	60 mg daily.	Counteracts immunosuppression of viral infection.
DMG (Gluconic from DaVinci Labs)	As directed on label.	Improves cellular oxygen concentration.
Germanium	200 mg daily.	Improves cellular oxygen, and is also good for discomfort and pain.
Lecithin	As directed on label. Take before meals.	Protects cells of the liver and is a fat mobilizer. Aids in preventing "fatty liver."
Superoxide dismutase (SOD) in Cell Guard from Biotec Foods	As directed on label.	A powerful antioxidant that neutralizes damaging superoxide free radicals.
Vitamin B complex in a multivitamin plus extra vitamin B$_{12}$ lozenges and	100 mg daily.	The B vitamins are absolutely essential for normal liver function. Injections may be necessary.
choline and	As directed on label.	
inositol and	As directed on label.	
niacin (B$_3$)	50 mg twice daily. Avoid higher amounts until healed.	*Caution:* Extremely high amounts of niacin may damage the liver.
Important		
Betaine HCl and multienzymes	As directed on label.	Important for proper digestion.
Calcium and	1,500 mg daily.	Essential for blood clotting, which is a problem in liver disease. Don't use bone meal.
magnesium (asporotate)	1,000 mg daily.	
L-Methionine and L-cysteine (amino acids)	500 mg twice daily on empty stomach with small amount of B$_6$ and C.	Detoxifies harmful hepatotoxins.
Protein (free form amino acids)	As directed on label.	Best for necessary supplemental protein. The liver breaks down protein and the "free form" takes the strain off the liver.
Unsaturated fatty acids (primrose oil, salmon oil, etc.)	As directed on label.	Combats inflammation of the liver and lowers serum fats.
Helpful		
Raw pancreas	As directed on label.	Aids in digestion and pancreatic function.
Vitamin A emulsion	25,000 IU daily.	Emulsion for easier assimilation and a safe form for liver problems. Be careful of "pill" form of vitamin A. The liver has to convert beta-carotene to vitamin A, which puts a strain on the liver. Emulsion form by-passes the liver.
Vitamin C plus bioflavonoids	3,000–5,000 mg daily.	A powerful antiviral agent.

HERBS

☐ Use black radish, dandelion, goldenseal, and red clover for hepatitis. Silymarin (a milk thistle weed extract) may help repair the liver.

RECOMMENDATIONS

☐ Eat a raw vegetable and fruit diet for two to four weeks. Drink "green drinks," carrot juice, and beet juice. *See* JUICING in Part Three. Start this diet with a cleansing fast (*see* FASTING in Part Three and follow the program).

☐ Avoid all fats, alcohol, sugar, and highly processed foods. Also avoid any drugs that have not been prescribed by your doctor. Drink only steam-distilled water. Avoid all raw fish and shellfish and eat no animal protein.

☐ Use chlorophyll enemas three times a week. Use one pint and retain for fifteen minutes. *See* ENEMAS in Part Three.

☐ Place warm castor oil packs over the liver area.

☐ A hepatitis B vaccine (Recombivax HB) is recommended by the American Medical Association for all homosexuals, drug users, pregnant immigrants from Asia, dental, and medical workers. FDA approval is expected in the near future.

CONSIDERATIONS

☐ A tragic indictment of the condition of the "life blood" of our nation is that 25 percent of those who receive blood transfusions develop hepatitis, according to researchers at the University of California.

☐ There is a new test that can spot a form of hepatitis that previously was undetectable. The test can pinpoint non-A and non-B hepatitis, which are caused by a virus and can be spread through transfusions. This type of hepatitis affects more than 150,000 Americans a year, and can also lead to cirrhosis, liver cancer, and other liver disorders. Clinical tests, devised by the Chiron Corporation of Emeryville, California, are to begin soon.

Hernia, Hiatal

Hiatal hernia is a condition that sometimes occurs when there is an opening or hole in the diaphragm muscles through which the stomach pushes, or herniates. Small hernias rarely cause any real trouble. About 50 percent of the population over forty years of age have a hiatal hernia.

Ulcers often accompany the hiatal hernia. The heartburn is due to the leakage of stomach acid back into the lower esophagus. This acid reflux may lead to ulceration of the esophagus. The ulcer can also occur in the duodenum or the stomach.

Symptoms include heartburn and belching. Often the acid comes up into the throat, causing a burning sensation, and there is frequently great discomfort behind the breastbone.

NUTRIENTS

SUPPLEMENT	SUGGESTED DOSAGE	COMMENTS
Important		
Proteolytic enzymes and	Take between meals.	For improved digestion. Avoid products containing hydrochloric acid (HCl).
pancreatin	Take with meals.	
Helpful		
Aloe vera juice	¼ glass in juice morning and night.	For healing of the intestinal lining.
Multivitamin and mineral formula	As directed on label.	Use a hypoallergenic formula.
Papaya enzyme	2 before meals.	Fresh papaya is good for digestion and healing.
Vitamin A emulsion	Take 50,000 IU for 1 month, then 30,000 IU for 2 weeks, and end with 20,000 IU.	Emulsion form enters the system quicker.
Vitamin B complex plus	100 mg B complex twice daily.	A hypoallergenic formula is best.
B₁₂ lozenges	1 lozenge dissolved under tongue between meals.	
Vitamin C	Limit to 500 mg daily.	A buffered form is best.
Zinc	50 mg daily.	Necessary for healing and repair of tissue.

HERBS

☐ Comfrey pepsin, goldenseal root, and red clover are beneficial for a hernia. Comfrey pepsin should not be used for extended periods.

RECOMMENDATIONS

☐ Eat several small meals daily. Include extra fiber in the diet.

☐ Do not lie down after consuming food, and avoid heavy lifting and bending. Give the stomach at least two hours to empty before lifting and other exertion.

☐ Do not consume spicy foods and do not take digestive enzymes that contain hydrochloric acid (HCl).

☐ Avoid fried foods (fats). They delay digestion and prolong the stomach's emptying time. Also avoid coffee, tea, alcohol, colas, and smoking. Do not wear tight belts or girdles.

☐ Avoid constipation and straining during a bowel movement.

CONSIDERATIONS

☐ Allergenic foods often magnify the symptoms and prolong healing. The hiatal hernia symptoms often clear up when allergenic foods are avoided. (*See* ALLERGIES in Part Two.)

☐ *See also* ULCERS and HEARTBURN, both in Part Two.

The Herpes Virus

There are two types of the herpes virus. Type I (herpes simplex) is recognized by cold sores and skin eruptions. It can also cause an inflammation of the cornea of the eye. If the eye becomes infected, see a doctor at once. This virus can cause encephalitis, an inflammation of the brain.

Type II (genital herpes) is sexually transmitted and is the most prevalent herpes infection. This viral infection can range in severity from a silent infection to a serious inflammation of the liver including fever, severe brain damage, and stillbirths. Babies can pick up the virus in the birth canal, risking brain damage, blindness, and death. A Cesarean section may be necessary to protect the baby.

After entering the body, the virus never leaves. It can only be kept under control so it will not break out in painful fluid-filled blisters that form around the mouth and genitals. These blisters are highly infectious for up to three weeks, until healed. The virus may lay dormant for long periods of time. Sickness, stress, and unknown factors can cause the virus to break out in open sores again.

After initial contact, the sores appear two to seven days after exposure. Recurrent eruptions are common. After a period of time, the virus burns itself out, rarely appearing after age fifty.

A mild tingling and burning in the vaginal area may be the first sign of genital herpes in women. Within a matter of a few hours, blisters develop around the rectum, clitoris, and cervix, and in the vagina. There is often a watery discharge from the urethra and pain when urinating.

In men blisters break out on the penis, groin, and scrotum, often with a urethral discharge and painful urination. Sometimes the penis and foreskin will swell.

Both men and women may have a low-grade fever and muscular aches. The male may also have tender swollen lymph nodes in the groin. After a few days, pus erupts from the blisters and forms large, painful ulcers. These sores crust over and dry while healing, usually leaving no scars.

NUTRIENTS

SUPPLEMENT	SUGGESTED DOSAGE	COMMENTS
Very Important		
L-Lysine	500–1,000 mg daily.	When the amount of lysine present exceeds the amount of arginine, the growth of the herpes virus is retarded.
Vitamin A emulsion or capsule form	50,000 IU daily.	Important for healing and prevents spreading of infection. The emulsified form is more easily assimilated.
Vitamin B complex	50 mg each and up 3 times daily.	Take a hypoallergenic form.
Vitamin C plus bioflavonoids	5,000–10,000 mg vitamin C; 30–60 mg bioflavonoids daily in divided doses.	Esterified or buffered form is best.
Zinc chelate	50–100 mg daily in divided doses.	For sores in and around the mouth, use zinc lozenges.

Important		
Acidophilus capsules or liquid	3 times daily on an empty stomach.	Needed for the production of the B vitamins. Prevents the growth of harmful microorganisms in the intestines.
Egg lecithin	As directed on label.	
Essential fatty acids (primrose or salmon oil)	As directed on product label.	Needed for cell protection.
Garlic capsules (Kyolic)	3 tablets 3 times daily with meals.	An immune system stimulant and a natural antibiotic.
Superoxide dismutase (SOD) from Biotec Foods	As directed on label.	Reduces infection and speeds healing. A powerful free radical destroyer.
Vitamin E	600 IU daily.	The emulsified form is more easily assimilated. Important in healing and prevents spreading of infection.

Helpful		
Calcium and magnesium	1,500 mg daily. 750 mg daily.	Chelated forms are best. Relieves stress and anxiety.
DMG (Gluconic from DaVinci Labs)	2 tablets twice daily, dissolved in mouth.	Enhances utilization of oxygen by tissue.
Multivitamin and mineral supplement	As directed on product label.	Take hypoallergenic form. Needed to enhance healing.
Proteolytic enzymes	2 tablets between meals.	Helps protect against infection; works on undigested food remaining in the colon.
Raw thymus concentrate	500 mg twice daily.	Enhances immune function.

HERBS

☐ Herpes treatment should include echinacea, myrrh, and red clover. Take two capsules of goldenseal three times daily or drink in tea form.

RECOMMENDATIONS

☐ Herpes infections in women increase the risk of cervical cancer. A pap smear should be done periodically.

☐ For type II sufferers: to ease swelling and pain in the genital area, use ice packs. Warm Epsom salts or baking soda baths will help itching and pain. Pat dry gently and keep lesions dry.

☐ Apply vitamin E alternately with vitamin A directly on sores. Or try L-lysine cream (LSO-1). Refrain from sexual intercourse until genital sores are completely healed for two weeks.

CONSIDERATIONS

☐ Avoid alcohol, processed foods, colas, white flour products, sugar, refined carbohydrates, coffee, and drugs to lessen the chance of an outbreak. Herb tea is beneficial; however, avoid all other teas.

☐ Wear cotton underwear. Practice good genital hygiene—keep clean and dry.

☐ Get plenty of rest. Stress reduction is important. Drink steam-distilled water.

☐ Eat the following in moderation during outbreaks: almonds, barley, cashews, cereals (grains), chicken, chocolate, corn, dairy products, meat, nuts and seeds, oats, and peanuts. These contain L-arginine, an amino acid that suppresses L-lysine, the amino acid that retards the growth of the virus.

☐ Refrain from citrus fruits and juices while the virus is active.

☐ A new virus, identified by the National Cancer Institute as the human B-cell lymphotropic virus (HBLV), is believed to be a member of the herpes virus family and may also be a factor in fatigue.

MEDICAL UPDATES

☐ The FDA has approved acyclovir, now marketed in oral form. This drug prevents outbreaks in 91 percent of patients. Caution should be practiced if the drug is taken on a regular basis. When stopped, a more serious outbreak than usual may occur.

This drug can be used for both oral and genital herpes, taken every four hours for ten days. Applying the lotion when sensing an outbreak will usually weaken the attack.

☐ Isotretinoin, a derivative of vitamin A, has had dramatic results with herpes simplex infections.

☐ Inter Vir (ointment) may bring quick relief. Isoprinosine, used in AIDS treatment, is being used successfully to treat herpes. This drug seems to have few side effects.

☐ Exovir-HZ Gel has been found to keep the virus from growing and spreading to new cells, reports the New York University Medical Center. This formula contains a spermicide called nonoxynol and an alpha-interferon drawn from white blood cells. Those using this drug had less severe recurrences and the pain was greatly decreased.

☐ Some physicians have used butylated hydroxytoluene (BHT) to treat this disease. This can have dangerous consequences, especially if taken on an empty stomach. Irritation and even perforation of the stomach can result. We do not recommend this treatment for herpes.

☐ *See also* COLD SORES, SEXUALLY TRANSMITTED DISEASES, and SHINGLES, all in Part Two.

Herpes Zoster

See SHINGLES.

High Blood Pressure (Hypertension)

When the heart pumps the blood through the arteries, the blood presses against the walls of the blood vessels. Those who suffer from hypertension have abnormally high blood pressure. Arteriosclerosis or atherosclerosis are common precursors of hypertension. Because the arteries are obstructed with cholesterol plaque in atherosclerosis, circulation of blood through the vessels becomes difficult. When the arteries harden and constrict in arteriosclerosis, the blood is forced through a narrower passageway. As a result, blood pressure becomes elevated.

In addition to arteriosclerosis, hypertension is often precipitated by cigarette smoking, stress, obesity, excessive use of stimulants such as coffee or tea, drug abuse, high sodium intake, and use of contraceptives. Because too much water retention can exert pressure on the blood vessels, those who consume foods high in sodium are at a greater risk for high blood pressure. Elevated blood pressure is also common in those who are overweight. Blood pressure can rise due to stress as well, which causes the walls of the arteries to constrict. In addition, those with a family history of hypertension may be more likely to suffer from high blood pressure.

Using a sphygmomanometer, the physician will take two types of blood pressure readings. The *systolic* pressure refers to the pressure exerted by the blood while the heart is pumping; this reading will indicate blood pressure at its highest. The *diastolic* pressure reads the blood pressure when the heart is at rest in between beats, when the blood pressure is at its lowest. Blood pressure readings are written in a ratio of systolic blood pressure to diastolic blood pressure. Both figures refer to the height that a column of mercury (Hg) reaches under the pressure exerted by the blood. Both the systolic and diastolic readings are important; neither should be high. A normal blood pressure reads 120 over 80 (120/80), with the systolic pressure measuring 120 mm Hg and the diastolic pressure measuring 80 mm Hg. Normal blood pressure readings can vary from 110/70 to 140/90, while readings of 140/90 to 160/90 or 160/95 indicate borderline hypertension. Any pressure over 180/115 is severely elevated. See the self-test and inset for how to take blood pressure.

An estimated 40 million Americans have high blood pressure. The heart must work harder to pump blood in those with high blood pressure, often leading to heart failure and stroke. High blood pressure is often associated with coronary heart disease, arteriosclerosis, kidney disorders, obesity, diabetes, hyperthyroidism, and adrenal tumors.

Hypertension often is asymptomatic. Advanced warning signs include headache, sweating, rapid pulse, shortness of breath, dizziness, and vision disturbances. Because hypertension often shows no signs, regular visits to your physician to check blood pressure are important, especially for those individuals in high risk categories. Have your blood pressure checked every four to six months.

BLOOD PRESSURE SELF-TEST

It is impossible to make a correct diagnosis of high blood pressure in a doctor's office with a single reading. The test needs to be repeated throughout the day to be accurate. Home testing is best because it enables the person to periodically monitor the condition. To take your blood pressure at home, purchase a sphygmomanometer—a device with an inflatable bladder inside a hollow sleeve that fits around the arm and is pumped up. There are electronic models available that are very easy to use.

The arm must be relaxed, supported, and held at chest level. The reading will be excessively high if the arm is too low. Do not speak while the pressure is being measured. Blood pressure usually rises when one talks. Slip the cuff on the upper arm and tighten. Pump up the bulb. Some units beep to indicate the systolic pressure (measured when the heart muscle contracts) and the diastolic pressure (measured when the heart muscle relaxes). Other sphygmomanometer units inflate and deflate the cuff automatically and either provide a digital read-out or give information in a computerized voice.

The sphygmomanometer measures the distance that mercury would move given the amount of pressure that the blood is exerting on it. A normal blood pressure

reading is 120 mm Hg systolic over 80 mm Hg diastolic (120/80). It can vary from a normal of 110/70 to 140/90. Borderline hypertension reads 140/90 to 160/90 or 160/95. Any pressure over 180/115 is severely elevated.

NUTRIENTS

SUPPLEMENT	SUGGESTED DOSAGE	COMMENTS
Essential		
Calcium and magnesium	1,500–3,000 mg daily. 750–1,000 mg daily.	Calcium deficiency has been linked to high blood pressure.
L-carnitine (amino acid)	500 mg twice daily on an empty stomach.	Transports long fatty acid chains. Together with L-glutamine and L-glutamic acid, this amino acid aids in preventing heart disease.
Selenium	200 mcg daily.	A selenium deficiency has been linked to heart disease.
Very Important		
Coenzyme Q$_{10}$	100 mg daily.	Improves heart function and lowers blood pressure.
Garlic capsules (Kyolic)	2 capsules 3 times daily.	This odorless garlic is beneficial in lowering the blood pressure.
Germanium	90 mg daily.	Improves tissue oxygenation.
L-Glutamine plus L-glutamic acid (amino acids)	500 mg daily.	Detoxifies ammonia. Aids in preventing heart disease.
Vitamin C	3,000–6,000 mg in daily divided doses.	Improves adrenal function; reduces blood-clotting tendencies.
Important		
Lecithin or lipotropic factors	As directed on label before meals.	Emulsifies fat, improving liver function and lowering blood pressure.
Vitamin E and/or octacosonol	Start at 100 IU; add 100 IU each month, increasing to 400 IU.	Improves heart function. Vitamin E emulsion can be taken for easier assimilation and in larger amounts.
Helpful		
Bromelin	As directed on label.	An enzyme that aids in the digestion of fats.
Kelp tablets	5 tablets daily.	A good source of minerals and natural iodine.
Kyo-Green	Take twice daily as directed on label.	This concentrated barley and wheatgrass juice contains important nutrients.
Multivitamin and mineral complex including vitamin A and zinc and potassium	As directed on label. 15,000 IU daily. 50 mg daily. 99 mg daily.	If taking cortisone, diuretics, or high blood pressure medication, take extra potassium.
Primrose or black currant or flaxseed or olive oil	Take as directed before meals.	These oils are good sources of unsaturated fats and are important for circulation and for lowering blood pressure.

How to Measure Blood Pressure

Your blood pressure measurement actually tells you how much pressure it takes to stop the flow of blood through your arteries. This is assumed to be equivalent to the pressure at the pump end, the heart.

Blood pressure is measured at two points in the heart's pumping rhythm: *systolic pressure* is taken when the heart is actually beating; *diastolic pressure* is taken when the heart is at rest between beats. The combined pressure is usually expressed as a fraction—120 (systolic)/80 (diastolic), for example. The normal systolic pressure for a healthy adult is 120 (100 for a child).

The figures refer to the height a column of mercury reaches under a certain pressure. The measurement is taken with a *sphygmomanometer*. This is a soft, inflatable cuff attached to a column of mercury (calibrated in millimeters). When the cuff is wrapped around your upper arm and inflated, the pressure in it pushes the mercury up the column. Systolic pressure is measured when there is no longer a pulse in the arm beyond the cuff; then the cuff is deflated and the diastolic pressure is taken when the blood flows freely once more.

Blood pressure should be taken with the person's arm bare. A tight sleeve may constrict the arm or make it impossible to apply the blood pressure cuff properly.

METHOD

The cuff should be placed around the person's arm about one inch above the bend in the elbow. Before beginning to work with the sphygmomanometer, check the following five items:

1. Be sure that the sphygmomanometer reads zero when there is no pressure in the system.
2. If you are using a mercury sphygmomanometer, be sure that there is sufficient mercury to pump to the top of the column.
3. Check to be sure that the mercury or needle (on the aneroid sphygmomanometer) will stay in place when the valve is closed.
4. Check the valve screw to make sure that it operates smoothly.
5. Inspect your stethoscope for cracks or leaks in the tubing, earpieces, bell, or diaphragm.

You should first feel for the blood pressure. Find the radial pulse. Then inflate the cuff 30 mm Hg beyond the point where the pulse is obliterated. Open the valve and release 2–3 mm Hg per second. When the pulsations of the radial pulse again become palpable, this is the systolic pressure. The diastolic blood pressure occurs when the vibrations in the artery cease. Diastolic pressure is much more difficult to obtain.

Now, you are ready to use the stethoscope to take the blood pressure. Follow this procedure:

1. Position the disc of the stethoscope snugly against the skin where the elbow bends—a little to the left of center on the right arm, and a little to the right of center on the left arm. There should be no gaps between the stethoscope and the skin, yet you should not apply any undue pressure. Make sure that the stethoscope is not touching the cuff at any point.
2. Position the earpieces of the stethoscope in your ears (with the earpieces directed forward).
3. Hold the stethoscope disc snugly in position with one hand while you pump the cuff with the other hand.
4. Pump the cuff until the mercury on the scale is about thirty points above the point where you felt the pulse disappear earlier, or about 200 mm Hg.
5. Loosen the valve slightly and permit the pressure to drop slowly. Listen carefully for the first sound of a beat—the number on the scale when you hear the first beat is the systolic pressure. (If you think that you missed the first beat or are unsure, tighten the valve again and pump the cuff up; repeat the method, listening carefully.)
6. Continue to deflate the cuff slowly until the last sound of blood is heard. When you hear no more blood flowing, the number on the scale is the diastolic pressure.

Proteolytic enzymes	Take between meals.	Aids in cleansing the circulatory system. Completes protein digestion.
Raw heart concentrate and Bio/Cardiozyme Forte from Biotics Research	As directed on label.	Strengthens the heart muscle.
Vitamin B complex with extra choline and inositol plus	100 mg each twice daily.	Important for circulatory function and for lowering blood pressure.
niacin (B₃)	3 times daily.	

HERBS

☐ Use cayenne, chamomile, fennel, hawthorn berries, parsley, and rosemary for high blood pressure. Drink three cups of suma herb tea daily.

RECOMMENDATIONS

☐ A salt-free diet is essential for lowering blood pressure. Lowering your salt intake is not good enough; eliminate all salt from your diet. Read all labels carefully and avoid those food products that have "soda," "sodium," or the symbol "Na" on the label. These indicate that the product contains salt. Some foods and food additives that should be avoided on a low-salt diet include Accent flavor-enhancer (monosodium glutamate); baking soda; canned vegetables; commercially prepared foods; certain dentifrices and over-the-counter medications that contain ibuprofen, such as Advil and Nuprin; diet soft drinks; foods with mold inhibitors, preservatives, and most sugar substitutes; meat tenderizers; softened water; and soy sauce. These products can cause the cells to swell and interfere with the effectiveness of diuretics used in the treatment of hypertension.

☐ A high-fiber diet and supplemental fiber are recommended. Oat bran is a good source of fiber. Eat plenty of fruits and vegetables, such as apples, asparagus, bananas, broccoli, cabbage, cantaloupe, eggplant, garlic, grapefruit, green leafy vegetables, melons, peas, prunes, raisins, squash, and sweet potatoes. The following juices are healthful: beet, carrot and celery, currant, cranberry, citrus fruit, parsley, spinach, and watermelon. Include seeded foods like brown rice, buckwheat, millet, and oats.

☐ Avoid foods such as aged cheeses, aged meats, anchovies, avocados, chicken liver, chocolate, fava beans, pickled herring, sour cream, sherry and wine, and yogurt. Bacon, corned beef, pork, sausage, and smoked or processed meats are prohibited. Eat only white fish and skinless turkey or chicken. The diet must be low in fats; avoid all animal fats, gravies, and bouillons.

☐ Keep your weight down. Regular moderate exercise is important to maintain proper circulation. Do not overexert yourself in hot or humid weather. Avoid excessive exercising and emotional stress.

☐ Do not take phenylalanine (found in NutraSweet) or L-tyrosine.

☐ Avoid antihistamines unless under a physician's direction.

☐ Take two tablespoons of flaxseed oil daily.

CONSIDERATIONS

☐ A periodic cleansing fast can help detoxify the body. Fast three to five days each month. See FASTING in Part Three.

☐ Drink steam-distilled water only.

☐ Be careful that you do not overexert yourself during sexual intercourse. Sexual intercourse can be dangerous for the hypertensive patient.

☐ If you are taking MAO inhibitors, which are drugs that are used to counter depression, lower blood pressure, and treat infections and cancer, avoid tyramine. Combining MAO inhibitors with tyramine causes the blood pressure to soar and could cause a stroke. Also avoid the amino acid tyrosine if on MAO drugs.

☐ Patients with hypertension often suffer apnea, in which they stop breathing. Apnea, which occurs while sleeping, is associated with loud snoring and restless sleep. It is not unusual for the apneic patient to feel excessively sleepy during the day. Evaluation and treatment of apnea can help reduce high blood pressure in these patients.

☐ People who snore heavily are much more likely to have high blood pressure or angina than silent sleepers. Researchers suggest that snorers may suffer from a slight malfunctioning of the part of the brain responsible for fluent breathing; this can put an unnatural strain on the heart and lungs due to oxygen shortage.

☐ Auriculin, a synthetic heart hormone, is being tested in twenty-five medical centers. It is very effective in lowering the blood pressure.

☐ Research has revealed that people with variations in two specific genes are twice as likely to develop high blood pressure from salt consumption. This discovery may enable doctors to identify children prone to high blood pressure; if these children could be identified at birth, their diets could be modified so that high blood pressure might be avoided in later life.

☐ See also ARTERIOSCLEROSIS and CARDIOVASCULAR DISEASE in Part Two.

High Cholesterol

Overindulgence in cholesterol-containing foods is dangerous, because these foods produce elevated blood cholesterol and triglycerides. In turn, these fats produce plaque-filled arteries that impede blood flow to the brain, kidneys, genitals, extremities, and heart. High cholesterol levels are the primary cause of heart disease, because cholesterol produces fatty deposits in arteries, fat accumulation, clogging of the arteries, and cerebrovascular and cardiac insufficiency. High cholesterol is also implicated in gallstones, impotence, mental impairment, and high blood pressure. Colon polyps and cancer have been linked to high serum cholesterol levels.

About 80 percent of total body cholesterol is manufactured in the liver, while 20 percent is from dietary sources. The body produces cholesterol because it is essential in building cell membranes and sex hormones, and it also aids digestion. Cholesterol becomes a problem when an excess of low-density lipoproteins (LDLs) are present in the body. It is this excess of LDLs that can trigger the formation of plaque on artery walls. High-density lipoproteins (called HDLs) are good because they sweep the body clean of excess cholesterol. If the body has too little HDL or too much LDL, there can be a problem. The levels of these substances are greatly influenced by diet. Vegetarians have low LDL, while exercise, vitamin C, and niacin elevate the "good guy"—HDL. (See the inset on cholesterol.)

CHOLESTEROL LEVEL SELF-TEST

A new test by Home Diagnostics of Edentown, New Jersey, that you can use to check your cholesterol levels is ready for home use, pending FDA approval. Keystone Medical Corporation of Columbia, Maryland, and Chem-Elec of North Webster, Indiana, will also seek FDA approval with the new finger-stick kits for testing cholesterol.

The tests contain pads that are the size of credit cards and have a chemical reagent zone. A drop of blood on the surface makes the reagents react with enzymes in the blood. Within about four minutes the zone changes color. Match the color zone against a color-coded chart to find the serum cholesterol level.

If you do have high cholesterol, follow the nutritional guidelines and recommendations that follow and see your doctor.

NUTRIENTS

SUPPLEMENT	SUGGESTED DOSAGE	COMMENTS
Very Important		
Choline and inositol and B complex and extra thiamine	100–300 mg 3 times daily.	The B vitamins, especially choline and inositol, are important in fat metabolism. Protects the liver from fat deposits.
Coenzyme Q$_{10}$	60 mg	Improves circulation.
Fiber or oat bran and/or guar gum		These help to lower cholesterol and supply needed fiber.
Garlic capsules (Kyolic)	2 capsules 3 times daily.	Odorless garlic that lowers cholesterol levels and blood pressure.
Lecithin	1 tbsp. 3 times daily before meals.	Lowers cholesterol.
Lipotropic factors	As directed on label.	Substances that prevent fat deposits (as in arteriosclerosis).

SUPPLEMENT	SUGGESTED DOSAGE	COMMENTS
Niacin (B$_3$)	500 mg daily.	Lowers cholesterol. Niacinamide is not effective.
Vitamin C plus bioflavonoids	3,000–8,000 mg daily in divided doses.	Lowers cholesterol.
Vitamin E emulsion	200–1,000 IU daily increasing dosage slowly.	Emulsion form offers rapid assimilation. Vitamin E and coenzyme Q$_{10}$ both improve circulation.
Helpful		
Chromium	200 mcg daily.	Necessary for fat synthesis.
Proteolytic enzymes	Take between meals.	Aids digestion.
Selenium	200 mcg	Selenium deficiency has been linked to heart disease.
Unsaturated fatty acids (black currant or borage oil and/or primrose oil)	As directed on label.	Unsaturated fatty acids reduce LDLs.

HERBS

☐ Cayenne, goldenseal, hawthorn berries, and kelp will help lower cholesterol.

RECOMMENDATIONS

☐ Research suggests that water-soluble dietary fiber is very important in reducing serum cholesterol. It is found in barley, beans, brown rice, fruits, glucomannan, guar gum, and oats. Oat bran and brown rice bran are the best foods for lowering cholesterol. Since fiber absorbs the minerals from the food it is in, take extra minerals separate from the fiber.

☐ Meat and dairy products are the primary offenders because they contain high levels of cholesterol. Coffee, stress, and sustained tension also raise the serum cholesterol. Alcohol, steroids, oral contraceptives, Lasix and other diuretics, and L-Dopa (prescribed for Parkinson's disease) are a few of the many drugs that elevate blood cholesterol.

☐ No salt, heated fats, or supermarket oils should be eaten. Stay away from red meat, animal products, non-dairy creamers, processed or refined foods, white bread, coffee, tea, alcohol, or tobacco. Reduce the amount of fats (including cholesterol) in your diet, making sure to take in plenty of fiber in the form of fruits, vegetables, and whole grains. A good all-around exercise program is important!

☐ A spirulina fast (*see* FASTING in Part Three), with carrot and celery juice or lemon and steam-distilled water, is most beneficial (monthly). Carrot juice helps to flush out fat from the bile in the liver and this helps lower cholesterol.

Understanding Cholesterol

Pick up just about any newspaper or magazine these days and you will probably find mention of cholesterol. Everyone is concerned with lowering his cholesterol level, and most people want to know how they can. It is first helpful to know how cholesterol is produced and used by the body.

Cholesterol is actually a crystalline substance consisting of fats. It is found naturally in the brain, nerves, liver, blood, and bile of both humans and vertebrate animals. This is why persons who wish to decrease their cholesterol levels are told to stay away from meat and other foods containing animal products or derived from animals.

Cholesterol is necessary for the proper functioning of the body and is produced mainly in the liver. It is used by cells to build membranes, and it is also used by sex hormones and in aiding digestion. This natural cholesterol travels from the liver through the bloodstream where it is delivered to the cells. The cells take what they need, and the excess cholesterol remains in the bloodstream. Excessive cholesterol often forms plaque, which sticks to artery walls and may eventually cause heart disease.

Researchers have discovered that there are two types of cholesterol: low-density lipoproteins (LDLs) and high-density lipoproteins (HDLs). LDLs are *bad* cholesterol; HDLs are *good* cholesterol. An analysis of the function of each will explain why.

Low-density lipoproteins are obtained by dietary means, from animal products. The body cannot use this type of cholesterol because it is in a form that the body does not want, and it often ends up as plaque formation on artery walls. No matter how much is obtained through diet, the body continues to produce its own natural or serum cholesterol, which it can use.

High-density lipoproteins remove excess cholesterol from the blood and tissues, which is why they are considered "good." Their exact function is not known, nor is it known if they work with other elements in the body to do this. Research continues on the function of HDLs. It is known that persons with high HDL levels and relatively low LDL levels have a low risk of heart disease. In those who already have clogged arteries or have had a heart attack, an increase in HDL levels and a decrease in LDL levels result in improvement of arterial obstruction. After HDLs have traveled through the bloodstream and collected the excess, they return it to the liver, where it is often—though it is not yet known how often—turned into LDLs. Because LDLs are undesirable, it is imperative that each of us realize the importance of diet in decreasing cholesterol levels.

The National Cholesterol Education Program has set the "safe" level of cholesterol at 200 mg/dl (mg/dl = milligrams per deciliter). This combines both HDL and LDL levels. A reading above 200 indicates potential for developing heart disease. A level of 200–239 is borderline, and those over 240 are at high risk.

The normal adult HDL level for men in the United States is 45–50, and 50–60 for women. It is suggested that higher levels such as 70 or 80 will protect against heart disease. An HDL level under 35 is considered risky. So if you have a cholesterol reading of 200 and your HDL level is 80 and LDL level is 120, you are considered low risk for heart disease. As your HDL decreases, your potential for heart problems intensifies, even if your total is on the low side.

It is only logical that we should decrease our intake of animal products and therefore decrease our overall cholesterol levels. There are, however, other sources that raise cholesterol: sugar and alcohol raise the level of *natural* cholesterol (that which the body produces). Although we do need this substance, we do not need to overproduce it, which is what happens when we consume sugar and alcohol. Stress also results in overproduction of natural cholesterol (*see* the inset in STRESS AND ANXIETY in Part Two). Therefore, we can fight off heart disease by avoiding the consumption of animal products, sugar, alcohol, and stress.

CHOLESTEROL COMMENTS

☐ Studies reveal that Third World diets, which consist of grains, fruits, and vegetables, yield a lower blood cholesterol. In the United States, Finland, and Norway, where people indulge heavily in dairy products and meat, extremely high rates of heart and circulatory disease are present. Even the children in these nations show progressive vascular disease due to hypercholesterolemia (an excess of cholesterol in the blood).

☐ Some people use margarine or vegetable oils because they contain no cholesterol. However, once these are heated and ingested, the system is overwhelmed by deadly fats. Other "experts" recommend fish oil to lower cholesterol, but fish oil is 100 percent fat, and the evidence is lacking that ingestion of fish oil reduces serum fats.

☐ A number of drugs lower blood cholesterol, but physicians have been warned by the drug companies of their serious side effects. Only as a last resort should these drugs be used.

☐ The *only* sensible way to keep the serum fats within a safe range is to follow a diet that excludes animal fats (e.g., milk and all dairy products) and includes ample amounts of fiber and bulk (e.g., whole grains, fruits, and vegetables). Vegetables and fruits are free of cholesterol!

☐ Cream substitutes (nondairy cream), unfortunately, are poor alternatives to cholesterol-heavy dairy products. Many contain coconut oil, which is a highly saturated fat. Soy or almond milk is preferred.

☐ Pure virgin olive oil helps reduce serum cholesterol.

A monosaturated acid-rich diet that includes olive oil may be the reason for the low cholesterol plasma levels found in Italy and Greece.

☐ Many fast-food restaurants use beef tallow (fat) in their hamburgers, fish, chicken, and French-fried potatoes. Not only do these fried foods contain high amounts of cholesterol, but this fat is rendered poisonous in the deep frying process, producing highly toxic chemical substances in these foods.

☐ There are good and bad fats, beneficial and harmful ones. Fats and lipids are needed for energy and are better sources than protein or carbohydrates. We need added fats in our diets because they also carry the fat-soluble vitamins A, D, E, and K. Vitamin K is easily destroyed by the use of mineral oil, heparin, dicumarol (blood thinners), many drugs, or aspirin. Most people overlook the need for vitamin K, but it has recently been linked to intestinal disorders. It is important in the treatment of arthritis. One rich source of vitamin K is alfalfa.

☐ Fats provide energy. They act as an intestinal lubricant and combine with phosphorus to form a substance that helps to build tissues and body cells. Fats stay in the digestive tract for longer periods, giving us a feeling of fullness. They also generate body heat. Fats soothe the nerves and coat them with a protective shield. Fat is found in all body cells in combination with other nutrients.

☐ Essential fatty acids are a very important link in our health chain. Essential fatty acids are substances that the body cannot manufacture and that must be supplied. The three types of essential fatty acids are linoleic, linolenic, and arachidonic.

☐ Good fats are polyunsaturated fats—all vegetable fats that are liquid at room temperature. Use cold-pressed oils only! Cold-pressed oils are those that have never been heated above 110°F during processing—at this temperature, enzyme destruction begins. The kinds of oils that should be used are polyunsaturated fats; all vegetable fats that are liquid at room temperature; those made from olive oil, nuts, seeds, soybeans, and flaxseed; primrose oil; and black currant oil.

☐ The right kind of fat is important, but most of us get too much of the wrong kind. Excess fat is stored in the liver, in the arteries, and around the heart and other tissues. The fats that should be avoided are saturated fats, which are of animal origin; hydrogenated fats such as coconut and palm kernel oils; and hardened fats and oils such as margarine, lard, and butter. Read labels carefully.

☐ Coffee drinkers should cut down or, better yet, avoid drinking coffee at all. Coffee in large amounts elevates cholesterol levels in the blood, more than doubling the risk of heart disease, say Norwegian scientists. A report published in *The New England Journal of Medicine* says that observation of 15,000 coffee drinkers revealed that as the intake of coffee rises, the amount of cholesterol in the blood goes up dramatically.

CONSIDERATIONS

☐ It is generally healthier to have a total cholesterol reading of less than 200, and the higher the HDL fraction, the better (see inset on cholesterol).

☐ There are claims that charcoal lowers the cholesterol level. Do not consume activated charcoal daily, as it also absorbs the good nutrients. Do not take charcoal with other medication.

☐ Gemfibroxil, a new cholesterol-lowering drug, may trigger psoriasis. Dermatologists suggest that the drug works well on cholesterol in the blood, but it can also provoke or worsen psoriasis.

☐ *See also* ARTERIOSCLEROSIS in Part Two and CHELATION THERAPY in Part Three.

HIV (Human Immunodeficiency Virus)

See AIDS.

Hot Flashes

See MENOPAUSE.

Human Immunodeficiency Virus (HIV)

See AIDS.

Hyperactivity

Hyperactivity is a disorder of certain mechanisms in the central nervous system. Various factors have been linked to hyperactivity including heredity, smoking during pregnancy, oxygen deprivation at birth, artificial additives in food, environmental pollutants, lead poisoning, and prenatal trauma. Preservatives and foods containing salicylates also contribute to this disorder. A low-protein diet may be a contributing factor.

Some of the symptoms of hyperactivity are head-knocking, lack of concentration, the disturbing of other children, self-destructiveness, temper tantrums, impatience, quick frustration, an inability to sit (even at mealtimes), clumsiness, sleep disturbances, and failure in school even though IQ is normal. Not all symptoms are present in any one child.

A hair analysis is important to rule out heavy metal intoxication. Lead, as well as copper, has been linked to behavioral problems. The latest finding is that phosphate additives may be responsible for hyperkinesis (exaggerated muscle activity). Learning disabilities and juvenile crime are present in 50 percent of the cases.

Although hyperactivity is primarily a problem of childhood, adults can be hyperactive too. The treatment program would remain the same.

In the following table, adjust the dosages according to age and severity.

NUTRIENTS

SUPPLEMENT	SUGGESTED DOSAGE	COMMENTS
Very Important		
Calcium plus magnesium	Use as directed on label and take a small amount at bedtime.	Needed for proper growth and has a calming effect.
Vitamin B complex with extra pantothenic acid (B$_5$) and	Dose depends on age and weight.	Needed for correct brain function and digestion. Enhances adrenal gland function.
B$_6$ (pyridoxine) and niacin (B$_3$)	Use as directed on label.	
Helpful		
Bio-Strath from Germany	As directed on label.	Contains yeast, herbs, and all B vitamins that have a calming effect.
Brewer's yeast	As directed on label.	A natural source of the B vitamins. *Caution:* Be careful of a possible allergy. Try ¼ tsp. and slowly increase while watching for reactions.
L-Cysteine (amino acid)	As directed on label.	Take if a hair analysis reveals a high level of metals.
Multivitamin and mineral complex	As directed on label.	High amounts of nutrients are needed.
Vitamin C	Use as directed according to age.	Antistress vitamin.

RECOMMENDATIONS

☐ Remove from the diet white sugar and its products, salt, soft drinks, teas, soy sauce, cider vinegar, milk, catsup, chili sauce, colored cheeses, chocolate, luncheon meat, salami, pork, sausage, meat loaf, hot dogs, bacon, ham, wheat, corn, mustard, colored butter, oleo margarine, ice cream (except all natural), candy (except homemade), cough drops, throat lozenges, antacid tablets, perfumes, and toothpaste. Use a natural toothpaste from a health food store.

☐ The hyperactive child should also not eat foods that contain artificial colors and flavorings, foods that contain the preservative BHT, processed and manufactured foods, and foods that contain natural salicylates. These include certain fruits and vegetables, almonds, apples, apricots, cherries, currants, all berries, peaches, plums, prunes, tomatoes, cucumbers, and oranges.

☐ Foods that the hyperactive child may eat are all fruits and vegetables that are not listed above and cereals, breads, and crackers that contain only rice and oats. To identify which foods are causing the child's hyperactivity, return those foods that have been eliminated from the diet one at a time for one week and watch for a change in the child.

☐ A low-phosphate diet is important. Carbonated beverages should be avoided. High levels of phosphorus and very low calcium and magnesium levels (which can be revealed through a hair analysis) usually indicate a potential for hyperactivity and seizures. Meat and fat are high in phosphorus. Excess copper is linked to behavioral dysfunction.

☐ The herb valerian root in extract form is being used for this disorder with a dramatic calming action and no side effects. Mix the extract in juice (as directed on label according to age) and drink two to three times a day.

CONSIDERATIONS

☐ Studies indicate that administration of GABA (gamma-amino butyric acid) decreases hyperactivity, as well as the tendency toward violence, epilepsy, mental retardation, and learning disabilities.

Hypertension

See HIGH BLOOD PRESSURE.

Hyperthyroid

This disorder occurs when the thyroid gland produces too much hormone, resulting in an overactive metabolic state. The body's processes, including digestion, speed up with this disorder. Malabsorption occurs, so a proper diet is important. The symptoms of hyperthyroidism are nervousness, irritability, increased perspiration, insomnia and fatigue, weakness, hair and weight loss, separation of the nails, hand tremors, intolerance of heat, rapid heartbeat, and sometimes protruding eyeballs. The condition is sometimes called thyrotoxicosis or Grave's disease.

The pituitary gland, parathyroid glands, and sex glands all work together and are influenced by thyroid function. If there is a problem in one place, they all may be affected.

This condition is not as common as an underactive thyroid (*see* HYPOTHYROID in Part Two). A malfunctioning thyroid can be the underlying cause of many recurring illnesses.

NUTRIENTS

SUPPLEMENT	SUGGESTED DOSAGE	COMMENTS
Very Important		
Multivitamin and mineral complex	As directed on label. Megadoses daily.	Increased vitamins and minerals are needed in this "hyper" metabolic condition.
Vitamin B complex with extra riboflavin (B_2) and thiamine (B_1) and B_6 (pyridoxine)	50 mg 3 times daily with meals.	Vitamin B injections may be necessary.
Helpful		
Brewer's yeast	1–3 tbsp. daily.	Rich in many basic nutrients, especially the B vitamins.
Essential fatty acids	As directed on label.	Needed for correct glandular function.
Lecithin	As directed on label.	Aids in digestion of fats and protects the lining of all cells and organs.
Vitamin C	3,000–5,000 mg daily.	Especially important in this stressful condition.
Vitamin E	400 IU daily. (Do not exceed this dosage.)	Avoid excessive amounts of vitamin E. This may stimulate the thyroid gland; however, a small amount is needed.

RECOMMENDATIONS

☐ Eat plenty of the following foods: broccoli, Brussels sprouts, cabbage, cauliflower, kale, mustard greens, peaches, pears, rutabagas, soybeans, spinach, and turnips. These help to suppress thyroid hormone production.

☐ Avoid dairy products for at least three months. Also avoid stimulants, coffee, tea, nicotine, and soft drinks.

CONSIDERATIONS

☐ Radioactive iodine (I-131) is used to treat this condition. Be wary of this. Severe side effects have been known to accompany the use of I-131.

☐ Also, don't rush into surgery! Try improving your diet first.

Hypoglycemia (Low Blood Sugar)

Oversecretion of insulin by the pancreas results in hypoglycemia, a condition in which there is an abnormally low level of glucose (sugar) in the blood. Heredity can be a cause, but the disease is most often precipitated by an inadequate diet. This is referred to as functional hypoglycemia (FH). Symptoms of FH have a direct relationship to the time and type of meal that was last eaten. A hypoglycemic may display any or all of the following symptoms: fatigue, dizziness, headache and irritability if meals are missed, depression, anxiety, cravings for sweets, confusion, night sweats, weakness in legs, swollen feet, tightness in chest, constant hunger, pain in various parts of the body (especially the eyes), nervous habits, mental disturbances, and insomnia.

Hypoglycemia mimics many diseases. Related disorders include allergies, asthma, hay fever, indigestion, obesity, nutritional deficiencies, malabsorption, colitis, constipation, and impaired memory. Abnormal protein and carbohydrate metabolism and poor adrenal function are part of hypoglycemia. Proper diet is a key factor for the hypoglycemic to maintain proper blood sugar levels. See the hypoglycemic diet below.

NUTRIENTS

SUPPLEMENT	SUGGESTED DOSAGE	COMMENTS
Very Important		
Chromium	300 mcg daily.	Vital in glucose metabolism; natural brewer's yeast is a good source. Picolinate is effective.
Vitamin B complex with extra	50–100 mg daily.	Important in carbohydrate metabolism.
thiamine (B$_1$) and	100 mg daily.	
niacin (B$_3$) and	100 mg daily.	
vitamin B$_{12}$ plus	300 mcg twice daily on an empty stomach.	
pantothenic acid (B$_5$)	1,000 mg daily in divided doses.	B$_5$ is important in adrenal gland function and conversion of glucose to energy.
Important		
Calcium plus	1,500 mg	Magnesium is important in carbohydrate (sugar) metabolism.
magnesium	750 mg Take both in divided doses after meals and at bedtime.	
L-Carnitine	Use as directed on label.	Converts stored body fat into energy.
L-Cysteine	Use as directed on label.	Blocks the action of insulin, which lowers blood sugar.
L-Glutamine with vitamin B$_6$ (pyridoxine) and vitamin C	1,000 mg on an empty stomach daily.	Reduces cravings for sugar.
Manganese	As directed on label.	Most hypoglycemics have low levels of this trace mineral in their blood.
Pancreatin (high potency)	Take with meals.	For protein digestion.
Proteolytic enzymes	Take between meals.	Hypoglycemics often fail to digest protein.
Spirulina or protein powder (free form amino acid)	Use as directed on label.	Works well between meals to balance blood sugar levels.
Vitamin C plus bioflavonoids	3,000–8,000 mg in divided doses.	For adrenal glandular insufficiency, common in hypoglycemia.
Vitamin E	400 IU daily and up.	Improves energy and circulation.
Zinc	50 mg daily.	Hair analyses reveal that most hypoglycemics are zinc deficient.
Helpful		
Aerobic Bulk Cleanse (ABC) with aloe vera juice	Take on an empty stomach in the morning without other supplements.	Drink quickly because it thickens. Aids in slowing down blood sugar reactions.
Dandelion root	Use as directed on label.	Excellent source of the B vitamins and calcium.
Liver injectables and B complex	2cc liver 1cc B complex	Needed to reduce stress, to promote absorption of nutrients, and to increase energy.
Mega- multiminerals and vitamin complex	Use as directed on label.	This disorder requires all nutrients for healing.
Royal jelly	Use as directed on label.	Contains natural pantothenic acid (B$_5$) to nourish the adrenal glands.

RECOMMENDATIONS

☐ The diet should include vegetables, brown rice, avocados, Jerusalem artichokes, seeds, grains, nuts, yogurt, raw cheese, cottage cheese, and kefir milk.

☐ Remove from the diet sugar, refined and processed foods such as instant rice and potatoes, white flour, soft drinks, alcohol, and salt. Avoid sweet fruits and juices such as grape and prune (mix with 50 percent water if used). Avoid macaroni, noodles, gravies, hominy, white rice, yams, and corn. Beans and baked potatoes twice a week is permissible.

☐ The hypoglycemic should not go without food. Instead, he should eat six to eight small meals throughout the day. Some hypoglycemics find that eating a small snack before bedtime helps. In addition, the diet should be rotated as food allergies are often linked to hypoglycemia. Food allergies aggravate both conditions, making the symptoms more pronounced.

☐ A high-fiber diet will help to stabilize the blood sugar swings. During a low blood sugar reaction, combine fiber with a protein food (i.e., bran or rice crackers with raw cheese or almond butter). Instead of eating applesauce, choose a whole apple. The fiber in the apple will inhibit fluctuations in blood sugar. Add a glass of fruit juice for a rapid rise in the blood sugar. Fiber alone (found in popcorn, oat bran, rice bran, crackers, and guar gum) will slow down a hypoglycemic reaction. Take fiber a half hour before meals to avoid a reaction. Spirulina tablets taken between meals will further stabilize the blood sugar.

CONSIDERATIONS

☐ Injections of B complex (1 cc) plus pyridoxine (1/2 cc) and liver (1 cc) have produced very good results. Injections should be taken twice weekly for three months, then decrease to once weekly for two months or more. This helps the hypoglycemic tolerate the foods that produce low blood sugar reactions. These injections are very important, especially for the elderly, because of common malabsorption problems.

☐ Fasting once a month with a series of lemon juice enemas is beneficial. (*See* FASTING and ENEMAS in Part Three.)

In order to prevent a low blood sugar reaction while fasting, spirulina or protein powder supplement should be used. After using this, patients start to feel better very quickly. They sleep better and have a sense of well being, and the frequent depression soon becomes a thing of the past.

☐ It is estimated that 50 percent of hypoglycemic individuals over fifty have reduced thyroid function and hypothyroidism. *See* HYPOTHYROID in Part Two.

☐ Caffeine, alcohol, and cigarette smoking result in profound swings (i.e., instability) of the blood sugar.

☐ *See also* ALLERGIES in Part Two.

Hypothyroid

Hypothyroidism is the underproduction of the thyroid hormone. This is a very common condition. Symptoms include fatigue, loss of appetite, overweight, painful premenstrual periods, muscle weakness, dry and scaly skin, a yellow-orange coloration in the skin (particularly on the palms), yellow bumps on the eyelids, hair loss (including eyebrows), recurrent infections, constipation, depression, slow speech, and myxedema (drooping, swollen eyes). The most frequent symptoms seen in those suffering from this disorder are intolerance to cold and fatigue. If a person is cold while others around him are hot, he is suffering from reduced thyroid function.

A condition called Hashimoto's disease is sometimes the cause of an underactive thyroid. In this disease, the body becomes allergic to the thyroid hormone. By measuring the hormone levels in the blood, it can usually be determined if the thyroid gland is working properly.

Problems with the thyroid can be the cause of many recurring illnesses and fatigue.

THYROID SELF-TEST

To test yourself for an underactive thyroid, keep a thermometer by your bed one night. When you awake the next morning, place the thermometer under your arm and hold it there for fifteen minutes. Keep still and quiet. Any motion can upset your temperature reading. A temperature of 97.6°F or lower may indicate an underactive thyroid. Keep a log! If your readings are in this category, see your doctor.

Treatment of a regular morning temperature of 96°F is three to four grains of Armour Thyroid Extract (by prescription). A person with a regular morning temperature of 97°F should take one to two grains. If you have side effects, speak to your physician about reducing the dosage.

NUTRIENTS

SUPPLEMENT	SUGGESTED DOSAGE	COMMENTS
Essential		
L-Tyrosine (amino acid)	500 mg twice daily on an empty stomach with small amounts of B₆.	Low plasma levels have been associated with a hypothyroid.
Sea kelp	10 tablets daily.	Contains iodine, the basic substance of the thyroid hormone.
Very Important		
Raw thyroid glandular (Armour Extract)	As directed by physician.	Available by prescription only. Synthetic thyroid hormones are often ineffective. *See* GLANDULAR THERAPY in Part Three.
Important		
Vitamin B complex including riboflavin (B₂) and	100 mg with meals. 50 mg twice daily.	Improves cellular oxygenation and energy. B₁₂ is absorbed better in lozenge form.
B₁₂ lozenges	15 mg dissolved under the tongue 3 times daily on an empty stomach.	
Helpful		
Brewer's yeast	As directed on label.	Rich in basic nutrients (B vitamins, etc.).
Iron chelate or Floradix formula	As directed on label.	Essential for enzyme and hemoglobin production.
Unsaturated fatty acids	As directed on label.	For proper functioning of the thyroid gland.
Vitamin A plus beta-carotene	15,000 IU daily.	Included in a multivitamin complex.
Vitamin C	500 mg 4 times daily.	Do *not* take extremely high doses—this may affect the production of the thyroid hormone.
Vitamin E	400 IU daily.	Avoid larger amounts.
Zinc	50 mg daily.	An immune system stimulant.

HERBS

☐ Bayberry, black cohosh, and goldenseal can help this thyroid condition.

RECOMMENDATIONS

☐ Eat molasses, egg yolks, parsley, apricots, dates, and prunes. Eat fish or chicken and raw milk and cheeses.

☐ Avoid processed and refined foods, including white flour and sugar.

☐ Eat these foods in moderation: cruciferous vegetables such as turnips, cabbage, broccoli, mustard greens, spinach, kale, Brussels sprouts, and peaches and pears. If you have severe symptoms, omit these foods entirely because they may further suppress thyroid function.

☐ Drink distilled water only! Avoid fluoride (including fluoride found in toothpaste) and chlorine (drinking water). Chlorine, fluoride, and iodine are chemically related. Chlorine and fluoride block iodine receptors in the thyroid gland, resulting in reduced iodine-containing hormone production and finally in hypothyroidism.

☐ Avoid sulfa drugs and antihistamines except under doctor's orders!

CONSIDERATIONS

☐ A study done at the University of Massachusetts reveals that levothyroxine, a drug commonly used to treat thyroid conditions, causes up to 13 percent bone loss. An estimated 19 million people take this drug for an overactive thyroid, enlarged thyroid, and thyroid cancer.

Hysterectomy

Hysterectomy is the surgical removal of the uterus. This is done for many different reasons. One common reason is fibroid tumors (these are benign), a condition that causes many problems. There are three different types of hysterectomy that are performed:

● *Total* hysterectomy in which the cervix is removed along with the uterus.
● *Partial* hysterectomy in which only the uterus is removed.
● *Pan* hysterectomy in which the ovaries, tubes, and uterus are removed.

Always seek a second opinion when hysterectomy is recommended. Check into alternative treatments before undergoing surgery.

After a pan hysterectomy, menopausal symptoms may appear, including hot flashes and emotional disturbances. When the ovaries are removed, the woman may almost instantly experience the "change of life."

If female hormones are required to control the symptoms, take the lowest dose possible. Ask your doctor for a combined hormone containing estrogen and progesterone to help reduce the risk of cancer.

The following supplements help counteract the side effects of hysterectomy.

NUTRIENTS

SUPPLEMENT	SUGGESTED DOSAGE	COMMENTS
Very Important		
Boron	3 mg daily.	Aids in calcium absorption and prevention of bone loss that sometimes occurs after a hysterectomy or menopause.
Calcium chelate and	2,000 mg daily.	Lack of estrogen hinders calcium uptake. Needed for
magnesium	1,000 mg daily. It is best to take these at bedtime.	the central nervous system.
Potassium	99 mg daily.	Needed when hot flashes occur to balance sodium lost through excess perspiration.
Raw thymus glandular	As directed on label.	Potentiates immune function.
Unsaturated fatty acids (primrose oil)	2 capsules 3 times daily.	Helps the body manufacture estrogen.
Vitamin B complex (high stress formula)	100 mg twice daily with meals.	Injections may be necessary.
Vitamin C	3,000–6,000 mg divided up daily.	An antistress vitamin also needed for tissue repair.
Vitamin E	Start with 400 IU; increase slowly to 1,200 IU.	Find the dosage that eases the hot flashes and maintain it. Important in estrogen production.
Important		
L-Arginine plus L-lysine (amino acids)	500 mg twice daily.	Two of the essential amino acids important in post-surgery recovery. L-Lysine is included to avoid an imbalance of the amino acids.
Helpful		
Gerovital H-3 (GH-3) tablets	1 tablet twice daily.	Minimizes menopausal symptoms.
Multiglandular (Cytozyme F from Henderson)	As directed on label.	Aids in glandular function.
Multivitamin and mineral complex	As directed on label.	Restores the essential vitamins and minerals to balance.

RECOMMENDATIONS

☐ If you have had recent surgery, take vitamin A and E emulsion and zinc in addition to the supplements in the table. Take 50,000 IU vitamin A and the amount of vitamin E that is included. Vitamins A and E are important in immune function. Also include 50 milligrams of zinc daily. Zinc is also important in immune function and promotes tissue repair.

☐ Avoid dairy products, caffeine, colas, sugar, red meat, and processed foods.

☐ *See* HYPOGLYCEMIA in Part Two and follow the diet.

CONSIDERATIONS

☐ There is a new laser treatment that *may* make the hysterectomy unnecessary. It is called a Yag type laser. It is available only in a few large cities. Ask your doctor about it.

☐ Vitamin E helps prevent incisional scarring and relieves itching and discomfort in the area surrounding the stitches. Open a vitamin E capsule and apply along the incision.

☐ *See also* MENOPAUSE in Part Two.

Immune System, Weakened

See WEAKENED IMMUNE SYSTEM.

Impotence

The inability to achieve or maintain an erection, premature ejaculation, and the inability to ejaculate makes it impossible for the male to impregnate the ovum of the female. This impotence may be psychological or organic in nature.

Some possible organic causes include low sperm count; peripheral vascular disease; diabetes; use of some medications, alcohol, or cigarettes; psychological factors; and having had mumps as an adult. There are many other causes of impotence. A qualified doctor's opinion is needed in most cases.

SELF-TEST

Purchase a kit called Snap-Gauge. This test is designed to detect and measure the rigidity of erections the male experiences while sleeping. Call (800) 328-1103 for more information.

NUTRIENTS

SUPPLEMENT	SUGGESTED DOSAGE	COMMENTS
Essential		
L-Arginine	As directed on label.	This amino acid increases the male sperm count.
Vitamin E	400–1,000 IU	Start with 200 IU and increase slowly.
Zinc	80 mg	Important in prostate gland function and reproductive organ growth.
Very Important		
Vitamin C	3,000–6,000 mg	Keeps the sperm from clumping and makes the sperm more motile.
Important		
Gerovital H-3 (GH-3) from Rumania or Zumba	As directed on label.	Both stimulate the sex hormones.
Liver injections	2cc twice weekly.	Found to be beneficial.
Octacosanol	1–2 capsules 3 times weekly.	Natural source of vitamin E. Good for hormone production.
Helpful		
Astrelin from Europe	As directed on label.	Has shown good results when taken in tablet form.
L-Tyrosine (amino acid)	500 mg twice daily. Take on an empty stomach.	Helps stabilize moods and alleviates stress.
Proteolytic enzymes	2 tablets between meals.	Enhances breakdown of foods so that nutrients can be absorbed.
Raw orchic substances	As directed on label.	These glandular extracts of the male reproductive organs promote their function. *See* GLANDULAR THERAPY in Part Three.
Vitamin A plus beta-carotene	15,000 IU 15,000 IU	Antioxidants that enhance immunity.
Vitamin B complex and vitamin B₆ (pyridoxine)	50 mg 3 times daily. 50 mg 3 times daily.	Needed for a healthy nervous system. Necessary for the synthesis of RNA and DNA, which contain the genetic instructions for cell reproduction.

HERBS

☐ Use ginseng and gotu kola.

RECOMMENDATIONS

☐ A balanced diet is important. Do not consume animal fats, fried foods, sugar, or junk foods. Do eat pumpkin seeds, bee pollen, or royal jelly.

☐ Avoid vigorous exercise, hot tubs, and saunas as this leads to reduced sperm counts. In fact, a University of

Michigan Medical Center study indicates that intense exercise may result in a drop in the production of hormones involved in potency, fertility, and sex drive.

☐ Do not smoke. Avoid being around cigarette smoke and avoid stress.

☐ Investigate the possibility of heavy metal intoxication. A hair analysis reveals possible heavy metal poisoning.

CONSIDERATIONS

☐ Keep in mind that sexual function changes with age. An older man may require more stimulation and a longer period of time to experience an erection.

☐ Alcohol intake decreases the body's ability to produce testosterone (a male hormone). New research at the Chicago Medical School reveals that drinking alcohol may cause "menopause" in men and put them at a higher risk of heart attack. Alcohol not only affects the sexual function in the male, but sets the stage for a heart attack and the potentially deadly side effects.

☐ Arteriosclerotic disease of the blood vessels, which restricts blood supply to the penis and to the nerves that otherwise would lead to sexual arousal, may result in a "failure to perform." *See* CIRCULATORY PROBLEMS in Part Two.

☐ A very common cause of impotence is the use of antihypertensive and tranquilizer drugs. The use of marijuana and cocaine also results in impotence. In addition, heavy smoking decreases sexual capabilities by damaging the tiny blood vessels that supply blood to the penis.

☐ Vasectomy for sterilization has been linked to prostate disease and even cancer.

☐ The drugs Tagamet and Zantac have significant side effects in some men. They may decrease the sperm count and even produce impotence. These drugs are frequently used in treating ulcers.

☐ The drug papaverine is used either alone or in combination with phentolamine to dilate the penile blood vessels, causing increased blood flow to the erectile tissue. The drug is deemed effective for both physiological and psychological impotence.

☐ Yohimex, a trade name for yohimbine, is taken by mouth. It increases parasympathetic activity, which increases sexual performance. This theoretically results in increased flow of blood to the penis.

Indigestion (Dyspepsia)

Indigestion may be a symptom of a disorder in the stomach or small or large intestine or it may be a disorder in itself. Symptoms can include gas, abdominal pain, heartburn, a bloated feeling, belching, nausea, vomiting, and a burning sensation after eating.

Chewing with the mouth open, talking while chewing, swallowing too much air by gulping down food, and washing down needed enzymes for digestion by drinking liquids with meals result in indigestion. Food allergies can also be the cause. They cause a fermentation of food in the colon that produces hydrogen and carbon dioxide. Carbohydrates are the main food source responsible for gas because of the bacteria they contain. It is important to find out which foods your body cannot digest. In addition, stay away from foods that cause this reaction (*see* ALLERGIES in Part Two). Stress and a lack of digestive enzymes can also cause intestinal problems.

STOMACH ACID SELF-TEST

Hydrochloric acid (HCl) is necessary for the breakdown and digestion of many foods. You can determine if you need hydrochloric acid with this simple test. Take a tablespoon of apple cider vinegar or lemon juice. If this makes your heartburn go away, then you need more stomach acid. If it makes your symptoms worse, then you have too much HCl and shouldn't take enzymes that contain HCl. If it helps the symptoms, sip pure apple cider vinegar and water with meals.

NUTRIENTS

SUPPLEMENT	SUGGESTED DOSAGE	COMMENTS
Very Important		
Aerobic 07 from Aerobic Life Products	9 drops in water once daily.	Controls putrefying bacteria in the bowel.
Aloe vera juice	¼ cup on an empty stomach in the morning and at bedtime.	Good for heartburn and other gastrointestinal symptoms. George's tastes like spring water.
High-fiber glucomannan or Aerobic Bulk Cleanse (ABC)	1 tbsp. in liquid upon arising. Drink down quickly before fiber thickens.	Colon cleansers that aid in normal stool formation.
Proteolytic enzymes from American Biologics or pancreatin	2 tablets with meals and 1 tablet with snacks.	Important for gas and bloating.

Important		
Acidophilus (Neo-Flora from New Moon Extracts)	½ hour before meals.	Necessary for normal digestion. Neo-Flora is a nondairy product.
Garlic capsules (Kyolic)	2 capsules with meals.	Aids in digestion and destroys unwanted bacteria in the bowel.
Vitamin B complex plus extra thiamine (B₁) and niacin (B₃) and B₁₂	100 mg with meals.	The B vitamins are essential for normal digestion.
Helpful		
Alfalfa (tablets or liquid)	As directed on label.	Supplies needed vitamin K and trace minerals.
L-Carnitine	As directed on label.	Carries fat into the cells for breakdown into energy.
Lipotropic factors (choline and inositol or lecithin)	Take before meals.	Fat emulsifiers that aid in the breakdown of fats.
L-Methionine	As directed on label.	Liver detoxifier.
Multidigestive enzymes	Take with meals.	Avoid products containing hydrochloric acid if heartburn or ulcers are present.
Pancreatin	3 after meals.	A helpful digestive enzyme.

HERBS

☐ Catnip, chamomile, comfrey, goldenseal root, fennel, fenugreek, mint teas, papaya, and peppermint are all good to use. Do not use comfrey over long periods of time. Slippery elm is good for inflammation of the colon; use as an enema for fast relief. (*See* ENEMAS in Part Three.)

RECOMMENDATIONS

☐ For upper gastrointestinal gas pancreatin is needed, and for lower gastrointestinal gas trace minerals are needed. Antacids are useless for gas and bloating. When having excess gas, use the juice of one fresh lemon in one quart lukewarm water as an enema to balance the body's pH. If gas is constant for days, use a bifidus enema. This will relieve the problem within hours.

☐ Acidophilus can also be used for indigestion, because a shortage of the "friendly" bacteria is most often the cause. Open ten capsules or one tablespoon powdered formula. Neo-Flora from New Moon Extracts is a nondairy product that can be used if reactions to dairy products occur. Acidophilus used as an enema hardly

ever results in a problem. You may experience some rumbling and slight disturbance for an hour or so, but it will subside.

☐ Consume well-balanced meals with plenty of fiber-rich foods such as fresh fruits, vegetables, and whole grain products.

☐ Avoid refined carbohydrates (sugar), bakery products, macaroni, dairy products, caffeine, citrus juice, tomatoes, pepper, carbonated beverages, potato chips, junk foods, fried and fatty foods, spicy foods, red meat, beans, snacks, and colas. Decrease salt consumption. Processed foods, junk foods, and all dairy products cause excess mucus formation, which results in inadequate digestion of protein. Limit your intake of peanuts, lentils, and soybeans. They contain an enzyme inhibitor.

☐ Food combinations are important. Protein and starches are a poor combination, as are vegetables and fruits. Milk should not be consumed with meals. Sugars must not be consumed with proteins or starches.

☐ Sipping one tablespoon of pure apple cider vinegar in a glass of water with meals aids digestion.

☐ Charcoal tablets are good for absorbing gas, but they interfere with other medication and nutrients. Do not take for long periods of time.

CONSIDERATIONS

☐ Drink the juice of a lemon in a cup of water first thing in the morning. This a good healer and blood purifier.

☐ If you have had abdominal surgery (such as a bowel shortened), pancreatin will help digest foods. Hypoglycemics (who have low blood sugar) also need pancreatin. After meals, if you have a stuffed feeling and a rumbling or gurgling with bloating and gas, use pancreatin.

☐ Rice and barley broth are good for disorders such as gas, bloating, and heartburn. Use five parts water to one part grain, and boil for ten minutes. Put the lid on and simmer for fifty-five minutes more. Strain, cool, and sip throughout the day.

☐ If stools are foul-smelling and are accompanied by a burning sensation in the anus, follow the fasting program. (*See* FASTING in Part Three.) This is often a sign that the colon contains toxic material.

☐ Exercise such as brisk walking and stretching and the herb formula Tum-Ease from New Moon Extracts enhance the digestive process.

☐ The elderly typically lack hydrochloric acid and pancreatin.

☐ Remember to chew food thoroughly; do not gulp it down in a hurry.

☐ See *also* ALLERGIES in Part Two and take the self-test.

Infertility

Infertility is the inability to become pregnant after a year or more of regular sexual activity during the time of ovulation. It is also the inability to carry a pregnancy full-term. Infertility is usually caused by a hormonal imbalance.

Some possible causes include pelvic inflammatory disease and chlamydia. Chlamydia is one of the leading causes of infertility, yet most women are unaware that they have the disease.

Some women develop antibodies to their partner's sperm due to an allergic reaction. This may be corrected by having the male use a condom for thirty days. The female's sperm antibodies decrease, and then intercourse without the use of a condom during the time of ovulation may lead to conception.

Because there are so many causes of infertility, in most cases a qualified doctor's opinion is needed.

OVULATION TIMING SELF-TEST

When planning for a baby, you can obtain a test that can help you determine the best time to conceive. Remember, however, that no test is 100 percent accurate. This test predicts the time of ovulation by measuring the corresponding rise in the level of luteinizing hormone (LH) present, which triggers the release of the egg.

A chemically impregnated dipstick detects the LH in urine samples. If the hormone has been released, it is indicated by a color change in the stick. After a positive result, ovulation takes place *within twelve to thirty-six hours*. Ovu-stick and another test kit called First Response can be purchased at your drugstore.

Most doctors must get your consent before performing diagnostic tests. There may be risks involved any time you penetrate the body using a tube, needle, or viewing instrument, or through radiation exposure, reactions to drugs, anesthetics, and dye materials used in certain imaging techniques. Risks vary depending on your age and health status, and the ability of your doctor.

NUTRIENTS

SUPPLEMENT	SUGGESTED DOSAGE	COMMENTS
Essential		
Vitamin E	400–1,000 IU. Start with 200 IU and increase slowly.	Needed for balanced hormone production.
Zinc	80 mg	Important for prostate gland function and reproductive organ growth.
Important		
Gerovital H-3 (GH-3) from Rumania or Zumba	As directed on label.	Both stimulate the sex hormones.
Liver injections	Twice weekly.	Found to be beneficial in promoting function of the sex organs.
Octacosanol	1 capsule 3 times daily.	The heart of wheat germ aids in hormone production.
Helpful		
Astrelin from Europe	As directed on label.	Has shown good results when taken in tablet form.
L-Tyrosine (amino acid)	500 mg twice daily. Take on an empty stomach.	Alleviates stress and aids in stabilizing moods.
Proteolytic enzymes	2 tablets between meals.	Aids in the breakdown of foods. Facilitates absorption of nutrients.
Raw ovarian concentrate	As directed on label.	A glandular product. *See* GLANDULAR THERAPY in Part Three.
Vitamin A plus	15,000 IU	Important in reproductive gland function.
beta-carotene	15,000 IU	
Vitamin B complex and	50 mg	Important in reproductive gland function.
vitamin B$_6$ (pyridoxine)	50 mg 3 times daily.	

HERBS

☐ Use dong quai and gotu kola.

RECOMMENDATIONS

☐ A balanced diet is important. Do not consume animal fats, fried foods, sugar, or junk foods. Do eat pumpkin seeds, bee pollen, or royal jelly.

☐ Avoid vigorous exercise, hot tubs, and saunas as this leads to changes in ovulation.

☐ Do not smoke. Avoid being around cigarette smoke, and avoid stress.

CONSIDERATIONS

☐ More women are waiting to bear children in later reproductive years. However, a woman's fertility begins to decrease when she reaches her thirties.

☐ PABA stimulates the pituitary gland and sometimes restores fertility to some women who cannot conceive.

☐ A recent study revealed that caffeine consumption may prevent women from becoming pregnant.

☐ Investigate the possibility of heavy metal intoxication, which may affect ovulation. A hair analysis reveals possible heavy metal poisoning.

☐ See IMPOTENCE in Part Two. The impotent male plays a significant role in infertility.

Inflammation

Inflammation occurs when a part of the body reacts to trauma or infection. It can be caused by arthritis, bacterial infection, or strain. The symptoms are swelling, heat, and pain. Sometimes the afflicted area turns red.

Any organ or tissue of the body, internal or external, can become inflamed. Internal inflammation is often caused by bacteria. Bacterial arthritis is usually associated with an infection elsewhere in the body, such as in the lungs, kidney, or gallbladder.

NUTRIENTS

SUPPLEMENT	SUGGESTED DOSAGE	COMMENTS
Essential		
Vitamin C plus bioflavonoids	3,000–6,000 mg divided up during the day.	Essential to the healing process and in reducing swelling.
Very Important		
Inflazyme Forte from American Biologics	2 tablets between meals and at bedtime.	Aids in controlling inflammation.
Proteolytic enzymes	4 tablets between meals and at bedtime. Take for 1 month.	Aids in controlling inflammation.
Superoxide dismutase (SOD) from Biotec Foods	As directed on label.	A high potency free radical scavenger.
Zinc	50 mg daily.	Helps to control inflammation and promotes healing.
Important		
Bromelin	Take on an empty stomach as directed on label. Take with a small amount of magnesium and L-cysteine to enhance results.	Has anti-inflammatory activity and increases the breakdown of fibrin, which forms around the inflamed area, blocking the blood and lymph vessels and leading to swelling. *Caution:* Do not take with other mineral supplements. Copper and iron counteract with bromelin.
Garlic capsules (Kyolic)	2 capsules with meals.	Anti-inflammatory odorless garlic.
Germanium	200 mg daily.	Stops free radical reactions. Provides relief from discomfort and pain.
Mineral complex (high in calcium) or bone complex	As directed on label.	Supplies important minerals, especially calcium. Needed to reduce stress.
Silica or horsetail extract	1 tablet twice daily.	Aids in absorption of calcium and repairs connective tissues.
Vitamin A and E emulsion or capsules	As directed on label.	Destroys free radicals and potentiates immune system. Vitamin E promotes healing by helping the body to use oxygen efficiently.
Helpful		
Kelp or alfalfa	5 tablets daily.	Contains a balance of essential minerals and chlorophyll, which cleanses the blood.
Raw thymus	As directed on label.	Improves thymus function—important for immune function.

HERBS

☐ Echinacea, goldenseal, pau d'arco, red clover, and yucca are all good for inflammation. Bilberry extract contains flavonoids, which reduce inflammation.

RECOMMENDATIONS

☐ Diet is very important! Eat 75 percent raw foods, and drink herb teas and juices. Avoid colas, sugar, white flour products, and junk foods.

☐ See FASTING in Part Three and follow the program for quick results.

☐ See HYPOTHYROID in Part Two and follow the program for quick results.

☐ The traditional methods for relieving inflammation are positioning the affected part properly (including splinting, if necessary), applying heat and/or ice (heat and cold therapies), taking medication along with nutritional supplements, and getting plenty of rest.

☐ See also ABSCESSES, ARTHRITIS, and SPRAINS, STRAINS, AND OTHER INJURIES OF THE MUSCLES AND JOINTS in Part Two.

Influenza

Influenza, also known as the "flu," is a highly contagious viral infection of the respiratory tract. Because this illness can be spread easily by coughing and sneezing, outbreaks of influenza are very common. Individual strains of the virus are constantly changing, so vaccinations against influenza have been only partly successful.

Influenza may appear suddenly after an incubation period of one to three days. The early signs of influenza are similar to those of the common cold—headache, weakness, and aching of the arms, legs, and back. The victim may feel feverish one moment, and then feel a chilling sensation the next. Most influenza sufferers have a dry throat and cough. The victim is often so tired that he does not feel like eating or doing anything else. Nausea and vomiting may occur as well. Although influenza is rarely fatal by itself, it does make the patient more susceptible to pneumonia, ear infections, and sinus trouble.

NUTRIENTS

SUPPLEMENT	SUGGESTED DOSAGE	COMMENTS
Essential		
Ascorbic acid flush or vitamin C	5,000–10,000 mg daily in divided doses.	*See* ASCORBIC ACID FLUSH in Part Three. For children, use a buffered C or calcium ascorbate.
Vitamin A plus beta-carotene	15,000 IU daily. 15,000 IU daily.	A powerful antioxidant and immunity booster.
Zinc gluconate lozenges	Dissolve 1 lozenge under the tongue every 2 hours.	Acts as a potent immunostimulant. Keep these tablets on hand and use at the first sign of the flu. Use until symptoms cease. Follow the same guidelines for children.
Important		
Garlic capsules (Kyolic)	2 capsules 3 times daily.	Odorless garlic that is important in immune function. Acts as an antibiotic and cleanses the system.
Protein (free form amino acids)	As directed on label.	Helps to repair tissue and control fever. Free form amino acids are rapidly absorbed and assimilated into the body.
Helpful		
Bifido Factor/ Life Start Two from Natren	As directed on label.	For infants and children. Replaces "friendly" bacteria and acts as an antibiotic.
Cold-Control Capsules (a Power Herb natural product)	As directed on label.	Can be purchased at a natural foods store.
Fenu-Thyme or Fenu-Comf (Nature's Way herb formulas)	As directed on label.	Helps rid the nose and sinuses of mucus.
Multiminerals or kelp	As directed on label. 5–10 tablets daily.	Minerals are vital for protection and healing.
Proteolytic enzymes	2–4 tablets between meals.	Has antiviral activity. Reduces inflammation.
Vitamin B complex in a multivitamin complex	100 mg daily.	Necessary in all cellular enzyme function.

HERBS

☐ Echinacea, ginger, pau d'arco, slippery elm, and yarrow tea are good for influenza. For fever, take catnip tea enemas and 1/4–1/2 teaspoon lobelia tincture every three to four hours until fever drops. This is for children also.

☐ Also helpful is one tablespoon slippery elm bark powder mixed with one part boiling water and half a cup honey for cough and sore throat. Put this in a jar and give one teaspoon every three to four hours.

☐ Eucalyptus oil is also beneficial. Put five drops in a hot bath or six drops in a cup of boiling water, put a towel over your head, and inhale the vapors.

☐ A tincture of echinacea and goldenseal is recommended for children. Put eight to ten drops in liquid every three hours until all symptoms are gone. This can also be obtained by contacting McZand Herbal, P.O. Box 5312, Santa Monica, CA 90405. Ask for their Zand Formula.

RECOMMENDATIONS

☐ Children who have flus frequently should be checked for thyroid malfunctions. Take the child's temperature rectally or under the arm.

☐ *See also* PNEUMONIA in Part Two.

Insect Allergy

The stings of a group of insects known as *hymenoptera*, such as bees, bumblebees, wasps, hornets, fire ants, and yellow jackets, cause an allergic reaction in 5 out of 1,000 people. Sometimes this reaction results in death. This reaction is known as an insect venom allergy.

Some biting insects, such as mosquitoes, can also cause allergic skin reactions that appear as scaly and itchy eczema. These problems are not allergies to the insect, but to the venom of the insect.

Allergic reactions to stings are often severe. The symptoms are difficulty in swallowing, hoarseness, labored breathing, weakness, confusion, severe swelling, and the feeling of impending disaster. A more severe reaction results in closing of the airway and/or shock (cyanosis and a drop in blood pressure), producing unconsciousness.

Using tweezers, immediately and carefully remove any stinger left in the skin. Reactions can occur within minutes or hours. If treatment is not sought immediately, death can result. If you have a known allergy to a particular venom, have a doctor prescribe an emergency treatment kit.

HERBS

☐ Sometimes brewer's yeast or garlic rubbed on the skin deters insects. Herbal pet collars that repel fleas contain oils of cedar, citronella, eucalyptus, pennyroyal, rue, and rosemary. These herbs may act as effective repellents.

RECOMMENDATIONS

☐ To avoid insect stings, wear plain, light-colored clothing—avoid wearing anything that is flowered or dark. Don't wear perfume, suntan lotion, hair spray, or shiny jewelry. Avoid wearing sandals or loose-fitting clothes.

☐ See ASCORBIC ACID FLUSH in Part Three and follow the directions.

☐ Soften charcoal tablets or capsules (these can be obtained from health food stores) in warm water and make a paste. Apply this paste to the bite. This helps draw out toxins and reduces swelling.

☐ Antihistamines given by injection or by mouth reduce later-appearing symptoms.

CONSIDERATIONS

☐ A venom extractor called "Lil Sucker" is available. It fits inside your pocket or purse. If you get stung, it produces a vacuum that sucks the venom out within two minutes. The end of the extractor can also be used to remove a honeybee stinger. For more information on this, call 1-(800) ITCHING.

Insect Bite

Some insect bites can be relatively harmless; others can be serious. Ticks can carry diseases such as Lyme disease or Rocky Mountain spotted fever and can infect their victims. Mosquitoes, although generally harmless, may carry malaria (although uncommon in the United States).

For *ant, mosquito, and chigger bites*, wash the area thoroughly with soap and water. Then, apply a paste made of baking soda and water. For chigger bites, use a brush and scrub. Use ice packs if swelling occurs.

For *tick bites*, try to remove the tick as quickly as you can using tweezers. The sooner the tick is removed, the less your chances of contracting Lyme disease. Put the tweezers as close to the skin as possible. Be gentle, and try not to leave the head or any other part of the tick imbedded in the skin. Do not touch the tick with your hands! Once it has been removed, scrub the bite with soap and water. Don't try to burn the tick out or use any home remedies like kerosene, turpentine, or petroleum jelly.

RECOMMENDATIONS

☐ Calamine lotion helps relieve itching. Calendula ointment is an excellent insect repellent and counterirritant. "Deet" stick repellent works on chiggers and mosquitoes.

☐ Sometimes brewer's yeast or garlic rubbed on the skin deters insects.

☐ Take a chlorine bleach bath before going out: one cup of bleach per tub of water. Insects dislike the smell. Swimming in a pool treated with chlorine also works.

☐ Avoid alcoholic drinks, as these cause the skin to flush and the blood vessels to dilate, which attracts mosquitoes and horseflies.

Insomnia

Habitual sleeplessness, repeated night after night, is classified as insomnia. It can result from drugs, hypoglycemia, muscle aches, indigestion, asthma, pain, and stress. A lack of the nutrients calcium and magnesium will cause you to wake up after a few hours and then not be able to return to sleep. All products containing caffeine make sleeping difficult.

Systemic disorders involving the lungs, liver, heart, kidneys, pancreas, digestive system, endocrine system, and brain all may affect sleep, as will poor nutritional habits.

There are some specific disorders that interfere with sleep. Sleep apnea is an absence of breathing several times a night. This is most common in adults, but can occur in children. Physical abnormalities of the chest, back, neck, or the base of the brain may be a cause. Obesity is a primary factor in sleep apnea. Endocrinological problems, hypothyroidism, acromegaly (a rare growth disorder), the use of alcohol, and sleep-inducing medications all affect one's ability to sleep soundly.

Narcolepsy sufferers will be drowsy and overcome with sleep during the day. Narcolepsy usually does not occur until after the age of fifteen. Brain infection, head trauma, and even a brain tumor may trigger this disorder.

NUTRIENTS

SUPPLEMENT	SUGGESTED DOSAGE	COMMENTS
Important		
Calcium lactate or	1,000 mg	Take after meals and at bedtime.
calcium chelate	1,500–2,000 mg daily in divided doses.	
Magnesium	1,000 mg	
Helpful		
Vitamin B complex plus extra pantothenic acid (B₅) and	As directed on label.	Helps promote a restful state.
B₆ (pyridoxine) and inositol	Take these alone or with added calcium.	

HERBS

☐ Catnip, EZ caps, hops, lady slipper, passionflower, skullcap, and valerian root (capsules or extract) are all good and will help the insomniac.

RECOMMENDATIONS

☐ Foods high in tryptophan promote sleep. At bedtime eat turkey, bananas, figs, dates, yogurt, tuna, and whole grain crackers or nut butter. A grapefruit half at bedtime also helps.

☐ Avoid caffeine, alcohol, sugar, tobacco, cheese, chocolate, sauerkraut, wine, bacon, ham, sausage, eggplant, potatoes, spinach, and tomatoes close to bedtime. These foods contain tyramine, which increases the release of norepinephrine, a brain chemical stimulant.

CONSIDERATIONS

☐ Research psychologist Dr. James Penland states that a large number of women may be suffering from a copper and iron deficiency. He believes this deficiency may be the cause of insomnia. A hair analysis will reveal whether there is a deficiency or not.

☐ Any of the following formulas are effective and safe:

● Calcium Night from Source Naturals.
● Silent Night from Nature's Way Products.
● Valerian Root Extract.

Irritable Bowel Syndrome

This inflammatory intestinal condition is a common gastrointestinal disorder. Twice as many women as men suffer from this disorder. IBS affects the large intestine. The muscular contractions of the intestine are irregular and uncoordinated, and this interferes with the movement of waste material through the bowel. The result is an excess of mucus and of toxins in the bowels and bloodstream.

The symptoms include constipation and/or diarrhea, abdominal pain, excess secretion of mucus in stools, nausea, flatulence, bloating, and anorexia. Because the symptoms are similar to cancer, consult your physician.

Check to see if you have food allergies—they are important factors in this disorder. Certain foods irritate the wall of the intestinal tract. Stress is also a factor. This syndrome can be substantially improved through proper diet.

NUTRIENTS

SUPPLEMENT	SUGGESTED DOSAGE	COMMENTS
Very Important		
Alfalfa tablets or liquid	1 tbsp. 3 times daily.	Contains vitamin K, needed to build the intestinal flora for proper digestion, and chlorophyll for healing and cleansing of the bloodstream.
Dioxychlor from American Biologics	As directed on label.	Destroys foreign bacteria in the digestive tract and carries oxygen to the tissues.

Important		
Acidophilus (nondairy)	As directed on label.	Use Neo-Flora from New Moon Extracts or DDS—to replenish the "friendly" bacteria. Needed for digestion and for the manufacture of the B vitamins.
Aloe vera juice	½ cup 3 times daily on empty stomach.	George's tastes like spring water. Use with Aerobic Bulk Cleanse (ABC), a colon cleanser. Aids in keeping the colon walls clean of excess mucus and in slowing down food reactions.
Fiber: oat bran or guar gum or rice bran or psyllium seed or Aerobic Bulk Cleanse (ABC)	As directed on label. Do not take fiber with other supplements or medications because fiber has great powers of absorption.	When mixed with George's Aloe Vera Juice, this combination has both a healing and cleansing effect. Avoid wheat bran, as it may be too irritating.
Garlic capsules (Kyolic)	As directed on label.	Liquid form is best. Aids in digestion and destruction of toxins in the colon.
Multivitamin and mineral complex (hypoallergenic)	As directed on label.	Supplies those nutrients lost or not absorbed.
Primrose or linseed oil	As directed on label.	Supplies essential fatty acids.
Protein (free form amino acids)	As directed on label.	Necessary for repair of mucous membranes of the intestines.
Proteolytic enzymes	As directed on label.	Use brand that is low in hydrochloric acid (HCl) and high in pancreatin for protein digestion and cleansing the bloodstream of undigested food. Aids in reducing inflammation.
Helpful		
Calcium and magnesium (chelate form)	2,000 mg 1,000 mg	Helps the "nervous stomach" and the central nervous system. Aids in preventing colon cancer.
Enteric-coated peppermint capsules	As directed on label.	This type capsule prevents the oil from being released in the stomach—it must be released in the colon. Aids in healing and digestion and also relieves upset stomach or that "too-full" feeling.

HERBS

☐ Cascara sagrada, chamomile, lobelia, pau d'arco, and rose hips are effective in the treatment of irritable bowel syndrome. Peppermint oil is used in Europe.

RECOMMENDATIONS

☐ A bland diet is recommended when an intestinal upset occurs. Put vegetables and fruits through a food processor or blender. A baby food diet is good because neither preservatives nor salt is added. If you are on a soft diet, fiber and a protein supplement should be added.

☐ Avoid animal fats, butter, margarine, all dairy products, fried foods, spicy foods, wheat bran and wheat products, nuts, seeds, all junk foods such as potato chips, ice cream, candy, all processed foods, sugar, coffee, soft drinks (all carbonated beverages), and pastries. These foods encourage the secretion of mucus by the membranes and prevent the uptake of nutrients. Also avoid alcohol and smoking; these irritate the linings of the stomach and colon.

☐ For excessive gas and bloating that lingers, read the section on ENEMAS in Part Three and follow the instructions for the *L. bifidus* retention enema. This will replace the "friendly" bacteria very quickly and will resolve the problem.

☐ Charcoal tablets purchased from your health food store will relieve gas and bloating. Take five tablets as soon as this problem arises. Do not use daily because charcoal tablets are very absorbent and will also absorb needed nutrients.

☐ *See* ACIDOSIS in Part Two and take the self-test for acidosis—significant acidosis may occur with IBS.

☐ *Also see* MALABSORPTION SYNDROME in Part Two for types of supplements needed.

☐ See *also* COLITIS and DIVERTICULITIS in Part Two.

Jaundice

Jaundice is a build-up of bilirubin in the blood. This yellow-brown substance is not removed in the normal way from the bloodstream by the liver and excreted as bile as it should be. This "back-up" of bilirubin in the blood produces a yellowing of the skin, urine, and whites of the eyes. The urine may also be darker than normal.

Jaundice is not in itself a disease, but is a sign of any one of several blood or liver disorders. It is usually an indication of cirrhosis of the liver, pernicious anemia, hepatitis, hemolysis of the blood, and neonatal jaundice.

Jaundice can also be a sign of obstruction to the flow of bile from the liver, through the bile ducts, to the gallbladder, and then to the intestinal tract. Because of the biliary tract obstruction, the bile then passes back into the bloodstream instead of into the digestive system, producing the jaundice. It can be caused by a tumor, a gallstone, or inflammation. In case of a tumor or stone, surgery may be necessary.

Neonatal jaundice occurs when the liver of a newborn baby does not function normally. This problem occurs most often in premature babies. Another form of jaundice in the newborn is obstructive jaundice. This is caused by a total absence of the baby's bile drainage ducts. However, slight jaundice in newborn babies is common and is not serious. It soon resolves itself.

NUTRIENTS

SUPPLEMENT	SUGGESTED DOSAGE	COMMENTS
Very Important		
Milk thistle extract (Liv-R-Actin from Nature's Plus)	Use as directed on label.	Known to repair damaged tissues in the liver. Liv-R-Actin from Nature's Plus has a good complex.

RECOMMENDATIONS

☐ *See* CIRRHOSIS OF THE LIVER in Part Two and follow the supplement program.

☐ Drink the following juices: lemon juice and water, beet tops and beet juice, and dandelion or black radish extract. All are good for rebuilding and cleansing the liver.

☐ Eat only raw vegetables and fruits for one week. Then eat 75 percent raw food for a month. Take fresh lemon enemas daily during this period. *See* ENEMAS in Part Three.

☐ Never consume raw or undercooked fish. Environmental Nutrition states that all raw fish carry the potential for infection from bacteria, parasites, and viruses.

☐ *See also* CIRRHOSIS OF THE LIVER and HEPATITIS in Part Two.

Kidney and Bladder Problems

There are several kinds of problems that may occur in the kidney and bladder. **Glomerulonephritis** (i.e., nephritis) occurs when the minute filtering units of the kidney become swollen and inflamed. There are two forms of glomerulonephritis that affect children. **Cystitis** is infection of the bladder (*see* BLADDER INFECTION in Part Two), and **pyelonephritis** is an infection of the kidney. Pyelonephritis can be chronic or acute. A kidney infection is often serious, requiring hospitalization.

Bright's disease involves nephritis, a chronic inflammation of the kidneys, and it is characterized by blood/protein in the urine with associated hypertension and edema. The kidney cannot properly excrete salt and other wastes, resulting in retention of salt and water (edema). When the bloodstream becomes toxic with wastes due to kidney malfunction, uremia develops.

The symptoms of urinary tract infections (kidney or bladder infections) are chills, fever, urgency and frequency of urination, back and abdominal pain, loss of appetite, nausea, and vomiting. The urine is cloudy and often bloody. Pain may be sudden and intense in the back just above the waist and running down the groin. If you have these symptoms, see your doctor. Antibiotics are sometimes needed. Omit iron supplements while the problem exists.

The following supplementation will aid in controlling urinary tract infection and will help maintain proper kidney and bladder function.

NUTRIENTS

SUPPLEMENT	SUGGESTED DOSAGE	COMMENTS
Essential		
Distilled water	A 6–8 oz. glass every hour while awake.	Extra fluids are very important. Quality water is essential for proper urinary tract function.
Very Important		
Acidophilus tablets or liquid	3 tablets daily or liquid 3 times daily.	Especially important if taking antibiotics.
Vitamin B₆ (pyridoxine) plus inositol and choline	50 mg 3 times daily.	Reduces fluid retention.
	1,000 mg	
Vitamin C plus bioflavonoids	2,000–4,000 mg daily.	Acidifies the urine. Potentiates immune function. Aids healing.
Important		
Dandelion root or extract and pumpkin extract	As directed on label.	Aids in excretion of the kidney's waste products. Needed for nephritis.
Helpful		
Calcium and magnesium	1,500 mg daily. 750 mg daily.	Magnesium is important in water absorption. Calcium and magnesium should be in a 2-to-1 ratio in the body. Do not use bone meal.

Hydrochloric acid (HCl) and digestive enzymes	As directed on label.	For the elderly. Necessary in digestion. Omit hydrochloric acid if you have a stomach ulcer.
L-Arginine	500 mg 4 times daily.	For kidney disease. Food sources are legumes, fish, soybeans, and seeds.
L-Methionine	As directed on label.	For improved kidney circulation.
Lecithin	1 tbsp. 3 times daily.	Needed for nephritis.
Multimineral complex (high potency)	As directed on label.	Mineral depletion is common in kidney disease.
Potassium	99 mg daily.	Needed for nephritis. Acts as a kidney stimulant. Omit if serum potassium is elevated.
Vitamin A emulsion	100,000 IU for 3 days; 50,000 IU for 5 days; then 25,000 IU daily.	Take emulsion form for safe, rapid assimilation of high doses. Do not take this high amount in pill form. Important in healing of urinary tract lining and in immune function.
Vitamin B complex (high potency) plus	100 mg daily.	Needed for nephritis.
riboflavin (B$_2$)	25 mg 3 times daily.	
Vitamin E emulsion or	800 IU emulsion daily.	Promotes immune function. An important free radical destroyer.
capsules	200 IU capsules, gradually increasing to 1,000 IU.	
Zinc	50–80 mg	An immunostimulant necessary for healing.

HERBS

☐ Goldenrod tea, juniper berries, marshmallow root, nettle, parsley, red clover, uva ursi, and watermelon seed tea are good for kidney and bladder problems. SP6 Cornsilk Blend from Solaray helps reduce water retention.

☐ Drink one quart of marshmallow tea daily. It will help to strengthen the bladder, to cleanse the bladder and kidneys, and to expel kidney stones.

☐ Buchu tea is good; do not boil it.

☐ KB combination from Nature's Way is a good herbal diuretic.

RECOMMENDATIONS

☐ Begin a low-protein diet, obtaining protein from vegetable sources. Quality vegetable sources for protein are peas, beans, lentils, mushrooms, and asparagus. High-protein diets cause the body to lose calcium, and when this is excreted, it passes through the kidneys and can cause painful kidney stones.

☐ Protein is broken down by the liver and kidneys. Accumulation of protein can result in uremia, which is the toxic build-up of protein waste (such as urea) in the blood. A protein source already broken down into free form amino acids is easiest to utilize.

☐ Drink three glasses of unsweetened cranberry juice daily. It inhibits the growth of bacteria by acidifying the urine.

☐ Consume 75 percent raw foods. Reduce your intake of potassium and phosphates. Do not use any salt or potassium chloride, a salt substitute. Also avoid fish, meat, eggs, spinach, rhubarb, Swiss chard, beet tops, tea, chocolate, and cocoa because of their high oxalic acid content. Excess oxalic acid may lead to kidney stones.

☐ Eat garlic, potatoes, asparagus, parsley, watercress, celery, cucumbers, papaya, and bananas. Watermelon and pumpkin seeds are also beneficial. Watermelon should be eaten alone. Eat seeds, sprouts, and green vegetables.

☐ Avoid dairy products except those that are soured such as yogurt, buttermilk, and cottage cheese.

☐ A goat's milk fast can be helpful. Try a raw goat's milk diet for two weeks, consuming nothing but four quarts of raw goat's milk, warmed to body temperature, each day. Add one tablespoon of crude blackstrap molasses to each quart. During this period, take 1,000 IU vitamin E and 75,000 IU vitamin A emulsion.

☐ Try a three-day cleansing and juice fast, and coffee or catnip tea enemas. See FASTING and ENEMAS in Part Three.

☐ Hot sitz baths are good for cystitis pain relief. Batherapy, which can be found in a health food store, is excellent.

☐ Women who suffer from recurrent bladder infections should not use tampons, and should always wear cotton underwear—never nylon.

CONSIDERATIONS

☐ A recent study at the Pharmaceutical Department of Chiba University in Japan found that spirulina reduced kidney poisoning caused by mercury and drugs. They discovered that adverse kidney side effects from pharmaceutical drugs may decrease when spirulina is combined with the use of drugs.

☐ Recurrent urinary tract infections indicate the possibility of a serious underlying problem—see your doctor!

☐ See also BLADDER INFECTION in Part Two.

Kidney Stones

Kidney stones are accumulations of mineral salts (combined mostly with calcium) which can lodge anywhere along the course of the urinary tract. Studies indicate that refined carbohydrates, including sugar, help precipitate kidney stones. The sugar stimulates the pancreas to release insulin, which in turn causes extra calcium to be excreted in the urine.

Symptoms of kidney stones include pain radiating from the upper back to the lower abdomen, frequent urination with pus and blood, and sometimes chills and fever.

Diet alone cannot remove the stones. See your doctor.

NUTRIENTS

SUPPLEMENT	SUGGESTED DOSAGE	COMMENTS
Very Important		
Magnesium oxide or magnesium chloride	500 mg daily.	Reduces calcium absorption.
Vitamin B$_6$ (pyridoxine)	100 mg twice daily.	Taken with magnesium, B$_6$ reduces oxalate, a mineral salt common in kidney stones.
Helpful		
Proteolytic enzymes	As directed on product label. Take between meals.	Aids normal digestion.
Raw kidney concentrate	500 mg daily.	Strengthens kidneys. *See* GLANDULAR THERAPY in Part Three.
Vitamin A emulsion or capsules	50,000 IU	Heals urinary tract lining often damaged by stones.
Vitamin C	3,000 mg daily in divided doses.	Acidifies urine. Most stones will not form in acid urine.

HERBS

☐ Ginkgo biloba extract and goldenrod are good.

RECOMMENDATIONS

☐ If you have a history of kidney stones or presently have kidney stones, avoid the amino acid L-cystine. A build-up can crystallize in the kidneys and form large stones that fill the interior of the kidney.

☐ Limit calcium intake and avoid dairy products. Milk and antacids may cause kidney stones.

☐ Avoid oxalic acid-containing or -producing foods such as asparagus, beets, parsley, rhubarb, sorrel, spinach, Swiss chard, and vegetables of the cabbage family. Also avoid alcohol, caffeine, chocolate, dried figs, lamb, nuts, pepper, poppy seeds, and black tea.

☐ Reduce intake of animal protein, because a high-protein diet leads to losses of calcium, which ends up in the urine. This produces excessive amounts of calcium in the kidney, often resulting in painful kidney stones.

☐ Increased fluid intake is extremely important.

☐ Reduce salt intake.

☐ Watermelon is a natural diuretic. Eat it alone and often. Melon has a cleansing effect, but when eaten with food, it will sour and become toxic.

☐ Use only distilled water for drinking and cooking. Also drink quality cranberry juice to help acidify the urine.

CONSIDERATIONS

☐ Sodium cellulose phosphate is effective on calcium-based stones. Potassium citrate is effective on stones not of calcium origin.

Lead Poisoning

Lead is one of the most toxic metal contaminants. It is a cumulative poison that is retained in the central nervous system, bones, brain, glands, and hair. Because it is one of the most widely used metals in the United States today, it is estimated that a large number of people have high levels of lead in their bodies. Sources of lead include lead-based paints, ceramic glazes, leaded gasoline, lead pipes and other piping using solder, lead-acid batteries used in automobiles, tobacco, liver, water, some domestic and imported wines, canned fruit (the lead from lead-soldered cans leaches out and is absorbed by fruits), garden vegetables, bone meal, and insecticides.

Up until the mid-1970s, the use of leaded gasoline was responsible for most of the lead in the environment. The amount of lead found in gasoline was significantly reduced after concern mounted about the environmental effects of lead from exhaust fumes. As a result, catalytic converters were installed in cars in 1973. Cars manufactured with catalytic converters take unleaded gasoline. Leaded gasoline has not been banned by the Environmental Protection Agency (EPA) and remains in use here in the United States and abroad. Although you can still find leaded gasoline, its availability is low. According to EPA spokesman Matthew McCarthy of the Air Programs Branch, the amount of lead currently allowable in one gallon of *leaded* gasoline is 1/10 of a gram.

Although vehicle emissions of lead were markedly reduced to 3,900 tons in 1986, an estimated 4 to 5 million metric tons of lead has accumulated in the soil due to the use of leaded gasoline in previous years. (Over 170,000 tons of lead were emitted into the environment yearly in the 1970s.) Those growing crops or garden produce near busy roads or highways should check the levels of lead present in the soil.

Lead poisoning was brought to our attention when many children were poisoned by lead paint peelings. Children are at higher risk for lead poisoning. A study by Dr. M. Erickson, published in *Pediatric Research*, revealed that pregnant women who have high levels of lead in their bodies could give birth to babies with high lead levels. An estimated 90 percent of the lead stored in the mother's body is free to cross the placenta to the fetus. Previous research indicates that low level lead exposure in young children may be associated with impaired intellectual development and behavioral problems. A recent study reported in *The New England Journal of Medicine* (January 1990) suggests that such low levels of lead in children may lead to lifelong problems, such as severe reading problems, poor eye–hand coordination, and slower reflexes. According to the Centers for Disease Control, 16 percent of all American children have lead blood levels that exceed the acceptable norm.

High levels of lead in the body have been implicated in hyperactivity. Psychologists at the University of Wyoming discovered a link between behavioral problems in children and their intake of lead. Children born to women who have toxic amounts of lead in their bodies generally suffer from growth retardation and nervous system disorders. In addition, Dr. M. Erickson reported in *Pediatric Research* (October 1983) that lead levels are significantly higher in infants who die of sudden infant death syndrome (SIDS) than in infants who die of other causes.

Another potential source of lead poisoning is water supplied through lead piping. Lead piping was used in homes built before 1930. Newer homes use copper plumbing; however, even if you have copper plumbing in your home, the chances are very good that it was assembled with solder, which is 50 percent lead. Solder leaches a significant amount of lead into the water supply, especially during the first few years after installation. Due to mounting concern over the amount of lead leaching into the water, the use of lead solder was banned in 1986.

Not only is the water supply at risk, but canned foods sealed with lead solder also represent a danger. The lead from lead-soldered cans leaches into the contents of the can, but acidic foods are especially susceptible. Canned fruit, fruit juices, and tomato sauce are primary targets for lead contamination. A newly opened can of juice will contain a lead concentration exceeding the maximum contaminant level, while an open can of juice remaining in the refrigerator for a few days will have dangerous levels due to oxidation. Despite these facts, the Food and Drug Administration (FDA) has not banned the use of lead solder in food cans. Instead, the FDA urged the domestic food canning and packaging industries in the mid-1970s to remove lead solder from cans on a voluntary basis. Since then, the percentage of cans using lead solder has been reduced from 90 percent in 1979 to 15.9 percent in 1987. Unfortunately, some manufacturers still continue to use old equipment and imported cans have no regulations regarding lead solder use.

Because lead used for glazing of ceramic products can also leach into food, the FDA restricted the amount of lead that could be leached from ceramic dinnerware in 1971, and then lowered the amount allowable again in 1980. Pottery manufactured in the United States should therefore be safe; however, there are no rules governing the glazing techniques of foreign producers. Due to the relatively large volume of imported ceramic products, the FDA is unable to check a significant number to insure safety.

Because lead accumulates in the body, toxic amounts can damage the kidneys, liver, heart, and nervous system. Those suffering from lead poisoning commonly have days of severe gastrointestinal colic. Gums typically turn blue and the victim may experience muscle weakness. Lead poisoning can eventually lead to paralysis of the extremities, blindness, mental disturbances, loss of memory, mental retardation, and even insanity. Chronic lead poisoning causes impotence in men, reproductive disorders, infertility, and anemia. High levels of lead in your body can cause a protein deficiency; those deficient in vitamin E will be more susceptible to lead toxicity as well.

TIPS FOR MAKING YOUR ENVIRONMENT LEAD-FREE

To avoid products containing lead:

1. Avoid cans sealed with lead solder, which leaches into foods. A lead-soldered can will often have

remnants of solder and indentations along the seam. Instead try to buy food in lead-free cans. These cans have been welded and have no side seem. Also be wary of imported canned foods, which have no regulations governing the use of lead solder.

2. Have your water tested to insure a safe level of lead and other minerals. WaterTest of Manchester, New Hampshire, will test your water for impurities. Call 1-(800) H20-TEST. Your state health department may also conduct tests for contaminants at a lower price. You may also call WaterWatch Hot Line at 1-(800) 792-0092, Monday to Friday from 9 a.m. to 5 p.m. You may also send away for the free booklet, "Water Quality Answers." Write to the Water Quality Association, 4151 Naperville Road, Lisle, IL 60532. Enclose a stamped, self-addressed envelope.

3. Be careful about buying imported ceramic products. Many foreign countries do not strictly regulate the amount of lead that is released into their ceramic products. The FDA is unable to check a significant number to insure safety.

NUTRIENTS

SUPPLEMENT	SUGGESTED DOSAGE	COMMENTS
Essential		
Calcium (chelated form with magnesium)	2,000 mg daily.	Calcium prevents lead from depositing in the body. Do not obtain calcium from dolomite, bone meal, or cow's milk; these all contain lead.
Garlic capsules (Kyolic)	2 tablets 3 times daily with meals.	Protects the body's immune system. Helps to bind and excrete lead.
Kelp and/or alfalfa	As directed on label.	Contains essential minerals, especially calcium and magnesium. Also removes unwanted metal deposits.
L-Lysine and L-cysteine and L-cystine (amino acids)	500 mg each on an empty stomach with water.	L-Lysine assists calcium absorption; L-cysteine and L-cystine are sulfur-containing amino acids that act as detoxifiers.
Vitamin C plus bioflavonoids with rutin	2,000–10,000 mg	Neutralizes the effect of lead. See ASCORBIC ACID FLUSH in Part Two.
Zinc	80 mg daily.	Low levels of zinc have been found in people having high lead levels.
Very Important		
Lecithin	Take with meals.	Protects all cell membranes.
L-Methionine and L-glutathionine (amino acids)	As directed on label; take these with a small amount of vitamins C and B6 for better assimilation.	These are powerful antioxidants that protect the liver, kidneys, heart, and central nervous system.
Selenium	200 mcg	A potent antioxidant.

Important		
Thiamine (B1) and vitamin B6 (pyridoxine) and B complex	100 mg	Vital in cellular enzyme function. Also important in brain metabolism. Help to remove lead from the brain.
Helpful		
Chromium	300 mcg daily.	Important in sugar metabolism.
Iron chelate or Floradix formula from Germany	As directed on label.	Take if iron-deficient.
Vitamin A and vitamin E capsules or vitamin A and E emulsion	Capsules: Start with 25,000 IU vitamin A and 400 IU vitamin E. Increase amount of vitamin E to 800 IU only and of vitamin A to 50,000 IU only for 2 months. Emulsion: As directed on label.	Free radical destroyers. The emulsified form enters the system rapidly.

RECOMMENDATIONS

☐ Make sure that your diet is high in fiber and that you supplement it with pectin (found in apples). Eat legumes, beans, eggs, onions, and garlic. These will help rid your body of lead.

☐ Chelation with EDTA can help prevent accumulation of lead. *See* CHELATION THERAPY in Part Three.

☐ Do not smoke!

☐ Drink steam-distilled water only.

CONSIDERATIONS

☐ If you suspect lead poisoning, a hair analysis will accurately indicate long-term accumulation of lead. Blood tests will reveal only the most recent exposure.

☐ You might want to try aloe vera gel or liquid. Take ½ cup in the morning and ½ cup before bedtime.

Legionnaires' Disease

This lung and bronchial tube infection is caused by bacteria (*Legionella pneumophilia*) and was first identified following an epidemic that affected 182 people attending an American Legion convention in 1976. The bacteria are transmitted through the air, and after exposure the incubation period is from two to ten days. The bacteria are sometimes found in excavation sites and newly plowed soil.

Symptoms of this disease include headaches, chills, fever up to 105°F, muscle aches, coughing, nausea, vomiting, diarrhea, and disorientation. The coughing begins without sputum but eventually produces sputum that is gray or blood-streaked.

Legionnaires' disease progresses rapidly and hospitalization may be necessary. It is probably *not* contagious. Laboratory blood studies and cultures of sputum will aid in diagnosing the disease.

NUTRIENTS

SUPPLEMENT	SUGGESTED DOSAGE	COMMENTS
Essential		
Beta-carotene	As directed on label.	The active ingredient in vitamin A that protects the lungs.
Garlic capsules (Kyolic)	2 capsules with meals.	Aids in destroying bacteria.
Vitamin C plus bioflavonoids	3,000 mg 3 times daily. 100 mg twice daily. Intravenous (IV) treatment may be beneficial. Consult your physician.	Powerful antioxidants that help to kill the bacteria.
Very Important		
Bulgaricum I.B. from Natren (*L. bulgaricus* culture)	As directed on label.	Aids digestion and destroys foreign bacteria.
L-Carnitine and L-cysteine (amino acids)	500 mg each daily.	Important in immune function.
Vitamin B complex	100 mg daily.	A complex of vital coenzymes needed for cellular function and protection.
Important		
Intenzyme from Biotics Research	3 times daily on an empty stomach.	Stimulates the immune system and reduces inflammation in the body.
Raw thymus extract and raw lung tissue	As directed on label.	Glandulars that potentiate thymus and lung function. Enhance immune function.
Vitamin A emulsion	Up to 100,000 IU daily.	Emulsified form allows you to exceed amounts that would normally be toxic because it bypasses the liver and will be readily available to the lungs and immune system to repair the lung tissues.
Vitamin E emulsion or capsules	Up to 400 IU twice daily.	An important antioxidant that protects the lung tissues.
Zinc	80 mg daily.	Zinc gluconate dissolved in the mouth is best. Important for immune response.

Helpful		
Coenzyme Q$_{10}$ plus germanium	60 mg daily. 200 mg daily.	Increases and regulates immunity. Carries oxygen to the cells.
Dioxychlor from American Biologics or Aerobic 07 from Aerobic Life Products	As directed on label.	Destroys infectious bacteria but not "good" bacteria.

HERBS

☐ Use echinacea, eucalyptus, and goldenseal for this disease. Drink catnip tea for fever.

RECOMMENDATIONS

☐ The diet should consist of 75 percent raw foods and slightly steamed vegetables.

☐ Avoid alcohol, dairy products, fried foods, sugar, and tobacco.

☐ Have the heating and cooling systems in your home cleaned and inspected regularly, and change the filters often. The infecting organism is often found in these areas.

☐ Use a cool mist humidifier. Keep warm—do not get chilled, as this will worsen the disease.

☐ Practice deep breathing exercises.

☐ Use a heating pad on the chest to relieve pain.

Leg Ulcers

Ulcers are open sores that develop on deteriorated patches of skin. When poor circulation in the legs restricts blood flow, the skin tissue begins to erode; it is thus more susceptible to the development of a running sore. The broken skin does not heal itself. Leg ulcers are more likely to develop in those with varicose veins. See your physician if you have this medical problem.

NUTRIENTS

SUPPLEMENT	SUGGESTED DOSAGE	COMMENTS
Important		
Coenzyme Q$_{10}$	60 mg daily.	Increases resistance to leg ulcers by increasing tissue oxygenation.

DMG (Gluconic from DaVinci Labs)	As directed on label.	Enhances utilization of oxygen.
Garlic capsules (Kyolic) or fresh garlic and onions	2 capsules 3 times daily.	Improves circulation and aids in healing process.
Germanium	200 mg daily.	Helps the immune system by stimulating the production of interferon. Improves tissue oxygenation and promotes healing.
Vitamin C and bioflavonoids	5,000–10,000 mg daily in divided doses.	Improves circulation and aids in healing process. Also keeps infection in check.
Vitamin E capsules or emulsion	400 IU up to 1,600 IU, increasing slowly. 800 IU daily of emulsion.	Helps the body use oxygen efficiently and speeds healing time. Use emulsion for rapid assimilation.

Helpful		
Folic acid	10 mg tablets 3 times daily plus injections twice weekly.	Vital for proper utilization of protein during the healing process. Add B complex for best results.
Iron (Floradix formula)	As directed on label.	Floradix formula is an excellent natural source.
Multivitamin and mineral formula	As directed on label with meals.	Necessary for proper healing.
Protein (free form amino acids)	As directed on label on an empty stomach.	Free form amino acids are rapidly absorbed and assimilated by the body. Repairs tissue and promotes healing.
Vitamin A capsules or emulsion	100,000 IU capsules daily for 1 month; then reduce to 25,000 IU. Take emulsion as directed on label.	Necessary for healing and protection of tissues. This formula enters the system quickly and is easily assimilated.
Vitamin B complex (high potency) with extra vitamin B$_{12}$	As directed on label.	Allows proper tissue enzyme function for healing and helps prevent anemia.
Vitamin K (alfalfa tablets)	As directed on label.	Obtain this important vitamin from alfalfa tablets or from food sources listed in recommendations section.
Zinc	50 mg daily.	For healing of tissue.

HERBS

☐ Use comfrey tea. This herbal tea can also be used as a poultice; soak a clean cloth in it and apply to aching, inflamed leg ulcers. Chaparral and red clover also are beneficial, and can be found in capsule form or may be used to prepare as a tea.

RECOMMENDATIONS

☐ In order to speed healing, apply vitamin E oil to the sores and bandage with sterile gauze pads. Change bandages daily until sores are healed. Vitamin E capsules can also be used. Cut open and apply to sores. Sometimes antibiotics are necessary in order for the sores to heal properly.

☐ Take acidophilus liquid or tablets. You can also obtain acidophilus from yogurt and soured products.

☐ Eat alfalfa sprouts and dark green leafy vegetables to obtain vitamin K.

☐ *See* FASTING in Part Three and follow the program.

☐ A raw foods diet for one month with slightly steamed vegetables benefits the healing process.

CONSIDERATIONS

☐ *See also* CIRCULATORY PROBLEMS and VARICOSE VEINS in Part Two and CHELATION THERAPY in Part Three.

Leukorrhea

Leukorrhea is a nonbloody white vaginal discharge. Leukorrhea is often caused by a one-celled microorganism called *Trichomonas vaginalis* or chlamydia, and is sometimes caused by a yeast (fungus) called monilia (i.e., *Candida albicans*). Other causes are excessive douching, a vitamin B deficiency, the use of antibiotics or oral contraceptives, or intestinal worms. Leukorrhea is common in diabetic and pregnant women.

The symptoms of leukorrhea are burning, itching, and vaginal discharge. When there is blood present in the discharge, it may indicate more serious disorders, including cancer. Any vaginal discharge should be evaluated by a physician.

NUTRIENTS

SUPPLEMENT	SUGGESTED DOSAGE	COMMENTS
Essential		
Garlic capsules (Kyolic)	2 capsules 3 times daily.	Odorless garlic that acts as a natural antibiotic and kills the fungus.
Unsaturated fatty acids	As directed on label.	Caprystatin is good. Effective as an antifungal substance.

Very Important		
Acidophilus or Maxidophilus or Megadophilus	2 capsules 3 times daily with meals.	Re-establishes normal bacterial flora. Especially needed if taking antibiotics. Has antifungal properties.
Vitamin B complex (high potency and yeast free)	100 mg 3 times daily.	Vitamin B deficiency is common in those with this infection.
Vitamin B₆ (pyridoxine)	50 mg 3 times daily.	Necessary for optimal immunity.

Important		
Vitamin C and bioflavonoids	3,000–8,000 mg	Vital in immune system function.

Helpful		
Calcium and magnesium (asporotate or chelate)	1,500 mg 750 mg	Relieves nervousness and irritability.
Vitamin A and beta-carotene	20,000 IU capsules daily for 1 month.	Aids healing of mucous membranes and enhances immunity.
Vitamin D	400 IU included in a multivitamin and mineral complex daily.	Necessary for calcium uptake.
Vitamin E	400 IU capsules daily.	Necessary for optimal immunity.

HERBS

☐ Drink three cups of pau d'arco tea daily. This herb is a natural antibiotic agent.

RECOMMENDATIONS

☐ Include yogurt and soured products in your diet.

☐ Douche with six capsules of acidophilus or plain yogurt. Also douche with Kyolic or the juice of fresh garlic and water. Keep clean and dry.

☐ Yeast-Gard vaginal suppositories, sold in some drugstores and most health food stores, are excellent for the treatment of vaginal candidiasis (i.e., yeast vaginitis).

☐ For itching, open a vitamin E capsule and apply to the area. A vitamin E or enzyme cream can also be used. Marigold Ointment from NatureWorks is good for severe itching.

☐ Wear white cotton underwear so that air can circulate freely.

☐ *See also* CANDIDIASIS in Part Two and follow the diet instructions!

☐ *See also* VAGINITIS and YEAST INFECTION in Part Two.

Lumbago

See BACKACHE.

Lupus

Lupus is a chronic inflammatory disease that affects many organs. It is an autoimmune disease—the body's own immune mechanism attacks itself. At least 80 percent of those who contract lupus are women.

There are two types of lupus: systemic lupus erythematosus and discoid lupus erythematosus. Systemic lupus erythematosus affects the organs and joints of the body, and the discoid type of lupus is a much less serious skin disease. Both types flare up and then go into remission.

The cause of systemic lupus remains obscure, but many believe that it is due to a virus that causes the immune system to develop antibodies that in turn attack the body's own organs and tissues. This produces inflammation of the blood vessels and/or joints, thereby affecting many parts of the body. The kidneys are usually involved. Fifty percent of those with systemic lupus develop nephritis. A kidney biopsy may be needed for the diagnosis.

Discoid lupus affects the skin. A rash forms over the nose and the cheeks in a butterfly pattern. The sun often causes the rash to flare up. This form of lupus is a disfiguring skin disease, a reaction sometimes related to infection with the tubercle bacillus. The lesions are a small, soft, yellowish group of lumps appearing on the skin. When they disappear, they often leave scars. The word "lupus" means wolf, chosen for this disease because the rash that appears on the face of those with the disease gives a wolflike appearance.

Ultraviolet rays from the sun can result in a flare-up of discoid lupus and may even induce the first attack. Fatigue, childbirth, infection, some drugs (drug-induced cases usually clear up when the drug is discontinued), stress, unidentified viral infections, and chemicals may also trigger an attack.

Some cases of lupus start as arthritis, with swelling and pain in the fingers and other joints. Serious cases can affect the brain, kidneys, and heart. When the central nervous system is involved, seizures, amnesia, psychosis, and deep depression may be present.

Many different treatments are used for lupus. Much of the medication used may have serious side effects.

Anti-inflammatory drugs are usually used first. Anti-malarial drugs, used to combat malaria, may alleviate the skin problems and sun sensitivity that afflict those who have lupus.

Corticosteroids are adrenal hormones that are considered important in the treatment of lupus. They must be used with caution and only for short periods of time. The side effects of steroids and other immunosuppressives include puffing or rounding of the face, facial hair, acne, weight gain, diabetes, cataracts, osteoporosis, peptic ulcers, and infection, which make prolonged use dangerous. Steroids may shut down the body's own adrenal hormone production.

Radiation treatment for lupus is still in the experimental stages. It involves using low doses of radiation to the lymph nodes to suppress the immune system. Anti-cancer drugs are sometimes used in treatment to decrease the immune system's responsiveness and the need for steroids. These anti-cancer drugs may be toxic to the bone marrow and must be used with caution. Plasmaphoresis filters the harmful anti-antigen complexes from the blood plasma. The use of this process in the treatment of lupus is still in the experimental stages.

According to the American Rheumatism Association, four of the following eight symptoms must be serially or currently present before a diagnosis can be made:

1. Abnormal cells in the urine.
2. Arthritis.
3. Butterfly rash on the cheeks.
4. Sun sensitivity.
5. Mouth sores.
6. Seizures or psychosis.
7. Low white blood cell count, low platelet count, or hemolytic anemia.
8. A specific antibody found in 50 percent of lupus sufferers or lupus erythematosus cells in the blood.

NUTRIENTS

SUPPLEMENT	SUGGESTED DOSAGE	COMMENTS
Very Important		
Calcium and magnesium	1,500–3,000 mg daily. 750 mg twice daily.	Necessary for pH balance and for protection against bone loss.
L-Cysteine and L-methionine (amino acids)	As directed on label.	Assists in cellular protection and preservation.
L-Cystine	As directed on label.	Important in skin formation and in white blood cell activity.
Proteolytic enzymes	As directed on label. Take with meals.	Powerful anti-inflammatory and antiviral agents.

Important		
Garlic capsules (Kyolic)	2 capsules with meals.	An immune system enhancer that protects enzyme systems.
Raw thymus and raw spleen	As directed on label.	Glandulars that enhance thymus and spleen immune function. See also GLANDULAR THERAPY in Part Three.
Unsaturated fatty acids	As directed on label.	Aids in arthritis prevention.
Vitamin C	3,000–8,000 mg	Aids in immune function.
Zinc	50–100 mg	Aids in immune function. Protects the skin and organs and promotes healing.
Helpful		
Acidophilus	As directed on label.	Use a nondairy type. Protects against intestinal bacterial imbalance.
Kelp or alfalfa tablets	5 tablets daily.	Supplies commonly deficient minerals.
Multimineral supplement containing the B complex (high quality, nonallergenic)	As directed on label. 50 mg with meals.	Supplies commonly deficient minerals. Heals mouth sores, protects against anemia, and protects the skin tissues. Important for correct brain function and for the digestion of foods.
Superoxide dismutase (SOD) from American Biologics or Cell Guard from Biotec Foods	As directed on label.	Powerful antioxidants; free radical scavengers.
Vitamin A emulsion and beta-carotene	25,000 IU 15,000 IU	Powerful antioxidant; free radical scavenger. Vitamin A is needed to heal skin tissues.
Vitamin E	400 IU and up.	Powerful antioxidant; free radical scavenger. Helps the body use oxygen more efficiently and promotes healing.

HERBS

☐ Echinacea, goldenseal, pau d'arco, and red clover are beneficial in treating lupus. Yucca is also good for arthritis.

RECOMMENDATIONS

☐ Mild cases of lupus respond well to supplements that build up the immune system. *See* WEAKENED IMMUNE SYSTEM in Part Two. A correct diet and rest are also important. In severe cases, physicians must often use cortisone and immunosuppressive agents to induce remission.

☐ A test for food allergies is helpful and often very revealing in cases of lupus. *See* ALLERGIES in Part Two for the self-test.

☐ Avoid eating alfalfa sprouts! They contain canavain (a toxic substance) which is incorporated into protein in place of arginine.

☐ Avoid strong sunlight and use protection from the sun.

☐ Rest is important. You should also exercise regularly.

☐ Avoid large groups of people and those with colds or other viral infections.

☐ Avoid using birth control pills. They may cause lupus to flare up.

☐ Eat a diet low in fat and salt—this kind of diet will be easy on the kidneys.

☐ See ARTHRITIS in Part Two and follow the program for diet, herbs, and fasting.

CONSIDERATIONS

☐ Up to 10 percent of lupus cases are caused by drug reactions, according to *The New England Journal of Medicine*. Lupus usually occurs in those taking certain drugs such as hydralazine for high blood pressure or procainamide for irregular heartbeat. There is a wide variety of drugs that can cause lupus. Other substances that are contributing factors in most cases of lupus are pollutants, chemicals, additives, and some foods. Some researchers believe that faulty genes are the culprit, but outside factors can still trigger lupus. Drug-related lupus usually does not affect the kidneys or nervous system. It is likely to be a milder case. The condition usually subsides when the drug is stopped, says Dr. Mark Totoritis of the Scripps Clinic in La Jolla, California.

☐ Many patients with lupus also have Raynaud's disease (see the entry for this disease in Part Two).

☐ Some lupus patients have been treated for many years for syphilis with penicillin because of false positive blood tests.

☐ What is the difference between AIDS and lupus? The AIDS virus destroys the immune system, while with lupus the body's own immune system overreacts and attacks itself.

☐ For more information on lupus, call the Lupus Foundation at 1-(800) 558-0121.

Lyme Disease

This disease takes its name from the town of Lyme, Connecticut, where it was first discovered. It is seen more often in Europe, although in recent years its prevalence in the United States has grown, especially in the areas where white-tail deer are found. Ninety percent of all known cases have occurred in California, Massachusetts, Minnesota, Connecticut, New York, Rhode Island, Wisconsin, and New Jersey. If you live in white-tail deer areas, you must use precaution when going near wooded areas. A tiny tick (*Ixodes dammini*) carried by the deer transmits the disease. Household pets like dogs and cats can carry the tick into the home where it can be transmitted to humans. In the eastern United States, the main host is the white-footed field mouse. In the West, lizards and jackrabbits carry the disease.

Tick bites often go undetected. The first sign of Lyme disease may be the appearance of a rash a few days after the tick bite, following a red papule on the skin. If this appears, see your doctor. Left untreated, Lyme disease can lead to arthritis and damage the cardiovascular and the central nervous systems.

Symptoms that accompany a tick bite include fatigue, flu-like symptoms, headache, stiff neck and backache, nausea, and vomiting. Enlargement of the spleen and lymph nodes, irregular heart rhythm, arthritis, and brain damage occur with the disease. Some of these symptoms slowly subside over two to three years. Often symptoms leave and recur without another tick bite.

Because tick bites are usually painless, Lyme disease may go unrecognized for weeks or even months. Doctors may fail to diagnose the disease before it is in its advanced stages. The disease resembles multiple sclerosis, gout, and Epstein Barr virus (chronic fatigue syndrome).

A test has been developed to identify Lyme disease. A blood sample is used to determine the number of specific antibodies present, which increases from three days to three weeks after infection. In addition, a urine test that may be more accurate will soon be made available. It will detect *Borrelia burgdorferi* bacteria, which cause Lyme disease.

Lyme disease usually occurs in three stages, although not everyone experiences all three:

1. Small raised bumps on the skin and/or a rash appears and may cover the entire torso for a day or two or several weeks and then fade. If a rash appears immediately, it may be a reaction to the

tick bite and not to the bacteria itself. Fever, chills, nausea, and vomiting may also occur.

2. Facial paralysis may occur weeks to months later. Enlargement of the spleen and lymph glands, severe headaches, enlargement of the heart muscle, and abnormal heart rhythm occur frequently.

3. Backache, stiff neck, joint pains that attack the knees, swelling and pain in other joints, and even degenerative muscle disease have been linked to Lyme disease.

The following nutrients help in the treatment of Lyme disease by strengthening the immune system. As yet, there is no specific antibiotic therapy for this disease.

NUTRIENTS

SUPPLEMENT	SUGGESTED DOSAGE	COMMENTS
Helpful		
Chlorophyll ("green drink")	Take daily.	A potent detoxifier.
Garlic capsules (Kyolic)	2 capsules 3 times daily.	A powerful immune system stimulator that acts as a natural antibiotic.
Germanium	100–200 mg daily.	Stimulates immune function.
Kelp	5 tablets daily.	Contains essential vitamins and minerals and aids in detoxifying the body.
Multivitamin and mineral complex (high potency)		For necessary vitamins.
Selenium	200 mcg daily.	A free radical scavenger (antioxidant).
Vitamin A	50,000 IU daily.	An important antioxidant.
Vitamin C	6,000–10,000 mg daily in divided doses.	Needed for adequate immune function.
Vitamin E	600 IU daily.	An important antioxidant.
Zinc gluconate lozenges	1 lozenge every 3 hours for 4 days. Dissolve under the tongue.	Necessary for immune function. Do not repeat lozenge regimen for at least 30 days.

HERBS

☐ Echinacea, goldenseal, milk thistle extract, red clover, and suma are good for Lyme disease.

RECOMMENDATIONS

☐ The following are precautionary measures to help prevent tick bites. Remember: Time is crucial because the longer the tick is attached, the greater the risk of Lyme disease.

- When near or in wooded areas, wear long pants tucked in socks, long sleeved shirts with high necks or a scarf, and a hat and gloves.
- Use Deet (N-diethyl metatoluamide) on clothing, neck, or any exposed area except the face. Deet lasts longer and is safer to use on clothing than on exposed skin, so cover as much of the body with clothing as you can.
- Do not use excessive amounts of Deet. Wash off as soon as you go indoors. Note: Deet could be fatal if ingested, so watch small children.
- Check yourself for any small raised bumps and for pinpoint size specks on clothing.
- Check pets after they have been outdoors and remove any ticks that you find.
- Check your children before going to bed during the summer if they spend a lot of time outdoors.
- Put suspicious clothing in the dryer for a half hour to kill ticks by dehydration. Washing clothes, even in hot water and bleach, will not necessarily kill ticks.
- In an overgrown area, try to stay near the center of the trails and out of wooded areas.

☐ If you find a bite, do the following:

1. Remove the tick with a pair of tweezers. Put the tweezers as close to the skin as possible and pull straight out. Don't twist as you pull and don't squeeze its bloated body or the bacteria may be injected into the skin. Thoroughly wash your hands and the bite area and apply rubbing alcohol to the bite area. Don't use a match to try to burn the tick out or any other home remedy like kerosene or petroleum jelly. If you suspect it is a deer tick, call your doctor. He may want to identify the tick.
2. Apply a topical antiseptic (rubbing alcohol).
3. For the next three weeks look for any of the symptoms listed in this section. See your doctor.

CONSIDERATIONS

☐ Heat relieves joint pain. Take hot baths or whirlpool treatments. Antibiotics may be needed. If prescribed, add some form of acidophilus daily.

Malabsorption Syndrome

This modern plague afflicts those who, over the course of time, have not eaten the correct diet or taken enough quality nutritional supplements. Besides being a serious condition itself, malabsorption also causes other problems, including osteoporosis and anemia.

How does this malfunction of the absorption mechanism occur? Some contributing factors are a poor diet deficient in needed nutrients; diseases of the pancreas, liver, and bile ducts that result in digestive disorders and a lack of bile and essential enzymes; an overconsumption of mucus-forming and processed foods; rapid intestinal transit time; an imbalance of intestinal bacterial flora (candidiasis); and diarrhea and/or constipation, which produce mucosal damage.

Treatments such as radiation therapy and digitalis and by-pass surgery severely reduce the absorptive area of the small bowel. Intestinal parasites, celiac disease (gluten enteropathy, nontropical sprue) from an intolerance to gluten in grains, diverticulitis and/or colitis, and an excessive use of alcohol, drugs, antacids, or laxatives all affect the absorption of essential nutrients from the intestine resulting in malabsorption syndrome.

Symptoms of poor absorption include weight loss, diarrhea, dry skin, hair loss, muscle weakness, fatigue, and anemia. These symptoms warrant immediate medical attention. The impaired absorption of protein induces swelling of the lower limbs (edema). The loss of potassium from diarrhea results in muscle weakness which, in turn, can cause serious heart disorders. Anemia results from lack of needed iron and folic acid. Calcium and vitamin D deficiency result in bone loss and tetany.

The body's inability to absorb B vitamins and to transfer amino acids across the intestinal mucosa results from malabsorption and causes further malabsorption, since these nutrients are essential in the absorption process itself. Therefore, a vicious circle occurs and perpetuates itself.

Treatment requires recognition of the cause and removal of the offending agent along with a healthful dietary regimen and supplementation. Appropriate medical consultation is needed in cases related to the use of drugs used to treat cancer, pancreatic insufficiency, and special problems associated with gastric or intestinal surgery.

Those suffering from malabsorption require more nutrients than the average person to treat and correct the problem. Nutrients in injectable form, powders, liquids, and lozenges are more easily assimilated. Many patients are unable to break down the supplements in pill form; some even discharge the pill whole in their stool. Sustained release and large, hard tablets should be avoided. A change of diet and a cleansing program that can heal and clean the colon are essential.

Regardless of how good your diet is or how many supplements you take, if you have any of the bowel disorders described previously, you may have nutritional deficiencies. Fecal matter that remains in the colon due to constipation decays and releases toxins and poisonous gases into the bloodstream. These toxins damage the tissues and organs. The bloodstream becomes poisoned and is unable to remove dead cells and waste. This results in fatigue, headache, nervousness, and insomnia.

Premature aging results from malabsorption. Malabsorption is also a significant factor in the overall aging process and may be why some of us age more rapidly than others. As we age, the intestinal tract gets "out of shape" and the lining becomes covered with hard fecal matter and mucus, which make absorption of nutrients difficult. The body needs nutrients to keep it youthful. Malabsorption is one reason why the elderly need higher amounts of nutrients.

If a change of diet and the correct supplements do not improve your health status in a few months, you may have a malabsorption problem. Those suffering from malabsorption need to bypass the intestinal tract when using supplements as much as possible in order to obtain the required nutrients and regain their health. Nutrients in the forms mentioned above should be used. Hard pills or sustained release type tablets should be avoided.

The fasting program should be followed once monthly. See FASTING in Part Three.

NUTRIENTS

SUPPLEMENT	SUGGESTED DOSAGE	COMMENTS
Very Important		
Acidophilis (nondairy) or Megadophilis	1 tsp. between meals 3 times daily.	Take on an empty stomach because stomach acid destroys the "friendly" bacteria. Needed for uptake and manufacture of many nutrients.
Dioxychlor from American Biologics	As directed on label.	Destroys harmful bacteria in the intestinal tract and cleanses the bloodstream.
Vitamin B complex plus vitamin B$_{12}$	2cc B complex. 1cc B$_{12}$ 3 times weekly.	Injections are the most effective. Consult your physician. Water-soluble vitamins such as the B vitamins are the most difficult to absorb and are lost in the urine.
Vitamin B$_{12}$ lozenges	1 lozenge under tongue on an empty stomach 3 times daily.	Needed for normal digestion and to prevent anemia.
Important		
Inflazyme Forte from American Biologics	2 with meals.	Needed to heal the colon and to aid protein uptake.
Kyolic liquid	As directed on label.	Aids digestion and promotes healing of the digestive tract. Works most effectively when taken with meals.

Protein (free form amino acids from Ecological)	3 times daily under tongue on empty stomach.	Needed because protein is not broken down properly into amino acids, which are needed for virtually all life functions.
Vitamin C buffered crystals with mineral chelates from Ecological	2,000–8,000 mg daily in divided doses with juice.	Needed to stimulate immune function and to aid uptake of nutrients.
Helpful		
Essential fatty acid complex in liquid form from Cardiovascular Research	As directed on label.	Needed to repair the cells along the intestinal walls and to assist in proper utilization of fats.
Liquid Liver Extract #521 from Enzymatic Therapy	As directed on product label.	Prevents anemia and supplies the necessary B vitamins in their natural form.
Proteolytic enzymes or multienzyme complex	Take 2 proteolytic enzymes between meals and 2 with meals or take 2 multienzymes with meals.	Needed for protein digestion.
Vitamin and mineral formula		Use powdered form that is yeast- and allergen-free to replace lost minerals.
Zinc gluconate lozenges	50 mg daily for 1 month.	Aids in the manufacture of digestive enzymes and in protein uptake.

RECOMMENDATIONS

☐ The following diet recommendations should be followed for a period of thirty days to give the colon a chance to heal and to cleanse its walls of hard matter and mucus. After thirty days, you may reintroduce the foods that you had eliminated back into your diet; however, do not add them back too quickly. Gradually add small amounts of these foods back into your diet.

☐ The diet should contain well-cooked brown rice; however, white rice should be excluded. Eat plenty of fruits, but limit your intake of citrus fruits. Oatmeal, steamed vegetables, and millet should also be part of the diet. Do not consume wheat products until healed. Eat broiled, steamed, or baked whitefish three times a week, but eliminate shellfish from the diet.

☐ Drink six to eight glasses of liquids including juice, quality water, and herb teas. (*See* HERBS in Part One for herbs that promote healing of the colon.) Use barley malt, a small amount of honey, and nut and soy milks for sweeteners.

☐ Avoid the following: butter and margarine, fried foods, and all types of oils and fats. These foods exacerbate malabsorption problems by coating the stomach and small intestines, which prohibits the passage of nutrients. Foods that encourage the secretion of mucus by the membranes should also be avoided because they interfere with absorption as well. These include all dairy products, processed foods, and instant foods, most of which are boxed or canned.

☐ Meats are difficult to digest and are acidic. Avoid products containing caffeine such as teas, coffee, colas, and chocolate; junk foods such as potato chips and candy; and products containing sugar, salt, MSG, and preservatives.

Manic-Depressive Disorder

This is a psychosis that is characterized by extreme mood swings. The typical manic-depressive individual will go from a period of unrealistic enthusiasm and elation to misery and the depths of depression. When he is in the depressive stage, he will demonstrate low self-esteem and have feelings of hopelessness. He will lack motivation to do anything, even to get out of bed. Some people in this stage sleep for weeks. They withdraw from social activities, avoid relationships with others, and are unable to work.

When in the manic stage, the manic-depressive individual will have what seems to be boundless energy. He will not want to rest or sleep for twenty-four hours or more.

The periods of mania start suddenly and without warning. They appear for no known reason and worsen rapidly. Some patients have these attacks frequently, and others have years between occurrences. Most people who suffer from this disorder seem relatively normal between stages. Approximately 3 percent of the population of the United States suffers from this disorder.

Some of the symptoms of manic-depressive disorder are changes in sleep pattern, withdrawal from society, extreme pessimism, failure to finish projects that were started with enthusiasm, chronic irritability, sudden attacks of rage, and lack of inhibition, especially in sexual behavior.

There are several theories for the causes of this disorder. It may be triggered by extreme stress. Some researchers believe that early experiences, such as the loss of a parent or other early childhood trauma, play an important role in its cause. There is also evidence of increased concentration of intracellular sodium during these mood swings, which returns to normal after recovery. In the depressed individual, monoamines are depleted in the brain.

NUTRIENTS

SUPPLEMENT	SUGGESTED DOSAGE	COMMENTS
Very Important		
L-Taurine (amino acid)	500 mg 3 times daily. Take with 50 mg vitamin B_6 and 100 mg vitamin C for better absorption.	L-Taurine deficiency results in hyperactivity, anxiety, and poor brain function.
L-Tyrosine (amino acid)	500 mg twice daily on an empty stomach. Add a small amount of vitamins B_6 and C for better assimilation.	Important in treating depression. Stabilizes mood swings.
Protein (free form amino acids)	Twice daily on an empty stomach.	Needed for normal brain function. Combats depression.
Vitamin B complex or		These can all be taken in one injection. The B vitamins are essential for normal brain function and a healthy nervous system.
liver injections and	2 cc twice a week.	
vitamin B_{12} and	1 cc twice a week.	
vitamin B_6 (pyridoxine) or	½ cc twice a week.	
vitamin B complex (hypoallergenic) capsules or tablets with	100 mg 3 times daily.	
B_{12} lozenges	1 tablet twice daily on an empty stomach.	Important in making myelin, the sheath covering the nerves.
Zinc	50 mg daily.	Protects the brain cells.
Important		
Lithium	By prescription only.	Alters the manic-depressive cycles, producing mood stability.
Helpful		
Multivitamin and mineral complex (high potency) containing	As directed on label.	Mineral imbalance may cause depression.
calcium and	1,500 mg	
magnesium	750 mg	
Unsaturated fatty acids	As directed on label.	Important for improved cerebral circulation and blood pressure stability.
Vitamin C	3,000–6,000 mg	A powerful immunostimulant. Aids allergic defenses.

RECOMMENDATIONS

☐ The patient should have no sugar or its by-products (read labels!). Dairy products, alcohol, soda, and caffeine should not be taken by persons with this disorder. Avoid foods with added chemicals, additives, or food colorings.

☐ The diet should consist of vegetables, fruits, nuts, seeds, beans, and legumes. Whole grains are recommended, but avoid excessive consumption of bread. Eat whitefish and turkey twice a week.

☐ High doses of B-complex vitamins are needed because the manic-depressive does not absorb the B complex easily.

CONSIDERATIONS

☐ *The New England Journal of Medicine* (1984) reported that individuals with depression and manic depression appear to be hypersensitive to acetylcholine, a chemical that carries messages to the brain. Therefore, *choline should not be taken in a dose that exceeds the amount in a multiple vitamin.*

☐ The *Journal of Orthomolecular Psychiatry* (1979) reported that manic depressives had deficiencies of the B-complex vitamins and that improvement in their conditions occurred with B_{12} injections and megadoses of the B vitamins. The B vitamins have a lithium-like effect on the brain. The trace metal lithium is known to alter the period of the rhythmic cycling and helps the manic depressive.

☐ The high doses used in lithium treatment may include the following side effects: nausea, vomiting, tremors, kidney dysfunction, and thyroid enlargement.

☐ Amino acids are important in the treatment of this disorder, especially taurine and tyrosine.

☐ See ALLERGIES in Part Two to determine if you have a food allergy. Certain foods may trigger an attack.

☐ See also DEPRESSION in Part Two.

Measles

Measles is a viral infection that attacks the respiratory system and causes a skin rash. Although it is typically a childhood disease, adults are also susceptible. It is very infectious and is spread by coughing and sneezing.

Red measles (rubeola virus) is a serious viral infection that infects the respiratory tract, eyes, and skin. This is one of the most contagious diseases. The incubation period after exposure is seven to fourteen days. Symptoms include sneezing, runny nose, cough, fever, red eyes that may be sensitive to light, tiny white spots in the mouth and throat, and a rash on the forehead and ears that spreads to all parts of the body.

Complications that could arise as a result of measles are a middle ear infection (especially if the sufferer has a history of repeated ear infections), bronchitis, croup, or pneumonia.

German measles (rubella) is a contagious but mild virus. However, if the disease is contracted in the first four months of pregnancy, it may cause serious birth defects. German measles affects the lymph glands in the neck and behind the ears. Symptoms are fever, fatigue, headache, muscle aches, and stiffness mainly in the neck. A rash often develops.

Dosages given in the following table must be adjusted according to age and weight.

NUTRIENTS

SUPPLEMENT	SUGGESTED DOSAGE	COMMENTS
Helpful		
Bio-Strath liquid from Germany	As directed on label.	Acts as a tonic. Contains the B complex.
Calcium and magnesium	As directed on label.	Magnesium is needed for tissue repair.
Proteolytic enzymes	Take on an empty stomach between meals.	*Caution:* For adult use only. Reduces infection and aids digestion.
Raw thymus	500 mg twice daily.	*Caution:* For adult use only. Stimulates the immune system.
Vitamin A and E emulsion	As directed on label.	Needed to reduce infection and to repair tissues. If child is over 10, use capsule form. If child is unable to swallow capsule, use cod liver oil.
Vitamin A or cod liver oil	10,000 IU for children twice daily for 1 week, then decrease to once daily.	Higher doses may produce eye damage.
Vitamin C	Children: 1,000–3,000 mg daily in divided doses. Adults: 3,000–10,000 mg daily in divided doses.	Very important for immune function. Controls fever and infection. Has antiviral properties. Use ascorbate or esterified form.
Vitamin E	200–800 IU	Neutralizes harmful free radicals, which would otherwise destroy the cell membrane. *Caution:* Not for use by children under 6 years of age.
Zinc gluconate lozenges	Dissolve 1 lozenge (15 mg) in the mouth 3 times daily. After 4 days, drop to 1 lozenge daily.	For immune response and tissue repair.

RECOMMENDATIONS

☐ If you have cancer or a weakened immune system, are on cortisone or anti-cancer drugs (radiation therapy), or have any type of illness with fever, you should not be immunized against measles.

☐ Catnip tea or garlic enemas help to lower fever. (*See* ENEMAS in Part Three.) Children and adults: Take a half teaspoonful of lobelia extract every four to five hours for pain.

☐ Drink plenty of fluids such as water, juices, and vegetable broths.

☐ Rest until rash and fever have disappeared.

CONSIDERATIONS

☐ Avoid processed foods.

☐ Keep lights dim. Do not read or watch television while eyes are sensitive to light.

☐ Antibiotics are not necessary unless complications occur.

Melanoma

See SKIN CANCER.

Memory Improvement

The B vitamins play an important role in maintaining memory, especially choline and B_6. The amino acids are also very important. A diet that is nutritionally deficient and high in processed foods, junk foods, and fried foods may cause poor memory and concentration. A hormone imbalance, as in menopause and certain glandular disorders, may also cause memory loss. The brain could also be affected by allergies to certain foods.

NUTRIENTS

SUPPLEMENT	SUGGESTED DOSAGE	COMMENTS
Very Important		
Choline	100 mg 3 times daily.	Increases amount of acetylcholine, the message carrier of the brain.
Niacin and niacinamide (B₃)	As directed on label.	Aids in function of the brain and blood flow.
Vitamin B complex plus extra	100 mg daily.	Injections may be necessary!
B₆ (pyridoxine) and	50 mg 3 times daily.	For improved memory.
pantothenic acid (B₅)	50 mg 3 times daily.	Helps transformation of choline to acetylcholine.

Vitamin C	3,000–10,000 mg	Powerful antioxidant. Improves circulation.
Important		
L-Glutamine and L-phenylalanine and aspartic acid (amino acids)	As directed on label.	Necessary for normal brain function.
Lecithin	1 tbsp. with meals or 2 capsules with meals.	Improves brain function (high in choline and inositol, important B vitamins).
Helpful		
Coenzyme Q₁₀	100 mg daily.	Improves brain oxygenation.
DMG (Gluconic from DaVinci Labs)	As directed on label.	Improves brain oxygenation.
Gerovital H-3 (GH-3) or Aslavital	As directed on label.	From Romania—good for the elderly.
RNA-DNA	As directed on label.	Increases energy production for memory transfer in the brain. *Caution:* Do not use if you have elevated serum uric acid or gout.

You may try one of these formulas if you are already taking multivitamin and mineral supplements:

- Brain Power Packs from BioSource.
- Cognitex 1-Life Extension Products.
- Fuel for Thought from Nature's Plus.
- Memo-Vites.

HERBS

☐ Anise, blue cohosh, ginkgo biloba extract, ginseng, rosemary, and bee pollen are helpful.

RECOMMENDATIONS

☐ The following foods should be consumed often: whole grains, tofu, farm eggs, legumes, wheat germ, soybeans, fish, brewer's yeast, nuts, millet, brown rice, and raw foods.

☐ Avoid dairy and wheat products for one month. If there is no memory improvement, slowly add these foods back to your diet.

☐ Do not consume refined sugars—these "turn off" the brain!

☐ An all-carbohydrate meal will adversely affect the memory. For a better memory, combine complex carbohydrates with foods comprised of 10 percent protein and 10 percent essential fats.

☐ Practice holding your breath for thirty seconds every hour for thirty days. This improves mental alertness.

☐ A hair analysis is recommended to rule out intoxication of heavy metals such as aluminum and lead.

☐ *See also* ARTERIOSCLEROSIS in Part Two and IMPROVING BRAIN FUNCTION in Part Three.

Ménière's Syndrome

Ringing in the ears, variable loss of hearing, loss of balance, dizziness, and nausea and vomiting are signs of Ménière's syndrome. The condition may affect one or both ears. This disorder often results from a metabolic disturbance, which is probably caused by a disturbed carbohydrate metabolism like that associated with hypoglycemia. Impaired blood flow to the brain from clogged arteries and poor circulation may be the cause. *See* CIRCULATORY PROBLEMS and ARTERIOSCLEROSIS in Part Two.

In the semicircular canals of the inner ear, increased fluid retention produces pressure in the inner ear which may disturb balance and hearing. Fluid retention during the premenstrual period in women, allergies, and spasms of blood vessels to the inner ear may cause this disorder.

NUTRIENTS

SUPPLEMENT	SUGGESTED DOSAGE	COMMENTS
Essential		
Manganese	5 mg daily.	A deficiency may be the cause of Ménière's syndrome.
Very Important		
Bio-Strath	As directed on product label.	A natural supply of the B complex. Acts as a tonic and enhances brain function.
Coenzyme Q₁₀	100 mg	Improves circulation.
Niacin (B₃)	200 mg 3 times daily.	If uncomfortable with flush caused by niacin, use part niacinamide.
Important		
Vitamin B complex (high stress) plus		Important for the nervous system.
vitamin B₆	100 mg 4 times daily.	
Vitamin C with extra bioflavonoids	3,000–6,000 mg daily in divided doses.	Esterified or buffered form is best.
Helpful		
Calcium and	1,500 mg	Chelated form is the most effective. Needed for stability of the nervous system and for muscle contraction.
magnesium	1,000 mg	

Lecithin	1 capsule or tbsp. before meals.	For cellular protection and brain function.
Unsaturated fatty acids (salmon or primrose oil)		Use salmon or primrose oil. Needed for metabolic disturbances.
Vitamin E	400 IU and up.	Promotes efficient oxygen use.

HERBS

☐ Use butcher's broom and ginkgo biloba extract or tablets.

RECOMMENDATIONS

☐ Avoid fats, caffeinated beverages, salt, sugar, and fried foods.

☐ *See* HYPOGLYCEMIA in Part Two for the hypoglycemic diet recommendations. Follow the program.

CONSIDERATIONS

☐ Do not exceed 200 milligrams of niacin if you are pregnant or have a liver disorder, gout, or high blood pressure.

Meningitis

Meningitis is an infection of the three membranes, called the meninges, that lie between the brain and the skull. The disease is contagious. It can be caused by poor nutrition and any number of viruses such as poliomyelitis and measles, fungi including yeast, or bacteria like meningococcus, pneumococcus, streptococcus, and tuberculosis. It may result from severe infection of the nose and throat or spread through the bloodstream. Meningitis is more common in children than in adults.

The early symptoms of meningitis include sore throat, red or purple skin rash, and signs of a previous, recent respiratory disorder. Other classic symptoms include stiff neck, headache, high fever, chills, nausea, vomiting, delirium, and sensitivity to light. Change in temperament and sleepiness signal changes in the cerebral fluid and frequently precede coma and death.

Symptoms of meningitis should be confirmed promptly by a medical doctor. If untreated, complications such as permanent brain damage and paralysis can

occur. Diagnosis is certain only after microscopic analysis and culture of the cerebrospinal fluid. Without complications, recovery from meningitis generally takes three weeks under a doctor's care.

The following recommendations are designed to support medical treatment, not replace it.

NUTRIENTS

SUPPLEMENT	SUGGESTED DOSAGE	COMMENTS
Helpful		
DMG (Gluconic from DaVinci Labs)	1 tablet twice daily dissolved in mouth.	Carries oxygen to the cells, relieving many symptoms.
Garlic capsules (Kyolic)	2 capsules with meals.	Odorless garlic. An immune system stimulant.
Germanium Ge-132	200 mg daily.	Enhances immune function.
Multivitamin and mineral supplement complex (high potency)	As directed on label.	Needed for tissue protection and healing.
Protein (free form amino acids)	As directed on product label.	Needed for tissue repair and protection of membranes. Free form amino acids are absorbed and assimilated quickly.
Raw thymus	500 mg twice daily.	Enhances immune response.
Vitamin A emulsion or capsules	100,000 IU emulsion or 75,000 IU capsules for the first 5 days, 50,000 IU for the next 7 days, and 25,000 IU thereafter.	A powerful antioxidant and immune booster. Needed for protection and healing of all membranes. The emulsion is easily absorbed.
Vitamin C with bioflavonoids	3,000–10,000 mg daily.	Reduces infection and aids in cleansing the bloodstream.
Zinc gluconate lozenges	1 tablet 3 times daily.	Dissolve lozenge in mouth. Do not chew.

HERBS

☐ For fever, use catnip tea enemas. (*See* ENEMAS in Part Three.) Catnip tea is also good for sipping.

RECOMMENDATIONS

☐ Eat a well-balanced diet including, but not limited to, fresh fruits and vegetables (50 percent raw), seeds, grains, nuts, yogurt, and soured products. Avoid the following foods, which encourage the formation of mucus: animal protein and its by-products, dairy products except for yogurt, salt, caffeine, and white flour products.

☐ Rest in bed in a dimly lit room. Drink plenty of high-quality liquids.

☐ Take cool sponge baths.

Menopause

Menopause, also referred to as "the change of life," is the point at which women stop ovulating. The menopausal period affects each woman differently. Some start early, some start and stop, but most experience the change around the age of fifty. Menopause usually lasts up to five years. Although estrogen levels drop during the postmenopausal period, the hormone does not disappear. Other organs take over in the production of estrogen and other hormones. The organs known as endocrine glands secrete hormones to maintain proper bodily functions.

The symptoms of hot flashes, dizziness, headache, difficult breathing, shortness of breath, heart palpitations, and depression may be caused by an estrogen deficiency. If one is hypoglycemic, the symptoms are often more pronounced. Stress puts a burden on the adrenal glands, causing them to overwork. Therefore, the adrenals produce smaller amounts of the hormones that are needed to help reduce the side effects of menopause. The hypothalamus is the area of the brain that regulates the heat-producing mechanism of the body. Hot flashes can be the result of widespread blood vessel dilatation.

To control severe symptoms in menopause, use the smallest possible dose of estrogen every other day. Estrogen combined with progesterone reduces the risk of uterine cancer. Estrogens may cause fluid retention and may increase the severity of asthma, heart disorders, kidney stones, epilepsy, or migraine headaches. Estrogens are important, but there is a risk in their use.

NUTRIENTS

SUPPLEMENT	SUGGESTED DOSAGE	COMMENTS
Very Important		
Enzymes with hydrochloric acid (HCl)	Take with meals.	Aids digestion.
Lecithin	1 capsule or 1 tbsp. before meals.	Important as an emulsifier for vitamin E.
Primrose oil or black currant oil	As directed on label.	Acts as a sedative and diuretic. Good for hot flashes. Important for production of estrogen.
Vitamin B₆ (pyridoxine) and	50 mg 3 times daily.	B₆ minimizes water retention and eases symptoms.
pantothenic acid (B₅)	100 mg 3 times daily.	B₅ is a powerful stress vitamin needed for adrenal function.
Vitamin E	400–1,600 IU daily.	Increase slowly until hot flashes cease.
Important		
Calcium and magnesium chelate	2,000 mg daily. 1,000 mg daily.	Relieves nervousness and irritability. Chelate form is the most effective.
Helpful		
Germanium	60 mg twice daily.	Aids in relieving discomfort. Makes oxygen more available to tissues.
L-Arginine and L-lysine (amino acids)	500 mg twice daily. 500 mg daily on an empty stomach.	Detoxifies the liver and ammonia. Aids liver function.
Multiglandular	As directed on label.	For hormonal stability. (*See* GLANDULAR THERAPY in Part Three.)
Multivitamin and mineral complex	Take with meals.	Needed in normal hormone production and function.
Potassium	99 mg daily.	Important in severe hot flashes and heavy perspiring.
Selenium	200 mcg daily.	An important trace mineral linked to normal hormonal balance.
Vitamin B complex	100 mg 3 times daily.	The B vitamins, especially B₅ and B₆, are very important in this stage of life. Injections have reduced hot flashes and have produced dramatic results in nervous disorders.
Vitamin C	3,000–10,000 mg daily.	For hot flashes.

HERBS

☐ Black cohosh, damiana, licorice, raspberry, sage, Siberian ginseng, and squaw vine are helpful in treating menopause. Licorice stimulates estrogen production.

☐ Ginseng aids in relieving depression and in the production of estrogen. Gotu kola and dong quai relieve hot flashes, vaginal dryness, and depression.

RECOMMENDATIONS

☐ Avoid dairy products—limit consumption to small amounts of yogurt or buttermilk. Dairy products, sugar, and meat cause most hot flashes. Diet should consist of 50 percent raw foods and protein supplements (for low blood sugar). Do not eat any animal products except for whitefish, and eliminate caffeine from the diet. Add blackstrap molasses, broccoli, dandelion greens, kelp, salmon with bones, sardines, and low-fat yogurt to your diet.

☐ Exercise is very important. Avoid stress when possible.

CONSIDERATIONS

☐ For itching in the vaginal area, use vitamin E cream (no fragrance added) or open a vitamin E capsule and apply. Marigold Ointment from NatureWorks stops the itching almost immediately.

☐ *See also* HYPOGLYCEMIA and HYSTERECTOMY in Part Two.

Menstrual Cramps

See PREMENSTRUAL SYNDROME.

Mercury Toxicity

Mercury is one of the most toxic metals—even more so than lead. This poison is found in our soil, water, food supply, fish, shellfish, sewage sludge, fungicides, and pesticides. Some grains and seeds are treated with methyl mercury chlorine bleaches, which seep into our food supply. Because methyl mercury contaminates our waters, large amounts are found in fish, particularly larger ones that are further along in the food chain. It is also used in many products, such as dental fillings, fabric softeners, cosmetics, laxatives containing calomel, some hemorrhoid suppository preparations and other medications, polishes, wood preservatives, latex, solvents, plastics, ink used by printers and tattooers, and some paints.

More than 180 million Americans have mercury amalgam fillings. When dentists refer to silver fillings, they are usually referring to amalgams, which contain 50 percent mercury. Minute amounts of methyl mercury are released from amalgam fillings while chewing; this mercury is absorbed into the mouth and air passages and transported in the blood. There is no barrier that prohibits mercury from reaching the brain cells. Mercury is extremely toxic and can do serious damage to the brain. The Swedish government has taken steps to ban the use of mercury amalgam fillings.

Mercury is a cumulative poison that is retained in the pain center of the brain and the central nervous system. Significant amounts of mercury in your body can produce insomnia, dizziness, fatigue, weakness, depres-

sion, memory loss, dermatitis, and hair loss. High levels can also interfere with enzyme activity, resulting in paralysis and blindness.

Signs indicative of a child suffering from mercury toxicity include behavioral changes, depression, irritability, and hyperactivity. Adults may display these symptoms as well. Victims may also experience allergic reactions or asthma; they may complain about a metallic taste in their mouth, and their teeth may loosen.

NUTRIENTS

SUPPLEMENT	SUGGESTED DOSAGE	COMMENTS
Essential		
L-Methionine and L-cysteine and L-cystine and L-glutathione (amino acids)	As directed on label; best taken on an empty stomach.	Needed for sulfur. Also helps to detoxify the harmful metals and toxins.
Selenium	200 mcg in divided doses daily.	Selenium neutralizes the effects of mercury.
Vitamin E	400–800 IU	Works with selenium to neutralize mercury.
Very Important		
Alfalfa and/or kelp	5 tablets daily.	Aids the body in removing toxins.
Garlic capsules (Kyolic)	2 capsules 3 times daily.	Odorless garlic. Acts as a detoxifier.
Vitamin A	50,000 IU for 1 month, decreasing to 25,000 IU.	Acts as a powerful antioxidant by destroying free radicals.
Vitamin C plus rutin	4,000–10,000 mg	Helps remove metals and strengthens the immune system.
Important		
Beta-carotene	15,000 IU	A powerful free radical scavenger.
Vitamin B complex	100 mg twice daily.	Important for the functioning and protection of the brain.
Helpful		
Brewer's yeast	As directed on label.	Good source of B vitamins.
Hydrochloric acid (HCl)	As directed on label.	Take if over 40 and deficient in hydrochloric acid.
Lecithin	1 tbsp. 3 times daily or 1 capsule 3 times daily.	Protects the cells of the brain from mercury poisoning.

RECOMMENDATIONS

☐ Eat organically grown foods, especially beans, onions, and garlic, for added sulfur. Supplement your diet with plenty of fiber (oat bran is a good source) and pectin (found in apples). Drink distilled water only. Drink plenty of pure fruit and vegetable juices.

☐ If you suspect mercury toxicity, confirm with a hair analysis. This can detect toxic levels of mercury. (*See* HAIR ANALYSIS in Part Three.) Because mercury accumulates in tissue, it does not show up in urine or blood samples.

☐ Broil fish; do not baste it in its juices. If there is mercury in the fish, it is primarily stored in the fat. By broiling the fish and draining the juices, you will get rid of much of the fat.

CONSIDERATIONS

☐ Hal A. Huggins, D.D.S., has written an informative book describing the dangers of dental amalgams called *It's All in Your Head.*

☐ High mercury levels have been linked with candidiasis. (*See* CANDIDIASIS in Part Two.)

☐ *See also* ENVIRONMENTAL TOXICITY in Part Two.

Migraine

The migraine begins with a throbbing headache that is usually centered above or behind one eye; or, it can begin at the back of the head and spread to one entire side of the head. It is usually accompanied by nausea, vomiting, blurred vision, and tingling and numbness in the limbs that can last up to eighteen hours. A classic migraine is preceded by an aura, which can consist of disturbances of vision, speech disorders, weakness, and sensory disturbances. An aura can also consist of brilliant stars, sparks, flashes, or simple geometric forms passing across the visual field.

Allergies are a common cause of migraine. It can also be caused by liver malfunction. Constipation, stress, environmental allergies, and lack of exercise should also be considered as possible underlying causes of migraine headache.

Seventy percent of migraine sufferers are women, and migraines often run in families. Many patients have abnormal levels of brain chemicals that cause excessive dilation and/or contraction of the brain's blood vessels.

NUTRIENTS

SUPPLEMENT	SUGGESTED DOSAGE	COMMENTS
Very Important		
DMG (Gluconic from DaVinci Labs)	Dissolve 1 tablet in mouth twice daily.	Improves brain oxygenation.
Multivitamin and mineral formula	As directed on label.	
Niacinamide plus niacin (B₃)	800 mg 200 mg 3 times daily.	Increases blood flow to the brain.
Rutin	200 mg	Removes toxic metals which may cause migraines.
Unsaturated fatty acids (EPA Pure/700 from Nature's Products) or salmon or primrose oil	As directed on product label.	Needed for brain cells and for fat metabolism.
Helpful		
Calcium plus magnesium	2,000 mg 1,000 mg	Chelate form is the most effective. Helps to control muscle contractions and to transmit nerve impulses throughout the body and to the brain.
Garlic capsules (Kyolic)	2 capsules with meals.	Odorless garlic. A potent detoxifier.
Pantothenic acid (B₅) or royal jelly from a natural source	100 mg twice daily.	Royal jelly is high in pantothenic acid. Needed by the adrenal glands when the body is under stress.
Vitamin B complex	As directed.	Needed for a healthy nervous system. Use hypoallergenic form. Injections may be necessary.
Vitamin B₆ (pyridoxine)	50 mg 3 times daily.	Required for normal brain function. Use hypoallergenic form.
Vitamin C	3,000–6,000 mg	Aids in producing the antistress adrenal hormones. Enhances immunity. Buffered or esterified form is best.

HERBS

☐ Feverfew, ginkgo biloba extract, peppermint, rosemary, and wormwood are effective in the treatment of migraine headaches. Feverfew helps to alleviate pain and ginkgo biloba enhances cerebral circulation.

☐ A study on the herb feverfew conducted at the University of Nottingham found that participants got an average of 24 percent fewer migraines, and vomiting was reduced, with no side effects.

RECOMMENDATIONS

☐ Avoid salt and acid-producing foods such as meat, cereal, bread, and grains. Also avoid fried foods and fatty and greasy foods. Omit from the diet dairy products, yellow cheese, and other cheeses that contain tyramine. Avoid the amino acids phenylalanine and tyramine, nitrites (preservatives found in hot dogs and luncheon meats), aspirin, and monosodium glutamate (MSG), a common seasoning.

☐ Chocolate and citrus fruits may precipitate an attack.

☐ Exercise is important. It also helps to massage the neck and back of the head daily.

☐ Take hypoallergenic supplements only.

CONSIDERATIONS

☐ The most commonly used drug, ergotamine, can be addicting and should not be taken more than two days weekly.

☐ Migraine headaches in women may result from hormonal changes during the menstrual cycle. After menopause the headaches usually decrease.

☐ Soft music has a calming effect and helps relieve migraines.

☐ Eat small meals and eat between meals to help stabilize wide swings in blood sugar that may precipitate a migraine. *See* HYPOGLYCEMIA in Part Two and follow the dietary guidelines. Include almonds, almond milk, watercress, parsley, fennel, garlic, cherries, and pineapple in the diet.

☐ *See also* HEADACHE in Part Two.

Mononucleosis

Mononucleosis (mono) is an infectious viral disease that affects the respiratory system and the lymph tissues and glands in the neck, groin, armpits, bronchial tubes, spleen, and liver. Symptoms include fever, sore throat, swollen glands, fatigue, headache, jaundice, and generalized aching. Mononucleosis is often mistaken for influenza. Bed rest is very important during the acute phase. Antibiotics are of no use unless there is a secondary infection.

Adequate rest, exercise, and nutrition are essential for the maintenance of general health and the prevention of mononucleosis. Protein is needed to stimulate the formation of antibodies, which protect against other infections such as jaundice and hepatitis that may accompany or follow mononucleosis.

NUTRIENTS

SUPPLEMENT	SUGGESTED DOSAGE	COMMENTS
Very Important		
Germanium	100 mg twice daily.	Essential for the immune system.
Megadophilus or Maxidophilus or a nondairy form of acidophilus	1 tsp. in liquid between meals.	"Friendly" bacteria are important, especially if taking antibiotics.
Proteolytic enzymes	2–3 tablets between meals and at bedtime on an empty stomach.	Reduces inflammation and aids in absorption of nutrients.
Vitamin A and E emulsion	100,000 IU vitamin A; slowly drop to 25,000 IU vitamin A. 400–800 IU vitamin E; slowly drop to 400 IU vitamin E.	For easy assimilation. Essential for the immune system.
Vitamin C plus bioflavonoids	5,000–10,000 mg daily in divided doses.	Ascorbic acid, buffered, or esterified form is best. Destroys the virus and boosts the immune system.
Important		
DMG (Gluconic from DaVinci Labs)	Dissolve 1 tablet in mouth twice daily.	Immune stimulant that enhances oxygenation.
Garlic capsules (Kyolic)	2 capsules with meals.	A powerful immune booster. Acts as a natural antibiotic.
Protein (free form amino acids)	¼ tsp. under tongue between meals on an empty stomach.	Free form amino acids from Ecological Formulas are recommended.
Vitamin B complex stress formula plus vitamin B$_{12}$ lozenges	1 lozenge twice daily.	Hypoallergenic form is best. Injections may speed recovery.
Helpful		
Multivitamin and mineral complex (high potency) with	As directed on label.	Necessary for normal cellular function and repair.
calcium and	1,000 mg	
magnesium and	750–1,000 mg	
potassium	99 mg	
Raw thymus plus raw glandular complex	500 mg 3 times daily.	Enhances immune response. *See* GLANDULAR THERAPY in Part Three.

HERBS

☐ Dandelion, echinacea, goldenseal, and pau d'arco may help mononucleosis.

RECOMMENDATIONS

☐ Plenty of rest and proper diet are essential for rapid healing. A diet of 50 percent raw foods is important.

☐ Use a protein supplement from a vegetable source. Spiru-Tein from Nature's Plus is a good protein drink for between meals.

CONSIDERATIONS

☐ Avoid sugar, processed foods, soft drinks, stimulants, coffee, tea, and white flour products. They are often toxic and depress the immune system.

☐ Drink daily eight glasses of distilled water plus fresh juice.

☐ Use chlorophyll in tablet form, or in a liquid form from vegetables, such as a "green" drink from leafy green vegetables or wheatgrass. Kyo-Green from Wakunaga of America Company is a highly concentrated natural barley and wheatgrass source of amino acids, vitamins, minerals, carotene, chlorophyll, and enzymes. It is also available in powder form and in this form contains chlorella, kelp, and brown rice.

☐ See also CHRONIC FATIGUE SYNDROME in Part Two.

Motion Sickness

People suffering from motion sickness experience symptoms that range from severe headache to nausea and vomiting while flying, sailing, or traveling long distances in automobiles or trains. The symptoms of motion sickness occur when excessive motion causes the vestibular apparatus of the ear, the eyes, and the sensory nerves to send conflicting signals to the brain, where the brain then misinterprets them. If severe, an attack can make the sufferer completely uncoordinated. Women are affected by this condition more frequently than men. Children under age two and the elderly are generally unaffected by excessive motion.

Other symptoms of motion sickness are loss of desire for food, excess salivation, cold sweats, sleepiness, and dizziness. Symptoms of nausea often indicate that the liver needs attention.

Natural remedies have been used with great success in cases of motion sickness. Prevention is the key to the problem. Do not eat heavily processed meals, consume alcohol, or eat junk foods. Take whole grain crackers with you and eat a few before and during the trip. Avoid smoke and food odors. Stay cool, if possible. If at sea, lie down and close your eyes at the first sign of motion sickness.

NUTRIENTS

SUPPLEMENT	SUGGESTED DOSAGE	COMMENTS
Essential		
Charcoal tablets	5 tablets 1 hour before trip.	A detoxifier. Purchase from a health food store.
Ginger capsules	2 tablets every 3 hours, beginning 1 hour before trip.	Good for nausea and upset stomach.
Magnesium	500 mg 1 hour before trip.	Acts as a nerve tonic.
Vitamin B₆ (pyridoxine)	100 mg 1 hour before trip. 100 mg 2 hours later.	Relieves nausea.
Helpful		
Cyclizine (trade name Marezine)	Take as directed.	Over-the-counter drug. Not always effective.
Dimenhydrinate (trade name Dramamine)	Take as directed.	Over-the-counter drug. Not always effective.
Meclizine (trade name Antivert)	As prescribed.	Sometimes helpful.
Meclizine (trade name Bonine)	As directed.	Over-the-counter drug. Not always effective.
Promethazine (trade name Phenergan)	As prescribed.	Prescription drug. Works well, but causes drowsiness.

RECOMMENDATIONS

☐ Liver homeopathic remedies may help reduce nausea. General nerve treatment with B-complex vitamins and phosphate salts may be needed.

Mouth and Gum Disease

See HALITOSIS; PERIODONTAL DISEASE.

Multiple Sclerosis

Multiple sclerosis (MS) is a progressive, degenerative disorder of the central nervous system. The disease is variable in its progression and affects various parts of the nervous system by destroying the myelin sheaths which cover the nerves, causing an inflammatory response. Its symptoms include a staggering gait, blurred vision, dizziness, numbness, breathing difficulty, weakness, tremors, slurred speech, bladder and bowel problems, emotional problems, sexual impotence in men, and paralysis.

There is no known cure for MS, primarily because the underlying cause is unknown; however, stress and malnutrition often precede the onset of the disease.

As in so many of the degenerative disorders, a strong immune defense system is essential in the treatment of MS. A strong immune system helps avoid infection, which can trigger this disease. Dr. Murray Bornstein, from the Albert Einstein College of Medicine in New York City, finds the drug Copolymer 1 to be an entirely new approach to the treatment of MS. It appears to present no risk to the patient, whereas the drugs currently used sometimes depress the immune system. This drug may prevent MS attacks.

MS usually occurs in persons between the ages of twenty-five and forty. The disease progresses slowly and may disappear for periods of time but usually returns intermittently, often in a more severe form. Long-term sufferers of MS may not benefit as well from supplements, but in the young patient just starting to exhibit symptoms, supplements may possibly slow or even stop the progress of the disease.

NUTRIENTS

SUPPLEMENT	SUGGESTED DOSAGE	COMMENTS
Very Important		
DMG (Gluconic from DaVinci Labs)	Dissolve 1 lozenge under tongue twice daily.	Enhances oxygen utilization by tissue. Reduces amount of free radicals in the body.
Kelp	5–10 tablets daily.	Supplies needed minerals and iodine.
Sulfur tablets from DaVinci Labs	500 mg 2–3 times daily.	Found in eggs, garlic, onions, and the amino acids L-cysteine and L-cystine.
Important		
Acidophilus or Megadophilus or Maxidophilus	1 tsp. twice daily on an empty stomach.	Replenishes "friendly" bacteria destroyed by stomach acid.
Calcium and magnesium	2,000–3,000 mg chelate. 1,000–1,500 mg chelate.	Chelate form offers best assimilation.
Inositol and choline	300–600 mg 150 mg	
L-Leucine, L-isoleucine, and L-valine combination from Carlson Labs	¼ tsp. twice daily on an empty stomach.	These amino acids should be taken together for correct balance. Aids in absorption of nutrients by the muscles.

Multidigestive enzyme	Take after meals.	
Potassium	300–1,000 mg	
Primrose oil	2 capsules 3 times daily.	Contains linoleic acid, which is needed.
Protein (free form amino acids)	¼ tsp under tongue between meals.	Free form amino acids are absorbed and assimilated quickly. (Ecological Formulas are good.)
Selenium	150–300 mcg	
Vitamin A plus beta-carotene	25,000 IU 15,000 IU	Use emulsion form for easier assimilation.
Vitamin B complex	100 mg 3 times daily.	Hypoallergenic form is best.
Vitamin B₆ (pyridoxine)	100 mg 3 times daily.	Hypoallergenic form is best.
Vitamin B₁₂	100 mcg twice daily.	Consider injections for all B vitamins. Consult your doctor.
Vitamin C	3,000–5,000 mg	Use buffered ascorbic acid form or esterified form.
Vitamin D	800–1,200 IU	
Vitamin E emulsion	Begin with 400 IU. Increase slowly to 1,800 IU.	Important for circulation, destroys free radicals, and protects the nervous system.
Vitamin K (alfalfa tablets)	200 mcg with meals.	Alfalfa tablets are helpful or take in liquid form.
Helpful		
Brewer's yeast	Start with a small amount and increase slowly.	
Coenzyme Q₁₀	30 mg twice daily.	Needed for improved circulation and tissue oxygenation. Strengthens the immune system.
Germanium Ge-132	200 mg	Strengthens the immune system.
Kyo-Green from Wakunaga of America Company	1 tsp. in liquid 3 times daily.	A good source of organic chlorophyll, live enzymes, vitamins, and minerals plus amino acids.
Lecithin	1 tbsp. 3 times daily or 1 capsule 4 times daily before meals.	Protects the cells. Needed for normal brain function.
Manganese	25 mg	
Multimineral formula (high potency)		
Phosphorus	900 mg	Needed for transfer of energy within cells.
Proteolytic enzymes	Take between meals 3 times daily.	Needed for digestion.
Raw thymus extract	500 mg twice daily.	Enhances immune function.

RECOMMENDATIONS

☐ A well-balanced diet is of great importance. All food eaten should be organically grown (no chemicals) including fruits, vegetables, grains, seeds (raw) and nuts, fertile eggs, and cold-pressed oils (never rancid). Plenty of raw sprouts, wheat, rye, and alfalfa are good as are lactic acid foods such as sauerkraut and dill pickles.

☐ Massage, exercise (especially swimming), and keeping mentally active are extremely valuable in bringing about remission of symptoms. Exercises that may increase body temperature can decrease the function of the nerves involved, and make symptoms worse. Exercises in cool water help by supporting the body's weight. Stretching exercises help to prevent muscle contractures.

☐ The family of an MS sufferer must learn about the disease. Emotional support is essential. Contact Multiple Sclerosis National Society by writing to 205 E. 42nd Street, Manhattan, NY 10017 or phone (212)986–3240. Physical therapy is often needed.

CONSIDERATIONS

☐ Fiber is important for avoiding constipation. Periodically take warm cleansing enemas with the juice of a fresh lemon. (*See* ENEMAS in Part Three.)

☐ Avoid extremely hot baths, showers, and overly warm surroundings, as these may trigger an attack.

☐ According to the New Jersey College of Medicine, x-ray irradiation to the lymph glands and the spleen has halted the progress of MS in 25 percent of the patients treated. However, radiation depresses the immune system.

☐ A two-year multicenter study reported in the *Archives of Neurology* that exacerbations of MS can be relieved by spinal injections of natural human fibroblast interferon.

☐ Do not consume sugar, coffee, chocolate, salt, highly seasoned foods, spices, or processed, canned, or frozen foods.

☐ Short fasts are helpful. *See* FASTING in Part Three.

☐ Lyme disease often mimics the symptoms of multiple sclerosis. *See* LYME DISEASE in Part Two.

Mumps

Mumps is a viral infection that typically infects children between the ages of three and sixteen. However, it can occur after puberty. When it does, it often causes complications (such as sterility) in the ovaries and testes. The average incubation period of the virus is eighteen

days. The mumps patient is contagious any time from forty-eight hours before the symptoms start to six days after the symptoms start. Symptoms include swelling of one or both of the parotid glands at the jaw angles below the ears, fever, sore throat, headache, and pain when swallowing or chewing. If the testicles are affected, they become swollen and painful; if the ovaries or pancreas is affected, abdominal pain results.

Mumps is not as contagious as measles, and one attack usually affords lifetime protection.

In the following table, dosages must be adjusted according to age. Unless otherwise noted, amounts listed are for adults.

NUTRIENTS

SUPPLEMENT	SUGGESTED DOSAGE	COMMENTS
Very Important		
Germanium Ge-132	200 mg daily.	Potentiates the immune system.
L. bifidus ("friendly" bacteria)	Use as directed on label.	Contains antibiotic substances that inhibit pathogenic organisms.
Vitamin C	3,000–10,000 mg daily in divided doses; 500 mg every 2 hours until improved.	Vitamin C destroys the virus. Use sodium ascorbate for children to lessen diarrhea.
Zinc lozenges	Dissolve in mouth every 4-6 hours.	Do not chew. Fast acting. Aids healing.
Important		
Maxidophilus or Megadophilus	Use as directed on label.	For adults or children. Contains antibiotic substances that inhibit pathogenic organisms.
Protein (free form amino acids) plus vitamin B complex with extra potassium	Use as directed on label. 100 mg 3 times daily.	Free form amino acids and B vitamins are important in healing.
Vitamin A emulsion and vitamin E	Adults: 50,000 IU. Children under 12: 15,000 IU. Adults: 400-800 for 1 week; then reduce dosage. Children under 12: 200 IU for 1 week.	Vitamins A and E potentiate the immune function.
Helpful		
Kelp	6 tablets daily.	Contains essential minerals, iodine, and all vitamins.

HERBS

☐ Echinacea helps reduce swelling. Make a tea with this herb and mix with a little juice and drink four times a day or more. Catnip tea enemas help reduce fever. (*See* ENEMAS in Part Three.) Lobelia extract is good for pain. Take a half teaspoon every three to four hours.

RECOMMENDATIONS

☐ Apply heat or ice, whichever feels best, to the swollen glands.

☐ Drink plenty of fluids. Avoid dairy products, white flour or sugar, tobacco, and coffee. Consume mostly raw fruits and vegetables that are juiced or softened.

CONSIDERATIONS

☐ A fast is helpful. *See* FASTING in Part Three.

☐ *See also* ASCORBIC ACID FLUSH in Part Three.

Muscle Cramps

Muscle cramping in different parts of the body is commonly caused by a calcium and magnesium imbalance and/or a vitamin E deficiency. Anemia, arthritis, and even arteriosclerosis may result in cramping.

Most muscle cramps occur at night when resting and affect the legs, especially the calf muscles, and the feet. These kinds of cramps occur more frequently in the elderly, the young, and persons with arteriosclerosis.

The use of diuretic drugs for high blood pressure or heart disorders may also be the cause of muscle cramping. If you are taking one of these drugs, be sure to add potassium to the program.

Poor circulation contributes to leg cramps. If you have cramps during the day while active, consult your doctor, as this may be a sign of impaired circulation. *See* CIRCULATORY PROBLEMS in Part Two.

NUTRIENTS

SUPPLEMENT	SUGGESTED DOSAGE	COMMENTS
Essential		
Calcium and magnesium (chelate or lactate)	1,500 mg daily. 750 mg and up daily.	Do not use the lactate form if you have a milk intolerance. A calcium and/or magnesium deficiency is most often the cause of cramping in the legs and feet at night.
Vitamin E	400–1,000 IU (Increase dosage slowly.)	Improves circulation. Vitamin E deficiency is linked to muscle cramps. A deficiency may cause leg cramps while standing or walking.
Very Important		
Potassium	99 mg daily.	Needed for proper calcium and magnesium metabolism.
Silicon	As directed on label.	Aids in calcium absorption.
Vitamin B complex with extra niacin (B$_3$) and thiamine (B$_1$)	100 mg daily.	For improved circulation and cellular function.
Vitamin C plus bioflavonoids	3,000 mg daily.	Improves circulation.
Vitamin D	400 IU daily.	Needed for calcium uptake.
Important		
DMG (Gluconic from DaVinci Labs)	As directed on label.	Improves tissue oxygenation.
Helpful		
Coenzyme Q$_{10}$	100 mg daily.	Improves heart function and circulation. Lowers blood pressure.
Lecithin	1–2 tbsp. with meals.	Reduces cholesterol.
Vitamin A	25,000 IU daily included in a multivitamin and mineral complex.	All are necessary nutrients.
Zinc	50 mg daily.	Needed for absorption of calcium and action of B vitamins.

HERBS

☐ Use Ca-T, dong quai, elderberry extract, ginkgo biloba extract, horsetail grass, saffron, and silica for circulation. Chaparral is especially good for leg cramps.

RECOMMENDATIONS

☐ Eat alfalfa, brewer's yeast, plenty of chlorophyll, cornmeal, kelp, and green leafy vegetables.

☐ Massage the muscles and use heat to relieve pain.

☐ If cramping occurs after walking and is relieved when you stop, suspect "claudication"—impaired circulation. *See* the self-testing section in ARTERIOSCLEROSIS, Part Two.

Muscle Injuries

See SPRAINS, STRAINS, AND OTHER INJURIES OF THE MUSCLES AND JOINTS.

Myocardial Infarction

When the coronary arteries that supply the heart with oxygen thicken, harden, and narrow, the heart is deprived of needed oxygen. This deprivation of oxygen often results in chest pain, called angina pectoris. When damage to the heart muscle is incurred, the individual suffers a heart attack or myocardial infarction. Because the coronary arteries cannot provide the heart with sufficient oxygen, physicians also commonly refer to a heart attack as a "coronary."

Common signs of an impending heart attack are chest pain that may extend to the left arm, the neck or jaw, or the area between the shoulder blades; heavy, substernal pressure that feels as if the chest is being squeezed; shortness of breath; sweating; nausea; and vomiting. In addition, insufficient blood flow to the heart can cause abnormal heartbeat rhythms called arrhythmias. These arrhythmias result in 500,000 sudden deaths each year in the United States, despite much-improved cardiac resuscitative techniques.

A coronary may be triggered by a partial or complete blockage of the coronary arteries, an emotional crisis, a heavy meal, or overexertion from exercise or heavy lifting.

NUTRIENTS

SUPPLEMENT	SUGGESTED DOSAGE	COMMENTS
Essential		
Choline and inositol and lecithin	As directed on label; up to 1,000 mg choline daily and 1 tbsp. lecithin with meals.	These substances aid in the removal of fat from the liver and bloodstream.
Coenzyme Q$_{10}$	100 mg daily.	Improves heart muscle oxygenation.
Selenium	300 mcg daily.	A deficiency of selenium has been implicated in heart disease.
Vitamin E capsules or liquid or vitamin E emulsion	Start with 200 IU, increasing slowly to 800 IU daily. As directed on label.	
Very Important		
Calcium and magnesium chelate	1,500 mg calcium daily. 1,000 mg magnesium daily. Divide up dosage between meals and at bedtime.	Important for maintaining proper heart rhythm and blood pressure.
Copper	3 mg daily.	A deficiency has been linked to heart disease.
Garlic capsules (Kyolic)	2 capsules 3 times daily.	This odorless form of garlic is beneficial for the heart and promotes circulation.
L-Carnitine and L-cysteine and L-methionine	500 mg each daily.	Prevents heart disease by reducing blood fat. High fat levels are a common precursor for "coronaries."
Multidigestive enzymes	Take with meals.	For proper digestion.
Proteolytic enzymes	2 tablets between meals.	Anti-inflammatory agents.
Unsaturated fatty acids (primrose or salmon oil)	As directed on label.	Protects the heart muscle cells.
Vitamin A emulsion	As directed on label.	An important antioxidant.
Zinc chelate	50 mg daily.	Zinc is necessary for proper balance with copper and for thiamine utilization.
Important		
DMG (Gluconic from DaVinci Labs)	As directed on label.	Improves oxygen utilization by the heart.
Vitamin C plus bioflavonoids	3,000–6,000 mg daily.	Aids in thinning the blood. Prevents blood clots.
Helpful		
Vitamin B complex with extra thiamine (B$_1$) and choline	50 mg B complex 3 times daily. Up to 1,000 mg choline daily.	Thiamine deficiency in the heart muscle leads to heart disease.

HERBS

☐ Helpful herbs are black radish, butcher's broom, celandine, cheonanthus, dandelion, fennel, ginkgo biloba, hawthorn berries, hops, horsetail, Irish moss, lobelia, parsley, red clover, and rose hips.

RECOMMENDATIONS

☐ Make sure your diet is high in fiber. Oat bran is a good source. Add the following to your diet: almonds, brewer's yeast, grains, raw goat's milk and goat's milk products, and sesame seeds.

☐ Minimize your intake of vitamin D; do not obtain from dairy products that are high in fat. Consumption of these will contribute to clogged arteries. Products that have been homogenized, such as milk and other dairy products, must be avoided. These homogenized products currently contain the enzyme xanthine oxidase, which damages the arteries and leads to arteriosclerosis.

☐ Refrain from alcohol use. Avoid cod liver oil, especially if drinking alcohol. Coffee, colas, tobacco, and other stimulants should be eliminated. Refrain from smoking.

☐ Barley water is beneficial. Boil one cup of barley in six pints of water for three hours. Sip barley water throughout the day for its health benefits.

☐ Do not eat red meat, highly spiced foods, sugars, or white flour. Refined sugars produce adverse reactions in all cells by causing wide variations in the blood sugar. The high surges are followed by hypoglycemic drops in the blood sugar, causing dangerous instability in the vital intracellular sugar levels.

☐ Sensible, moderate exercise and a proper diet with nutritional supplements can prevent arteriosclerosis of the coronary arteries and myocardial infarction.

CONSIDERATIONS

☐ Drink steam-distilled water only.

☐ A fasting program can be beneficial. Fast three days a month. See FASTING in Part Three, and follow the program.

☐ See also CHELATION THERAPY in Part Three.

☐ See also ARTERIOSCLEROSIS, CARDIOVASCULAR DISEASE, and CIRCULATORY PROBLEMS in Part Two.

Nail Problems

The fingernails protect the nerve-rich fingertips from injury. Nails are composed of protein, keratin, and sulfur. The nail bed is the skin on top of which the nails grow. Nails grow from .05 to 1.2 millimeters a week.

Nail changes or abnormalities are often the result of nutritional deficiencies or specific conditions.

Deficiencies produce the following changes in the nails:

- Lack of vitamin A and calcium causes dryness and brittleness.
- A vitamin B deficiency causes fragility, with horizontal and vertical ridges.
- Insufficient intake of vitamin B_{12} leads to excessive dryness, very rounded and curved nail ends, and darkened nails.
- Lack of protein, folic acid, and vitamin C causes hangnails. White bands are also an indication of protein deficiency.
- If there is insufficient "friendly" bacteria (lactobacillus) present in the body, fungus forms under and around nails.
- Lack of hydrochloric acid (HCl) contributes to splitting nails.

- "Spoon" nails and/or vertical ridges may indicate iron deficiency.

NUTRIENTS

SUPPLEMENT	SUGGESTED DOSAGE	COMMENTS
Very Important		
Protein (free form amino acids)		The building materials for new nails. Free form amino acids are rapidly absorbed and assimilated by the body.
Vitamin A or	25,000 IU daily.	The body cannot utilize protein without vitamin A. The emulsion form is more readily assimilated.
vitamin A emulsion	50,000 IU daily.	
Helpful		
Brewer's yeast	As directed on label.	Contains all the needed nutrients; high in protein.
Calcium and magnesium and vitamin D	As directed on label.	Necessary for nail growth.
Gelatin	As directed on label.	Foundation for nails.
Iron (Floradix formula)	As directed on label.	Iron deficiency produces "spoon" nails and/or vertical ridges.
L-Cysteine and L-methionine (amino acids)	As directed on label.	Contains sulfur, which is necessary for skin and nail growth.
Silicon (oat straw tea and horsetail)	As directed on label. Available also in tablet form.	Needed for hair, bones, and strong nails.
Vitamin B complex plus extra riboflavin (B_2) and vitamin B_{12} and folic acid		Vitamin B deficiency results in fragile nails.
Vitamin C	3,000 mg daily.	Hangnails and inflammation of the tissue surrounding the nail (i.e., paronychia) are linked to vitamin C deficiency.

RECOMMENDATIONS

☐ A high-protein diet with a protein supplement is necessary for healthy nails. Egg yolk is a good source of protein. Eat oatmeal, nuts, seeds, grains, and a 50 percent fruit and vegetable diet.

☐ If you expose your hands to too much water and soap, the nail may become loose from the nail bed. Water causes the nails to swell, and they shrink when dry, resulting in loose and brittle nails.

☐ Do *not* cut cuticles. Uncovering the nails this way is harsh and irritating, causing infection. Use baby oil or cream and gently push them back. If you have diabetes,

Disorders That Show Up in the Nails

Nail changes may signify a number of disorders elsewhere in the body. These changes may indicate illness even before the rest of the body does. Seek medical attention if any of the following symptoms are suspected.

- *Thick nails* may indicate that the vascular system is weakening and the blood is not circulating properly.
- *Lengthwise grooves or ridges* may indicate a kidney disorder and is associated with aging. An iron deficiency may also cause ridges.
- *If the white moon area of the nail turns red*, it may indicate heart problems; *if it turns slate blue*, then it indicates overexposure to silver or lung trouble.
- *Brittle nails* signify possible iron deficiency and thyroid problems, impaired kidney function, and circulation problems.
- *Flat nails* can denote Raynaud's disease.
- *Yellow nails* can indicate internal disorders long before other symptoms appear. Some of these are problems with the lymphatic system, respiratory disorders, diabetes, and liver disorders.
- *White nails* indicate possible liver or kidney disorders and/or anemia.
- *Dark nails and/or thin, flat, spoon-shaped nails* are a sign of vitamin B_{12} deficiency or anemia.
- *Deep blue nail beds* show pulmonary obstruction such as asthma or emphysema.
- *Nail beading* is a sign of rheumatoid arthritis.
- *Pitted red-brown spots and frayed and split ends* indicate psoriasis; vitamin C, folic acid, and protein are needed.

- *Nails that chip, peel, crack, or break easily* show a nutritional deficiency and insufficient hydrochloric acid and protein. Minerals are also needed.
- *Brittle, soft, shiny nails without a moon* may indicate an overactive thyroid.
- *White lines across the nail* may indicate a liver disease.
- *Thinning nails* may signal an itchy skin disease (lichen planus).
- *Nails separated from the nail bed* may signify a thyroid disorder.
- *A half-white nail with dark spots on the tip* points out a possible kidney disease.
- *Raised nails at the base with small white ends* show a respiratory disorder such as emphysema or chronic bronchitis. This nail condition may also be hereditary.
- *Red skin at the bottom of the nail* may indicate a connective tissue disorder.
- *Ridges* can signify a possible infection such as the flu.
- *Downward curved nail ends* may denote heart, liver, or respiratory problems.
- *White lines* show possible heart disease, high fever, or arsenic poisoning.
- *Ridges running up and down the nails* indicate a tendency to develop arthritis.
- *Nails that resemble hammered brass* indicate a tendency toward partial or total hair loss.
- *Unusually wide, square nails* can suggest a hormonal disorder.
- *White nails with pink near the tips* are a sign of cirrhosis.

see your doctor if the cuticles become inflamed, because the infection can spread. Do not repeatedly immerse your hands in water that contains detergents or chemicals; this results in split nails. Discolored nails can be caused by prolonged illness, stress, nicotine, allergies, or diabetes.

☐ Use a base coat before using nail polish to prevent yellowing. If nails are green, it could be a bacterial infection or a fungal infection which separates the nail from the bed. Acidophilus is needed.

☐ Wear cotton-lined gloves when doing housework such as dishes and laundry or when using furniture polish. This protects your hands against harsh chemicals.

☐ *See* HYPOTHYROID in Part Two and take the temperature test to determine thyroid function. Poor thyroid function may be reflected in the nails.

CONSIDERATIONS

☐ Physicians prescribe 250 milligrams of griseofulvin (Fulvicin), four times daily, for a fungus infection of the nails. The white blood cells must be monitored during this treatment. A new antifungal agent will be marketed soon called ketoconazole.

Nephritis

See KIDNEY AND BLADDER PROBLEMS.

Nervousness

See STRESS AND ANXIETY.

Neuritis

Neuritis is the inflammation or deterioration of a nerve or group of nerves. Symptoms can include pain, tingling, and loss of sensation in the affected nerve area; swelling and redness; and, in severe cases, convulsions. The causes of neuritis are varied and can include a nutritional deficiency (B vitamins); a metabolic imbalance; a direct blow or nearby bone fracture; infection involving a nerve; diseases such as diabetes, gout, and leukemia; ingestion of methyl alcohol; and toxic levels of metals such as lead and mercury.

Optic neuritis occurs when inflammation affects the optic nerve in the eye, causing gradual or sudden blurred vision. In severe cases, temporary blindness may occur in a few days. The eye may also be painful.

NUTRIENTS

SUPPLEMENT	SUGGESTED DOSAGE	COMMENTS
Essential		
Lecithin	Take with meals.	Important in nerve protection and repair.
Multivitamin and mineral complex (high potency) containing vitamin A		Nutritional deficency is common. Neuritis is often the first sign.
Thiamine (B$_1$)	100 mg twice daily.	Thiamine deficiency is common in neuritis.
Vitamin B complex (high stress) plus vitamin B$_{12}$	100 mg and higher daily.	Injections are best. Vitamin B deficiency is common.
Very Important		
Calcium chelate	2,000 mg daily.	Important in nerve impulse conduction.
Magnesium chloride	400–1,000 mg daily.	Important in nerve impulse conduction.
Protein (free form amino acids)	As directed on label.	Necessary in nerve repair and function. Free form amino acids are easily absorbed and assimilated by the body.
Important		
Proteolytic enzymes or Inflazyme Forte from American Biologics	3 times daily on an empty stomach.	Potent anti-inflammatory agents.
Helpful		
Brewer's yeast or Bio-Strath	As directed on label.	Contains all essential nutrients and protein.
Vitamin C plus bioflavonoids	3,000–6,000 mg daily in divided doses.	Has antiviral and anti-inflammatory potential.
Zinc	50–80 mg daily.	Important in immune function.

RECOMMENDATIONS

☐ Increase fluid intake and avoid stimulants such as coffee, carbonated beverages, caffeine, and cigarettes.

☐ A diet of fruits, vegetables, nuts, seeds, and grains is good.

Nickel Toxicity

Although toxic levels of nickel have not been established, it is known that small amounts of nickel are useful in certain bodily functions. Minute amounts of nickel are important in DNA and RNA stabilization. Nickel also helps to activate certain enzymes such as trypsin, arginase, and carboxylase.

Excess amounts of nickel may cause skin rashes (dermatitis) and respiratory illness and interfere with enzymes in the Kreb's cycle. Significant levels of nickel may also contribute to myocardial infarction, a disease of the coronary vessels.

Cooking utensils containing nickel may add to your dietary intake of nickel and should be avoided. Nickel can also be found in hydrogenated fats and oils, refined and processed foods, stainless steel cookware, superphosphate fertilizers, and tobacco smoke. You should beware of stainless steel cookware, especially when preparing acidic foods.

Many natural foods contain nickel as well. These include buckwheat, legumes, oats, and cabbage. A nickel deficiency may affect iron and zinc metabolism.

You may wish to reconsider having your child's ears pierced. A high incidence of allergic reactions to earrings and posts containing nickel have been reported in youngsters who have had their ears pierced. Nickel toxicity may result from nickel alloys used in dental surgery.

RECOMMENDATIONS

☐ A hair analysis will detect toxic levels of nickel and other minerals.

☐ *See also* CHELATION THERAPY in Part Three.

Nosebleeds

Nosebleeds are commonly caused by physical injury, such as a blow to the nose. Excessive dryness (causing the nasal membranes to crack, form crusts, and bleed), sudden change in atmospheric pressure, scratching with the fingernail, or blowing the nose too forcefully can also cause injury to the nasal lining.

There are two types of nosebleeds: anterior and posterior. A posterior nosebleed primarily affects the elderly, especially if they have high blood pressure. This nosebleed comes from the rear of the nose and runs down the back of the mouth into the throat no matter what position the person is in. If severe, it can flow in both directions. This nosebleed requires the care of a physician.

The anterior nosebleed is the common type and flows from the front part of the nose. If one stands or sits, the flow of blood comes out of one or both nostrils. When lying down, it may go back into the throat. This nosebleed can be frightening, but is not serious. To stop an anterior nosebleed:

1. Blow all the clots out of both sides of the nose.
2. Sit up in a chair and lean forward (do not tilt the head back).
3. Put a small piece of gauze inside the nostil(s), then pinch all the soft parts of the nose together between your thumb and index finger. Hold for five minutes.
4. Apply crushed ice or cold washcloths to the nose, neck, and cheek.
5. Lie back and refrain from any activity for a few hours and any vigorous exercise for at least two days.

RECOMMENDATIONS

☐ When bleeding is controlled, apply a small amount of vitamin E—open a capsule and apply inside the nose. If unavailable, use a small amount of petroleum jelly and pack with gauze.

☐ Vitamin K is essential for normal blood clotting. Sources are alfalfa, kale, and all dark green leafy vegetables.

☐ When the nasal membranes become sore from dryness, use comfrey ointment or aloe vera.

☐ If you have recurrent nosebleeds, see your doctor.

CONSIDERATIONS

☐ Try increasing the environmental humidity.

☐ Sometimes a blood thinner such as Coumadin, Heparin, or aspirin may cause nosebleeds.

Obesity

Obesity is, quite simply, an excess of body fat. Anyone who is 20 percent over the norm for their age, build, and height is considered obese. Those who are obese are more likely to experience kidney trouble, heart disease, diabetes, high blood pressure, complications of pregnancy, and psychological problems. Liver damage is also common in overweight persons. Some of the causes of obesity are glandular malfunctions, malnutrition, emotional tension, boredom, habit, and love of food.

Obesity has been linked to food sensitivity/allergy. Changing your eating habits is important in losing weight. Malnutrition may be another important factor in obesity. When there is inadequate intake of all the essential nutrients, fat is not easily or adequately burned.

NUTRIENTS

SUPPLEMENT	SUGGESTED DOSAGE	COMMENTS
Very Important		
Aerobic Bulk Cleanse (ABC) or	As directed on label.	Especially good for high or low blood sugar problems and also provides fiber. Gives a "full feeling," cutting down hunger feelings. Do not take within an hour of medication or vitamins.
glucomannan	3 tablets ½ hour before meals with large glass of liquid.	
Essential fatty acids (primrose or linseed oil)	Use as directed on label.	Used with a low-fat diet to replace essential fatty acids.
Kelp	6 tablets daily.	Balanced minerals and iodine. Aids in weight loss.
Lecithin	Take with meals as directed on label.	A fat emulsifier; breaks down fat.
Protein (free form amino acids)	Use as directed on label.	Free form amino acids are better utilized.
Spirulina or Spiru-Tein from Nature's Plus	3 tablets between meals.	Excellent source of usable protein. Contains needed nutrients, stabilizes the blood sugar, and can replace a meal.
Vitamin C	3,000–6,000 mg daily.	Necessary for normal glandular function.

Helpful		
L-Arginine and L-ornithine and L-lysine	500 mg each or as directed on label before bedtime.	Not for children or diabetics. Do not take without lysine; it may cause an imbalance. These amino acids decrease body fat.
L-Carnitine	As directed on label.	Aids in fat metabolism and weight loss.
L-Phenylalanine	As directed on label.	An appetite suppressant that tells the brain you are not hungry. *Caution:* Do not take in high doses if you have high blood pressure or diabetes, or are pregnant.
Multivitamin and mineral supplement		Obesity and nutritional deficiency are parts of the same syndrome.
Vitamin B_6 (pyridoxine) and B complex with vitamin B_{12}	50 mg 3 times daily.	Vitamin B_6 removes excess water.
Vitamin E	400 IU daily.	Important in fat metabolism.

RECOMMENDATIONS

☐ Be active—take a brisk walk before breakfast to burn off fat. Do not worry as much about the number of calories you consume as you do about eating the proper foods in the diet. Remember: Exercise is the best way to control your weight, not an overly strict diet. Exercise is the best way to rid the body of fat and to maintain good muscle tone.

☐ Follow the fasting program once monthly. (*See* FASTING in Part Three.)

☐ Remember to rotate your foods and to eat a variety of foods.

☐ Drink six to eight glasses of liquids daily, such as distilled water and herb teas. They are nonfattening fillers.

☐ Make sure your bowels move daily.

☐ Use extra fiber daily. Take fiber with a large glass of liquid one-half hour before meals.

☐ Put less food on your plate. Chew slowly. Undereat and do not chew gum. Gum starts the gastric digestive juices flowing and will make you feel hungry sooner in addition to overworking your digestive system.

☐ Never consume animal fat (found in butter, cream, ice cream, whole milk, rich dressings, mayonnaise, and fried foods). However, do not eliminate sources of "good" fat (containing unsaturated fatty acids) such as avocados, olive oil, and nuts. Use these foods in moderation—no more than twice a week.

☐ Do not use any white flour products, salt, white rice, or processed foods. Also, avoid fast food restaurants and all junk foods. Do not consume sweets such as soda, pastries, pies, cakes, doughnuts, and candy. Omit all forms of sugar from the diet.

☐ Eat more complex carbohydrates that also offer protein such as tofu, lentils, plain baked potatoes (no toppings), sesame seeds, beans, brown rice, whole grains, and whitefish (no shellfish).

☐ Never do grocery shopping on an empty stomach. You will be tempted to buy forbidden foods and will often buy more food than you need or can use before it loses its freshness.

☐ Eat fresh fruits and an abundance of raw vegetables. Make one meal each day entirely of vegetables and fruits. Use low-calorie vegetables such as broccoli, cabbage, carrots, cauliflower, celery, cucumbers, green beans, kale, lettuce, onions, radishes, spinach, and turnips. Low calorie/low carbohydrate fruits include apples, cantaloupe, grapefruit, strawberries, and watermelon. The following are the highest in carbohydrates and calories and should be consumed in moderation: bananas, cherries, corn and hominy, figs, grapes, green peas, pears, pineapple, sweet potatoes, white rice, and yams. While raw foods are preferable, foods that are being heated should either be baked, broiled, steamed, or boiled. Never consume fried or greasy foods.

☐ Make lunch your main meal instead of dinner. Some people have had excellent results consuming no food after 3 p.m.

☐ Consume healthy snacks and desserts:
- Celery and carrot sticks.
- Low-fat cottage cheese topped with fresh applesauce and walnuts.
- Crackers topped with sesame butter and sesame seeds.
- Unsweetened gelatin made with fruit juice in place of sugar and water.
- Natural whole grain, sugar-free muffins.
- Freshly made, unsalted popcorn.
- Rice cakes topped with nut butters (but not peanut butter).
- Watermelon, fresh fruits, and frozen fruit popsicles.
- Unsweetened yogurt topped with granola or nuts and fresh fruit.

☐ Herb teas mixed with unsweetened fruit juice are very satisfying low-calorie drinks and are also very filling. Use between meals and when a desire for sweets hits you.

☐ Use barley malt sweetener instead of sugar. This is

highly concentrated, but is not dangerous. It contains only three calories to one gram (two teaspoons). This sweetener is particularly beneficial to the diabetic or hypoglycemic patient.

☐ Yellow vegetables, chestnuts, corn, white potatoes, brown rice, oatmeal, apples, grapes, and buckwheat all contain a small amount of essential fatty acids and should be part of the diet in moderation. Nuts, seeds, avocados, olives, coconuts, and wheat or corn germ are high in vegetable fatty acids and should not be overused.

CONSIDERATIONS

☐ A weight-loss diet research center in England reported using one part vegetable oil to two parts apple cider vinegar in massage to rid the body of fat. We recommend using pure virgin olive oil because it needs no refrigeration. Knead lightly but firmly over the fat areas at least three times weekly for quick results. It is also good for sore and stiff joints.

☐ College students have lost up to fifteen pounds in less than two weeks consuming only baby foods, fiber (guar gum or glucomannan), and spirulina. This diet should not be harmful. It contains no salt, fat, sugar, or chemicals. Earth's Best baby foods are organic and can be found in health food stores. There are many good fruits, cereals, and vegetables to choose from. Be sure and add plenty of liquids and some form of fiber. A dieter can stay on this diet until the desired weight is obtained. Guar gum adds fiber to the diet, and spirulina supplies protein and needed vitamins and minerals. The baby food also contains needed nutrients and should be rotated. The meat varieties of baby food— lamb, veal, beef, turkey, and chicken—can also be added if desired.

☐ Researchers have found that weight reduction can be improved with the use of a combination of the amino acids L-ornithine and L-arginine enhanced by L-lysine (see table for dosages). L-Ornithine helps to release a growth hormone, lacking in adults, that burns fat and builds muscle. This combination works best while the body is at rest. Never take an amino acid formula that does not contain L-lysine with L-arginine. Without L-lysine, an imbalance can result, possibly causing an outbreak of cold sores or previously dormant herpes.

☐ A recent study revealed that one third of those patients who went on crash diets of 500 calories or less developed gallstones.

☐ The drug Dimitrophinol, used for weight loss, may cause cataracts. The American Cancer Society found that those who used artificial sweeteners gained weight. They seem to increase the appetite.

Osteoporosis

A lack of calcium is the major cause of osteoporosis, the gradual loss of bone mass resulting in increased fractures, loss of height, pain in the hip and back, and spinal curvature. Osteoporosis primarily affects women, as bone mass is approximately 30 percent greater in men than in women. The risk of developing osteoporosis increases with age, as the peak bone mass is achieved at about thirty-five years of age. It affects 25 percent of postmenopausal women. Estrogen deficiency is the leading cause of osteoporosis in the menopausal female. Today osteoporosis affects as many as 15–20 million people in the United States.

Other causes of osteoporosis are an inability to absorb sufficient amounts of calcium through the intestine, a calcium-phosphorus imbalance, a lack of exercise, prolonged jaundice, a gastrectomy, and a lactose intolerance.

A diet that is adequate in protein, calcium, magnesium, phosphorus, vitamin C, and vitamin D is the best prevention and treatment for osteoporosis.

NUTRIENTS

SUPPLEMENT	SUGGESTED DOSAGE	COMMENTS
Essential		
Calcium	1,500–2,000 mg daily.	Injections may be necessary. Calcium is the largest and most difficult molecule to utilize.
Magnesium complex	1,000 mg daily.	Important in calcium uptake.
Silica tablets (silicon)	Use as directed on label.	Contains high amounts of calcium in a form that is easily absorbed. Necessary for calcium utilization and bone strength.
Very Important		
Boron	3 mg daily; do not take higher amounts.	Improves calcium absorption.
L-Lysine and L-arginine (amino acids)	As directed on label.	Aids calcium absorption and connective tissue strength.
Multidigestive enzymes with betaine hydrochloride and proteolytic enzymes	Take with meals. Take between meals.	Needed for proper absorption of calcium and all nutrients.

Phosphorus complex	As directed on label.	Important in bone formation.
Sulfur tablets	As directed on label.	Necessary for calcium uptake. Increases bone and connective tissue strength. Sulfur food sources are eggs, onions, garlic, and asparagus.
Vitamin A, D, and E emulsion	50,000 IU vitamin A for 1 month, then decrease to 25,000 IU; continue with 400 IU vitamin D and 400 IU vitamin E.	Important in retarding the aging process. Vitamin D has a special role in calcium uptake.
Zinc	50 mg	Important for calcium uptake and immune function.
Helpful		
Bone complex from Biotics Research	As directed on label.	Raw bovine tissue is found in these products: Cytogland, F-Cytozyme, and M-Cytozyme PT/BT.
Cod liver oil	3 tsp. twice daily.	A natural source of vitamins A and D. *Note:* Avoid cod liver oil if diabetic.
Kelp	10 tablets daily.	A rich source of important minerals.
Manganese	As directed on label.	Do not take calcium and manganese together—they compete for absorption. Vital in mineral metabolism.
Multivitamin and mineral supplement with high mineral content	As directed on label.	Contains essential minerals.
Vitamin B$_{12}$	1,000 mcg daily.	Promotes normal growth. Consider injections.
Vitamin C	3,000 mg and up daily.	Important for collagen and connective tissue.

HERBS

☐ Try feverfew, horsetail (silicon), oatstraw (a form of silica), and shavegrass if you have osteoporosis.

RECOMMENDATIONS

☐ The elderly lack sufficient stomach acid and should include calcium lactate (if not allergic to milk) or calcium phosphate to their diet.

☐ Keep active, and exercise regularly. Calcium loss results from lack of exercise, but can be reversed with sensible exercise.

☐ DLPA (DL-Phenylalanine), found in health food stores, is good for bone pain. Take on an empty stomach with vitamin B$_6$ and vitamin C. However, do not use if suffering from high blood pressure or if you are pregnant.

☐ Recently approved by the FDA, the prescription drug calcitonin is said to have no side effects even with long-term range. Do not use if you have a history of kidney stones. Studies show that calcitonin prevents further loss of bone mass in 70 percent of patients.

☐ If taking diuretics, thyroid supplements, or blood-thinning drugs, increase the amount of calcium prescribed. The use of thiazide diuretics is dangerous and can cause kidney stones. Do not use this diuretic with calcium and vitamin D.

☐ Consume whole grains at a different time than calcium because whole grains contain a substance that binds the calcium and prevents its uptake. Calcium is best absorbed at bedtime and also aids in sleeping.

CONSIDERATIONS

☐ Good sources of easy to assimilate calcium are buckwheat, buttermilk, cheese, dandelion greens, flounder, kefir, kelp, molasses, nuts and seeds, oats, seaweed, tofu, most vegetables, wheat germ, whole wheat products, and yogurt. Broccoli, kale, and turnip greens are also good vegetable sources without high levels of oxalic acid, which inhibits calcium absorption. Also good to eat are sardines and salmon with bones.

☐ Certain characteristics increase your risk for osteoporosis. Consult your doctor if you are concerned about any of the following factors, which can contribute to bone loss. Women who are most likely to have excess bone loss are those who:

- Have a fair complexion.
- Are thin and have small bones.
- Have experienced an early menopause naturally.
- Have a family history of osteoporosis.
- Have never been pregnant.
- Smoke.
- Are not physically active.
- Drink excessive amounts of alcohol.
- Have a high intake of coffee, tea, or cola.
- Have a low dietary calcium intake.
- Regularly use cortisone, anti-seizure medication, or anticoagulants.
- Do not exercise.
- Have chronic liver or kidney disease, or overactive endocrine glands.
- Have a low calcium intake and a high phosphorus diet.
- Have digestive disorders.
- Have had their ovaries removed.

☐ Avoid phosphate-containing drinks and foods such as soft drinks, high-protein animal foods, and alcohol.

In addition, citrus fruits and tomatoes may inhibit calcium intake. Also avoid smoking, sugar, and salt. Limit the intake of almonds, beet greens, cashews, chard, rhubarb, and spinach because they are high sources of oxalic acid.

OSTEOPOROSIS COMMENTS

☐ A study conducted by *The Journal of Clinical Nutrition* reports that women who are vegetarians have less bone loss (around 7 percent), while women who consume meat have bone loss of 35 percent.

☐ Studies indicate that caffeine is linked to calcium loss. Adults given 300 milligrams of caffeine excreted more than the normal amount of calcium in their urine. Another study revealed that caffeine is associated with decreased bone minerals in women.

☐ Indomethacin, ibuprofen, and other nonsteroidal anti-inflammatory drugs used for pain relief weaken the hip joints.

☐ Scientists at Stanford University believe a hormone found in salmon may slow the progress of osteoporosis.

☐ Bone disintegration with pain in the hips, lower back, or legs and vertebral fractures (usually affecting people over fifty years of age) are commonplace. Only x-rays can reveal bone loss, and then only after 30 percent or more of the loss has occurred.

☐ The cost of osteoporosis in the United States has been estimated at 3.8 billion dollars annually.

Pancreatitis

Pancreatitis is an inflammation of the pancreas. It is caused by an obstruction of the pancreatic duct from stones, scarring, or cancer. Alcoholism, viral infection, abdominal injury, obesity, poor nutrition, and drugs increase your risk of developing pancreatitis.

The disease can be either acute or chronic. Acute pancreatitis is indicated by nausea, vomiting, and pain around the umbilicus radiating to the back (an extremely critical condition). Chronic pancreatitis is often related to gallbladder infections and gallstones.

Other symptoms include abdominal swelling, excessive gas, upper abdominal pain described as burning or stabbing, vomiting, fever, hypertension, muscle aches, and abnormal fatty stools.

The pancreas is a gland that produces the hormones insulin and glucagon to control blood sugar and digestive enzymes. For this reason, pancreatitis often causes diabetes and digestive difficulties.

NUTRIENTS

SUPPLEMENT	SUGGESTED DOSAGE	COMMENTS
Essential		
GTF (chromium)	300 mcg daily.	Important in maintaining stable blood sugar levels.
Very Important		
Calcium chelate	1,500 mg daily.	Calcium and magnesium work closely together.
Magnesium chelate	1,000 mg daily.	Magnesium counteracts glandular disorders.
Pancreatin	Take with meals.	Pancreatic enzyme deficiency is common in pancreatitis.
Proteolytic enzymes	Between meals on an empty stomach and at bedtime.	Aids in reducing inflammation. Reduces strain on the pancreas by helping to digest proteins.
Raw pancreas concentrate	As directed on label.	Contains certain proteins needed to repair the pancreas.
Vitamin B complex with extra pantothenic acid (B_5) and	100 mg 3 times daily.	Antistress vitamins. Pantothenic acid and niacin are important in fat and carbohydrate metabolism.
niacin (B_3)	50 mg 3 times daily.	
Important		
Lipotropic factors (choline, inositol, and/or lecithin)	As directed on label.	Fat emulsifiers that aid in fat digestion.
Vitamin C (ascorbic buffered)	1,000 mg 4 times daily and up if needed.	A potent free radical scavenger (antioxidant). Follow program for ASCORBIC ACID FLUSH in Part Three.
Helpful		
Coenzyme Q_{10}	75 mg daily.	A powerful antioxidant and oxygen carrier.
Germanium	200 mg daily.	A powerful antioxidant and oxygen carrier. Aids in relieving discomfort.
Vitamin E	400–800 IU daily and up. In capsule form, begin with 200 IU and increase slowly to desired dosage.	A powerful antioxidant and oxygen carrier. Important in tissue repair.

RECOMMENDATIONS

☐ Use Echinaforce Extract from Bioforce of America. Take 200 drops twice a day. Antibiotics may be necessary. Be sure to consume buttermilk, kefir, and yogurt. Add some form of acidophilus to the program.

CONSIDERATIONS

☐ Diet is very important. *See* DIABETES in Part Two and follow the dietary guidelines—see your doctor.

☐ Cancer of the pancreas is the fourth leading cause of cancer deaths in the United States.

Parkinson's Disease

Also called shaking palsy or paralysis agitans, Parkinson's disease is a degenerative disease affecting the nervous system. Its cause is unknown, but symptoms appear when there is an imbalance of two chemicals, dopamine and acetylcholine, in the brain. Scientists found a deficiency of dopamine in certain brain cells. This chemical carries messages from one nerve cell to another. When the brain is not able to manufacture dopamine, Parkinson's disease results. Malnutrition is believed to be a major underlying factor.

Symptoms of this disease include muscular rigidity, drooling, loss of appetite, a stooped, shuffling gait, tremors that include a characteristic pill-rolling movement of the thumb and forefinger as they rub against each other, impaired speech, and a fixed facial expression. The disease may start with a tremor of the hands while at rest. The body gradually becomes rigid and the limbs stiffen.

The drug most often used to treat this disease is levodopa; however, it isn't effective alone and can have serious side effects, including paranoia and hallucinations. If taking this drug, do not take vitamin B_6. Taken together, vitamin B_6 and levodopa elevate brain dopamine. Using vitamin B_6 alone is probably safer and is as effective. Digested protein prevents this drug from reaching the brain, where it is needed for effectiveness. Eat protein only at dinner, not when taking the drug. In addition, the drug Sinemet reduces stiffness.

NUTRIENTS

SUPPLEMENT	SUGGESTED DOSAGE	COMMENTS
Very Important		
Calcium and magnesium	1,500 mg daily. 750 mg	Needed for nerve impulse transmission. These important minerals work together.
GABA (gamma-amino butyric acid)	As directed on label.	Functions as a neurotransmitter in the central nervous system by stabilizing neuron activity.
Lecithin and/or phosphatidyl choline	1 tbsp. 3 times daily.	Important in transmission of nerve impulses.
L-Glutamic acid (amino acid)	As directed on label.	Improves nerve impulse transmission.
L-Tyrosine (amino acid)	Use only as prescribed by physician.	Mood regulator.
Vitamin B complex (high potency)	100 mg three times daily with meals. Consider IV administration—consult your physician.	Extremely important in brain function and enzyme activity.
Vitamin B_6 (pyridoxine)	Up to 1,000 mg	Injections are best. Brain dopamine production depends on vitamin B_6.
Vitamin C plus bioflavonoids	3,000–8,000 mg	Improves cerebral circulation. Potent antioxidants and antistress substances.
Vitamin E	600–1,000 mg Start with smaller amounts and increase dosage slowly.	Protects important vitamins and minerals from free radical destruction. An antioxidant.
Helpful		
Brewer's yeast or Bio-Strath	As directed on label.	Contains B vitamins and balanced minerals needed by the central nervous system.
Gerovital H-3 (GH-3) from Rumania	As directed on label.	Improves memory and brain function.
Multidigestive enzymes	Use as directed on label.	Aids in digestion.
Multivitamin and mineral complex	Use as directed on label.	Malnutrition is common in Parkinson's disease.
Niacin (B_3)	100 mg 3 times daily with meals.	Improves brain circulation. Flushing may occur from niacin use—this is normal.
Raw brain concentrate	Use as directed on label.	A glandular extract that directly improves brain function.

RECOMMENDATIONS

☐ The diet should contain 75 percent raw foods with seeds, grains, nuts, and raw milk.

☐ Fasting and chelation are both helpful. (*See* FASTING and CHELATION THERAPY in Part Three.)

☐ If on the drug levodopa, consume in moderation only bananas, beef, fish, liver, oatmeal, peanuts, potatoes, and whole grains. These foods contain vitamin B_6 and interfere with the drug's potency.

Pellagra

Pellagra is a vitamin deficiency disease. It is caused by a long-term shortage of B vitamins, particularly niacin, riboflavin, and thiamine. It is prevalent in populations that eat diets high in corn. Pellagra rarely occurs here in the United States, thanks to our more varied diet. But it continues to threaten Americans who suffer from diseases that deplete the body of niacin, riboflavin, and thiamine, such as chronic gastrointestinal disturbances or alcoholism.

The symptoms of pellagra include an inflamed and sore red tongue, loss of appetite, diarrhea, loss of weight, weakness, depression, anxiety, headaches, and dizziness. Itchy dermatitis on the hands and neck is a prominent characteristic of the disease. Symptoms of subclinical pellagra have been misinterpreted as mental illness. For this reason, schizophrenic and hyperactive problems in children might signal niacin and vitamin B deficiency.

A diet adequate in niacin, thiamine, riboflavin, folic acid, vitamin B_{12}, and protein will prevent pellagra. A diet rich in niacin, thiamine, riboflavin, folic acid, and vitamin B_{12} will cure the disease.

NUTRIENTS

SUPPLEMENT	SUGGESTED DOSAGE	COMMENTS
Essential		
Vitamin B complex plus extra	100 mg daily.	B vitamins work best when taken together. Injections may be necessary. If so, combine 2 cc B complex and ½ cc each of B_1, B_2, and B_{12}.
niacin (B_3) and	100 mg daily.	
thiamine (B_1) and	50 mg taken with meals.	
riboflavin (B_2) with	50 mg taken with meals.	
vitamin B_{12} lozenges containing	1 tablet on an empty stomach twice daily.	
folic acid or	400 mcg	
brewer's yeast or	As directed on label.	Natural sources of the B complex.
Bio-Strath	As directed on label.	

RECOMMENDATIONS

☐ Consume white skinless breast of chicken and turkey, halibut, salmon, sunflower seeds, tuna, and swordfish. A diet rich in the amino acid tryptophan is necessary. Tryptophan helps manufacture niacin in the body.

CONSIDERATIONS

☐ B vitamins are found in avocados, bananas, broccoli, collards, figs, legumes, nuts and seeds, peanut butter, potatoes, prunes, tomatoes, and whole grain or enriched bread and cereal.

Periodontal Disease

Periodontal means "located around a tooth." The term refers to any disorder of the gums or other supporting structures of the teeth. Treatment with natural methods stresses nutrients that fight infection and rebuild bone.

Gingivitis (inflammation of the gums) is considered to be an early stage of periodontal disease caused by sticky deposits of bacteria, mucus, and food particles called plaque. Researchers believe that plaque accumulation causes the gum to become infected and swollen, and to bleed. As the gum swells, it forms a pocket between the teeth, causing a trap for more plaque. The gum becomes red, soft, and shiny. Other possible causes of gingivitis include breathing through the mouth, badly fitting fillings which irritate surrounding gum tissue, and a diet consisting of too many soft foods that rob the teeth and gums of much needed "exercise."

If left untreated, gingivitis can lead to a condition called pyorrhea (periodontitis). This is an advanced stage of periodontal disease often related to a deficiency of vitamin C, bioflavonoids, calcium, folic acid, or niacin. It occurs when bacteria get between the gum and teeth, causing infection. Pyorrhea causes halitosis, with painful and bleeding gums. This slowly eats away the bone in the jaw. Abscesses are common. Severe cases will require surgery to remove the infected tissue from the gum and reshape the bone.

Causes of pyorrhea include poor nutrition, improper brushing, wrong foods, sugar, chronic illness, glandular disorders, blood disease, smoking, drugs, and excessive alcohol.

NUTRIENTS

SUPPLEMENT	SUGGESTED DOSAGE	COMMENTS
Essential		
Coenzyme Q_{10}	100 mg	Used successfully in Japan for mouth and gum disease.
Vitamin C plus bioflavonoids	4,000–10,000 mg	Promotes healing, especially of bleeding gums.
Very Important		
Calcium	1,500 mg	Helps prevent bone loss around the gums.
Magnesium	750 mg	Take the chelate form.
Vitamin A	Start with 100,000 IU for 1 month. Decrease to 50,000 IU for 2 weeks. End with 25,000 IU. Or take vitamin A emulsion in same amounts for better assimilation.	Needed for healing of the gum tissue.

Vitamin E	400 IU and increase slowly to 1,000 IU.	Needed for healing of the gum tissues. Also open up a capsule and rub on the gums.
Important		
Proteolytic enzymes	2 tablets between meals and at bedtime.	Helps break down food particles, especially those left in the colon.
Vitamin B complex with extra	50 mg with meals.	For digestion.
folic acid and	100 mg with meals.	
niacin	100 mg with meals.	
Zinc	50–80 mg	Needed to prevent infection and for healing.

RECOMMENDATIONS

☐ Brush teeth with goldenseal herb powder every day for at least one month. After one month, change brands of toothpaste. Don't stay on the same brand; some brands may irritate the gums. Change toothbrushes every month to keep the disease in check. Bacteria live on the toothbrush. A bacteria-destroying toothbrush sanitizer can be purchased that has been proven effective in tests conducted by the University of Oklahoma School of Dentistry. The device automatically turns on every half-hour for two minutes to provide thorough sanitization of the bristles twenty-four hours a day. Call 1-(800) 543-3366 for more information. Also helpful: take baking soda and make a paste with hydrogen peroxide and pack around the teeth overnight.

☐ Use dental floss daily. A wooden toothpick called Stim-U-Dent works well. Use between meals to clean and stimulate the gums with a massaging motion. Use faithfully every day.

☐ Try a dental rinse called Plax to help loosen plaque. Listerine also helps to remove plaque.

☐ An automatic toothbrush called Interplak helps to remove plaque. For more information, call 1-(800) 537-1600 and ask for operator #11.

☐ Use a *very* soft toothbrush. Be sure to brush the gums and tongue. The most effective way to get under the gums is to tilt the toothbrush upward with the bristles at an angle to the gum and to brush in a forward and backward motion using short strokes. There is a tablet you can purchase at most drugstores that, when chewed after brushing, shows up as colored areas where you missed brushing. Brush until the color is gone.

☐ Open a capsule of vitamin E oil and rub on inflamed gums. This is very healing and helps soreness.

☐ In addition to the products described above, we recommend the following tooth and gum products. Most of these can be bought at health food stores.

- *Dentie*. Black toothpaste that originated in Japan; a mixture of charred eggplant powder and sea salt. Dentie combines the eggplant powder with clay, seaweed cellulose, glycerine, and natural peppermint essence.
- *Nature de France (Pierre Cattier)*. Contains a clay base for healing.
- *Nature's Gate*. Contains baking soda and sea salt, which is effective against plaque and gum disease. Contains vitamin C.
- *Meswak*. Produced from the meswak tree, this product has antibiotic and anti-inflammatory properties.
- *Peelu*. Contains a natural tooth whitener derived from the diminutive peelu tree, native to the Middle East and Asia. People have chewed its branches for centuries to keep their teeth white. Also contains natural flavor, fruit pectin, sodium lauryl sulfate (from coconut oil), and vegetable glycerine.
- *Tom's Natural Toothpaste*. Contains natural calcium base. Features myrrh (an astringent herb) and propolis.
- *Weleda Salt Toothpaste*. Contains baking soda and salt formulation with medicinal herbs and silica.
- *Vicco Pure Herbal Toothpaste*. Contains extracts from plants, bark, roots, and flowers used in the Ayurvedic medicine of India.

CONSIDERATIONS

☐ Diabetes and several kinds of blood disorders put the sufferer at high risk for developing gum disease.

☐ Applying ice to the gums can relieve the pain of a toothache until you can get to your dentist. Rubbing clove oil on the tooth can also help.

☐ Although all vitamins and minerals are essential for the proper formation and continued health of the teeth, an adequate vitamin C intake is especially helpful for the prevention of gingivitis and pyorrhea, while a deficiency of it causes teeth to loosen and deteriorate. Vitamin A seems to control the development and general health of the gums; a lack of this vitamin often results in gum infection. Vitamin A is also necessary for the formation and maintenance of tooth development in children. The minerals important for healthy teeth are sodium, potassium, calcium, phosphorus, iron, and magnesium. A varied diet of fresh fruits, green leafy vegetables, meat, and whole grain bread will provide the teeth and gums with needed exercise and supply the body with the vitamins and minerals that are essential for dental health.

Fluoride Update

In his *Report on Water*, H.W. Holderby, M.D., discusses the effects of fluoride on health. Fluoride, which is derived from the deadly chemical fluoride, is not dangerous in small amounts; however, a government investigation of 156 cancer deaths over the past three years suggests that fluoride accumulates in the human body and may eventually cause cancer and/or other fatal illnesses. Although both animal and human epidemiology studies have been conducted with fluoride, they have not been extensive enough to arrive conclusively at whether or not fluoride is a carcinogen. Water is the number one source of fluoride, and toothpaste is the second. A copy of Dr. Holderby's report is available from Natural Food Associates, Atlanta, TX 75551. Enclose thirty-five cents.

Pneumonia

Pneumonia is an inflammation in the lungs caused by different bacteria, viruses, and fungi. The tiny air sacs in the lung area become inflamed and fill with mucus and pus. It is unlikely to be contagious.

Although symptoms can vary in intensity, they usually include fever, chills, cough, muscle aches, fatigue, sore throat, enlarged lymph glands in the neck, bluish nails (cyanosis), pains in the chest, and rapid, difficult respiration.

Typical contributing factors to pneumonia are the common cold, influenza, seizure or stroke, aspiration under anesthesia, alcoholism, smoking, kidney failure, sickle cell disease, malnutrition, foreign bodies in the respiratory passages, bacteria, viruses, chemical irritants, and even allergies.

Vitamin A is necessary for maintaining the health of the lining of the respiratory passages. A deficiency of the vitamin increases susceptibility to respiratory infections, which in turn can lead to pneumonia.

Bacterial pneumonia is very dangerous. Symptoms usually include shaking, chills, and a high temperature. The cough is dry at first, then a rust-colored sputum is produced, and breathing becomes rapid and labored. Children under twelve most often contract this type of pneumonia.

Weakness will remain for four to eight weeks after recovery. A positive diagnosis can be made only with a chest x-ray.

In the following table, the suggested dosages are for those over 100 pounds. Adjust dosage according to your age and weight.

NUTRIENTS

SUPPLEMENT	SUGGESTED DOSAGE	COMMENTS
Essential		
Beta-carotene	15,000 IU daily.	Protects the lungs from free radical damage.
Vitamin A emulsion	Up to 100,000 IU daily.	Emulsified A is safe in higher doses because it bypasses the liver. It is more readily available for repair and immune function.
Vitamin C plus bioflavonoids	3,000–10,000 mg daily in divided doses. 100 mg twice daily.	Very important for immune response and for reducing inflammation. Bioflavonoids are needed to activate vitamin C. *See* ASCORBIC ACID FLUSH in Part Three and administer accordingly.
Very Important		
Bulgaricum I.B. from Natren	On an empty stomach as directed on label.	For replacement of "friendly" bacteria.
L-Carnitine and L-cysteine (amino acids)	As directed on label.	Protects the lungs from free radical damage.
Protein (free form amino acids)	As directed on label.	Important in tissue repair.
Vitamin B complex	100 mg 3 times daily.	Needed for normal digestion, production of antibodies, and formation of red blood cells, and for healthy mucous membranes.
Important		
Raw thymus extract and raw lung tissue	500 mg each twice daily.	Stimulates immune response and promotes healing of lung tissue.
Vitamin E emulsion or capsules	1,500 IU emulsion or 400 IU twice daily before meals in capsule form.	A potent antioxidant that protects the lung tissues and enhances oxygen utilization.
Zinc	80 mg daily.	Needed for tissue repair and immune function. Zinc gluconate dissolved in the mouth is very effective.
Helpful		
Coenzyme Q$_{10}$	100 mg daily.	Enhances cellular oxygen utilization.
Germanium	200 mg daily.	Aids in relieving discomfort. Promotes immune response.
Inflazyme Forte from American Biologics	2 tablets between meals and at bedtime on an empty stomach.	Helps keep the infection in check.
Proteolytic enzymes	3 times daily on an empty stomach.	Aids in absorption of nutrients and reduces inflammation.

HERBS

☐ Ginger and Green Farms Herbal C are recommended for pneumonia.

RECOMMENDATIONS

☐ See your doctor if you suspect pneumonia. If taking antibiotics, take acidophilus capsules or two table-spoons of liquid three times each day.

☐ The diet should consist of raw fruits and vegetables. Take a protein supplement from a vegetable source (free form amino acids). Include chlorophyll in a "green drink" or take in tablet form.

☐ Exclude from the diet dairy products, sugar, white flour products, coffee, all tea except herb tea, and cigarettes.

☐ Drink plenty of juices. Liquids help to thin the lung secretions. Fast on pure juices, fresh lemon juice, and distilled water. (See FASTING in Part Three.)

CONSIDERATIONS

☐ A cool mist from a humidifier or vaporizer is helpful. A heating pad on the chest will relieve pain.

☐ See also INFLUENZA and COMMON COLD, both in Part Two.

Poison Ivy

When the sap of the poison ivy plant makes contact with uncovered skin, it produces redness, rash, swelling, blistering, and intense, persistent itching in sensitive people. Exposed areas such as the hands, arms, and face are most frequently the first to be affected. Scratching transmits the inflammation, via the hands, to other parts of the body.

The irritating substance in poison ivy is the oily sap in its leaves, flowers, fruit, stem, bark, and roots. The plant is poisonous even after long drying, but is particularly irritating in the spring and early summer when it is full of sap.

The first symptom of poison ivy is a burning and itching sensation. This is followed by a rash, swelling, and oozing blisters. Symptoms appear within a few hours to seven days after contact.

The poisons can be conveyed to the skin in ways other than direct contact. Some have contracted poison ivy simply by petting an animal that has been in contact with it. Those that are highly sensitive to poison ivy can be infected by inhaling smoke from a nearby brush fire in which the plant is burning. Severe cases of mouth poisoning have been reported when children have eaten the leaves or grayish berries of the poison ivy plant.

If you suspect that you have accidentally handled poison ivy or brushed against it, wash your skin immediately. Yellow laundry soap is best for this purpose. Lather several times and rinse in running water after each sudsing. Wash clothing, gear, or pack material in plenty of soapy water. Note that stubborn cases that do not respond to proper treatment are often due to repeated contact with contaminated clothing.

Mild cases of poison ivy are signalled by a few small blisters that occur on the hands, arms, or legs. Treat mild cases by applying compresses of very hot, plain water for brief intervals. Or, apply compresses soaked in a dilute Burrow's solution (one pint to fifteen pints of cool water). Purchase Burrow's solution at your drugstore.

Severe cases of poison ivy are signalled by many large blisters, acute inflammation, fever, or inflammation on the face or genitals. If severe poison ivy is suspected, contact a doctor to relieve discomfort and guard against secondary infection until the attack subsides.

The best treatment for poison ivy is prevention. Learn to recognize, and avoid, this harmful plant. Its leaves always grow in clusters of three, one at the end of the stalk, the other two opposite each other. Memorize the poison ivy rhyme: "Leaflets three, let it be."

Those whose activities take them into forests and through thick underbrush should wear appropriate protective clothing: trousers, long sleeves, shoes, socks, and gloves. Once in contact with poison ivy, these are not safe to re-wear until they have been laundered or dry cleaned.

Poison ivy grows in many parts of the United States. It is responsible for more than 350,000 cases of skin poisoning each year. In all, there are sixty varieties of poisonous plants indigenous to the United States. Apart from poison ivy, the most common are oak-leaf poison ivy, western poison oak, and poison sumac. Other botanical skin irritants include goldenrod, crabgrass, nettle, table grass, dog fennel, hollyhock, and Indian mallow.

The dosages given in the following table are for adults only. Adjust the dosage according to age.

NUTRIENTS

SUPPLEMENT	SUGGESTED DOSAGE	COMMENTS
Important		
Vitamin C	3,000–8,000 mg	To prevent infection and spreading.
Helpful		
All-Purpose Bacteriaside Spray from Aerobic Life Products	As directed on label.	Destroys bacteria. Prevents spreading.

Calamine lotion	As directed on label.	Contains calamine, phenol, and zinc oxide. Has drying properties for faster healing.
Marigold Ointment from NatureWorks or aloe vera gel	As directed on label.	May relieve itching.
Other good lotions: Antivy lotion Calamatum aerosol Surfadil lotion	As directed on labels.	Prevents spreading and aids healing.
RUS-TOX (homeopathic remedy or lotion)	As directed on label.	Relieves itching and promotes healing.
Vitamin A	25,000 IU daily.	Needed for healing of skin tissues. Also boosts the immune system.
Vitamin E or enzyme cream	As directed on label.	Aids in healing and prevents scarring.
Zinc	80 mg daily.	Needed for repair of skin tissues.

HERBS

☐ The following herbs are good for poison ivy or poison oak: bloodroot, echinacea, goldenseal, lobelia, myrrh, and Solomon's seal. A strong tea made of equal parts of white oak bark and lime water is very good for poison ivy or poison oak. Apply a bandage wet with this solution and change it as often as it becomes dry.

RECOMMENDATIONS

☐ See a doctor if a fever occurs, or if a widespread rash involving the eyes, mouth, or genitals occurs.

☐ If you are aware of contact, remove all clothing and shoes, and immediately use laundry soap and water or alcohol to deter the attack. This procedure is useless if not done immediately.

Poisoning

See ALUMINUM TOXICITY; ARSENIC POISONING; CADMIUM TOXICITY; CHEMICAL ALLERGIES; CHEMICAL POISONING; COPPER TOXICITY; DDT POISONING; ENVIRONMENTAL TOXICITY; LEAD POISONING; MERCURY TOXICITY; NICKEL TOXICITY.

Polyps

Polyps are benign (not cancerous) growths of varying sizes, which are found on stalk-like structures growing from the epithelial lining of the large intestine, cervix, bladder, or other mucous membranes. They are common in the rectum and sigmoid colon.

Familial polyposis is hereditary. A large number of growths, which can become cancerous, develop in the colon. A surgical procedure called a colectomy, which often is necessary, requires the removal of the entire colon. In some cases the rectum is left in place and connected to the small intestine so as to allow for a bowel evacuation. However, in most cases, polyps return in the rectum. Rectal bleeding or a mucus drainage are common symptoms.

Jerome J. DeCosse, M.D., Ph.D., and his colleagues in Wisconsin's Department of Surgery and Pathology discovered that when vitamin C was added to the treatment, five out of eight patients either had a reduction in the number of polyps or had complete elimination of the polyps.

Cervical polyps line the inside of the cervix of the uterus. Symptoms indicative of cervical polyps include a heavy, watery, bloody discharge from the vagina. Bleeding may occur after sexual intercourse, between periods, and after menopause. Polyps are more common in women who have not had children. A pap smear may or may not detect cervical polyps. They rarely return once removed.

Bladder polyps produce blood in the urine. Unless they are removed, cancer of the bladder may follow.

NUTRIENTS

SUPPLEMENT	SUGGESTED DOSAGE	COMMENTS
Essential		
Beta-carotene	15,000 IU daily.	An important antioxidant. Protects the epithelial linings (mucous membranes) of the body cavities.
Calcium included in multivitamin and mineral complex	1,000–1,500 mg daily.	Calcium protects against colorectal polyps.
Vitamin A	25,000 IU daily.	Protects the membranous linings. The emulsified form is very effective.
Vitamin C	5,000–10,000 mg in daily divided doses.	Reduces the number of polyps, and may eliminate them altogether.

Very Important		
Vitamin E	400 IU increasing slowly to 800 IU.	A potent antioxidant. Promotes a vital chemical process called lipid peroxidation. If vitamin E deficiency occurs, the membrane linings are vulnerable to damage.

Important		
Aerobic Bulk Cleanse (ABC)	Use with aloe vera juice. Drink down quickly before it thickens.	Cleanses the colon, assisting in normal stool formation.
Aerobic 07 from Aerobic Life Products	As directed on label.	Destroys unwanted bacteria in the colon.

Helpful		
Coenzyme Q$_{10}$	60 mg daily.	An important antioxidant. Increases cellular oxygen levels.
Garlic capsules (Kyolic)	2 capsules between meals.	Odorless garlic that acts as a natural antibiotic. Enhances immune function.
Germanium	200 mg daily.	An important antioxidant and potent immune system enhancer.
Superoxide dismutase (SOD) complex from American Biologics or from Biotec Foods	Use as directed on label.	An important antioxidant and free radical destroyer.

RECOMMENDATIONS

☐ A high-fiber diet with no animal fats is important. (*See* the diet in CANCER, Part Two.) Include in the diet apricots, broccoli, brown rice, cabbage, cantaloupe, carrots, cauliflower, garlic, oatmeal, onions, green peppers, sweet potatoes, sesame seeds, spinach, and sunflower seeds. Eat some form of fiber daily. Oat bran and rice bran are good sources of fiber. Exclude from the diet fried foods, highly processed foods, caffeine, tobacco, and alcohol.

Pregnancy Planning and Testing

OVULATION TIMING SELF-TEST

When planning for a baby, there is a test available that can help you determine the best time to conceive. Remember, however, that no test is 100 percent accurate. This test predicts the time of ovulation by measuring the corresponding rise in the level of luteinizing hormone (LH) present, which triggers the release of the egg.

A chemically impregnated dipstick detects the LH in urine samples. If the hormone has been released, it is indicated by a color change in the stick. After a positive result, ovulation takes place *within twelve to thirty-six hours*. Ovu-stick and another test kit called First Response can be purchased at your drugstore.

Most doctors must get your consent before performing diagnostic tests. There may be risks involved any time you penetrate the body using a tube, needle, or viewing instrument, or through radiation exposure, reactions to drugs, anesthetics, and dye materials used in certain imaging techniques. Risks vary depending on the mother's age and health status, and the ability of the doctor.

PREGNANCY SELF-TEST

To determine if you are pregnant, there are two basic tests available.

1. A positive result is indicated in one test kit when a ring forms at the bottom of the test tube after mixing your morning urine with specific chemical agents in the tube.
2. In another test morning urine is collected, a small quantity is placed in a test tube, and an indicator stick is placed in the tube with the urine sample for fifteen minutes. The indicator stick is then placed into another tube for an additional fifteen minutes. If the stick changes color, you should assume that you are pregnant and confirm this positive test result with your physician.

Studies show that these in-home pregnancy tests are only 77.1 percent accurate. See your doctor to confirm positive results.

Pregnancy-Related Problems

Pregnancy is the very happy time between conception and childbirth in which a fetus grows and matures for nine months (approximately 280 days) inside a female's womb until it is ready to be born. Unfortunately, there are many common problems that can occur during a pregnancy which may be as life threatening as a miscarriage or as simple as stretch marks. Most of these problems occur due to hormonal changes within the body, nutrient deficiencies in the mother, or a shift in weight distribution due to the sudden weight gain. Following is a description of these various problems including natural remedies as well as helpful hints and suggestions that the pregnant woman can follow to maintain maximum health during pregnancy. It is important to remember that it is necessary to consult and work with a health care provider, be it a doctor, a nurse, a nurse practitioner, or a midwife.

BACKACHE

☐ To minimize back pain during pregnancy, the mother should not stay in any one position for long periods of time, should not wear high-heeled shoes as they increase the likelihood of backache, and should not do any forward bending or strong upward stretching exercises. She should also learn to include two to three minutes of stretching in her daily routine.

☐ Another helpful hint for eliminating backache is to soak a small towel in cider vinegar. Squeeze off any excess and lay down in bed on your side. Spread the towel directly across your back. Relax this way for 15–20 minutes.

BLEEDING GUMS

☐ To avoid excessive bleeding gums during pregnancy, the mother should floss her teeth daily, brush her teeth at least three to four times daily (remembering to rinse her mouth well), and massage her gums with clean fingers when necessary.

☐ Be sure the diet contains enough calcium and high-quality, complete proteins. Increase the intake of vitamin C rich foods as a deficiency in this vitamin can contribute to bleeding gums. In addition, the smoking mother is draining an additional amount of vitamin C from her body. If you are pregnant and smoke, quit or at least cut down drastically.

☐ See your dentist at least once during the pregnancy, but do not have any x-rays taken.

CONSTIPATION

☐ To relieve this problem, add more fresh and dried fruit such as prunes, raisins, and figs to the diet. Eat fresh vegetables and salads containing a variety of raw green and colored vegetables daily. It is important to drink six to eight glasses of liquid, including water, each day. Whole grain breads, cereals, and whole bran flakes are helpful. Begin with two teaspoons of bran in a glass of apple juice twice a day. Keep in mind that the bran may cause some gas until the system is used to it.

☐ Do not take over-the-counter laxatives without a health care practitioner's permission.

☐ Walking at least a mile a day is very helpful in addition to setting a regular time each day for bowel movement. The feet and legs should be elevated during elimination to relax the anal muscles. Remember that increasing progesterone in the system makes the bowels less efficient.

☐ If all else fails, an enema, using body temperature water, may be used occasionally.

DIZZINESS

☐ The mother's blood pressure may drop due to the pressure of the uterus on major blood vessels, causing dizziness. Do not change positions quickly. The mother should take her time and focus on what she is doing.

GAS (FLATULENCE)

☐ Keep a food diary in order to determine what foods or food combinations are causing the gas. Eat four to five small meals a day, instead of three big meals. Chew food slowly and well. Cook your foods quickly using a perforated steamer instead of boiling food for long periods of time. Walking a mile a day should help digestion and elimination, in addition to setting a regular time for bowel movement.

☐ To reduce gas-causing sulfur compounds in beans (e.g., baked, garbanzo, pinto, navy), bring one cup of beans to a boil in five cups of water. Boil for one minute. Drain and add five fresh cups of water. Bring to a second boil and cook according to directions.

GROIN SPASM, STITCH, OR PRESSURE

☐ This problem is often felt as a "stitch" on the right side. The round ligaments connecting the corners of the uterus to the pubic area will kink and go into a spasm. In the later months of pregnancy, lower groin pressure may develop. Exercising daily (with a health care provider's recommended exercises) can help to alleviate this condition.

☐ Breathe deeply during the spasm. Bend toward the point of pain in order to allow the ligament to relax. Rest in bed on one side until the spasm is over.

HEARTBURN

☐ Heartburn occurs more often during pregnancy due to the re-entrance of stomach fluids into the esophagus (food tube) because of the expanded size of the uterus. Do not consume spicy or greasy foods, alcohol, coffee, baking soda, or Alka-Seltzer antacid tablets.

☐ Drink one tablespoon of cream, milk, or buttermilk before eating to coat and soothe the stomach. Eat four to six small meals a day.

☐ Remain active.

HEMORRHOIDS

☐ When suffering from hemorrhoids, it is important to increase the intake of roughage in the diet with such foods as raw vegetables, fruits, dried fruits, whole bran flakes, and whole grain breads. This helps to soften stools and make elimination easier. Hard stools may be very painful and cause bleeding. Also, drink six to eight glasses of liquid a day including water, juices, and herbal teas.

☐ Keep feet and legs elevated on a high footstool while eliminating. This helps to move the bowels by relaxing the anal muscles. Do not strain and do not stay on the toilet bowl for too long.

☐ Cold witch hazel compresses will help shrink the hemorrhoids.

☐ Walking one mile a day helps digestion and elimination.

☐ *See also* HEMORRHOIDS in Part Two.

INSOMNIA

☐ Insomnia is very common during the last weeks of pregnancy, when finding a comfortable sleeping position is difficult. Also, a vitamin B deficiency can often cause insomnia. Therefore, increase intake of vitamin B-rich foods.

☐ Do not force yourself to sleep if you are not really tired. Read or do nonstrenuous chores until you feel sleepy.

☐ Herb teas such as chamomile, marjoram, and lemon balm are known for their sleep-inducing qualities. Try a hot cup of tea with honey or lemon before bed or in the middle of the night.

☐ Arranging pillows behind or under your tummy to relieve breathlessness can be very helpful. Also keep in mind that this is a natural way to prepare for the 3 a.m. feeding.

LEG CRAMPS

☐ During pregnancy, it is wise to increase calcium and potassium intake by eating foods such as bananas, grapefruit, oranges, cottage cheese, yogurt, salmon, sardines, soybeans, almonds, and sesame seeds to help avert leg cramps. However, if they do occur, the following suggestions may help:

- While sleeping or sitting, elevate the legs higher than the heart.
- Do not stand in one place for too long. Shift your weight from one leg to the other.
- Do not point your toes outward; point your toes upward instead to relieve cramps.
- Walk one mile a day to circulate the flow of blood through the legs.
- When experiencing a cramp, apply a hot water bottle or heating pad to the cramping area and apply pressure (using your hands).

MISCARRIAGE AND SPONTANEOUS ABORTION

☐ Some women cannot carry a baby to full term and experience a miscarriage or spontaneous abortion. There are many reasons for this, including emotional stress, malnutrition, general malaise, and illness such as infection and glandular disorder.

☐ Women with this problem can boost their chances of a full-term pregnancy with a new immunization procedure. Doctors at the University of Michigan inject two vaccines of white blood cells from the father into the mother. This prevents an abnormal reaction in the woman's immune system that results in rejection of the growing fetus as a "foreign transplant."

MOOD CHANGES

☐ Quite common during pregnancy, mood changes are thought to be caused by hormonal changes and a deficiency of B vitamins. While for the most part these mood changes must simply be endured, the mother should increase her intake of foods rich in the B vitamins and iron. Inadequate iron intake causes anemia, which can make the mother feel tired, irritable, and unhappy.

MORNING SICKNESS

☐ Approximately 50 percent of all pregnant women experience some degree of nausea and vomiting during the first three months of pregnancy. This is commonly called morning sickness, but it can occur at any time of day.

☐ Do not go without eating or drinking because of the nausea. Mothers suffering from morning sickness should eat small, frequent meals and snack on whole grain crackers with nut butters or cheese. These crackers or whole wheat toast can be kept near the bed and eaten before arising. In addition, during this time the mother should take 50 milligrams of vitamin B₆ every four hours, and in the morning take 400 milligrams of magnesium. However, she should not take these supplements over an excessively long period of time.

☐ The herb ginger, taken in capsule form, is also beneficial. The following herbs, taken in tea form, also help relieve nausea: red raspberry leaf, basil, ginger, and peppermint.

NOSEBLEEDS AND NASAL CONGESTION

☐ During pregnancy, increased blood volume often causes some capillaries to rupture, causing a nosebleed. And, inner nasal passages normally swell. A lack of vitamin C may be a contributing factor. Fortunately, these conditions will disappear with the birth of the baby.

☐ Do not use nasal sprays or nose drops. Instead, use an empty nasal spray container filled with warm water to spray into the nose. This will help to moisten the nose and shrink the membranes.

☐ A humidifier will be helpful at this time.

☐ Increase your intake of vitamin C rich foods such as broccoli, cabbage, grapefruits, lemons, oranges, peppers, and strawberries.

☐ Dairy products tend to stimulate the secretion of mucus. Supplement the diet with dolomite, calcium and magnesium, or bone meal while decreasing dairy product consumption.

SCIATICA

☐ The sciatic nerve is the largest nerve in the body arising from the sacral plexus, leaving the pelvis through the greater sciatic foramen, running through the hip joint and down the back of the thigh. Irritation of this nerve is common during pregnancy and usually disappears with the birth of the baby.

☐ A registered physical therapist or a chiropractor who has been specially trained to deal with pregnancy problems is best able to deal with this problem. Have your health care provider recommend someone.

SKIN PROBLEMS

☐ Common skin problems during pregnancy are pimples, acne, red marks, and mask of pregnancy (dark blotches on the skin of the face). These skin changes will, however, disappear with the birth of the baby.

☐ Five milligrams of folic acid before each meal may help the pregnancy mask to disappear.

☐ Do not use make-up if skin is broken out.

SORENESS IN THE RIB AREA

☐ This soreness often disappears in the last six weeks of pregnancy, once the baby drops into position to be born.

☐ When experiencing this problem, change positions often.

STRETCH MARKS

☐ Stretch marks are wavy reddish stripes appearing on the abdomen, buttocks, breasts, and thighs that gradually turn white. They are caused by the excessive and rapid weight gain typically associated with pregnancy, and appear when the skin becomes overstretched and the fibers in the deep layers tear. Unfortunately, once they appear they are permanent, but they do become much less noticeable.

☐ Stretch marks can be prevented, however, by applying the following recipe externally to the places in which they commonly appear.

½ cup virgin olive oil
¼ cup aloe vera gel
6 capsules vitamin E or vitamin E oil, cut open
4 capsules vitamin A or vitamin A oil, cut open

Mix all ingredients in a blender, store in a jar, and refrigerate. Apply daily.

☐ Elastin cream is also very good for stretch marks.

SWEATING

☐ At this time, your body is making sure that its temperature is perfect for your baby's development. You should dress accordingly by wearing loose, light, comfortable clothing.

☐ Do not use a hot tub during pregnancy. This increase in body temperture can often cause the baby to go into fetal distress.

Tests Performed During Pregnancy

There are many tests that can be performed during pregnancy to determine the health of the unborn child. However, many of these tests bring risk to the mother and the baby. Therefore, they should be applied only when medically indicated and not routinely for the mother's or the doctor's convenience. If a test is suggested, be sure that you are fully aware of why it is needed and of any dangers that may be involved before making a decision.

AMNIOCENTESIS

This medical procedure is performed during pregnancy to determine the health of an unborn baby. A local anesthetic is given to the mother and then a long, hollow needle is inserted into the pregnant uterus to remove amniotic fluid for cellular analysis. This is a highly risky procedure both to the unborn baby and to the mother. Risks include some chance of blood exchange between the mother and the baby, infection of the amniotic fluid, peritonitis, blood clots, placental hemorrhage, injury to the baby, and premature labor. Therefore, great care must be taken in recommending and then in performing the amniocentesis.

This test can determine the sex of the baby, but should definitely not be performed only to find this out. This test should be performed only if you plan to terminate the pregnancy if an abnormality is found, or if this knowledge will alter your prenatal care.

CHORIONIC VILLI SAMPLING (CVS)

The chorionic villi are finger-like projections of the embryonic sac that contain cells that have the same genetic composition as the embryo. This new test takes a small sample of this chorionic tissue to determine genetic abnormalities in the fetus. It can be performed earlier than amniocentesis, usually between the eighth and tenth weeks of pregnancy, and takes about a half hour to complete.

Possible risks from CVS include infection, maternal or fetal bleeding, spontaneous abortion, Rh immunization, birth defects, and perforation of the membrane surrounding the embryo. Advantages of this test are the quickness of the results and the ability to perform it early in pregnancy. Again, as with all tests, the pluses and minuses must be carefully weighed before making a decision.

ULTRASOUND

Ultrasound is a procedure in which sound is projected off objects through the use of high frequency sound waves. This was originally developed for the space program, but later found uses in prenatal care.

One form of ultrasound, the sonogram or B-scan, directs intermittent sound waves toward the pregnant woman's abdomen. An outline of the baby, placenta, and other structures involved in pregnancy are transmitted to a video screen. In this way, the doctor can determine fetal position, estimate the maturity of the baby, confirm a multiple pregnancy, find the location of the placenta, check the baby's heart rate, and estimate the baby's due date.

Ultrasound, though effective and safer than x-ray, has not yet been determined by the U.S. Food and Drug Administration as safe for routine use and should be used only when medically indicated.

ESTRIOL EXCRETION STUDIES, NON-STRESS TEST, OXYTOCIN CHALLENGE TEST

These tests are also used to determine the baby's health. The Estriol Excretion Study determines the best time for delivery of the baby in cases of diabetes or other difficulties in pregnancy. The Non-Stress Test determines fetal well-being, and the Oxytocin Challenge Test helps determine how well the baby will undergo the stress of labor.

Your health care provider will discuss all of these tests in depth with you if it is determined that any of them are necessary. Remember that it is your body and your baby. You should be fully informed as to anything that will occur or that might possibly happen.

SWELLING (EDEMA) OF THE HANDS AND FEET

☐ A rise in estrogen in the body causes swelling of the hands and feet. Some swelling is to be expected and is acceptable. However, tell your health care provider about the condition as soon as you notice any swelling. It can be the first stage of toxemia, a serious disease of pregnancy.

☐ Your hands, legs, and feet may get puffy and swollen. Be sure to remove your rings when this happens. Do not wait, or the rings may have to be cut off.

☐ Avoid all highly processed foods, while maintaining a well-balanced high protein diet. Do not take diuretics (water pills).

☐ Wear loose, comfortable clothing. Be sure to wear properly fitting shoes, which may be larger than your normal size. However, once the baby arrives, your feet will return to normal. In addition, do not sit with a weight, such as another child, on your lap, as this impedes circulation.

☐ Walking one mile a day helps to keep this condition under control.

URINATION (FREQUENT)

☐ Frequent urination is a natural by-product of the early and late months of pregnancy and, as a side benefit, prepares you for the upcoming nightly trips to the baby's room.

☐ Do not cut down on fluid intake. Drink six to eight glasses of fluid a day.

VARICOSE VEINS

☐ Varicose veins are enlarged veins close to the surface of the skin which usually disappear after the birth of the baby. The following suggestions will help alleviate the condition:

● Do not wear restrictive knee socks, garters, belts, or high-heeled shoes.
● Do not stand for long periods of time or sit in cross-legged positions. Change positions frequently.
● As often as you can, sit with your feet up higher than your heart.
● Wear support hose if your health care provider recommends them. Keep them near your bed and put them on before you get out of bed.
● Walking one mile a day is very helpful.

☐ *See also* VARICOSE VEINS in Part Two.

NUTRITIONAL HEALTH IN PREGNANCY

It is important to have a balanced diet high in nutrients and fiber and low in bad fats and cholesterol. The following is a list of nutrients for maintaining health in pregnancy.

NUTRIENTS

SUPPLEMENT	SUGGESTED DOSAGE	COMMENTS
Very Important		
Folic acid	800 mcg	
Iron (Floradix formula)	30 mg	Floradix formula is a good source of iron.
Protein supplement from a vegetable source		Lack of protein has been linked to deformities in the baby.
Vitamin B complex		
Vitamin C	2,000–4,000 mg	Larger doses taken before delivery may help reduce labor pain by 50 percent.

Helpful		
Acidophilus or some form of "friendly" bacteria		
Calcium and	1,500 mg	
magnesium	750 mg	
Kelp	5 tablets daily.	
Multimineral and trace minerals		
Selenium	3 mcg per lb of body weight.	May play a role in protecting the lung tissue in the infant.
Vitamin A	25,000 IU	Take in beta-carotene form.
Vitamin D	1,000 IU	
Vitamin E	400 IU	Premature and low birth weight infants are often deficient in vitamin E.
Vitamin K (alfalfa tablets)		Take for excessive bleeding.

Herbs

☐ Red raspberry leaf tea helps the uterus contract more effectively. Drink more of this tea during the last six weeks of pregnancy. Shepherd's-purse helps uterine contractions at birth. Nettle leaves is a good tonic to use also during pregnancy.

☐ We also recommend as an herbal combination, squaw vine (aids in childbirth), licorice, and damiana.

Recommendations

☐ Consult your doctor about the use of any supplements and medications. When pregnant, avoid the following medications, which stunt fetal growth: Alka-Seltzer, antihistamines, cold pills, cough remedies, Datril, decongestants, Di-Gel, estrogens, Gelusil, Maalox, mineral oil (blocks the absorption of the fat-soluble vitamins), Pepto-Bismol, Rolaids, Tums, and Tylenol.

☐ The drugs Dilantin and phenobarbital, used for epileptic seizures, have four times the usual risk of producing babies with heart defects. In addition, the drugs ampicillin and tetracycline may cause fatal heart malformations.

☐ Aspirin has been linked with fetal deformities, bleeding, and death.

☐ Asparatame (*see* the NutraSweet inset in CHEMICAL ALLERGIES, Part Two) and phenylalanine may alter brain growth in the fetus (Medical World News).

☐ Accutane, used for acne, can cause birth defects (Harvard Medical School Health Letter). Also avoid Tegison, which is used for psoriasis.

☐ Large quantities of caffeine cause birth defects.

☐ A well-balanced, nutritious diet plus moderate exercise, fresh air, and rest should be maintained.

☐ Do not consume junk food, highly seasoned or fried foods, alcohol, or coffee. Do not smoke or use drugs, except as prescribed.

Considerations

☐ Three to five percent of all pregnant women develop gestational diabetes. This occurs during the second half of pregnancy. A screening between the twenty-fourth and twenty-eighth weeks of pregnancy should, therefore, be performed for gestational diabetes.

☐ Lack of zinc, manganese, and folic acid and an imbalance of proteins have been linked to fetal deformities and mental retardation.

Premenstrual Syndrome

Premenstrual syndrome (PMS) is a disorder that affects menstruating women one to two weeks before the menstrual cycle begins. Symptoms can include any or all of the following: depression, cramps, water retention, skin eruptions, headaches, bloated abdomen, backache, breast swelling and tenderness, insomnia, fatigue, nervousness, joint pain, fainting spells, and changes in personality (such as outbursts of anger, violence, and thoughts of suicide). PMS has been linked to food allergies, candidiasis, and malabsorption.

Unfortunately, some women have been diagnosed as mentally ill when vitamin therapy, exercise, and change of diet was all that was needed. One of the causes of PMS is a hormone imbalance—excessive estrogen levels and inadequate progesterone levels. Low blood sugar (hypoglycemia) is also an important factor. Fluid retention affects the blood flow, reducing the oxygen in the uterus, ovaries, and brain.

NUTRIENTS

SUPPLEMENT	SUGGESTED DOSAGE	COMMENTS
Very Important		
Calcium with magnesium chloride	1,500 mg 1,000 mg	Relieves cramping, backache, and nervousness.
Primrose oil	2 capsules 3 times daily.	Contains GLA, an essential fatty acid.
Vitamin B complex plus extra	100 mg 3 times daily.	
vitamin B$_6$ (pyridoxine) and	50 mg 3 times daily.	B$_6$ reduces water retention.
pantothenic acid (B$_5$) and	100–200 mg	B$_5$ reduces stress and is needed by the adrenal gland.
B$_{12}$ lozenges	200 mcg twice daily.	B$_{12}$ reduces stress.
Vitamin E	Start with 400 IU; increase slowly to 800 IU.	Good for sore breasts. Improves oxygen utilization and limits free radical damage.
Important		
Corn silk or KB herbs	2 with meals.	An herbal formula that removes excess water from the tissues.
Helpful		
Choline plus inositol and methionine	1 g each.	Aids in nerve impulse transmission. Prevents estrogen-related cancers.
Chromium	200 mcg daily.	Stabilizes blood sugar levels.
Iron (Floradix formula)	As directed on label.	Easily assimilated iron formula.
Kelp	4 tablets daily.	A good mineral source.
L-Lysine	500 mg daily.	Start 5 days before menstrual period for those who suffer from hypoglycemia and/or herpes.
L-Tyrosine	500 mg twice daily.	Needed to reduce anxiety, depression, and headache.
Multivitamin and mineral complex with manganese	As directed on label.	Needed for relief of symptoms.
Vitamin C with bioflavonoids	3,000 mg in divided doses.	Aids in relief of discomfort and breast swelling. Also boosts the immune system.
Vitamin D	As directed on label.	Needed for uptake of calcium and magnesium.

HERBS

☐ Dong quai relieves PMS symptoms including pain, bloating, vaginal dryness, and depression. Blessed thistle, cayenne, kelp, raspberry leaves, sarsaparilla, and squaw vine are also good for PMS. Siberian ginseng effectively alleviates premenstrual symptoms; however, do not use if you are hypoglycemic.

RECOMMENDATIONS

☐ Do not consume salt, caffeine, alcohol, red meats, dairy products, sugar in any form, processed foods, or junk or fast foods. Do not smoke.

☐ The thyroid gland's function should be evaluated. A significant number of women who suffer with PMS have some sort of thyroid dysfunction. *See* the self-test in HYPOTHYROID, Part Two.

☐ The effectiveness of oral contraceptives is sharply reduced when taking antibiotics. Estrogen-type hormones should not be used if any of the following are present: breast cancer, pregnancy, abnormal vaginal bleeding, or phlebitis (inflammation of leg veins).

CONSIDERATIONS

☐ A few days of fasting using fresh juice and spirulina before menstruation begins will help alleviate the PMS symptoms. (*See* FASTING in Part Three.)

☐ Eat plenty of fresh fruits and vegetables, whole grains, cereals and breads, beans, peas, lentils, nuts and seeds, and broiled chicken, turkey, and fish. Have high-protein snacks between meals.

☐ A food allergy test and a hair analysis to rule out heavy metal intoxication are recommended.

☐ Drink one quart of distilled water daily, starting a week before the menstrual period and ending one week after.

☐ *See also* ALLERGIES in Part Two and HAIR ANALYSIS in Part Three.

Prostate Disorders

The prostate is the most common site of disorders in the male genitourinary system. The most significant of these disorders are prostatitis, benign hypertrophy of the prostate, and cancer. Frequent and increased urination (especially at night), difficulty in urinating, lessening of the force of flow, and an accompanying burning sensation are all symptoms of prostate problems.

The prostate is a doughnut-shaped male sex gland, positioned beneath the urinary bladder. It encircles the urinary outlet, or urethra. Contraction of the muscles in the prostate squeeze fluids into the urethral tract during ejaculation. These prostatic fluids are ingredients in semen.

Prostatitis, common in men of all ages, is the acute or chronic inflammation of the prostate gland. The usual cause is a bacterial infection from another area of the body which has invaded the prostate. Prostatitis can partially or totally block the flow of urine out of the bladder, resulting in urine retention. This causes the bladder to become distended, weak, tender, and suscep-

tible to infection as a result of the increased amount of bacteria in the retained urine. Infection in the bladder is easily transmitted up the ureters to the kidneys.

Symptoms of acute prostatitis are pain between the scrotum and rectum, fever, frequent urination accompanied by a burning sensation, and blood or pus in the urine. Symptoms of chronic prostatitis are frequent and burning urination with blood in the urine, lower back pain, and impotence. As prostatitis becomes more advanced, urination becomes more difficult.

Benign hypertrophy of the prostate occurs in approximately one third of all men over fifty years of age. It is the result of gradual enlargement of the prostate. While not cancerous, benign hypertrophy of the prostate can cause disability and even serious illness if left untreated. When the prostate becomes too large, it presses against the urethral canal. This interferes with normal urination and backs up in the kidneys. As a result, the kidneys become damaged by both the pressure and the contaminated urine. Kidney infection is likely to occur when the kidneys are filled with this contaminated urine. Bladder infections such as cystitis, which are associated with prostatitis, are likely as well.

Symptoms of enlargement of the prostate include the need to pass urine frequently during the night, with frequency increasing as time goes on. There can be pain, burning, and difficulty in starting and stopping urination, as well.

Cancer of the prostate is the third most common malignancy in men, following cancers of the lung and colon. It rarely occurs in men under sixty years of age. Because symptoms are vague, nearly 90 percent of prostatic cancer remains undetected until it has spread beyond the most easily treated stage.

Symptoms of early cancer of the prostate are similar to symptoms of benign hypertrophy of the prostate. They are blood in the urine, or reddish or pink urine; difficulty in starting urination; increasing frequency of arising at night to pass urine; and a burning sensation during urination. A history of venereal disease or repeated prostatic infections has been linked to developing cancer of the prostate. Family history does not appear to play a part. Cancer of the prostate changes the way the prostate feels when it is examined rectally. The usual rubbery firm consistency hardens to a wood-like firmness. Confirmation of cancer of the prostate must be done by a physician. All men over forty-five years of age should have a thorough prostate examination every three years.

In cases of prostatitis and benign hypertrophy of the prostate, treatment with antibiotics and analgesics may be necessary. Treatment of cancer of the prostate may require surgery.

NUTRIENTS

SUPPLEMENT	SUGGESTED DOSAGE	COMMENTS
Essential		
Zinc	80 mg daily.	A zinc deficiency has been linked to prostatitis.
Very Important		
Bee pollen	6 tablets or 2 tsp. raw bee pollen.	Begin with a small amount; increase gradually.
Essential fatty acids	2 capsules 3 times daily.	Important in prostate function.
Garlic capsules (Kyolic)	2 capsules 3 times daily.	Odorless garlic that acts as a natural antibiotic.
Prostate tablets (raw glandular)	As directed on label.	Normalizes prostate function.
Vitamin A	25,000 IU (At least 15,000 IU beta-carotene.)	Potent antioxidant and immune system enhancer.
Vitamin E	600 IU	Potent antioxidant and immune system enhancer.
Helpful		
Brewer's yeast and/or pumpkin seeds	As directed on label.	Good sources of zinc.
Kelp	6 tablets daily.	Supplies necessary minerals for improved prostate function.
Lecithin	Take before meals.	For prostate cellular protection.
Magnesium plus calcium	As directed on label.	Supplies necessary minerals for improved prostate function.
Vitamin B$_6$ (pyridoxine) plus B-complex vitamins	50 mg twice daily.	B$_6$ has anti-cancer properties.
Vitamin C	1,000–5,000 mg daily.	Promotes immune function and aids healing.

HERBS

☐ Acute inflammation or enlargement of the prostate gland will often respond to certain herbal teas, but if no improvement takes place or if the symptoms recur, consult a urologist.

☐ A decoction of equal quantities of gravel root, sea holly, and hydrangea root, of which three to four tablespoonfuls are taken three times daily, will ease inflammation and reduce the discomfort of urination. Marshmallow leaves may be added to this mixture for their demulcent properties if burning and heat persist. Other helpful teas are made from the diuretic herb buchu (do not boil) and from corn silk.

☐ Horsetail is astringent and can be used if small amounts of blood are passed and for frequent urination at night. Combine it with hydrangea for greater effect on an enlarged gland. Other helpful herbs for these symptoms are goldenseal root (diuretic and antiseptic); parsley, juniper berries, uva ursi, and slippery elm bark (diuretics and genitourinary tract tonics); and ginseng (a tonic for male reproductive organs).

RECOMMENDATIONS

☐ For prostatitis increase fluid intake. Drink two to three quarts of spring or distilled water daily to stimulate urine flow. This prevents retention, cystitis, and kidney infection.

☐ Prostate cancer is one of several common cancers that have been confirmed in the laboratory as being diet related. Therefore, diet is important in prevention. Maintain a whole food diet. Regular intake of zinc (15 milligrams daily) and polyunsaturated fatty acids (three to six capsules daily) in later life may help prevent development of problems. Use cold-pressed oils such as sesame seed, safflower, or olive oils to obtain fatty acids. Consume more nuts and seeds, raw vegetables, fruits, fresh juices, dried beans, peas, and brown rice. Avoid refined carbohydrates, coffee, strong tea, and alcohol. These have been linked to cancer of the prostate. Too much fat in the diet may result in prostate cancer as well. Chemical reactions occur when fat is cooked, leading to the production of free radicals. It is believed that these reactions play a major role in this cancer.

☐ Exercise is important, but do not ride a bicycle. Walking is good exercise. Avoid exposure to very cold weather.

☐ Hydrotherapy effectively increases circulation in the prostate region. One method involves sitting in a tub that contains the hottest water tolerable for fifteen to thirty minutes once or twice a day. Another form of hydrotherapy involves spraying the lower abdomen and pelvic area with warm and cold water, alternating three minutes hot, one minute cold. Another technique using hydrotherapy involves sitting in hot water while emersing the feet in cold water for three minutes, and then sitting in cold water while emersing the feet in hot water for one minute.

☐ Eat one ounce of pumpkin seeds or take pumpkin seed oil capsules as directed daily. Raw pumpkin seeds eaten daily are helpful for almost all prostate troubles because they are rich in zinc.

CONSIDERATIONS

☐ Sexual intercourse while the prostate is infected and irritated may further irritate the prostate and delay recovery.

☐ Vasectomy has been linked to prostate disorders and cancer.

☐ Zinc deficiency has been linked to enlargement of the prostate. Soil used for farming is often deficient in zinc, and unless we eat husks of cereals or brewer's yeast, it is difficult to get much zinc in the diet.

☐ The new drug leuprolide may shrink enlarged prostates. Some of the side effects that can occur with the use of leuprolide are impotence, decreased libido, and even hot flashes. This drug should be taken only by men who are not concerned with potency.

☐ According to the August 1989 issue of the *Medical Tribune*, the risk of prostate cancer for males who have undergone a vasectomy is three times greater than that of males who have not had a vasectomy.

Psoriasis

Psoriasis appears as patches of silvery scales or red areas on legs, knees, arms, elbows, scalp, ears, and back. The toes and fingernails lose their luster and develop ridges and pits. Often hereditary, it is linked to a rapid growth of cells in the skin's outer layer. It may result from a faulty utilization of fat. Psoriasis is most common between the ages of fifteen and twenty-five, and is not infectious. Attacks can be triggered by nervous tension and stress, illness, surgery, cuts, poison ivy, several viral and bacterial infections, sunburn, or the drugs lithium, chloroquine, and beta-blockers.

Only the scales and skin debris, which are quite itchy, can be removed. There is presently no known cure. The disease seems to lessen during the summer months. It may go away on its own, but once you have had psoriasis, it is always possible that it will return.

NUTRIENTS

SUPPLEMENT	SUGGESTED DOSAGE	COMMENTS
Essential		
Unsaturated fatty acids (primrose oil)	1 capsule 3 times daily.	Unsaturated fatty acids are important for all skin disorders. Aids in preventing dryness.
Very Important		
Proteolytic enzymes	Take between meals.	Stimulates protein synthesis and repair.
Vitamin A emulsion	100,000 IU for 1 month; then decrease to 50,000 IU or capsules.	Essential for healthy skin and nails. Emulsion form allows quicker absorption. Essential for normal skin and nails.
Vitamin B complex plus B₁₂ lozenges and folic acid and thiamine (B₁) and pantothenic acid (B₅) and B₆ (pyridoxine)	50 mg 3 times daily.	Necessary in all cellular functions. An antistress vitamin. Helps to maintain healthy skin.
Vitamin C	2,000–10,000 mg	Important for collagen and connective tissue.
Vitamin D	400–1,000 IU	Needed for healing of skin and for calcium uptake.
Vitamin E emulsion	As directed on label.	Neutralizes free radicals that damage the skin. Emulsion form allows quick absorption.
Important		
Kelp	5 tablets daily.	Supplies balanced minerals. Good source of iodine.
Zinc	50–100 mg daily.	Protein metabolism depends on zinc. Protein is needed for healing.
Helpful		
Lipotropic factors or lecithin	1 tbsp. with meals or 2 capsules.	These are fat emulsifiers. Lecithin protects the cells.
Multivitamin and mineral complex containing magnesium and calcium chelate	Use as directed on label.	Needed for basic vitamins and minerals.

HERBS

☐ Use dandelion, goldenseal, sarsaparilla, and yellow dock. Lavender is excellent to use in a sauna or steam bath because it stimulates new cell growth. Poultices made from chaparral, dandelion, and yellow dock can help psoriasis.

RECOMMENDATIONS

☐ Avoid fats (milk, cream, butter, eggs), sugar, processed foods, white flour, and citrus fruits. Fish oil or primrose oil interferes with the production and storage of arachidonic acid (AA), a natural inflammatory substance that makes the lesions of psoriasis turn red and swell. Avoid red meat and dairy products because they contain AA.

☐ Eat a 50 percent raw foods diet. Oils made from sesame seeds, flaxseed, or soybeans are important. Fish should be added to the diet.

☐ Apply sea water with cotton several times a day to affected areas. Linseed oil has helped many people—take one tablet or three capsules daily for unsaturated fatty acid. If a tar shampoo is prescribed, do *not* use for a long period of time. Add two teaspoons of ginger to bath water.

MEDICAL UPDATES

☐ The drug methotrexate is effective and popular with patients. Another drug, hydroxyurea, and drugs called retinoids are under study but also have side effects. Cyclosporine drug therapy is being tested with good results. A study of a new drug called Rocaltrol by Boston University reported improvement in patients when applied directly to the skin. *All of these drugs have potentially serious side effects.*

☐ The freezing of moderately sized psoriasis lesions using liquid nitrogen is being tested, with good results. Moderate sunlight also usually helps.

☐ A skin patch called Actiderm is being manufactured by ConvaTec/Squibb. This makes the most common psoriasis medication and steroid (cortisone) ointments more effective. The patch gives better results with milder steroids and fewer doses. Steroids may have adverse side effects.

☐ Activated vitamin D, available by prescription only, helps those with severe forms of the disease. For more information send a self-addressed stamped envelope to: Dr. Michael Holick, Boston University Medical School, Building M, Room 1013, 80 East Concord Street, Boston, MA 02118.

☐ The drug Legison, used for stubborn cases of psoriasis, can cause bone spurs in the knees and ankles. One study found that 84 percent of those using this drug for five years had bony build-ups causing stiffness and restriction of movement.

☐ Long-wave ultraviolet light (UVA) has been effectively used to treat psoriasis, but skin cancer may be a side effect. Oxsoralen-Ultra, a liquid drug, is also widely used.

Radiation Poisoning

The human body must be protected from radioactive particles found in the air and in contaminated food and water. Radioactive substances are made up of unstable atoms that can harm the body. Even if only one cell were exposed to radiation, the radiation could destroy, damage, or alter the make-up of that cell. When the energy released by the radioactive element is strong enough to dislodge electrons from other atoms or molecules in its path, it will damage living tissue. This type of radiation is called ionizing radiation. Alteration of cell structure by radioactive particles can lead to the development of cancer. Because all cells carry DNA material, mutated cells can be passed to offspring through reproduction.

A radioactive element is structurally similar to its nonradioactive counterpart, differing only in the number of neutrons it contains. If you do not obtain sufficient amounts of calcium, potassium, and other nutrients in your diet, the body will absorb the radioactive elements that are similar in structure to these nutrients. For example, if an individual is not obtaining proper amounts of calcium, his body will absorb radioactive strontium-90 or other elements that are similar in structure to calcium instead. If the body obtains sufficient amounts of potassium in the diet, it will not retain radioactive cesium-137, which is similar to potassium. If the cells are able to obtain all the nutrients they need from the diet, they will not need to absorb their radioactive substitutes; the radioactive substances are more likely to be discarded from the body.

Many patients are injected with radioactive elements designed to trace a problem area so that more accurate diagnoses can be made. Common sources of radiation are medical and dental x-rays (see the section on x-ray radiation at the end of this entry), building materials containing radon or uranium, cellular phones, computers with video display terminals, electronic games, microwave ovens, radar devices, satellite dishes, smoke detectors, and tobacco. Symptoms associated with the use of these products include cataracts, dizziness, fatigue, severe headache, and nausea.

RADIATION THERAPIES

In order to protect the body from radioactive elements, it is necessary to obtain the proper amounts of nutrients, so that their radioactive counterparts will not be needed. Certain foods and nutritional supplements, which act as chelating agents, can also help by drawing these radioactive elements out of the body.

Radioactive Iodine-131

Because iodine is needed by the thyroid to produce hormones, it helps to regulate body processes. If the amount of iodine in the diet is insufficient, the body

---

Free Radicals

One of the dangers of radiation is that it encourages the formation of free radicals. A free radical is an atom or group of atoms that has at least one unpaired electron. Because another element can easily pick up this free electron and cause a chemical reaction, these free radicals can effect dramatic changes in the body. Hydrogen peroxide is an example of an unstable substance involved in free radical reactions. Because these free radicals are highly volatile, they can cause a lot of damage.

Free radicals are normally present in the body in small numbers. Biochemical processes naturally lead to the formation of free radicals, and under normal circumstances the body can keep them in check; however, exposing the body to ionizing radiation activates the formation of free radicals. The formation of a large number of free radicals stimulates the formation of more free radicals, leading to greater instability.

Damage is incurred due to excessive radical formation. The presence of a dangerous number of free radicals can alter the way in which the cells code genetic material. Changes in protein structure can occur as a result of errors in protein synthesis. The body's immune system may then see this altered protein as a foreign substance and try to destroy it. The formation of mutated proteins can eventually damage the immune system and lead to leukemia and cancer, as well as a host of other diseases.

In addition to damaging genetic material, free radicals can destroy the protective layer of fat in the cell membrane. The formation of free radicals can also lead to retention of fluid in the cells, which is involved in the aging process. Calcium levels in the body may be upset as well.

In addition to radiation, the diet can also contribute to the formation of free radicals. When the body obtains nutrients through the diet, it utilizes oxygen and these nutrients to create energy. In this oxidation process, oxygen molecules containing unpaired electrons are released. These oxygen free radicals can cause damage to the body if produced in extremely large amounts. A diet that is high in fat can increase free radical activity. Oxidation occurs more readily in fat molecules than it does in carbohydrate or protein molecules. Cooking fats at high temperatures, particularly frying foods in oil, can produce high numbers of free radicals. Supplementing the diet with antioxidants such as the enzymes superoxide dismutase and glutathione peroxidase, vitamins A, C, and E, and the trace minerals selenium and germanium can inhibit the formation of these free radicals by pairing up their free electrons. By preventing free radical formation, antioxidants help to detoxify the body. *See* ANTIOXIDANTS in Part One for information on supplements that act as antioxidants.

---

will supply the thyroid with radioactive iodine-131 instead. The body is exposed to radioactive iodine-131 due to atmospheric contamination of food and water. The presence of radioactive iodine-131 in the thyroid can damage nearby cells, decrease the functioning ability of the thyroid, and lead to cancer.

Many were exposed to radioactive iodine fallout as a result of the nuclear disaster in Chernobyl. In order to protect the body from this dangerous radioactive element, victims of the incident were given large amounts of iodine. If the thyroid was in need of iodine, it would absorb the radioactive iodine salts; however, if the body was saturated with iodine, there would be no need for iodine, and less radioactivity would occur in the thyroid gland. Iodine-131 is prevalent in milk due to exposure of cows and goats to radioactive (and acid) rain in the fields.

NUTRIENTS

SUPPLEMENT	SUGGESTED DOSAGE	COMMENTS
Very Important		
Calcium and magnesium	1,500 mg 750 mg	Protects against radiation.
Coenzyme Q$_{10}$	60 mg daily.	Japanese research has found that this substance protects against many chemicals and radiation.
Germanium	200 mg daily.	A potent anti-cancer substance.
Kelp	5–10 tablets or 2 tsp. granules daily.	All the essential minerals, especially iodine, protect against radiation poisoning.
Vitamin C plus bioflavonoids and rutin	2,000–10,000 mg daily.	A powerful free radical scavenger. *See* ASCORBIC ACID FLUSH in Part Three.
Vitamin E	Start at 400 IU; increase slowly to 800 IU.	Neutralizes harmful free radicals.
Important		
Garlic capsules (Kyolic)	2 capsules 3 times daily.	Odorless garlic that acts as a powerful immunostimulant and protector.
L-Cysteine and L-methionine (amino acids)	500 mg each of L-cysteine and L-methionine taken on an empty stomach with juice. Vitamins B$_6$ and C enhance absorption of these amino acids. Do not take with milk.	Potent detoxifiers that help protect the liver. Important for protection against radiation and pollution.

275

Lecithin	1 tbsp. 3 times daily or in capsule form, taken before meals.	Necessary for cell protection.
Raw thyroid extract or tablets	As directed on label.	A glandular for thyroid protection.
Vitamin B complex	100 mg with meals twice daily.	For cellular function and protection.
Helpful		
Brewer's yeast or Bio-Strath	As directed on label.	Contains a balance of nutrients, B vitamins, and important minerals.
Multivitamin and mineral complex	As directed on label.	For cellular protection.

Recommendations

☐ Supplement your diet with pectin, found in apples, and kelp (seaweed). Kelp is an iodine-rich food. The element sodium alginate, which is also found in seaweed, acts as a chelating agent. It protects the body from the harmful effects of radiation by binding with the radioactive elements, and then excretes them from the body. Also eat plenty of broccoli, Brussels sprouts, cabbage, and cauliflower.

☐ Use soured milk products such as yogurt, buttermilk, and kefir milk. These contain the friendly *lactobacillus* bacteria that protect the gastrointestinal tract. They have also been found to protect against radiation.

Strontium-90 Radiation

Strontium-90 is a radioactive element that is similar in structure to calcium. Due to nuclear testing, strontium-90 has contaminated the earth. Tragically, this radioactive element has accumulated in our bones and teeth. Making sure that the diet contains adequate amounts of calcium can protect the body from strontium-90 radiation poisoning; studies indicate that the body will retain and use strontium-90 only if sufficient amounts of calcium are not available. Radioactive contamination with strontium-90 is associated with anemia, bone cancer (sarcoma) and many other forms of cancer, and leukemia. To protect against strontium-90 radiation poisoning, include the following supplements in your radiation therapy program.

NUTRIENTS

SUPPLEMENT	SUGGESTED DOSAGE	COMMENTS
Helpful		
Brewer's yeast or Bio-Strath	As directed on label.	Contains important basic nutrients.

Calcium and magnesium (chelate)	2,000 mg daily. 1,000 mg daily.	Counteracts strontium-90. Calcium and magnesium should be taken in a 2-to-1 ratio.
Coenzyme Q$_{10}$ and germanium	60 mg daily. 200 mg daily.	Coenzyme Q$_{10}$ and germanium are important free radical scavengers.
Garlic capsules (Kyolic)	2 capsules 3 times daily.	Odorless garlic. A potent immunostimulant.
Kelp	5 tablets daily.	Contains necessary minerals, especially iodine and calcium, for protection against accumulation of strontium-90.
L-Cysteine and L-methionine (amino acids)	As directed on label.	Protects against the harmful effects of radioactivity and pollution.
Lecithin	1 tbsp. with meals or 2 capsules daily.	Protects the cell membrane.
Multivitamin and mineral complex (high potency formula)	As directed on label.	Essential to basic radiation protection.
Selenium	200 mcg daily.	An important antioxidant.
Superoxide dismutase (SOD) from Biotec Foods	As directed on label.	A powerful free radical scavenger.
Vitamin B complex (high stress formula)	100 mg daily.	Needed for all cellular enzyme systems.
Vitamin C	2,000–10,000 mg daily in divided doses.	Vitamins C and E neutralize and destroy free radicals formed by radiation.
Vitamin E	Start at 200 IU; increase slowly to 800 IU.	Protects the cells from free radical formation.

Recommendations

Supplement the diet with pectin (found in apples), seaweed, and sunflower seeds. Pectin binds with strontium-90. Eliminate all dairy products, except for yogurt and soured products. Milk and dairy products are major sources of dietary strontium-90 in the United States. Crops fed to cows have often been irrigated with water contaminated with strontium-90.

X-Ray Radiation

Today a dental check-up typically includes x-rays to locate cavities. Physicians take x-rays to determine whether a bone is broken, to check cardiovascular and respiratory health, and to locate brain tumors and areas of dysfunction. Women are urged to have regular mammograms for early detection of breast cancer. Despite the widespread use of x-rays, dentists, physicians, chiropractors, and hospitals have often ignored the potential danger and long-term effects of small amounts of radiation. Sterility, tissue damage, cancer, and leukemia are among the risks for those exposed to low levels of radiation from x-rays. Women who are exposed to x-rays while pregnant are at a higher risk of having a miscarriage or delivering a baby with birth defects.

Cancer research indicates that a significant percentage of women in the United States have inherited a gene, oncogene AC, that is sensitive to x-ray exposure; in these women, even short periods of x-ray exposure can lead to the development of cancer.

The dosage of x-ray exposure is measured in units called roentgens (pronounced rent-kins). The National Academy of Science has reported that exposure to ten milliroentgens from x-rays increases the cancer rate. This is the same amount of radiation that the chest is exposed to during a tuberculosis chest x-ray. Mammography uses a much lower dose of x-rays. Because mounting evidence suggests that there may be *no* safe level of radiation, avoid x-rays unless absolutely necessary. Prolonged exposure to radiation destroys the body's immune system.

To protect against radiation from x-rays, follow the supplement program below.

NUTRIENTS

SUPPLEMENT	SUGGESTED DOSAGE	COMMENTS
Very Important		
Coenzyme Q$_{10}$	100 mg daily.	Researchers in Japan have found that coenzyme Q$_{10}$ protects the body from harmful radiation.
Kelp	6 tablets daily or obtain from a seaweed food source.	Protects against radiation.
L-Cysteine and L-methionine and L-glutathione (amino acids)		Detoxifies harmful substances. Protects against the harmful effects of radiation.
Important		
Garlic capsules (Kyolic)	2 tablets 3 times daily.	Stimulates and protects the immune system.
Germanium	200 mg daily.	Enhances immune function.
Oxy-5000 from American Biologics	As directed on label.	This antioxidant is high in SOD.
Pantothenic acid (B$_5$)	200 mg before and after x-ray exposure; 50 mg daily thereafter.	Protects against the harmful effects of radiation.
Selenium	200 mcg daily.	A free radical scavenger that protects against cancer.
Vitamin C	3,000–10,000 mg daily.	Vitamin C complex, which is high in rutin (200 mg), is best. Vitamin C protects the immune system.
Helpful		
Brewer's yeast	As directed on label.	A natural source of pantothenic acid, as well as the other B vitamins.
Inositol plus	100 mg daily.	Protects against the harmful effects of radiation.
B-complex vitamins	50 mg 3 times daily.	
Lecithin	1 tbsp. with meals.	Protects cell membranes from radiation.
Vitamin A	25,000 IU daily.	Vitamins A and E protect and strengthen the immune system.
Vitamin E	400–1,000 IU daily.	
Zinc	50–80 mg daily.	Helps increase immunity. Research has shown that doses of up to 100 mg zinc aid the immune system, while doses greater than 100 mg depress the immune system.

Herbs

☐ The herb chapparal helps protect against harmful radiation.

Recommendations

☐ Include apples in the diet; they are a good source of pectin, which binds with radioactive particles. Also use buckwheat, which is high in rutin, a part of the vitamin C complex that protects against radiation. Cold-pressed safflower and olive oils, avocados, and lemons are also beneficial. These supply essential fatty acids.

Considerations

☐ *See also* WEAKENED IMMUNE SYSTEM, Part Two.

☐ Drinking distilled water is healthful.

Raynaud's Disease

Raynaud's disease affects the circulatory system and results in hands and feet that are hypersensitive to the cold. The small arteries that supply the toes and fingers become very sensitive to cold and suddenly contract. Lack of oxygenated blood causes the fingers or toes to become a whitish or bluish hue. Symptoms come on quickly and result in the affected area's shrinking. Ulcers form, damaging the tissues and resulting in chronic infection under and around the fingernails and toenails. Gangrene may result from prolonged contraction of the arteries.

Causes include Buerger's disease (a nerve disorder) and certain drugs that affect the blood vessels such as channel blockers, ergot preparations, antihypertensives, and alpha- and beta-adrenergic blockers.

NUTRIENTS

SUPPLEMENT	SUGGESTED DOSAGE	COMMENTS
Essential		
Coenzyme Q_{10}	60 mg daily.	Improves tissue oxygenation.
Vitamin E emulsion or capsules	Start with 200 IU, and increase slowly to 1,000 IU.	Use emulsified form for rapid and safe assimilation. Improves circulation. Acts as an anticoagulant, dissolving clots in the legs, heart, and lungs.
Very Important		
Chlorophyll (Kyo-Green)	Liquid or pill form; a fresh green drink made from green leafy vegetables.	Kyo-Green helps reduce the infection and supplies nutrients that enhance blood flow.
Choline and inositol	Use as directed on label.	Lowers cholesterol and helps circulation.
DMG (Gluconic from DaVinci Labs)	1 tablet 3 times daily.	Improves tissue oxygenation.
Germanium	200 mg daily.	Makes oxygen available to tissues and relieves discomfort.
Lecithin	1 tbsp. with meals.	Lowers blood fat.
Vitamin B complex (high potency) plus extra folic acid and vitamin B_6 (pyridoxine) and niacin (B_3)	100 mg daily.	Necessary for metabolism of fat and cholesterol. Niacin dilates small arteries, improving circulation.
Important		
Aerobic 07 from Aerobic Life Products	Use as directed on label.	Improves tissue oxygenation.
Bee propolis or royal jelly		Strengthens the cardiovascular system and acts as a natural antibiotic.

HERBS

☐ Treat with butcher's broom, cayenne, garlic, ginkgo biloba extract, and pau d'arco.

RECOMMENDATIONS

☐ Keep hands and feet warm. A warm climate is best. Wear comfortable shoes and do not go barefoot out-doors. Always wear gloves in cold weather. Avoid stress when possible.

☐ Avoid fatty and fried foods. Include 50 percent raw foods in your diet. *See* NUTRITION, DIET, AND WELLNESS in Part One, and follow the dietary guidelines.

☐ Avoid drugs that constrict the blood vessels such as birth control pills and migraine headache medicine. Drug therapy may be necessary; calcium-channel blockers are currently being used.

☐ Do not smoke.

Reye's Syndrome

Reye's syndrome is a disease that strikes children between the ages of four and fifteen. It occurs after a viral infection, most often the flu or chicken pox. After the child has the infection, he will run a fever and vomit. Convulsions and even coma may follow. This disease may result in brain damage and death. About one-quarter of those who acquire Reye's syndrome die from the disease.

A study done by the Atlanta Center found that 96 percent of the children who had Reye's syndrome had been given aspirin. The study also indicated a correlation between the amount of aspirin taken and the severity of the disease. The greater the amount of aspirin taken, the more severe the disease. The makers of aspirin are now required to alert users to the link between aspirin and this fatal condition.

The symptoms of Reye's syndrome are confusion, seizures, vomiting, weakness and paralysis in the arms or legs, double vision, speech impairment, hearing loss, and coma.

The three warning signs of Reye's syndrome are:

1. Prolonged and heavy vomiting, followed by drowsiness that appears just as the child is starting to recover from the flu or chicken pox.
2. Agitation and delirium.
3. Fatigue and confusion.

Within four days the child may go into a coma. No child has to die of this disease. Awareness of the warning signals and prompt treatment are most important. If the child receives an intravenous solution of glucose (sugar) and electrolytes (salts) within twelve to twenty-four hours after the heavy vomiting starts, he has an excellent chance of survival. This treatment is safe.

Dr. James Huibi, Associate Professor of Pediatrics at the University of Cincinnati, notes that this simple yet

278

highly effective treatment must be given promptly. Parents should be made aware of these serious signs and symptoms.

RECOMMENDATIONS

☐ Some doctors may not be aware of these critical signs and will tell you to give the child aspirin and call him if he doesn't improve. *Don't* be put off. Take the child to the hospital immediately. *Do not give your child aspirin when he has a fever!*

CONSIDERATIONS

☐ The British aspirin industry withdrew all children's aspirin products from the British market last year in response to the aspirin/Reye's link.

☐ *See also* CHICKEN POX, COMMON COLD, and INFLUENZA, all in Part Two.

Rheumatic Fever

Rheumatic fever is an infection resulting from a streptococcal bacteria in the body. It often develops as a complication of the same infection that causes strep throat, tonsillitis, scarlet fever, or ear infection. It most often affects children aged three to eighteen. Left untreated, rheumatic fever may affect one or several parts of the body such as the heart, brain, and joints. The first signs of rheumatic fever are typically pain, inflammation and stiffness in any large joint such as the knee, and fever. The pain and swelling travel from one joint to another. There may be an accompanying skin rash. After one occurrence, there is a tendency for recurrence of the disease.

Antibiotic therapy should be taken to prevent heart damage, so a form of acidophilus is needed to replace the "friendly" bacteria.

The suggested dosages listed in the following table are for those who weigh 100 pounds and over. Adjust the dosage according to weight and age.

NUTRIENTS

SUPPLEMENT	SUGGESTED DOSAGE	COMMENTS
Important		
Garlic capsules (Kyolic)	2 capsules 3 times daily.	A natural antibiotic.
Maxidophilus or Megadophilus or Life Start	As directed on label.	Especially important with antibiotic use. Life Start by Natren is for children.
Vitamin C	*See* ASCORBIC ACID FLUSH in Part Three for correct amounts.	Potentiates immune function and aids in reducing pain and swelling.
Helpful		
Calcium chelate plus magnesium	1,500 mg daily. 1,000 mg daily.	Important nutrients that work together.
Coenzyme Q$_{10}$	100 mg	Potentiates immune system.
Germanium	200 mg	Helps reduce pain and swelling and potentiates the immune system.
Kelp	5 tablets daily.	Contains essential minerals.
Proteolytic enzymes	4–6 tablets between meals.	An important antioxidant. Omit if under age 10.
Vitamin A	25,000 IU daily.	Important antioxidant. Consider the emulsion form for rapid assimilation.
Vitamin B complex	50 mg 3 times daily.	For healing and improved immune function.
Vitamin D or cod liver oil	400 IU or more daily.	Needed for healing and absorption of minerals, especially calcium.
Vitamin E emulsion or capsules	800 IU in emulsion form or in capsules, start with 200 IU daily and increase slowly to 800 IU daily.	Increases tissue oxygenation and reduces fever. Consider vitamin E emulsion for quicker assimilation.

HERBS

☐ Birch leaves help reduce pain.

☐ Catnip tea enemas will reduce fever. (*See* ENEMAS in Part Three.) Drink catnip tea, lobelia, and dandelion. An extract of this herbal combination can be purchased at a health food store to put into juice.

RECOMMENDATIONS

☐ Drink plenty of fresh juices and distilled water. No solid food should be consumed until there is improvement, and then keep to a light diet, including fresh fruits and vegetables with yogurt, cottage cheese, and fruit juices.

☐ *See also* ARTHRITIS, BURSITIS, and FEVER, all in Part Two.

Rheumatoid Arthritis

See ARTHRITIS.

Rickets

This disease of malnutrition is caused by a deficiency of calcium, phosphorus, and vitamin D. This causes the bones to become soft, resulting in deformity. Symptoms include decaying teeth, beads felt along the ribs, bowed legs, a narrowed rib cage, a protruding breast bone, and knock knees. Early signs include nervousness, tetany, leg cramps, and numbness in extremities.

Adults can exhibit rickets (called osteomalacia) when pregnant or breastfeeding or when absorption problems exist. It may also occur in those who do not get enough sunshine or if the diet is so low in fats that adequate bile cannot be manufactured and vitamin D cannot be absorbed.

Be watchful if your child has severe allergies, celiac disease, asthma, bronchitis, or colon disturbances because these conditions often result in absorption problems. This may be difficult to detect at first because growth and weight are normal with these conditions.

Follow the program below. Because of wide age spans, no dosage schedule is given for most supplements. Consult your doctor.

NUTRIENTS

SUPPLEMENT	SUGGESTED DOSAGE	COMMENTS
Essential		
Calcium		Do not use bone meal or dolomite.
Very Important		
Vitamin D		Necessary for utilization of calcium and phosphorus.
Important		
Boron	3 mg daily.	Enhances calcium absorption. For adults only.
Silicon (Silica)	500 mg daily.	Strengthens bones and connective tissue. Aids calcium absorption.
Helpful		
Betaine HCl (hydrochloric acid)		May be needed for proper digestion. For adults only.
Cod liver oil		Good source of vitamins A and D.
Multivitamin and mineral complex with extra vitamin B_{12}		If malabsorption is a problem, take higher amounts of all vitamins and minerals.
Phosphorus		Needed for bone and tooth formation.
Proteolytic enzymes	2 tablets between meals.	Important in digestion. For adults only.
Vitamin A		Necessary for growth.
Zinc		Needed for calcium absorption.

RECOMMENDATIONS

☐ Have a hair analysis done to see what minerals are needed. Food allergy testing may prove beneficial.

☐ Change your diet. Eat more raw fruits and vegetables, raw nuts and seeds, yogurt, and cottage cheese. A diet high in calcium is essential. Do not eat sugar, junk foods, or soda.

Schizophrenia

The two kinds of mental illness are mood disorders and schizophrenic disorders. Those who suffer from mood disorders seem to be normal between episodes. This is not true for victims of schizophrenia, who very seldom behave normally between episodes. The symptoms of schizphrenia are tension, depression, personality problems, fatigue, mental derangement, and hallucinations.

Because it is difficult to diagnose a patient as schizophrenic, treatment proceeds by trial and error, using the dominant symptoms as a guide. When drugs fail as treatment, electroconvulsive treatment (ECT) is used. The drug lithium is often used to treat schizophrenia, and some patients who have used it have shown improvement.

The mildest schizophrenic disorder is paranoid or schizotypal personality, and the most severe is chronic deteriorating schizophrenia. Some researchers believe that schizophrenia is hereditary, or that it results from complications during birth, head injuries, a reaction to a virus, or environmental poisons that have reached the brain. Childhood head injuries and birth complications do appear at a high rate in schizophrenic patients.

Schizophrenia and pellagra (niacin—vitamin B_3—deficiency) have been linked by psychiatrists. *See* PELLAGRA and CELIAC DISEASE in Part Two for information on gluten intolerance. Undiagnosed celiac disease may cause symptoms similar to schizophrenia. Gluten intolerance can also alter the mind and cause severe depression. Schizophrenia is often associated with high copper levels in tissues. Some cases have been linked to food allergies, so consider a food allergy test. Many patients improve after fasting. Medical schools often fail to teach that food affects body and mind, and most disorders go unrecognized because of failure to perceive this connection between food allergies and mood.

(*See* ALLERGIES in Part Two and FASTING in Part Three.) A wide range of drugs can also cause schizoid-type symptoms.

There is good scientific evidence that schizophrenia is the result of a defect in body chemistry—a defect that is most often inherited. Chemicals carrying messages to the brain function abnormally in those with this defect.

NUTRIENTS

SUPPLEMENT	SUGGESTED DOSAGE	COMMENTS
Essential		
Ginkgo biloba extract	2 capsules 3 times daily.	Improves brain function and cerebral circulation.
Very Important		
Germanium	200 mg daily.	Makes oxygen more available to the brain.
Niacin or niacinamide (B$_3$)	100 mg 3 times daily. 1,000 mg daily.	Niacin deficiency is linked with schizophrenia. Under supervision, several grams a day have been administered with good results. Injections are best, daily or three times a week.
Protein supplement (free form amino acids)	3 times daily on an empty stomach.	Needed for normal brain function. Free form amino acids are rapidly absorbed and assimilated by the body.
Vitamin B complex plus vitamin B$_{12}$ injections or vitamin B complex capsules	1 cc injection of each 3 times a week (under doctor's supervision only). 100 mg 3 times daily.	Vitamin B deficiency is related to brain malfunction.
Vitamin B$_6$ (pyridoxine)	100 mg twice daily.	Pyridoxine is required by the nervous system and is necessary for normal brain function.
Vitamin E emulsion	800 IU or capsules to 1,000 IU, increasing slowly, starting with 200 IU.	An antioxidant that improves brain circulation. Emulsion form enters the system quicker.
Important		
Coenzyme Q$_{10}$	75 mg daily.	Improves cerebral circulation.
DMG (Gluconic from DaVinci Labs)	As directed on label.	Enhances cerebral oxygen utilization.
Essential fatty acids (primrose oil)	2 capsules 3 times daily.	Helps cerebral circulation and supplies needed essential fatty acids, such as linoleic acid.
L-Glutamine	1–4 g daily. Take with vitamins B$_6$ and C on an empty stomach.	A neurotransmitter needed for normal brain function.
Lecithin	1 tbsp. or 1 capsule before meals.	Improves brain function. Contains choline and inositol. Works well with vitamin E.
Vitamin C	5,000–10,000 mg	Improves brain function and enhances the immune system.
Helpful		
Bio-Strath	As directed on label.	A tonic that also supplies organic iron from food sources.
Kelp	8 tablets daily.	Contains balanced essential minerals.
Lithium	By prescription only.	Helps depression.
Multivitamin and mineral complex	As directed on label.	Needed for normal brain function.
Thyroid glandular	As directed on label.	Reduced thyroid function results in poor cerebral function. *See* HYPOTHYROID in Part Two and GLANDULAR THERAPY in Part Three.
Zinc and manganese	As directed on label.	Important minerals. Zinc balances excess copper. Manganese enhances the B vitamins necessary for brain functions.

RECOMMENDATIONS

☐ A hair analysis could reveal mineral imbalance.

☐ Follow the diet listed under HYPOGLYCEMIA in Part Two.

☐ The diet should include breast of chicken, turkey, brewer's yeast, halibut, peas, sunflower seeds, and tuna. Also include foods rich in niacin such as broccoli, carrots, corn, eggs, fish, potatoes, tomatoes, and whole wheat.

☐ Sometimes extremely high doses of certain vitamins are needed to keep the mind functioning.

CONSIDERATIONS

☐ Good results have been obtained with the following injection program: 1 cc liver extract, 1 cc B complex, and ½ cc vitamin B$_6$. Administer three times a week for three weeks, then drop to twice weekly for three months. After this three-month period, reduce frequency of injections to once weekly.

☐ Many suicides among the young may be related to undiagnosed schizophrenia, says a doctor from Queens Hospital in New York.

Seborrhea

Seborrhea is a disorder of the sebaceous glands, the glands that secrete oil. Seborrhea occurs on the scalp, face, and chest most often, but can appear on other parts of the body. It is characterized by greasy patches on the body that form scales and crusts. Seborrheic skin is prone to such conditions as alopecia, seborrheic dermatitis, and acne.

Zinc	50–80 mg	For tissue repair and enhances immunity.

HERBS

☐ Dandelion, goldenseal, and red clover are good. Chaparral may be used as a rinse.

RECOMMENDATIONS

☐ Eat 50–75 percent raw foods and soured products such as yogurt. Avoid chocolate, dairy products, flour, fried foods, nuts, seafood, and sugar. Follow the fasting program once a month (*see* FASTING in Part Three).

☐ Don't pick at or squeeze the infected skin. Avoid using irritating soaps, but make sure you keep the affected areas clean. Avoid greasy ointments and creams. Keep your hair clean and make sure you use a non-oily shampoo.

☐ Try changing your hair products—use one without chemicals. Sometimes this helps.

☐ *See also* DANDRUFF in Part Two.

Senility (Senile Dementia)

Senility occurs in old age but it is really not very common in the elderly. Many of those diagnosed as senile are actually suffering from the effects of drugs, depression, deafness, brain tumors, thyroid problems, or liver or kidney problems. Nervous disturbances, stroke, and cerebral dysfunction are considered symptoms of the "senility syndrome." Often, a nutritional deficiency is the cause.

There are several types of seborrhea:

- *Cap'itis*. Located on scalp.
- *Congestive*. *See* LUPUS in Part Two.
- *Corporis*. Located on the trunk.
- *Facier*. Located on the face.
- *Nigra or Nigricans*. Dark-colored seborrhea.
- *Oliosa*. Seborrhea with an oily content.
- *Rosacea*. Middle-age seborrhea that reappears.
- *Sicca*. Dry form of seborrhea with scales.

Seborrhea may be caused by a vitamin A deficiency. The advice of a competent physician should be sought early. It is best not to use over-the-counter ointments to treat it—this can cause an overload on the skin. A dermatologist usually prescribes cleaning lotions containing a drying agent with sulfur and Resorcin and/or Deprosone cream. If antibiotics are prescribed, don't fail to take extra B-complex vitamins and either acidophilus or Megadophilus to replace the "friendly" bacteria destroyed by the antibiotics.

NUTRIENTS

SUPPLEMENT	SUGGESTED DOSAGE	COMMENTS
Essential		
Unsaturated fatty acids (primrose oil)	As directed on label.	Important for many skin disorders; contains needed linoleic acid.
Important		
Vitamin A	Up to 50,000 IU	Vitamin A deficiency may cause seborrhea.
Vitamin B complex extra high stress formula plus extra vitamin B6	As directed on label.	The B vitamins, especially B6, are needed for protein metabolism (i.e., healing and repair).
Vitamin E	400–800 IU daily.	Speeds healing. Increases oxygen intake.
Helpful		
Acidophilus	As directed on label.	Take daily in some form, especially if antibiotics are used.
Coenzyme Q10	60 mg daily.	An important free radical scavenger that supplies oxygen to the cells.
DMG (Gluconic from DaVinci Labs)	As directed on label.	Increases tissue oxygen.
Kelp	5 tablets daily.	Contains balanced minerals. Good iodine source.
Lecithin	Take with meals.	For cellular protection.
Multivitamin and mineral complex	As directed on label.	
Protein supplement (free form amino acids)	As directed on label.	For healing and repair. Take in the free form for quicker absorption and assimilation.

NUTRIENTS

SUPPLEMENT	SUGGESTED DOSAGE	COMMENTS
Essential		
Bio-Strath	As directed on label.	This is a tonic that has demonstrated good results.
Protein (free form amino acids)	As directed on label.	A protein deficiency is common in the elderly. Protein is needed for normal brain function.
Vitamin B complex and vitamin B12	100 mg 3 times daily. 2,000 mcg daily. Injections with added B6 and B12 are best in severe cases! Sublingual form is also effective.	The elderly cannot absorb the B vitamins efficiently.

Very Important		
Choline	500 mg twice daily.	Important in brain function. Improves memory and mental capacity.
Niacin (B₃)	100–500 mg daily. Take with niacinamide to reduce flushing. The flush is harmless.	Improves cerebral circulation and lowers cholesterol.
Vitamin C	3,000–10,000 mg daily.	Reduces blood clotting tendency, improving cerebral circulation.
Vitamin E	600–1,000 IU daily. Start with 200 IU; increase slowly.	Boosts immunity, which declines during aging. Improves cerebral circulation.
Important		
Gerovital H-3 (GH-3) from Rumania	As directed on label.	Consider injections. It has produced good results.
Helpful		
Coenzyme Q₁₀	60 mg daily.	Potent free radical scavenger and immunostimulant. Supplies needed oxygen to the cells.
Germanium	100 mg daily.	Potent free radical scavenger and immunostimulant. Supplies needed oxygen to the cells.
L-Glutamine	As directed on label. Take on an empty stomach with 50 mg vitamin B₆ and 500 mg vitamin C.	Needed for normal brain function.
Lecithin	3 tbsp. or 6 capsules daily in divided doses before meals.	For brain cell protection and function.
Multivitamin supplement (high potency)	As directed on label.	For necessary vitamins.
Zinc	50–80 mg daily.	Aids in heavy metal detoxification and enhancing immunity.

*Note: Avoid heavy coated or sustained release vitamins! These are difficult for the elderly to break down.

HERBS

☐ Use blue cohosh and anise, which appear to sharpen brain power. Ginkgo biloba improves cerebral circulation, enhancing brain function and memory. Take 400 milligrams three times daily.

RECOMMENDATIONS

☐ Diet is extremely important. The diet should consist of 50-75 percent raw foods along with seeds, whole grain cereals and breads, raw nuts, and yogurt and soured products. Eat Swiss cheese, brown rice, and

plenty of fiber daily. Drink plenty of liquids, even if you are not thirsty—as we grow older, our "thirst system" does not work well.

☐ Bowels should move daily—enemas may be needed (See ENEMAS in Part Three). Oat bran, rice bran, and a high-fiber diet are important. ABC (Aerobic Bulk Cleanse), a colon cleanser, is very helpful.

☐ Exercising and walking, keeping mentally active, and doing things you enjoy like keeping a hobby are important. Some elderly people withdraw and keep to themselves because it seems easier. Many have trouble accepting aging. Some withdraw out of loneliness. They need love and family around them.

☐ One cc each of B-complex and liver injections plus ½ cc (50 mg) vitamin B₆ (pyridoxine) are important for the elderly and should be given at least once weekly. They are prone to absorption problems, and therefore are lacking in nutrients, especially the water-soluble vitamins.

☐ A hair analysis will reveal whether the body is incurring damage due to the presence of toxic levels of metals like aluminum and lead. *Also see* ALLERGIES in Part Two to rule out food allergies.

☐ *See also* ALUMINUM TOXICITY and ALZHEIMER'S DISEASE, both in Part Two.

Sexually Transmitted Diseases

Sexually transmitted diseases are those that are passed on during sexual intercourse or other intimate contact with the sex organs. The two most common types of sexually transmitted diseases are gonorrhea and syphilis. However, there are many other sexually transmitted diseases. They include chancroid, lymphogranuloma venereum, granuloma inguinal, genital herpes, chlamydia, trichomoniasis, candidiasis, and AIDS.

In females, gonorrhea is often asymptomatic. When there are symptoms, they include frequent and painful urination, vaginal discharge, abnormal menstrual bleeding, acute inflammation in the pelvic area, and rectal itching.

Males usually do experience symptoms of gonorrhea. These symptoms include a yellow discharge of pus and mucus from the penis and slow, difficult, and painful urination.

The symptoms usually appear seven to twenty-one days after sexual contact. Penicillin or another antibiotic is the usual treatment. Be sure to add some

Easy Reference Guide to Detect Sexually Transmitted Diseases (STDs) in Their Early Stages

It is vital that a sexually transmitted disease be caught in its early stages so that severe, irreparable damage to the body does not occur. Familiarize yourself with the beginning stages of the STDs for early detection and treatment.

Disease	Beginning Stages
AIDS (Acquired Immunodeficiency Syndrome)	Early symptoms include headache, night sweats, weight loss, fatigue, swollen lymph glands, fever, heavily coated white tongue (oral thrush—candidiasis), diarrhea, and lung infections.
Candidiasis	Itching in the genital area, pain when urinating, and a thick odorless vaginal discharge are frequently present. Candidiasis is unusual in the male and indicates a weakened immune system.
Chlamydia	Often there are no symptoms. Some females experience a white vaginal discharge that resembles cottage cheese, a burning sensation when urinating, itching, and painful intercourse. A clear watery urethral discharge in the male probably is a chlamydia infection.
Genital Herpes	Symptoms include itching, burning in the genital area and discomfort urinating, and a watery vaginal or urethral discharge. A weeping vesicular eruption in the vagina or on the penis is an early sign.
Genital Warts	Single or clusters of soft, cauliflower-like growths in and around the vagina, anus, penis, groin, and scrotal area.
Gonorrhea	Often without symptoms. Females become silent carriers. If there are symptoms in the female, they include frequent and painful urination, cloudy vaginal discharge, vaginal itching, inflammation of the pelvic area, and abnormal uterine bleeding. If the male has a purulent urethral discharge, he should assume he has gonorrhea until proven otherwise.
Pelvic Inflammatory Disease (PID)	A purulent vaginal discharge with fever and lower abdominal pain.
Syphilis	Symptoms in the early contagious stages are a sore on the genitalia, a rash, patches of flaking tissue, fever, a sore throat, and sores in the mouth or anus.
Trichonomiasis	Vaginal itching and pain, with a watery foamy greenish or yellow odorless discharge, are frequently present. A clear urethral discharge is an early sign in the male.

acidophilus to your diet if you are taking one of these antibiotics.

If left untreated, the gonorrhea organism (gonococcus) can enter the rest of the body through the bloodstream and go into the bones, joints, tendons, and other tissues. At this stage the disease is difficult to detect and is often misdiagnosed as simple arthritis.

There is a new strain of gonorrhea that has spread rapidly since it was first identified in 1985. This strain is resistant to the drug tetracycline and some forms of penicillin, but it can be cured.

Syphilis is caused by a bacterium called *Treponema pallidum*. This disease can be contracted through physical contact such as kissing, as well as through sexual intercourse. If left untreated, it will progress for years in three stages. In the first stage a sore (chancre) appears, and in the second stage a rash and patches of flaking tissue appear in the mouth or genital area. If the disease progresses to its third stage, which is rare today, brain damage, hearing loss, heart disease, and/or blindness can occur.

Doctors in many countries are calling cervical dysplasia (the formation of abnormal tissue in the cervix, a precancerous condition of the cervix), the newest sexually transmitted epidemic. They believe that it is caused by the same virus (*papilloma* virus) that causes venereal warts.

NUTRIENTS

SUPPLEMENT	SUGGESTED DOSAGE	COMMENTS
Very Important		
Acidophilus	3 capsules or 1 tbsp. liquid 3 times daily.	Important when taking antibiotics.
Garlic capsules (Kyolic)	2 capsules 3 times daily.	A natural antibiotic and immune system stimulant.

284

Protein (free form amino acids)	As directed on label.	Needed for tissue repair. Use free form for quicker absorption and assimilation.
Vitamin C	3,000–10,000 mg daily divided into 4 daily doses.	Potentiates immune function. Is an antiviral agent.
Zinc	100 mg daily.	
Important		
Kelp	6 tablets daily.	Supplies balanced vitamins and minerals.
Vitamin B complex	50 mg 3 times daily.	Necessary in all cellular enzyme system function.
Helpful		
Coenzyme Q$_{10}$	30–60 mg daily.	Powerful free radical scavenger.
Germanium	100 mg daily.	Speeds healing and reduces pain or discomfort.
Multivitamin and mineral complex (high potency)	As directed on label.	
Raw glandular complex plus extra thymus	As directed on label.	Promotes immune function.
Vitamin K (alfalfa)	100 mcg daily in tablet form as directed on label.	Antibiotics destroy bowel bacteria that produce vitamin K which is necessary for blood clotting. Alfalfa is a good source.

HERBS

☐ Echinacea, goldenseal, pau d'arco, and suma may alleviate symptoms. Alternate teas and consume three cups daily or take in capsule or extract form.

RECOMMENDATIONS

☐ These diseases are highly contagious. *The Journal of the American Medical Association* suggests that you protect yourself with condoms. Condoms should be used, but they are no guarantee of protection against venereal disease!

☐ *See also* AIDS, CANDIDIASIS, CHLAMYDIA, WARTS, and YEAST IN-FECTION in Part Two.

Shingles (Herpes Zoster)

Shingles, caused by the same virus that causes chicken pox, affects the nerve endings in the skin. It usually occurs on the skin of the abdomen under the ribs leading toward the navel, but can appear anywhere on the body. An attack of shingles is often preceded by three or four days of intense pain in the affected area. Then numerous and excruciatingly painful and itchy blisters develop, normally lasting between seven and fourteen days. These blisters eventually form crusty scabs and drop off.

The virus may lie dormant in the spinal cord and nerve ganglia for years until triggered. Risk of shingles increases with the use of anti-cancer drugs, Hodgkin's disease and other cancers, stress, and immune system deficiency. If shingles develop near the eyes, the cornea can become affected and blindness may result. See an ophthalmologist if the shingles appear on the forehead near the eyes or on the tip of the nose.

After an attack of shingles, the pain may continue even after the blisters have disappeared, especially in the elderly. The pain can sometimes last for months or years. This post-herpetic syndrome can be even more painful than the original infection.

NUTRIENTS

SUPPLEMENT	SUGGESTED DOSAGE	COMMENTS
Essential		
L-Lysine (amino acid)	500 mg twice daily.	Important for healing.
Vitamin C plus bioflavonoids	2,000 mg twice daily.	Aids in destroying the virus and boosting the immune system.
Very Important		
Cayenne capsules	Use as directed on label.	Contains capsaicin. Relieves pain and aids in healing.
Vitamin B complex plus extra vitamin B$_{12}$	100 mg 3 times daily. Injections, under doctor's recommendation and supervision only, may be necessary.	Needed especially for malnutrition.
Zinc chelate	80 mg for 1 week, then reduce to quicker absorbing 50 mg zinc lozenges.	Enhances immune system and protects against infection.
Important		
Calcium chelate plus magnesium	1,500 daily. 750 mg daily.	For nerve function and healing. Antistress formula.
Vitamin A emulsion	75,000 IU for 2 weeks, then drop to 50,000 IU or take 25,000 IU in capsule form.	Potentiates immune system and protects against infection. Emulsion form enters the system quickly.
Vitamin D	1,000 IU twice daily for 1 week, then drop to 400 IU.	Aids in healing of the tissue, and needed for calcium absorption.
Vitamin E	400–800 IU daily.	Helps prevent scar tissue. You may also open a capsule and apply directly to infected skin.

Helpful		
Coenzyme Q$_{10}$	60 mg daily.	Free radical scavenger. Potentiates immune function.
Germanium	200 mg daily.	Free radical scavenger. Potentiates immune function.
Multivitamin and mineral complex		Especially necessary in malnutrition.
Proteolytic enzymes	Take with and between meals.	Antioxidant properties. Neutralizes free radicals.

RECOMMENDATIONS

☐ The diet must include raw fruits and vegetables, brewer's yeast, brown rice, and whole grains. A cleansing fast is very important. (*See* FASTING in Part Three.)

☐ Avoid drafts. Allow sunlight on the affected area for short intervals. Gently wash the blisters when bathing and avoid touching or scratching them. Avoid Tylenol-type medications (those that contain acetaminophen), as they will prolong the illness.

CONSIDERATIONS

☐ Shingles is now being treated with acyclovir or Inter Vir. Capsaicin, an ingredient in cayenne, provides relief for some sufferers of chronic pain. Capsaicin is also the active ingredient in Zostrix, a topical cream.

Sinusitis

Sinusitis is an inflammation of the nasal sinuses that accompanies upper respiratory infection. More than 50 percent of all cases of sinusitis are caused by bacteria. The sinuses affected by this infection include those above the eyes, inside each cheekbone, behind the bridge of the nose, and in the upper nose.

Acute sinusitis is frequently caused by colds or bacterial and viral infections of the nose, throat, and upper respiratory tract. Chronic sinusitis problems may be caused by small growths in the nose, injury of the nasal bones, smoking, and irritant fumes and smells. Allergenic sinusitis may be caused by hay fever and food allergies, especially allergies to milk and dairy products.

Symptoms of sinusitis include headache, earache, toothache, facial pain, cranial pressure, loss of sense of smell, tenderness over the forehead and cheekbones, and occasionally a high fever. Sometimes sinusitis produces a swollen face followed by a stuffy nose and thick discharge of mucus. Antibiotics may be necessary. If drainage is clear after a week, you probably do not have an infection; if mucus is greenish or yellowish, you do. If drainage is clear without a cold, you probably have allergies.

Swelling around the eyes is a serious sign. If left untreated, sinusitis can lead to asthma, bronchitis, pharyngitis, laryngitis, pneumonia, or other respiratory disorders.

NUTRIENTS

SUPPLEMENT	SUGGESTED DOSAGE	COMMENTS
Very Important		
Bee pollen	Start with a small amount and increase slowly.	Increases immunity and speeds healing.
Fenu-Thyme from Nature's Way Products or Bronc-Ease from Nature's Herbs (herb formulas)	2 capsules 3 times daily.	Relieves nasal and sinus congestion.
Vitamin B complex with extra vitamin B$_6$ (pyridoxine) and pantothenic acid (B$_5$)	125 mg and up twice daily.　　　　　　　100 mg 3 times daily.	Megadose formula is needed.
Vitamin C plus bioflavonoids	2,000–10,000 mg daily in divided doses.	Potentiates immune function and destroys viruses.
Helpful		
Coenzyme Q$_{10}$	60 mg daily.	Valuable immune system stimulant. Increases cellular oxygenation.
Garlic capsules (Kyolic)	2 capsules 3 times daily.	Odorless garlic. Valuable immune system stimulant. A natural antibiotic that keeps the infection in check.
Germanium	100 mg daily.	Valuable immune system stimulant. Increases cellular oxygenation.
Proteolytic enzymes	Take with and between meals.	Destroys free radicals. Also aids in digestion of foods.
Zinc gluconate lozenges	Dissolve in mouth every 2–4 hours.	Antiviral agent and immunity booster. Use at first sign of a cold.

HERBS

☐ The following herbs are effective in the treatment of sinusitis: anise and horehound, brigham tea, echinacea, fenugreek, goldenseal root, lobelia, marshmallow, mullein, red clover, and rose hips. The herbal combination PSI by Terra Maxa is also good.

RECOMMENDATIONS

☐ Do not use force when blowing your nose, as this forces mucus back into the sinus cavities. Instead, draw the secretion to the back of the throat by sniffing, then expel. The use of a vaporizer is helpful. However, do not use decongestants for long periods of time, if at all, and do not use them if you have high blood pressure or heart problems as they may dangerously elevate the blood pressure.

☐ A diet of 75 percent raw foods should be maintained. Reduce salt intake. A cleansing fast is very important. (*See* FASTING in Part Three.) Drink plenty of distilled water and juices. Do not eat dairy foods, except for soured products like yogurt and cottage cheese, because they increase mucus formation.

☐ Hot liquids help the mucus to flow, relieving congestion and sinus pressure.

Skin Cancer

There are three forms of skin cancer. The two most common and curable forms are squamous cell and basal cell carcinoma. With early detection and treatment, these types of skin cancer are curable. Melanoma is a more rare type of skin cancer that is much more serious. Sun exposure is not only the major cause of wrinkles; it is responsible for 90 percent of most forms of skin cancer.

In squamous cell carcinoma, the underlying skin cells are damaged and this leads to the development of a tumor or lump under the skin. In most cases, the ears, hands, face, and lower lip are affected. The lump may resemble a wart or an ulceration that never heals.

If detected early, treatment is effective. The tumor is cut away. If the growth is large, a skin graft may be necessary. Other treatments are cryosurgery (when the affected area is frozen), chemosurgery, and radiation therapy. Most patients recover, but regular checkups for at least the next five years are advised.

Basal cell carcinoma is the most common of the three types of skin cancer. Unlike other malignant growths, it does not spread until it has been present for a long period of time. Again, overexposure to strong sunlight is the major factor. The cell damage results in an ulcer-like growth that spreads slowly as it destroys tissue. A large pearly looking lump is the first sign, and this lump usually occurs on the face by the nose or eyes. After about six weeks, the lump becomes an ulcer with a raw, moist center and a hard border that may bleed.

Scabs will continually form over the ulcer. The scabs come off, but the ulcer never heals. Sometimes basal cell carcinomas show up on the back or chest as flat sores that grow slowly. This type of skin cancer is treated the same way as squamous cell carcinoma. If these carcinomas return, the same treatment is repeated.

The most dangerous form of skin cancer, malignant melanoma, can be life threatening if not treated at an early stage. With this type of skin cancer, a tumor arises from the pigment-producing cells of the deeper layers of the skin. Melanoma can be cured if discovered and treated early. It often begins as a lesion that looks like a mole. Most people have moles—this does not make them a cancer risk. Most moles appear early in life. Beware of new moles that appear after age forty. Any mole that appears unusual or that changes in size or color should be looked at by a doctor as soon as possible.

Some families are genetically at higher risk to suffer melanoma. At birth they often have odd moles, called "congenital nevi," or later develop moles called "dysplastic nevi" that may be precursors to skin cancer.

Those who have a family history of melanoma should avoid the sun and always use a sunscreen cream protection. Further, a close watch must be kept on any suspicious skin lesions, and they should be checked regularly by a physician. Melanomas occur most frequently on the upper back and on the lower legs. They may occur under the nails and on mucous membranes. *Mycosis fungoides* is a rare type of slow-growing cancer. It is preceded for years by itching skin lesions. Eventually the lesions become firmer and ulcerate. A skin biopsy will enable the doctor to make the diagnosis. If left untreated, these lesions ulcerate and involve the lymph nodes and even other organs in the form of lymphoma.

As stated before, skin cancers are most often caused by overexposure to the sun's ultraviolet (UV) rays. These rays disrupt the genetic material (DNA) in the skin cells, causing severe tissue damage and cancer. This disease is also linked to sun exposure. People who have had severe or blistering sunburns are twice as likely to develop the disease. People with fair skin, who sunburn easily, are at the greatest risk for skin cancer, because they have less protective pigment in their skin. See SUNBURN in Part Two.

The warning signs of skin cancer are:

1. An open sore that bleeds, crusts over, and will not heal properly.
2. A reddish, irritated spot that is usually on the chest, shoulder, arm, or leg. It may itch, hurt, or cause no discomfort at all.

3. A smooth growth with an elevated border and a center indentation. As it becomes bigger, tiny blood vessels develop on the surface.
4. A shiny scar-like area that may be white, yellow, or waxy with a shiny, taut appearance.
5. An enlarging, irregular, "angry" appearing lesion on the face, lips, or ears.

You should see a doctor about any of these growths. Excisional biopsy often cures the problem in its early stages; more radical surgery may be necessary if excision is delayed.

NUTRIENTS

SUPPLEMENT	SUGGESTED DOSAGE	COMMENTS
Essential		
Coenzyme Q₁₀	100 mg daily.	Improves cellular oxygenation.
DMG (Gluconic from DaVinci Labs)	As directed on label.	Improves cellular oxygenation.
Essential fatty acids (primrose oil)	2 capsules before meals.	For cellular protection.
Garlic capsules (Kyolic)	2 capsules 3 times daily.	Enhances immune function.
Germanium	200 mg daily.	Improves cellular oxygenation, deterring cancer growth; potent immunostimulant.
Proteolytic enzymes or Wobe-Mugos-N-Dragees	2–6 tablets with meals. 2–6 tablets between meals.	Powerful free radical scavengers.
Selenium	200 mcg daily.	Powerful free radical scavenger.
Superoxide dismutase (SOD)	As directed on label. Consider injections under the supervision of your doctor.	Destroys free radicals.
Vitamin A emulsion	50,000–100,000 IU daily for 10 days or for as long as on program.	The emulsion form is readily absorbed.
and beta-carotene	15,000 units	A powerful antioxidant that destroys free radicals.
Vitamin B complex and/or brewer's yeast	100 mg daily. 3 times daily.	B vitamins are necessary for normal cell division and function.
Vitamin C plus bioflavonoids	5,000–10,000 mg daily in divided doses.	Powerful anti-cancer agent. *See* ASCORBIC ACID FLUSH, Part Three.
Vitamin E emulsion	Up to 1,000 IU daily.	Emulsion form is easily assimilated. Places less stress on the liver.
Helpful		
Aerobic 07 from Aerobic Life Products or Dioxychlor from American Biologics	As directed on label.	Antimicrobial agents.
Comprehensive mineral and trace element supplement, rich in potassium and calcium and magnesium	2,000 mg daily. 1,000 mg daily.	Essential for normal cell division and function.
L-Cysteine and L-methionine (amino acids)	As directed on label.	Detoxifies harmful substances.
L-Taurine (amino acid)	As directed on label.	Functions as foundation for tissue and organ repair.
Megadophilus or Maxidophilus or Primadophilus DDS	As directed on label.	Has an antibacterial effect on the body. A milk-free brand is available.
Multiple enzyme digestive formula	Take with meals as directed.	Aids digestion.
Multivitamin	Take with meals as directed on label.	Should not be sustained release. Take a formula that is iron free.
Niacin and folic acid and choline	100 mg daily. 500–1,000 mg daily.	B vitamins that improve circulation, build red blood cells, and aid liver function.
PABA	Less than 400 IU daily.	Protects against skin cancer.
Raw glandular complex with extra raw thymus	As directed on label.	Stimulates glandular function, especially the thymus (site of T-lymphocyte production).
Seaweed or kelp	5 tablets daily.	For mineral balance.
Vitamin B₁₂	Injections (under doctor's supervision only) or by sublingual route are recommended.	Prevents anemia.

RECOMMENDATIONS

☐ Everyone should take protective measures while in the sun. The sun's ultraviolet rays are strongest between 10 a.m. and 2 p.m. Stay out of the sun as much as possible between these hours.

☐ Wear lightweight clothing that is made of tightly woven material. Ultraviolet rays may cause skin cancer of the eyelids and even cataracts. They are also harmful to the retina, so wear sunglasses that will block the UV rays. There are sunglasses that will block up to 95 percent of these UV rays.

☐ Always use a sunscreen! Use one that has a sun protection factor (SPF) of at least 15. Eighty-five percent of the UV rays penetrate through the clouds; therefore, sunscreen should be applied every day, even when it is overcast. Be sure to protect the lips with a lip balm or lip block that has an SPF of 15, too.

☐ Check for discharge from moles. Be alert to moles that are irregularly shaped or that change in size or color; those that have ridges around the edges, spread, bleed, or itch; or lesions that are constantly irritated by rubbing clothes.

CONSIDERATIONS

☐ Certain medications may make the skin more susceptible to sun damage. These include antibiotics, antidepressants, diuretics, antihistamines, sedatives, estrogen, and acne medications such as retinoic acid. Others may result in severe sunburn after only a short period of time in the sun. Ask the doctor or pharmacist if such a reaction could occur with any medication that you take.

☐ Suntanning beds (those used in tanning salons) were once considered safer than the sun. The equipment in the beds emits only UV-A rays, which are the sun's cool rays. Hot B rays (UV-B) were considered primarily responsible for tanning, burning, and skin cancer. Now there is evidence that the UV-A rays may cause the same damage as the UV-B rays. Beware of tanning salons!

☐ It may be possible to contract skin cancer without even being in the sun. The ozone layer once acted as a protective atmospheric sunscreen. As the ozone layer diminishes, people will be more prone to skin cancer as well as radiation.

☐ A June 1988 article from the *British Journal of Surgery* suggests that essential fatty acids, found in evening primrose oil and fish oil, may have a beneficial role in the prevention and treatment of malignant melanoma.

Skin Problems

The skin is the body's largest organ. It consists of three layers—the epidermis (outer layer), the dermis (middle layer), and the subcutaneous layer (inner layer). Because the skin acts as a shield between the body and the millions of foreign substances that exist in our environment, it often reacts with acne, rashes, bumps, scales, redness, and other skin problems. Skin irritations are characterized by scaling, flaking, thickening, color changes, itching, cracking, and dryness. The skin excretes toxins and poisons that are present in the body, as do the kidneys and bowels.

There are many reasons for skin reactions. They include allergies to molds, foods, chemicals, cosmetics, and other substances; insect bites; reactions to plants, as in poison ivy; diaper rash in infants; reactions to the sun and wind; rashes from parts of the body rubbing together (this often occurs in the inner thighs); reactions to drugs; reactions to detergents; reactions to alcohol; and literally thousands of other causes.

SPECIFIC SKIN CONDITIONS

Rosacea is reddening of the skin, usually the forehead, nose, cheekbones, and chin. Most often pustules do not appear except on the nose. They can be very tender. A thickening of the skin can occur. The cause of rosacea is unknown, but often spicy foods, hot liquids, alcohol, stress, excessive heat or cold, and sunlight may set off a reaction. Tetracycline is used to control rosacea along with topical medication applied to the inflammation.

Intertrigo is an eruption of the skin caused by two skin surfaces rubbing together causing friction. The groin, breasts, underarms, and inner thighs are the areas usually involved. These areas provide an environment for the growth of bacteria or yeast (see CANDIDIASIS, Part Two). These organisms may cause ulcerations. Treatment of this disorder involves keeping the skin surface clean, dry, and free of friction. A hair dryer on a cool setting may be helpful when used several times a day along with baby powder. Add garlic, soured products, and acidophilus to the diet.

Sebaceous cysts develop as a small swelling on the face, scalp, or back. These subcutaneous nodules of sebum often become chronically infected. If the growth becomes large or infected, it should be removed to prevent the spread of infection.

NUTRIENTS

SUPPLEMENT	SUGGESTED DOSAGE	COMMENTS
Very Important		
Primrose oil	2 capsules 3 times daily.	A good healer for dermatitis, acne, and most other skin disorders. Contains linoleic acid, which is needed by the skin.
Vitamin A	25,000 IU daily for 3 months, dropping to 15,000 IU daily.	Necessary for healing and construction of new skin tissue.
Vitamin B complex with extra vitamin B₁₂	As directed on label.	The antistress and anti-aging vitamins.
Important		
Kelp	5 tablets daily.	Supplies balanced minerals. Needed for good skin tone.
Vitamin E	400 IU increasing slowly up to 800 IU.	Protects against free radicals.

Zinc	50 mg daily.	For tissue repair. Enhances immune response.
Helpful		
Ageless Beauty from Biotec Foods	As directed on label.	Protects the skin from free radical damage.
Aloe vera gel	As directed on label.	Apply on dry skin. Has excellent healing properties.
Cocoa butter	As directed on label.	Good for stretch marks.
Collagen	As directed on label.	Good for very dry skin. A nourishing cream.
Elastin	As directed on label.	Helps stretch marks and wrinkling.
Gerovital H-3 (GH-3) cream	As directed on label.	Excellent for the prevention of wrinkles. Good for acne or any discoloring of the pigment in the skin.
Linseed oil	1,000 mg capsules or 1 tsp. liquid.	Supplies the needed essential fatty acids.
Retinoic acid	By prescription only. Take as directed by physician.	Gives the same effect as a "chemical peel." Takes around 6 months of use; removes the top layer of skin, leaving new, baby-like skin. Test on a small spot to determine any reaction. Removes fine wrinkles. Excellent for age spots, precancerous lesions, and sun-damaged skin. Avoid sun exposure to the face while using retinoic acid.
Superoxide dismutase (SOD)	As directed on label.	A free radical destroyer. Also good for brown age spots.

HERBS

☐ For *oily skin*, apply an herbal formula of licorice root, lemon grass, and rose buds. Use a sauna for fifteen minutes two or three times a week. Simmer the herbs in a pan with distilled water, and hold your face over the pan, with a towel over your head. Be sure your face is clean before the sauna, and finish by splashing cold water on your face. Air dry or pat with a towel. The herbs mentioned above can be used with a cotton ball and dabbed on the face after the herbal formula has been made. This combination may also be used in sauna steam.

☐ *Combination of oily and dry skin* is most common. Use the herbs lavender, peppermint, and chamomile. A sauna is also good for this condition.

☐ For *dry skin*, follow the same as for combination skin, and add unsaturated fatty acids to the diet.

☐ For *acne*, use the herbs red clover, strawberry leaves, and lavender. Drink the red clover daily as a tea in addition to using it in a sauna. Lavender is excellent in the sauna for killing germs and stimulating new cell growth.

☐ The herb chaparral works well for skin cancer. Take as a tea or in pill form. It aids in healing, softens the skin, and makes the skin's texture smooth.

☐ For ringworm (skin infection), put raw garlic over the ringworm and cover. You can also use black walnut extract.

RECOMMENDATIONS

☐ Drink plenty of water and liquids. Cuts and cracks in the nails indicate a need for more liquids.

☐ Avoid fried foods, animal fat, and heat-processed supermarket oils. Use cold-pressed oils only. Beware of rancid oils.

☐ Sun in excess is most damaging to the skin, and causes dryness, wrinkles, and even rashes and blisters.

☐ Do not drink soft drinks or eat sugar, chocolate, potato chips, or other junk foods.

☐ For cracking and dry skin on the fingers, use calendula cream or oil with comfrey, vitamin E, and aloe vera at bedtime, then wear plastic gloves overnight.

☐ A skin rash in children may be caused by consumption of eggs, peanuts, milk, wheat, fish, chicken, pork, or beef. Eggs, peanuts, and milk account for 75 percent of skin rashes in children. Cocoa butter is a good skin cream and isn't expensive. It also helps reduce skin wrinkling. Keep in the refrigerator after opening.

☐ Smoking increases wrinkles, especially around the mouth. It can also make the skin dry and leathery.

☐ Many doctors use hydrocortisone cream for minor irritations, poison ivy, insect bites (those that itch), and diaper rash.

☐ Skin irritations can be caused by an allergy to a mold. Have a test to rule out allergies or *see* the self-testing in ALLERGIES, Part Two.

☐ *See* HYPOTHYROID in Part Two and take the self-test to make sure the thyroid is functioning properly.

☐ Sulfur keeps the skin smooth and youthful. It is found in garlic, onions, eggs, asparagus, and the amino acid L-cysteine, which can be purchased in pill form.

☐ Use benzoyl peroxide for a few weeks—avoid putting it around the eyes and mouth.

☐ *Enlarged pores* are caused by smoking and too much sugar over a period of years.

☐ *Puffy eyes* are caused by excess salt; check for food allergies.

☐ *Scabies* causes a persistent, itchy rash. See your doctor and have him take a scraping of the skin to be examined under a microscope. The parasite, the itch mite, can be removed with application of the drug lindane. Scabies is a problem of elderly patients in nursing homes and children in day care centers. It is highly contagious.

☐ Most *moles* are harmless. Those that are larger than the top of a pencil eraser, are flat or nearly flat, have jagged edges, or have a mottled color should be checked. If a new mole appears or an existing mole turns blue, white, or red and begins to bleed or develops a crust, have it checked immediately. (*See* SKIN CANCER, Part Two.)

☐ *See also* ACNE and DERMATITIS in Part Two.

Smoking Dependency

Today, tobacco smoking is the cause of one-third of all cancer deaths and one-fourth of all fatal heart attacks in the United States alone. In fact, many degenerative diseases and illnesses are directly linked to cigarette smoking, such as lung cancer, chronic bronchitis, heart disease, emphysema, respiratory ailments, and others such as cancer of the mouth and throat (from smokeless tobacco), cancer of the bowel, angina, diarrhea, heartburn, and peptic ulcers. Cancer of the lip, larynx, esophagus, and pharynx is related to chewing smokeless tobacco. And, cancer of the tongue has almost doubled because of the increase in the use of smokeless chewing tobacco.

Cigarettes are a factor in 17.2 percent of all deaths in the United States each year. Eighty-five percent of lung cancer is smoking related, and 85 percent of deaths from chronic obstructive pulmonary disease is a direct result of smoking. The American Lung Association reports that 350,000 Americans die every year from smoking. This is more than the combined deaths from alcohol, illegal drugs, traffic accidents, suicide, and homicide.

It is a proven fact that smoking is deadly. If you smoke, you are shortening your life span by as much as ten to fifteen years. For example, 40 percent of heavy smokers die before they reach retirement age. In addition, in psychological terms smoking is considered a form of suicide. The smoker knows the risks of smoking yet he continues to smoke.

The ingredients that make up a cigarette should be an immediate signal to the smoker or would-be smoker that the habit is dangerous. Along with traces of certain gases with unknown effects, tobacco smoke contains nicotine, carbon monoxide, carcinogens, and irritant substances. Although nicotine is a stimulant, in large doses it acts as a depressant. Nicotine makes the heart pump faster and work harder, increasing the likelihood of heart disease. And, although smokers claim that smoking relaxes them, nicotine actually causes palpitations and a generalized feeling of anxiety. Carbon monoxide, when combined with the body's hemoglobin, prevents oxygen from being transported throughout the body. Carbon monoxide also allows for the development of cholesterol deposits on artery walls. These two factors increase the risk of heart attack and stroke. Hydrogen cyanide, a chemical contained within the smoke, causes bronchitis by inflaming the lining of the bronchi.

Research on addiction indicates that nicotine works much like heroin, cocaine, and alcohol. In fact, when nicotine was intravenously administered to volunteers, many of them could not tell the difference between the effects of nicotine and cocaine. Nicotine produces pleasurable sensations and physical dependency because it operates through the central nervous system. Unpleasant withdrawal symptoms usually occur when smokers refrain from smoking. They typically feel irritable, depressed, and anxious, and experience a phlegmy cough, stomach cramps, and headaches. These symptoms, however, usually last no longer than a few weeks.

Cigarette smoking poses a serious threat to the female. Studies indicate that females who smoke have the following consequences: they reach menopause early because of toxic chemicals in the tobacco that affect the hormone-producing cells in the ovaries; they face a greater risk of osteoporosis after menopause; and, in addition to the higher risk of lung cancer, the female smoker has a much higher risk of cancer of the cervix or the uterus. Women who smoke are less fertile and have more difficulties with their pregnancies. They have more spontaneous abortions, stillbirths, and premature deliveries. The babies are smaller and at much higher risk than the babies of nonsmokers.

In addition, men who have smoked for years are more likely to have abnormally low penile blood pressure, which contributes to the inability to have an erection. Smoking damages the tiny blood vessels that supply the penis.

If you cannot stop smoking or are in jeopardy as a passive smoker, the following nutrients will help protect against the dangers of smoking.

NUTRIENTS

SUPPLEMENT	SUGGESTED DOSAGE	COMMENTS
Essential		
Oxy-5000 from American Biologics	2 tablets 3 times daily.	A powerful antioxidant. Destroys free radicals produced in the smoke.
Vitamin B complex plus extra vitamin B$_{12}$ and folic acid	100 mg daily.	Necessary in cellular enzyme systems damaged in the smoker.
Vitamin C	3,000–7,000 mg daily.	Important antioxidant. Smoking drastically depletes vitamin C.
Very Important		
Vitamin A and beta-carotene	25,000 IU daily. 15,000 IU daily.	Antioxidants that aid in the healing of mucous membranes. Beta-carotene is important for lung protection.
Zinc	50–80 mg daily.	Important in immune function.
Helpful		
Coenzyme Q$_{10}$	30 mg daily.	Free radical scavenger. Improves tissue oxygen levels.
Germanium	30 mg daily.	Free radical scavenger. Improves tissue oxygen levels.
L-Methionine and L-cysteine and L-cystine (amino acids)	Use as directed on label.	Potent detoxifiers that protect the lungs, liver, brain, and tissues from cigarette smoke.
Multivitamin and mineral complex and beta-carotene including selenium	25,000 IU daily. 200 mcg daily.	Necessary for immune function. Selenium helps to prevent cell damage.
Raw thymus	As directed on label.	A glandular that improves immune function.
Vitamin E	800 IU daily. Start with 200 IU and increase 200 IU each month until up to 800 IU.	An important antioxidant needed to protect all cells from damage by the smoker.

RECOMMENDATIONS

☐ The urge to smoke lasts only from three to five minutes. Although it is difficult, wait it out; it will get easier and easier. However, do not just sit and do nothing while you are having the craving. Take a walk or do some sit-ups—anything to take your mind off the cigarettes.

CONSIDERATIONS

☐ Fresh carrot juice daily is the best preventive measure against lung cancer. A proper diet is most important.

Avoid stress as much as possible. Consume more asparagus, broccoli, Brussels sprouts, cabbage, cantaloupe, cauliflower, spinach, sweet potatoes, and turnips. *See* CANCER in Part Two.

☐ A lack of beta-carotene and the vitamin B complex has been linked to lung and throat cancer.

☐ George Papanicolaou, inventor of the cervical pap smear (for detection of uterine cancer), has also invented a test for the detection of lung cancer. It is called a sputum cytology test. Sputum is coughed up from the lungs and the bronchial tubes and is examined for signs of cancer. There has been controversy among doctors disputing the method and the accuracy of this test. However, there is hope that this method will detect the presence of cancer a few years before chest x-rays can.

Snake Bite

The victim of a snake bite may exhibit mild to severe symptoms because there are many varieties of poisonous snakes and the strength of their venoms differs. All snake bite victims should be seen by a doctor immediately. In the meantime, the victim should remain as still as possible.

Some of the symptoms of snake bite include swelling or discoloration of the skin and a racing pulse. The victim will become weak and possibly short of breath. Nausea and vomiting may occur. In extreme cases, there will be severe pain and swelling. The pupils will dilate, and shock and convulsion may occur. The victim may twitch and his speech may become slurred. In the most severe cases, paralysis, unconsciousness, and death will result.

After seeing a doctor, the following suggestions can be implemented to help alleviate pain and symptoms.

NUTRIENTS

SUPPLEMENT	SUGGESTED DOSAGE	COMMENTS
Helpful		
Calcium gluconate	500 mg every 4–6 hours.	To relieve pain. Acts as a sedative.
Pantothenic acid (B$_5$)	500 mg every 4 hours for 2 days.	Antistress vitamin.
Vitamin C	5,000–15,000 mg (10,000 mg every hour).	A powerful detoxifier. Relieves pain and discomfort and lessens infection. *See* ASCORBIC ACID FLUSH in Part Three.

HERBS

☐ Echinacea should be taken in tea and capsule form. Drink yellow dock tea or take two capsules of yellow dock every hour until the symptoms are gone.

☐ Poultices of white oak bark leaves and bark, comfrey, or slippery elm can be used. Plantain poultice, plantain salve, or comfrey salve can be used. (*See* POULTICE in Part Three.) If you live in an area where there are rattlesnakes, eat plantain. It grows near rattlesnake dwellings, and will supply some protection.

RECOMMENDATIONS

☐ If medical help is not immediate, apply a constricting band two to four inches above the bite. Keep calm and immobilize the affected area, keeping below heart level if possible. Cold therapy such as an ice pack is not recommended. If rapid swelling or severe pain develops, a half-inch incision should be made directly below the fang marks, and suction should be performed. The cut should be made along the long axis of the limb with a sharp, sterilized blade just through the skin, and suction should be done for thirty minutes with a suction cup or with the mouth (spit out the blood!). Never make cuts on the head, neck, or trunk.

☐ In a life-threatening situation, massive doses of vitamin C may save the victim's life.

CONSIDERATIONS

☐ If you spend much time outdoors, you may want to purchase a one-handed vacuum pump to extract the poison from insect bites. This pump is painless, and in an experiment done with this pump, 94 percent of the participants had either no reaction or a minor one from the bite. For information, contact: Tecnu Enterprises, 828 E. First Avenue, Department LL, Albany, OR, or call 1-(800) ITCHING.

Sore Throat

A sore throat can be caused by anything that irritates the sensitive mucous membranes at the back of the throat and mouth. Some irritants include viral and bacterial infections, allergic reactions, dust, smoke, fumes, extremely hot foods or drinks, tooth or gum infections, and abrasions. Chronic coughing and excessive loud talking also irritate the throat. Hoarseness is a common side effect.

Typically, a sore throat is an extension of the common cold, tonsillitis, sinusitis, or a viral infection. An acute sore throat should run its course within a few days to a few weeks.

NUTRIENTS

SUPPLEMENT	SUGGESTED DOSAGE	COMMENTS
Helpful		
Acidophilus capsules or liquid	Use as directed on label.	Especially important if taking antibiotics.
Bee propolis	Use as directed on label.	Protects mucous membranes of the mouth and throat.
Garlic capsules (Kyolic or Kyo-Green)	2 capsules with meals. 3 times daily.	Odorless garlic. For improved immune function. Contains live enzymes, amino acids, vitamins, minerals, and chlorophyll for healing.
Vitamin A emulsion	Take 100,000 IU for 1 week, reduce to 50,000 IU for 1 week, and end with 25,000 IU. Or use 50,000 IU in capsule form daily.	Enters system rapidly. Aids healing. Potentiates immune function.
Vitamin C	10,000 mg daily.	Has antiviral properties. *See* ASCORBIC ACID FLUSH in Part Three.
Zinc gluconate lozenges	1 every 2 hours until pain is relieved. Take in high dosages for no longer than 1 week.	For pain relief, healing, and improved immune function.

RECOMMENDATIONS

☐ Liquid vitamin C is good to sip. Allow it to drip down the throat slowly. Gargle alternately with chlorophyll and sea salt (a half teaspoon in a glass of warm water) every few hours. Drink plenty of liquids—fresh juices are best. *See* FASTING in Part Three, and follow the program. Raw honey with lemon juice is good for coating the throat.

☐ Catnip tea enemas will reduce fever. *See* ENEMAS in Part Three.

CONSIDERATIONS

☐ If a sore throat is recurrent or lasts for long periods, suspect mononucleosis.

☐ A constant tickle or chronic irritating cough could be an indication of food allergies.

☐ If antibiotics are taken, eat yogurt and take acidophilus to replace the destroyed "friendly" bacteria.

☐ Many sore throats and infections may be the result of bacteria on toothbrushes. It takes seventeen to thirty-five days to infect a toothbrush, so change once monthly.

☐ *See also* COMMON COLD, MONONUCLEOSIS, SINUSITIS, and TONSILLITIS, all in Part Two.

Spider Bite

The stings of some spiders, as well as scorpions and centipedes, can be dangerous, and most are painful. In case of spider bite, see your doctor immediately. Keep in mind that rattlesnake and black widow venom are almost the same, so they should be treated similarly. Try to rid the body of as much poison as possible by encouraging bleeding. This can be done by suction (*see* SNAKE BITE in Part Two).

If there is swelling or pain after a spider bite, apply a constricting band two to four inches *above* the bite. Keep calm. Immobilize the affected area, keeping it below the heart level if possible. The victim should lie down and be kept warm. Pack ice around the wound to slow down the spread of the poison.

NUTRIENTS

SUPPLEMENT	SUGGESTED DOSAGE	COMMENTS
Helpful		
Calcium gluconate	As directed on label.	Helps relieve pain.
Pantothenic acid (B₅)	500 mg	Has anti-allergy properties.
Vitamin C	5,000–15,000 mg (10,000 mg every hour).	Very important in crisis allergy situations! See ASCORBIC ACID FLUSH, Part Three.
Vitamin C and pantothenic acid (B₅)	Injections should be administered in life-threatening cases by a medical professional.	Needed for protection from the venom. Aids in detoxifying the venom from the body.
Vitamin E capsule and vitamin E oil	Cut open 1 capsule, and apply daily.	Aids healing and relieves discomfort.

HERBS

☐ Echinacea can be taken as a tea or in capsule form. Drink as much yellow dock tea as you can, or take two capsules of yellow dock every hour until symptoms are relieved. Apply poultices of white oak bark and leaves, comfrey, slippery elm, or plantain.

RECOMMENDATIONS

☐ *See also* BEE STING, INSECT ALLERGY, and SNAKE BITE in Part Two.

Sprains, Strains, and Other Injuries of the Muscles and Joints

If an individual stresses a muscle beyond its capability, the muscle will become strained; it may knot up instead of relaxing. Putting undue weight on the muscles and using the muscles for prolonged periods without rest can create muscle strain.

When the ligament connecting bone to muscle is stretched beyond its capability, the ligament may tear, causing a sprain. The soft tissue surrounding the joint may be sore, swollen, and bruised. The joints most often injured are the ankles, back, fingers, knees, and wrists. Sprains may result from unexpected movement or twisting of the affected area or from a hard fall. These types of injuries are common in athletes.

The following supplement program can help these injuries heal.

NUTRIENTS

SUPPLEMENT	SUGGESTED DOSAGE	COMMENTS
Very Important		
Proteolytic enzymes	3 tablets between meals.	Destroys free radicals that are released during injury.
Helpful		
Protein (free form amino acids) plus vitamin B₁₂ and vitamin B₆ (pyridoxine) and vitamin C	As directed on labels.	Helps to repair and strenthen connective tissue, ligaments, and tendons. Free form amino acids reduce body fat and help maintain a positive nitrogen balance for increased energy.
Calcium (gluconate and chelate forms) plus magnesium	1,500–2,000 mg daily. 750–1,000 mg daily.	Both forms of calcium are needed to assure assimilation. Needed for repair of bone and connective tissue. Magnesium is also very important for the skeletal system.
DMG (Gluconic from DaVinci Labs)	As directed on label.	Increases tissue oxygenation.
Liver (from Argentine beef only)	As directed on label.	Injections should be considered.

Mixed raw bovine neonatal tissue from Biotics Research or	As directed on label.	Stimulates healing of muscles and bones.
Osteoblast from Arteria	As directed on label.	
Multimineral formula	As directed on label.	Vital to tissue repair.
Potassium	99 mg daily.	Vital to tissue repair.
Silica (silicon)	500 mg daily.	Needed for connective tissue repair and calcium absorption.
Unsaturated fatty acids		
Vitamin B complex (high potency) with additional pantothenic acid (B₅)	100 mg daily. 500 mg daily.	All the B vitamins are important during stressful situations, especially B_5.
Vitamin C	3,000–5,000 mg daily.	Calcium ascorbate is the best source for these injuries.
Vitamin E	400–1,000 IU daily.	A free radical scavenger.
Zinc	50 mg daily.	Important in tissue repair.

RECOMMENDATIONS

☐ Do not use heat immediately following the injury. Apply cold packs to the injured area immediately, especially if a sprain may be involved. The cold will help reduce swelling and inflammation. Use this method of cold therapy for twenty-four to thirty-six hours following the injury. If an ankle or muscle is injured, keep it elevated. After the initial cold therapy, alternate between hot and cold treatments every twenty minutes to help relieve pain.

☐ For possible sprain, see your physician immediately. To eliminate the possibility of a fracture or broken bones, have x-rays taken immediately following the injury.

☐ In order to provide support, an elastic bandage can be used to wrap the sprained part for two to four weeks following the injury. Make sure that the bandage allows adequate circulation. Refrain from using the injured part for a few days or until swelling and pain is relieved.

☐ Soaking the affected area in warm or hot water may help relieve prolonged pain; however, do not do so until the swelling subsides.

☐ Combine turmeric and a little hot water. Smooth into a paste. Apply this mixture to the injured area with a gauze dressing. This treatment is good for bruises and helps to reduce swelling. Clay poultices can also be used. Fresh mullein leaves are beneficial when used in a poultice. *See* POULTICE in Part Three.

CONSIDERATIONS

☐ *See also* FRACTURE in Part Two.

Sports Nutrition

Carbohydrates and fats—not proteins—are the main sources of energy used by the muscles. If you consume more carbohydrates than you use, you will add extra pounds to your body weight. The body can convert dietary fat to body fat more easily than it can convert excess carbohydrates to body fat, so limit your fat intake. If there are insufficient carbohydrates available, the body will need to use protein, which is needed for tissue and structural repair, for energy. When the body must use its protein for energy, losses of lean tissue and muscle occur.

Since the body uses carbohydrates and fats for energy, its need for protein does not increase with exercise. It requires larger amounts of carbohydrates or fats to exercise than it does to sit at a desk; however, it does not require more protein. Excess protein intake increases elimination of urine by the body. This may cause dehydration and hinder your performance and endurance. You may faint if you become dehydrated. Because excess protein is not stored, it puts a strain on the liver and kidneys.

The following nutritional guidelines will enhance your performance while exercising and should be followed for optimum health:

- Avoid the following foods before a workout: bananas, celery, grapes, peaches, and shrimp. Severe reactions to them have occurred after exercising.
- Solid foods should be consumed four hours before competition or vigorous exercise, and any liquids should be consumed two hours prior to exercising.
- Limit consumption of roughage before exercising. It requires energy to digest it, and will make you feel full and sluggish.
- If you have any known food allergies, exercise may increase the absorption of the allergenic food by the body, resulting in a more severe reaction to it.
- Drink fluids before exercising or running regardless of whether or not you feel thirsty. A combination of half unsweetened juice and half water is beneficial. You will lose moisture even in the wintertime when you inhale and exhale vigorously during exercise. You can lose 25 percent more fluids in the winter due to the cold. Wear a face mask if jogging in the winter; it will help decrease dehydration.

In addition to the guidelines for good nutrition, you should exercise the following precautions to avoid injury and promote fitness:

- Always stretch and warm up the muscles first before exercising to avoid injury to the muscles. Before the muscles have been worked, they are at a temperature of 98°F and are stiff. After a five-minute warm-up, their temperature rises several degrees and loosens them up. After a workout, also be sure to cool your body temperature to normal before taking a shower. Providing for a cool-down period will prevent abnormal muscle contractures and even heart attack.
- If you have heart problems, avoid lifting weights. While lifting, you stop breathing for a moment and the chest muscles and abdomen tighten, exerting undue pressure on the lungs and heart. Circulation to the brain and heart is also decreased.
- Long-term use of steroids such as cortisone and anabolic steroids leads to osteoporosis, shrinkage of the testicles, cancer, sterility, and breast enlargement. Steroids taken by women can result in shrinkage of the breasts, excess facial and body hair, breast cancer, and deepened voices. Anabolic steroids may cause heart attacks. You can use sarsaparilla or saw palmetto to replace natural and synthetic testosterone instead of steroids. Don't gamble—it may cost you your life!
- Gravity boots and the back swing should be avoided by the following persons: those with glaucoma, heart disorders, hernias, artery disorders, and spinal instability, and anyone using blood thinners such as aspirin or anticoagulants.

The following supplements will promote good health in those involved in physical conditioning.

NUTRIENTS

SUPPLEMENT	SUGGESTED DOSAGE	COMMENTS
Essential		
DMG (Gluconic from DaVinci Labs)	Take in sublingual form.	Use before and during workouts to increase oxygen supply to the cells.
Important		
Potassium	99 mg daily.	Needed to replace potassium lost through sweat during exercise.
Selenium	200 mcg	Works synergistically with vitamin E.
Vitamin C (ascorbic acid) plus bioflavonoids and rutin	3,000 mg	Increases energy.
Vitamin E	400–1,000 IU	Supplies oxygen to the cells and increases energy levels.
Helpful		
Bee pollen	1,000 mg daily.	Increases energy and endurance.
Betaine HCl plus amylase and lipase and papain and trypsin	50 mg daily with meals.	For complete digestion and absorption of nutrients.
Calcium chelate or asporotate and magnesium oxide	1,000 mg daily. 500 mg daily.	For a healthy heart and bones.
Chromium (GTF)	200 mcg daily.	Stabilizes the blood sugar.
Coenzyme Q$_{10}$	60–100 mg daily.	Increases tissue oxygenation.
Copper	3 mg daily.	For bone formation and healing.
Garlic capsules (Kyolic)	2 capsules 3 times daily.	For energy and detoxification.
Germanium	100 mg daily.	Increases tissue oxygenation.
Iron	18 mg daily.	For hemoglobin production.
Kelp	150 mg daily.	High in iodine.
Liver	As directed on label.	Use only Argentine liver.
L-Arginine and L-carnitine and L-lysine and L-ornithine (amino acids)	250 mg daily. 200 mg daily. 500 mg daily.	Use amino acids in place of steroids. L-Carnitine carries fat to the muscles for energy. Arginine and ornithine stimulate the growth hormone that helps to burn fat and to build muscle tissues. L-Lysine is especially helpful if prone to cold sores and herpes outbreak.
Manganese	10 mg daily.	Bran is an excellent source of this vital trace mineral.
Octacosanol	1,000 mg daily.	Found in wheat germ. Reduce dosage of vitamin E if using octacosanol.
Omega-3 fatty acids	As directed on label.	Omega-3s are polyunsaturated. They lower cholesterol and triglyceride levels.
RNA complex	As directed on label.	For tissue and organ repair.
Silicon	25–100 mg	For normal growth and bone repair.
Vitamin A plus beta-carotene	10,000 mg 15,000 mg	Destroys free radicals formed during exercise.
Vitamin B complex with extra vitamin B$_{12}$ plus folic acid and niacin and pantothenic acid	100 mg daily in sublingual form. 800 mcg daily. 100 mg daily. 100 mg daily.	All B vitamins improve energy and help stress during exercise.
Vitamin D	1,000 IU daily.	Important in calcium (i.e., bone) metabolism.
Zinc gluconate	50 mg daily.	For stress and tissue repair.

HERBS

☐ Drink fenugreek tea. Ginseng and horsetail also aid in physical conditioning.

CONSIDERATIONS

☐ Canned oxygen, complete with a mask, is available for five dollars. This product is manufactured by the Japanese.

STD

See SEXUALLY TRANSMITTED DISEASES.

Strained Muscle

See SPRAINS, STRAINS, AND OTHER INJURIES OF THE MUSCLES AND JOINTS.

Stress and Anxiety

Stress can result from many things: a high-pressure job, relationships, financial problems, loneliness, crowds, and traffic jams. Because of the complexity of today's world, stress is experienced by everyone at one time or another.

Long-term stress often occurs when the situation that causes anxiety is not relieved. For example, a person who must care for and live with a family member who is physically or mentally ill experiences stress on a daily basis. Families whose economic status is far below what they need, who must worry about where the next meal will come from or where they will sleep that night, suffer from extreme stress.

Even those who are financially well-off, well-educated, and healthy experience stress. No one, no matter how content they seem, is exempt. Some people even create their own stress; there may be nothing wrong, but they will find something to worry about. Today, most of us are exposed to the most mentally taxing, stressful environment ever.

Although everyone experiences stress, not everyone handles it constructively. The body can handle some stress, whether it is physical or mental. It must be coped with, and most people have the ability to do this. If stress is short-term, then the chances are good that it will be dealt with. It is long-term stress that causes the body to break down.

Many people attribute their stress-related symptoms to "nerves," and, in fact, stress first affects the parts of the body that are related to the nervous system, especially through the digestive and intestinal systems. Initial symptoms of stress-related digestive disorders may be an ulcer attack or colitis. Irritability, high blood pressure, headaches and neckaches, diarrhea, dizziness, and loss of appetite are other disorders precipitated by stress. If the stress that produces these symptoms is not handled properly, then more serious illnesses may result.

Researchers at the University of Texas believe that when the brain is under stress, it produces an excess of the hormone ACTH. This hormone inhibits the manufacture of white blood cells so vital in fighting disease.

Relaxation is often difficult for the person suffering from anxiety, but it is necessary to alleviate the stress. A proper diet is also extremely important. The disorders that arise from stress are often the result of nutrient deficiencies; the body does not handle nutrients well during these times. The B-complex vitamins are very important for proper functioning of the nervous system. Vitamin B-complex injections are helpful, reducing the damage to the immune system. They also aid in improving brain function and reducing anxiety.

NUTRIENTS

SUPPLEMENT	SUGGESTED DOSAGE	COMMENTS
Essential		
Vitamin B complex plus	1 cc	Results can be seen quickly with intramuscular injection.
liver and	1 cc	
B₆ (pyridoxine) injections	½ cc 3 times weekly for 2 months, dropping to once weekly for 2 months, and then weekly as needed.	
or vitamin B complex in tablet form and	100 mg daily.	Take along with injection described above, or if unable to take injections, use alone.
pantothenic acid (B₅)	100 mg 3 times daily.	B₅ is the antistress vitamin.
Very Important		
Calcium and	2,000 mg daily.	Take chelate or lactate form of calcium. Do not take lactate if you are allergic to milk products.
magnesium	1,000 mg daily.	
L-Tyrosine (amino acid)	1,000 mg in divided doses (500 mg in daytime, 500 mg at bedtime on an empty stomach). Take with 50 mg vitamin B₆ and 500 mg vitamin C for better assimilation.	Helps reduce stress to the body. Effective and safe sleeping aid.
SP 14 combination from Solaray	As directed on label.	An antistress preparation.
Vitamin C with bioflavonoids	3,000–10,000 mg	Stress depletes the adrenal gland hormones, the antistress hormones. Vitamin C is essential to adrenal gland function.

Dealing With Stress

Stress is an unavoidable part of life. Everyone experiences stress and everyday small stresses are not harmful. In fact, they are often just stimulating enough to make life enjoyable, or at least interesting.

Some people handle stress well. Others are more negatively influenced by it. They are often driven and ambitious, and put themselves into situations that less driven people tend to avoid. Those who are driven are often said to have type "A" personalities, and the more relaxed personality is labeled type "B."

A study was done at the University of Washington Medical School that scientifically rated stressful situations by their negative effects on the physical and mental health of persons. Rated highest is the death of a spouse, and divorce is next, followed by other stressful circumstances such as marriage, personal illness, etc. They found that the larger the number of these situations that are experienced by a person, the higher the chance of illness.

Dr. Hans Selye, stress expert and author of *Stress Without Distress*, says that it is not stress that is harmful—it is *dis*tress. Distress occurs when emotional stress is prolonged and not dealt with in a positive way. The physical and emotional state that results from distress can lead to illness. The less serious conditions that are stress-related are fatigue, headache, heartburn, indigestion, insomnia, and even hair loss. The more serious conditions and diseases are acidosis, backache, cancer, Crohn's disease, depression, diarrhea, diverticulosis, hypertension, impotence, migraine headaches, pancreatic disease, and ulcers.

When faced with a high degree of stress, the body reacts this way: digestion shuts off and heart rate increases, with a resulting increase in blood pressure and breathing. Fats and sugars are released from stores in the body, cholesterol levels rise, and the blood prepares for clotting (necessary in case of injury) by changing in composition. In primitive times, these changes in the body prepared man to flee or fight. Now, we rarely use this response. A state of continual stress eventually tires the body, weakens the immune system, creates states of hypertension, raises cholesterol levels, and initiates conditions such as headaches, pains, sleeplessness, indigestion, and depression, which can turn into much more serious problems.

What should you do about stress? There are many different ways to relieve stress; choose the ones that work best for you. The following is a list of suggestions.

- Physical activity can clear your mind and keep stress under control. Some people like to run or walk by themselves; others prefer team sports such as basketball or soccer. Any type of exercise will do the trick, if a *regular* exercise program is followed. Exercising once a month will not do much to relieve stress.
- Some people find that meditation helps them relax and handle stress.
- Try to rest and to get enough sleep. This may be difficult, because stress often keeps you up at night, although there are some people who welcome sleep as an escape. The less sleep you get, the more stressful you will feel, and the higher your chance of becoming ill will be, because your immune system will weaken.
- Deep breathing is good and can be done when you are faced with a stressful situation at home, at work, while in your car, or elsewhere.
- Take a day off—that's what weekends are for! Take a drive or go to the beach. If you prefer, stay home and work in the yard or read. Try to control your thoughts during this time so that you don't think about work or whatever problems are causing the stress.
- Hobbies are great for relieving stress. What do you enjoy doing? Take the time to do it and enjoy yourself. Don't feel guilty for spending time and money doing something for yourself! Your health is worth it.
- Try not to take life so seriously. Learn to laugh.
- If you cannot handle the stress, you may need professional help. There is nothing wrong with resorting to therapy to help you handle your problems. It is often enlightening to talk about your problems with someone who can remain totally objective.
- Avoid caffeine, which aggravates stress, and smoking, alcohol, and drugs. While drugs and alcohol may offer temporary relief from stress, the stressor is still there the next day, and your health suffers with their use. Remember, there is no escape from stress. You must—and can—learn to handle it.

One of the most important ways that anyone can remain in good health during stressful times is by following a correct diet. Along with avoiding caffeine and alcohol, you should also stay away from sugar, white flour products, preserved meats, and heavy spices and seasonings. Do not eat junk foods! A good diet will give you the strength you need and keep your nervous system and immune system in great shape.

Helpful		
Brewer's yeast or Bio-Strath	As directed on label.	Bio-Strath is a tonic full of needed concentrated yeast, enzymes, amino acids, vitamins, and minerals.
Extra fiber (Aerobic Bulk Cleanse (ABC) or oat bran)	As directed on label.	For bowel cleansing and improved bowel function.
GABA (amino acid) combined with inositol	As directed on label.	Acts as a tranquilizer.
Kelp	5 tablets daily.	A balanced vitamin/mineral preparation.
Lecithin	2 capsules with meals.	Coats the nerve fibers. For cellular protection and brain function.
L-Lysine plus vitamin C and zinc gluconate	As directed on label.	For cold sores, which are often the first indicator of stress. Reduces stress so better handled.
Multivitamin and mineral complex containing vitamin A and potassium	25,000 IU daily. 99 mg daily.	Especially necessary during stress. Potassium is needed for adrenal gland function.
Proteolytic enzymes	Take between meals.	Destroys free radicals released during stress.
Raw adrenal plus raw thymus		Stimulates adrenal and thymus glands, so important in the body's stress reaction.
Vitamin E	400 IU	For needed immune function.
Zinc	50 mg	For needed immune function.

HERBS

☐ Use catnip, chamomile, hops, lady slipper, passionflower, pau d'arco, rose hips, rosemary and melissa, Siberian ginseng, skullcap, and valerian root.

RECOMMENDATIONS

☐ Diet is so important. Stay away from foods that create stress on the system such as colas, fried foods, junk foods, sugar, white flour products, and potato chips. Eat a 50 to 75 percent raw foods diet. Eliminate dairy products for three weeks; reintroduce slowly and observe the return of symptoms of your "nervous" condition. A quality diet, exercise, and proper rest are very important! You'll be amazed at the results.

☐ A hair analysis can rule out heavy metal intoxication as the cause of depression. Look into this, and *see* ALLERGIES in Part Two to rule out food allergies. For quick results, follow the fasting program in Part Three.

Sunburn

Sunburn is caused by excessive exposure to ultraviolet rays. The amount of exposure that will cause a burn depends on the individual, the place, the time, and the atmospheric conditions.

Avoid the sun when the ultraviolet rays are at their strongest, between the hours of 11 a.m. and 2 p.m. Reflections from water, metal, sand, or snow may double the amount of rays you absorb.

Burns are classified in three degrees. A first-degree sunburn reddens the skin. A second-degree sunburn causes reddening of the skin with some water blisters. *A third-degree sunburn requires the immediate care of a physician* and causes lower cell damage and the release of fluid, resulting in eruptions and breaks in the skin where bacteria and infection can enter.

Remember that ultraviolet rays can penetrate clouds—you can burn without realizing it on hazy days. *See* SKIN CANCER in Part Two.

NUTRIENTS

SUPPLEMENT	SUGGESTED DOSAGE	COMMENTS
Important		
Potassium	99 mg daily.	Potassium loss must be replaced.
Protein (free form amino acids)	Use as directed on label.	Needed for tissue repair. Free form amino acids are easily absorbed and assimilated.
Vitamin A and E emulsion or		Emulsion enters the system more rapidly.
vitamin A capsules and	Start with 100,000 IU for 2 weeks, then decrease to 50,000 IU until healed.	Destroys free radicals released from burning the skin.
vitamin E capsules	Start with 100 IU and increase slowly to 1,600 IU for third-degree burns.	Aids in tissue repair and healing of scar tissue.
Vitamin C plus bioflavonoids	10,000 mg and up.	Use ascorbates. Needed for tissue repair and healing. Also reduces scarring.
Helpful		
All-Purpose Bacteriaside Spray from Aerobic Life Products	Use as directed on label.	Destroys bacteria on the skin, reducing infection.
Aloe vera gel	Apply 3–4 times daily.	Good on burn after healing starts. Reduces pain and scarring.
Calcium and magnesium	2,000 mg 1,000 mg	Necessary for pH balance and potassium utilization. Also reduces stress on tissues.
Silicon	Use as directed on label.	Horsetail extract is good. Repairs connective tissue.

Unsaturated fatty acids	Use as directed on label.	Needed for tissue healing.
Vitamin B complex/PABA	100 mg daily.	Important for serious burns. PABA is good for protecting the skin.
Vitamin E ointment or capsule	Use ointment on burn after healing starts or open a capsule and apply.	Prevents scarring.
Zinc	100 mg daily for 1 month; then reduce to 50 mg daily.	Used for tissue healing.

RECOMMENDATIONS

☐ For third-degree burns, your doctor may prescribe Silvadene Cream, antibiotics, and/or debridement to remove dead tissue, and possibly hydrotherapy to loosen dead skin. Keep muscles flexible. Muscle contracture can result from overlying skin damage and contraction.

☐ Diet for second- and third-degree burns is very important. Eat high-protein foods for tissue repair. Plenty of fluids should be consumed as the sun can quickly dehydrate the body.

☐ Cold clay poultices are very good. Apply cold-water compresses immediately.

☐ Some suggestions for treating sunburned skin are:

● Make a large pot of strong tea and let it cool. Soak cotton in the tea and apply to the affected areas. Leave on for up to thirty minutes.
● Dissolve one pound of baking soda into a tub of cool water. Soak in the tub for about thirty minutes.
● Massage aloe vera juice on the sunburned area. Reapply every hour. *Note*: Aloe vera will also help moisturize and relieve the skin of dryness. Use pure products without mineral oil, paraffin waxes, alcohol, or coloring.

CONSIDERATIONS

☐ Retinoic acid (vitamin A), the active ingredient in a prescription medication, helps to repair skin that has been sun-damaged from years of tanning.

Temperomandibular Joint Syndrome (TMJ)

As estimated 10 million Americans suffer from TMJ. Temperomandibular joint syndrome produces pain in the muscles and joints of the jaw that sometimes radiates to the face, neck, and shoulder. There may also be difficulty opening the mouth all the way, and clicking, grinding, and popping noises occur during chewing and movement of the joint.

Another cause of pain in the joints of the jaw is rheumatoid arthritis. In this disorder, the symptoms are more severe in the morning. This is usually not the case with TMJ.

After a careful examination, the doctor may use techniques such as arthrography, in which an opaque dye is injected into the joint and then viewed with fluoroscopy. There are also other ways to diagnose the problem. Often, the doctor will make a bite plate for the patient to wear at night to prevent clenching the teeth and compressing the joint and to correct the bite.

TMJ may have a number of causes. The two most common causes are a poor bite, with clenching and grinding of the teeth (bruxism), especially at night, and stress. (*See* BRUXISM and STRESS AND ANXIETY, both in Part Two.) Stress management, combined with heat and muscle relaxants, may often relieve the symptoms. A correct diet and the proper supplements, with or without a bite adjustment, often solve the problem.

NUTRIENTS

SUPPLEMENT	SUGGESTED DOSAGE	COMMENTS
Essential		
Calcium chelate and	2,000 mg	For proper muscular function and sedation effect. Prevents
magnesium	1,500 mg in divided doses after meals and at bedtime.	bond softening and relieves stress.
Vitamin B complex with extra	100 mg 3 times daily.	Antistress vitamins.
pantothenic acid (B$_5$)	100 mg twice daily.	
Helpful		
Coenzyme Q$_{10}$	60 mg daily.	Protects during stress.
L-Tyrosine (an amino acid) plus	500 mg on an empty stomach.	Improves quality of sleep. Relieves anxiety and depression.
vitamin B$_6$ and	50 mg at bedtime.	
vitamin C	500 mg	
Multivitamin and mineral complex	As directed on label.	Hypoallergenic product is best.
Vitamin C	4,000–8,000 mg	Combats stress. Necessary in adrenal gland function.

HERBS

☐ Hops, passionflower, skullcap, valerian root extract, and SP-14 from Solaray will help.

RECOMMENDATIONS

☐ Diet is very important. Avoid high-stress foods: all forms of sugar, all white flour products, all junk foods, candy, colas, potato chips, pies, and fast foods.

☐ The diet should include slightly steamed vegetables, fresh fruits, whole grain products, clear water fish, skinless chicken and turkey, brown rice, and homemade soups and breads.

☐ See FASTING in Part Three and fast at least once a month to give the body and jaws a rest.

☐ See also BRUXISM in Part Two.

Thrush

See CANDIDIASIS; YEAST INFECTION.

Thyroid

See HYPERTHYROID; HYPOTHYROID.

TMJ

See TEMPEROMANDIBULAR JOINT SYNDROME.

Tonsillitis

Tonsillitis is an inflammation of the tonsils, the glands of lymph tissue located on either side of the entrance to the throat. The inflammation is typically caused by viruses and other bacteria, often streptococcal organisms, which are present when the body's resistance is lowered. Tonsillitis can also be caused by an improper diet that is high in carbohydrates and low in protein and other nutrients. The more repeated bouts of tonsillitis a person has, the more difficult it is to cure. Each time the tonsils become inflamed, scar tissue accumulates on the tonsils.

A doctor should be consulted to determine what type of sore throat you have. Symptoms of tonsillitis include soreness, redness, pain and swelling of the tonsils, difficulty in swallowing, hoarseness, and coughing. Other possible symptoms are headache, earache, fever and chills, nausea and vomiting, nasal obstruction and discharge, and enlarged lymph nodes throughout the body.

Tonsillitis affects not only children. People of all ages can be afflicted with inflammation of the tonsils.

NUTRIENTS

SUPPLEMENT	SUGGESTED DOSAGE	COMMENTS
Important		
Vitamin C	3,000–5,000 mg	See ASCORBIC ACID FLUSH in Part Three.
Zinc gluconate lozenges	Dissolve in mouth every 2–3 hours.	An immunostimulant that aids healing.
Helpful		
Acidophilus capsules or liquid	As directed on label.	Necessary if antibiotics are used.
Chlorophyll		Use as a gargle.
Cod liver oil	As directed on label.	Aids immune response and healing of tissue.
Proteolytic enzymes	Take between meals.	Aids in reducing inflammation.
Vitamin A emulsion	10,000 IU for 5 days; 50,000 IU for 1 week; end with 25,000 IU.	Needed for repair of tissue. Aids healing.
Vitamin B$_6$ (pyridoxine) and pantothenic acid (B$_5$) plus B complex		Helps reduce swelling.
Vitamin E capsules	400 IU	

HERBS

☐ Chamomile, echinacea, pau d'arco, sage, and thyme are good in treatment of tonsillitis.

☐ Catnip tea enemas are especially good for fever. (*See* ENEMAS in Part Three.) For fever, pain, and swelling use a quarter teaspoon of lobelia extract every two hours until the fever is down. Make echinacea tea and drink as much as you can. Rest and drink plenty of fluids.

RECOMMENDATIONS

☐ A cleansing juice fast for three days with vegetable broth is helpful. *See* FASTING in Part Three.

☐ Use a warm salt-water gargle. Do not smoke.

Toxicity

See ALUMINUM TOXICITY; ARSENIC POISONING; CADMIUM TOXICITY; CHEMICAL ALLERGIES; CHEMICAL POISONING; COPPER TOXICITY; DDT POISONING; ENVIRONMENTAL TOXICITY; FOOD POISONING; LEAD POISONING; MERCURY TOXICITY; NICKEL TOXICITY.

Tuberculosis

Tuberculosis (TB) is a highly contagious disease caused by the bacteria *Mycobacterium tuberculosis*. It primarily affects the lungs, but can spread to the bones, kidneys, intestines, spleen, and liver.

The symptoms may be slow in developing and initially resemble influenza. Tuberculosis often begins with a cough that is frequently accompanied by bloody sputum. As the condition worsens, the victim experiences fever, severe night sweats, chronic fatigue, weight loss, chest pain, shortness of breath, and infected urine. In advanced cases, TB of the larynx occurs, making the patient unable to speak above a whisper.

The risk of contracting TB increases with unsanitary conditions, close contact with someone infected, impaired immune system function from chronic illnesses such as AIDS, an unbalanced diet, and a sedentary lifestyle.

NUTRIENTS

SUPPLEMENT	SUGGESTED DOSAGE	COMMENTS
Very Important		
Coenzyme Q$_{10}$	75 mg	Helps carry oxygen to tissues for healing.
Garlic tablets (Kyolic)	2 tablets with meals.	Odorless garlic that acts as a natural antibiotic. Keeps infection in check and stimulates immune function.
L-Cysteine and L-methionine (amino acids)	500 mg twice daily.	Protects the lungs and liver by detoxifying harmful toxins.
Protein (free form amino acids)		Needed for tissue repair. Free form amino acids are rapidly absorbed and assimilated by the body.
Selenium	200 mcg daily.	Protects against free radicals and promotes a healthy immune system.
Vitamin A emulsion or vitamin A capsules	200,000 IU emulsion. 25,000 IU in capsule form.	Vital for healing of lung tissue.

Vitamin B complex (high stress) plus brewer's yeast and extra pantothenic acid (B$_5$) and vitamin B$_6$ (pyridoxine)	Injections may be necessary. Consult physician. 100 mg 3 times daily. 50 mg 3 times daily.	Needed for production of red blood cells and antibodies. Aids in utilization of oxygen.
Vitamin C	*See* ASCORBIC ACID FLUSH in Part Three; find your dose and follow instructions.	Strengthens immune response. Promotes healing.
Vitamin D capsules	Start with 1,000 IU daily. Decrease slowly to 400 IU daily.	Essential for utilization of calcium and phosphorus. TB victims need sunlight daily and/or vitamin D for healing.
Vitamin E capsules	Start with 400 IU daily. Increase slowly until taking 1,600 IU daily.	Powerful free radical scavenger. Protects the lung tissues and provides oxygen to the cells. *Caution:* If you have high blood pressure, take 400 IU daily and increase slowly to 1,600 IU daily.
Important		
Germanium	200 mg	Absorbs excess hydrogen ions and removes them from the body, making oxygen more available to the tissues.
Multimineral supplement (high potency) containing calcium and magnesium	Take with meals. Do not take sustained release formula. 1,000 mg 750 mg	All nutrients are needed for strength and healing.
Kelp	10 tablets daily.	For a natural supply of minerals. Rich in iodine.
Oxy-5000 from American Biologics	As directed on label.	An antioxidant with superoxide dismutase (SOD).
Proteolytic enzymes and multidigestive enzymes	Take between meals. Take with meals.	Needed to keep inflammation down, to digest essential nutrients, and to improve absorption.
Zinc	50–80 mg	Promotes immune function and healing.

HERBS

☐ Drink three cups daily of echinacea and pau d'arco tea, or use the extract form of both and add the drops to water.

RECOMMENDATIONS

☐ The diet should consist of at least 50 percent raw vegetables and fruits. Eat two fertilized eggs daily. Also eat yogurt, buttermilk (and all soured forms of milk), fish, fowl, raw cheeses, raw seeds and nuts, whole grains, and garlic.

☐ Drink pineapple juice and fresh carrot juice daily with a "green drink." Kefir milk and fresh sugar-free yogurt should become part of the daily diet.

CONSIDERATIONS

☐ A chest x-ray or a tuberculosis skin test can detect the disease. See a doctor.

☐ Avoid stress. Rest, sunshine, and fresh air are most important. A dry climate is recommended.

☐ Specific anti-tuberculosis medications are available. Be aware of their side effects.

Tumors

A tumor is a swelling or abnormal growth of tissues having no useful function in the body. Tumors may either be benign or malignant. Benign tumors are isolated growths that can occur anywhere in the body. They generally do not spread to other parts of the body and usually do not return after being surgically removed. Although benign tumors are generally limited in growth, they usually should be removed; a small percentage of these benign tumors later become malignant. Fibroids are benign tumors that most often occur in the uterus. Hundreds of thousands of hysterectomies are performed each year due to the presence of fibroid tumors in the uterus.

Unlike benign tumors, malignant tumors are cancerous and must be treated as early as possible. They tend to spread to other parts of the body and are likely to recur after surgical removal. *See* CANCER in Part Two for more information.

Environmental factors and diet seem to play an important role in the development of tumors. Some tumors have decreased in size and others have actually disappeared after victims changed their dietary program and supplemented their diets with vitamins and minerals. The dietary changes and supplements that follow enhance immune function, suppressing the growth of tumors—both benign and malignant.

NUTRIENTS

SUPPLEMENT	SUGGESTED DOSAGE	COMMENTS
Important		
Coenzyme Q$_{10}$	30 mg daily.	Promotes immune function; carries oxygen to the cells.
Garlic capsules (Kyolic)	2 capsules with meals.	Studies conducted in Japan have shown good results. The size of tumors was reduced in many using Kyolic.
Germanium	200 mg daily.	Promotes immune function.
Proteolytic enzymes	As directed on label.	Helps the immune system. Aids in the breakdown of undigested foods.
Vitamin C	3,000–10,000 mg daily in divided doses.	Promotes immune function.
Helpful		
Kelp tablets	6 tablets daily.	Promotes immune function. Supplies balanced minerals.
Lecithin	Take with meals as directed on label.	For necessary vitamins and minerals.
Multivitamin and mineral supplement (high potency)	Take with meals as directed on label.	For necessary vitamins and minerals.
Raw thymus extract or glandular	As directed on label.	Stimulates the thymus gland, which is important for immune function. *See* GLANDULAR THERAPY in Part Three.
Vitamin A and vitamin E	50,000 IU daily. Start at 400 IU; increase gradually to 1,200 IU.	Powerful immunostimulants and antioxidants. Emulsion formula is the best for easier assimilation.
Vitamin B complex plus brewer's yeast Vitamin B$_6$ (pyridoxine) and pantothenic acid (B$_5$)	As directed on label. 50 mg 3 times daily.	B vitamins are vital in intracellular metabolism and normal cell multiplication. Consult a physician about possible injections.

HERBS

☐ Use barberry, dandelion, Jason Winters and pau d'arco teas, and red clover. Many people with tumors have responded well to poultices made from comfrey, pau d'arco, ragwort, and wood sage. *See* POULTICE in Part Three.

RECOMMENDATIONS

☐ *See* FASTING in Part Three and follow the program.

☐ Raw fruits and vegetables should comprise 50 percent of the diet. Nuts and seeds, whole grains, and yogurt and yogurt products should be included in the diet. *Also see* the diet in CANCER in Part Two.

☐ Eliminate animal protein, dairy products, salt, sugar, white flour, and white flour products from the diet. Also avoid processed and packaged foods. These types of foods contain no enzymes, are hard to digest, and cause toxic substances to form in the colon and bloodstream.

CONSIDERATIONS

☐ Those with breast tumors may benefit from a poultice made of poke root. *See* POULTICE in Part Three for directions on how to prepare one. Primrose oil is specifically useful for breast tumors. Take two capsules before meals.

☐ Iron deficiency has been linked to tumors. Before taking iron, have a blood test done to determine if a deficiency is present. Use caution when taking iron.

☐ A study conducted by scientists of the University of California at Los Angeles School of Medicine reported in the December 1988 issue of *Prevention* magazine that sodium linoleate, which is comprised of linoleic acid (an essential acid), has demonstrated its ability to fight cancer cells in laboratory tests. Mice with tumors that were injected with sodium linoleate survived from eighteen to forty-eight days longer than mice not given the injection. In addition, tumor growth was prevented altogether in more than 40 percent of the mice.

☐ *See also* FIBROCYSTIC DISEASE OF THE BREAST in Part Two.

Ulcers

Ulcers occur along the gastrointestinal tract, especially in the stomach (called a gastric ulcer), duodenum, and colon. Ulcers can also appear as bedsores (*see* BEDSORES in Part Two).

An ulcer results when, during stress, the body's defense of the lining of the stomach is damaged and the stomach cannot secrete sufficient mucus to protect it against the strong acid essential for digestion. The ulcer is aggravated by the level of anxiety of the individual before eating.

Aspirin and vitamin C may create more acid. When aspirin is taken over a period of time, it can cause ulcers. Steroids taken for arthritis and even nonsteroidal anti-inflammatory drugs may contribute to stomach ulcers. Heavy smokers have trouble healing an ulcer.

The varied symptoms of an ulcer can include stomach pain, lower back pain, headaches, choking sensations, and itching.

STOMACH ACID SELF-TEST

Hydrochloric acid (HCl) is necessary for the breakdown and digestion of many foods. You can determine if you need hydrochloric acid with this simple test. Take a tablespoon of apple cider vinegar or lemon juice. If this makes your heartburn go away, then you need more stomach acid. If it makes your symptoms worse, then you have too much HCl and shouldn't take enzymes that contain HCl. If it helps the symptoms, sip pure apple cider vinegar and water with meals.

NUTRIENTS

SUPPLEMENT	SUGGESTED DOSAGE	COMMENTS
Important		
L-Glutamine	500 mg daily on an empty stomach.	Important in the healing of peptic ulcers.
Pectin	As directed on label.	A controlled study reported good results with supplementation of pectin for duodenal ulcers.
Vitamin E	400 IU daily and up.	Aids in reducing stomach acids and in relieving pain.
Helpful		
Aloe vera juice or gel	4 oz. daily.	Aids in pain relief and speeds healing.
Iron (ferrous fumarate from Freeda vitamins or chelated form or Floradix formula from Germany)	As directed on label.	Helps prevent anemia, which may occur with bleeding ulcers.
L-Histidine	As directed on label.	Significant in healing.
Proteolytic enzymes	Take between meals.	Works on undigested food remaining in the colon, and helps reduce inflammation. *Caution:* Use a brand that doesn't contain hydrochloric acid (HCl).
Unsaturated fatty acids (Salmon or primrose oil or MaxEPA)		Protects the stomach and intestinal tract from ulcers.
Vitamin A emulsion or capsules	100,000 IU for 1 month; decrease to 50,000 IU for 1 month; end with 25,000 IU or take 25,000 IU daily in capsule form.	Needed for healing. Protects the mucous membranes of the stomach and intestines.
Vitamin B complex plus extra B₆ (pyridoxine)		Avoid high amounts of niacin (over 25 mg).
Vitamin E emulsion or capsule	400–800 IU	A potent antioxidant.
Vitamin K	100 mcg daily.	Found in alfalfa and dark green leafy vegetables.
Zinc	50–80 mg daily.	Promotes quicker healing.

HERBS

☐ Use bayberry, chamomile tea, catnip tea, goldenseal root, myrrh, sage, and slippery elm. Cayenne (also known as capsicum) is especially good for ulcers. Use it to stop the bleeding. Licorice is also beneficial for gastric and duodenal ulcers.

RECOMMENDATIONS

☐ Do not smoke or take aspirin.

☐ Try to relax and avoid stressful situations.

☐ Freshly made cabbage juice is beneficial for ulcers. Drink immediately after juicing—do not store. For ulcer pain, drink a large glass of water. This dilutes the gastric hydrochloric acid and flushes it through the stomach and duodenum.

☐ Do not drink milk, even though it neutralizes stomach acid. The calcium and protein in milk stimulates the production of more acid; milk has a rebound effect. Almond milk is a good substitute.

☐ Avoid fried foods, caffeine, tea, alcohol, salt, chocolate, strong spices, animal fats of any kind, and carbonated drinks. Instead of drinking soda, sip lemon juice and water.

☐ Eat small and frequent meals. Eat well-cooked millet, cooked white rice, raw goat's milk, and soured milk products such as yogurt, cottage cheese, and kefir. If symptoms are severe, eat soft foods such as avocados, bananas, potatoes, squash, and yams daily. Put all vegetables through a blender or processor. Eat well-steamed vegetables like broccoli and carrots occasionally. For bleeding ulcers, consume baby foods and add nonirritating fiber such as guar gum and psyllium seed. Great results have been reported after thirty days on this diet. The foods are easy to digest, nutritious, and without chemicals.

☐ Keep the colon clean—take enemas periodically. (See ENEMAS in Part Three.)

CONSIDERATIONS

☐ A new drug, Misoprostol, is being used in twenty-three countries for peptic ulcers. This drug may be best for smokers.

☐ Pain in the upper abdomen and blood in the stool may indicate an ulcer. Pulsebeat Enterprises has introduced the Hemacolon Kit, which is designed to detect blood in the stool. Each kit contains three tests, which can be conducted in the convenience of your home. For more information, write to Pulsebeat Enterprises, 2600 Netherland Avenue, Bronx, NY 10463.

☐ Blue grapes are used in Europe for ulcers.

☐ *See also* BEDSORES in Part Two.

Underweight

This section is for use in treating undernourished people who require nutritional rehabilitation or those who have increased nutrient requirements. This would include victims of hepatitis, burns and trauma, and anorexia that results from cancer and its treatment.

To stimulate a poor appetite, the diet must be individualized to accommodate the patient's tolerances and intolerances. Undernourished people may become anorexic at the sight of large amounts of food. Therefore, small frequent feedings may be better tolerated; gradually increase the amount of food. Consideration of the appearance and smell of the food, as well as the eating environment, is also important when trying to stimulate a poor appetite. The color red helps to stimulate taste buds.

NUTRIENTS

SUPPLEMENT	SUGGESTED DOSAGE	COMMENTS
Essential		
Liver extract (liquid)	As directed on label.	Excellent source of B vitamins and minerals. Easily assimilated.
Vitamin B complex	100 mg daily. Take with meals. Injections under the supervision of your doctor may be necessary.	Increases the appetite. Aids in digestion of fats, carbohydrates, and protein.
Zinc	80 mg daily.	Improves senses of taste and smell.
Important		
Bio-Strath	As directed on label.	Yeast and herbs from Germany. Appetite stimulant.
Garlic capsules (Kyolic)	2 capsules with meals.	Provides protection against free radicals. Contains many essential nutrients.
Helpful		
Floradix formula	As directed on label.	Increases appetite and helps digestion.
Multidigestive enzymes	As directed on label.	Aids digestion. Omit hydrochloric acid (HCl) if you have ulcers.
Multivitamin and mineral supplement (high potency)	As directed on label.	Supplies balanced vitamins and minerals.

Spiru-Tein from Nature's Plus	Take between meals as directed on label.	A safe protein supplement.

HERBS

☐ Fenugreek has long been used as an appetite stimulant, especially for the elderly. It also aids digestion.

RECOMMENDATIONS

☐ Have a complete medical examination to rule out any physical disorder. *See* the thyroid test in HYPOTHYROID, Part Two, to determine thyroid function. Rule out anorexia nervosa or bulimia—*see* ANOREXIA NERVOSA and BULIMIA, both in Part Two.

☐ The diet should consist of at least 300 grams of complex carbohydrates, 100 grams of protein, and from 2,500 to 3,000 calories a day. Include starchy vegetables such as potatoes and beans, grains, turkey, chicken, fish, eggs, avocados, olive oil, safflower oil, raw cheeses, nuts, and seeds. Eat only whole grain breads, rolls, macaroni, crackers, and hot and cold cereals.

☐ Use soy-based cream soups that are nondairy as desired. (Soy milk can be purchased in health food stores and can be used in the same ways as dairy milk.) These cream soups are usually higher in protein than broth soups and should be used as tolerated. Drink herb teas, fruit and vegetable juices, and Perrier or mineral water. Bananas are good for infant weight gain.

☐ If you smoke, stop. Avoid junk foods, coffee, soft drinks, and fried foods. Eat these high-calorie snacks between meals or before bedtime: raw cheese; banana soy pudding; turkey, chicken, or tuna sandwiches with cheese; rice crackers; iced herb tea with juice; yogurt; nut butters; yogurt fruit shakes; carob soy milk; almond milk; buttermilk; custard; nuts; and avocados.

☐ Walking and/or moderate exercise is important if possible, but avoid strenuous exercise. Some exercise helps in the assimilation of nutrients and in increasing the appetite.

☐ Eat in relaxed surroundings and never eat when upset or nervous.

☐ *See also* APPETITE, POOR.

Urinary Tract Infections

See CYSTITIS; KIDNEY AND BLADDER PROBLEMS; VAGINITIS.

Vaginitis

Vaginitis may be caused by bacteria, a yeast infection, excessive improper douching, a vitamin B deficiency, or intestinal worms.

Symptoms include burning and itching with vaginal discharge. This condition is more common in diabetic or pregnant women. The most common cause of vaginitis seems to be taking antibiotics, which destroy the "good" bacteria in the body. Oral contraceptives often produce vaginal inflammation.

NUTRIENTS

SUPPLEMENT	SUGGESTED DOSAGE	COMMENTS
Very Important		
Acidophilus capsules (Maxidophilus or Megadophilus)	2 capsules 3 times daily with meals.	Replenishes normal "friendly" bacteria.
Garlic capsules (Kyolic)	1 capsule with meals.	Garlic has antifungal properties.
Unsaturated fatty acids	As directed on label.	Aids healing.
Vitamin B complex (high potency)	100 mg	Often deficient in vaginitis.
Yeast-Gard vaginal suppositories	As directed on label.	Excellent antifungal agent. Reduces pain.
Helpful		
Maxidophilus	1 tsp. with 1 quart warm water for douche.	Can alternate with apple cider vinegar douche.
Vitamin A and vitamin E capsules	50,000 IU capsule daily. 400 IU capsule daily.	Aids healing. Powerful antioxidant.
Vitamin B$_6$ (pyridoxine)	50 mg 3 times daily.	Estrogen use increases need for B$_6$.
Vitamin C	2,000–5,000 mg	Important immune system stimulant. Necessary for tissue healing.
Vitamin D with calcium and magnesium	1,000 mg 1,500 mg 1,000 mg	Relieves stress. Women need these extra supplements at this time.

RECOMMENDATIONS

☐ Diet is important. Follow the diet in CANDIDIASIS, Part Two, until healed.

☐ Avoid sweet-smelling douches. Instead, you can douche with two capsules of acidophilus or plain yogurt. You can also add one teaspoon of fresh garlic juice.

☐ Wear white cotton underwear so that air can circulate freely.

☐ For itching, open vitamin E capsules and put on the inflamed area, or use vitamin E or enzyme cream.

☐ Add three cups of pure apple cider vinegar to your bath water to treat vaginitis. Soak in the tub for twenty minutes. Spread your legs open to allow water to flow into the vagina for douching.

CONSIDERATIONS

☐ The drug ketoconazole is used by many doctors, with no apparent adverse side effects. Mycelex-G is also used.

☐ Avoid taking zinc and iron supplements until healed. Bacterial infections require iron for growth. The body will store iron in compartments in the liver, spleen, and bone marrow when a bacterial infection is present in order to prevent further growth of the bacteria.

☐ *See also* CANDIDIASIS, CYSTITIS, KIDNEY AND BLADDER PROBLEMS, and YEAST INFECTION, all in Part Two.

Varicose Veins

Varicose veins are abnormally enlarged, swollen veins that occur most often in the legs. They are the result of a breakdown of the valves inside the veins that allow blood to flow back to the heart. If the valves do not work properly, blood accumulates in the veins, stretching them and causing varicosity.

Because lack of circulation contributes to the formation of varicose veins, they are common in people who sit for prolonged periods of time without movement (usually at their job), who sit with their legs crossed, who lack proper amounts of exercise, who are overweight or pregnant, or whose family exhibits a tendency toward varicose veins. People who are overweight or who engage in heavy lifting, and women who are pregnant, will be more prone to varicose veins because they put increased pressure on the legs.

These prominent, bluish, bulging veins are often accompanied by dull, nagging aches and pains. Swelling, leg sores, leg cramps, and a feeling of heaviness in the legs are characteristic of varicose veins. See your doctor if you have any of these symptoms. Do not be concerned if you have spider veins; they are harmless and should not cause any problems.

Hemorrhoids are a particularly painful type of varicose veins. Hemorrhoids are varicose veins of the anus or rectum. Symptoms of hemorrhoids include rectal itching, pain, and blood in the stool. Besides lack of circulation, hemorrhoids are usually caused by constipation, improper diet, and liver damage. *See* HEMORRHOIDS in Part Two for further information.

NUTRIENTS

SUPPLEMENT	SUGGESTED DOSAGE	COMMENTS
Very Important		
DMG (Gluconic from DaVinci Labs)	50 mg 3 times daily.	Improves oxygen utilization in the tissues.
Important		
Vitamin C plus	3,000–6,000 mg daily.	Vitamin C aids circulation by reducing blood clotting tendencies. Bioflavonoids promote healing and prevent bruising.
bioflavonoids complex	100 mg daily.	
Helpful		
Brewer's yeast	As directed on label.	Contains needed protein and B vitamins.
Lecithin liquid or capsule	1 tbsp. with meals or equal amount in capsule form.	Fat emulsifier that aids circulation.
Multivitamin complex (high potency)	As directed on label.	Needed for healing.
Potassium	99 mg daily.	Constipation is common for those with a potassium deficiency.
Vitamin B complex with extra vitamin B$_{12}$ and B$_6$ (pyridoxine)	3 times daily.	Needed to help in digestion of foods and relief of hemorrhoids.
Vitamin D	1,000 mg daily taken with 1,500 mg calcium chelate and 750 mg magnesium at bedtime.	Helps relieve leg cramps when combined with calcium and magnesium.
Vitamin E	Start at 400 IU and increase to 1,000 IU slowly.	Improves circulation and aids in preventing heavy feeling in the legs.
Zinc	80 mg daily.	Aids healing.

HERBS

☐ We recommend using any of these herbs: buckthorn bark, butcher's broom, collinsonia root, padma 28, parsley, red grapevine leaves, stone root, and uva ursi.

RECOMMENDATIONS

☐ Regulate your diet carefully. Your diet should be low in fat and refined carbohydrates, and contain plenty of fish and fresh fruits and vegetables. Avoid animal protein, processed and refined foods, sugar, ice cream, fried foods, cheeses, peanuts, junk foods, tobacco, alcohol, and salt. Make sure that your diet contains plenty of fiber. You want to keep the bowels clean. Aerobic Bulk Cleanse (ABC) is effective.

☐ To increase your circulation, it is important that you exercise. Avoid long periods of standing or sitting. Change your daily routine to allow more time for exercise and movement for your legs. Take rest periods several times during the day to elevate your legs. Avoid crossing your legs, heavy lifting, and putting any unnecessary pressure on your legs. Wear loose clothing that does not restrict blood flow. It is a good idea for women to wear supportive elastic stockings; these will help support varicose veins and help prevent them from becoming more swollen.

☐ Take a sitz bath daily. (*See* SITZ BATH in Part Three.) Mineral bath therapy can be very therapeutic.

☐ Vitamin K can help bleeding hemorrhoids. Good sources are alfalfa, blackstrap molasses, and dark green leafy vegetables.

CONSIDERATIONS

☐ Bathe your legs or other affected area in white oak bark herb tea three times a day, if possible, to help stimulate the blood flow. Heat this strong tea, but do not boil. Also apply directly to the affected areas.

☐ Holistic Rectal Ointment has been shown to give relief from the itching and pain of hemorrhoids.

☐ Some doctors use the Micro-Cure process, in which a sodium tetradecyl sulfate solution is injected into the infected vein. The solution fuses the vein walls together permanently, closing the defective vein. Your body will compensate by finding an alternative route for blood flow.

☐ You can use raw potato suppositories or cayenne and garlic enemas to help heal hemorrhoids and relieve pain. Peel potatoes and cut them so that they are shaped like small cones.

☐ *See also* CIRCULATORY PROBLEMS and HEMORRHOIDS in Part Two.

Venereal Disease

See SEXUALLY TRANSMITTED DISEASES.

Vertigo

Vertigo is the sensation of dizziness, faintness, or lightheadedness. It is related to the sense of balance and equilibrium. Dizziness occurs when the central nervous system receives conflicting messages from the inner ear, eyes, muscles, or skin pressure receptors.

Those who suffer from vertigo feel that they are sinking or falling, that the room and its objects are spinning around, and sometimes that they are spinning too. It can be caused by brain tumors, high and low blood pressure, allergies, head injuries, lack of oxygen to the brain, anemia, infections, nutritional deficiencies, neurological disease, psychological stress, change of atmosphere, blockage of the ear canal or eustachian tube, middle ear infections, excess wax in the ear, or moving too quickly from lying or sitting to a standing position. Poor cerebral circulation can also cause dizziness and the inability to maintain balance. Vertigo is sometimes accompanied by nausea and hearing loss.

NUTRIENTS

SUPPLEMENT	SUGGESTED DOSAGE	COMMENTS
Very Important		
DMG (Gluconic from DaVinci Labs)	As directed on label.	Increases brain oxygen.
Niacin (B₃)	100 mg 3 times daily.	Improves cerebral circulation and lowers cholesterol.
Vitamin B complex injections with B₆ (pyridoxine) and vitamin B₁₂ or vitamin B complex (high stress)	100–400 mg daily.	Necessary for normal brain and central nervous system function.
Vitamin C	3,000–10,000 mg daily in divided doses.	An antioxidant that also improves circulation.
Vitamin E	400–800 IU daily, increasing dosage slowly.	Improves circulation.
Important		
Choline or inositol and/or lecithin	3 times daily as directed on label.	Necessary in nerve function. Lecithin prevents hardening of the arteries and improves brain function.

Coenzyme Q$_{10}$	60 mg daily.	Improves circulation to the brain.
Ginkgo biloba extract	120 mg daily.	Improves brain function by supplying oxygen.

Helpful		
Brewer's yeast	Start with a small amount and work up.	Contains balanced B vitamins.
Calcium with magnesium	1,500 mg daily. 750 mg daily.	Aids in circulation (heartbeat).
Germanium	100 mg	Makes oxygen more available to the brain.
Kelp	5 tablets daily.	For necessary balanced minerals and vitamins.
Multivitamin and mineral supplement	As directed on label.	For necessary balanced minerals/vitamins.

HERBS

☐ Butcher's broom, cayenne, chaparral tea, dandelion extract or tea, and ginkgo biloba extract are beneficial for vertigo.

RECOMMENDATIONS

☐ Avoid nicotine, caffeine, salt, and fried foods. Avoid extreme or rapid head movements and rapid changes in body position.

Viral Infections

The viruses that cause infections are smaller than bacteria and can pass through the smallest cellular filters of the body. When viruses enter the body, they live on the body's cell enzymes. Viral infections are characterized by fever, headaches, muscular aching, and chills. The common cold is a viral infection, as are some forms of croup, mononucleosis, influenza, polio, tonsillitis, infectious hepatitis, encephalitis, measles, some bladder infections, and asthma.

Drugs relieve only the symptoms—they do not kill the virus. Antibiotics are not effective against viral infections; they kill bacteria but not the virus. When a viral infection gets out of hand and bacterial complications set in, antibiotics help. The body's defense system reaction against these infections is the same for all viral infections, no matter what organ is affected.

NUTRIENTS

SUPPLEMENT	SUGGESTED DOSAGE	COMMENTS
Very Important		
Inflazyme Forte from American Biologics or proteolytic enzymes	Take 2 capsules between meals.	Has antiviral capacity.
Vitamin C with bioflavonoids	3,000–10,000 mg daily in divided doses.	Powerful antiviral agent. See ASCORBIC ACID FLUSH in Part Three.
Zinc	50–100 mg daily.	Important in antiviral immune function.
Important		
DMG (Gluconic from DaVinci Labs)	As directed on label.	Improves tissue oxygen that neutralizes viral effects.
Maxidophilus or some form of acidophilus	¼ tsp. 3 times daily.	Inhibits pathogenic organisms. Especially needed if taking antibiotics.
Raw thymus	As directed on label.	Important in immune function, stimulating the thymus gland.
Vitamin A emulsion or capsule form	As directed on label.	A powerful antioxidant and free radical scavenger. Emulsion form enters the system quickly.
Helpful		
Garlic capsules (Kyolic)	2 capsules 3 times daily.	Potentiates immune function.
Germanium	200 mg daily.	Potentiates immune function.
Kelp	6 tablets daily.	Contains needed balanced vitamins and minerals.
L-Cysteine (amino acid)		An antioxidant that protects against viruses.
Vitamin B complex (high potency) and pantothenic acid (B$_5$)	As directed on label. 100–200 mg	Antistress vitamins. Needed if taking antibiotics.

HERBS

☐ Drink echinacea and pau d'arco teas daily. Catnip tea is also good. To relieve a fever, use a catnip tea enema.

RECOMMENDATIONS

☐ Do not eat dairy products, meat, white flour products, or sugar. Try a diet of raw fruit and vegetables.

☐ Go on a juice fast for three days or more, with cleansing enemas. (See FASTING and ENEMAS in Part Three.)

☐ Get plenty of rest.

☐ If you have infections that recur, check for low thyroid function—*see* the self-test in HYPOTHYROID in Part Two. Also test yourself to see what food allergies exist that may be destroying the immune system.

Vitiligo

This is a skin condition, also called leukoderma. It is characterized by white patches surrounded by a dark border. For some reason, the skin can no longer produce melanin, which is a skin pigment. Often, malfunction of the thyroid may be behind this disorder. (To check thyroid function, *see* the thyroid self-test in HYPOTHYROID in Part Two.) Proper nutrition is necessary along with good supplementation.

NUTRIENTS

SUPPLEMENT	SUGGESTED DOSAGE	COMMENTS
Very Important		
PABA	100 mg and up, 3 times daily.	Aids in stopping discoloration of the hair.
Pantothenic acid (B₅)	300 mg in daily divided doses.	Antistress vitamin; important in skin pigmentation.
Important		
Essential fatty acids (primrose oil)	Use as directed on label.	Stimulates hormone function and contains all the needed essential fatty acids.
Vitamin B complex	50 mg and up, 3 times daily.	Needed for proper skin tone and texture. An antistress vitamin.
Helpful		
Ageless Beauty from Biotec Foods	As directed on label.	A powerful antioxidant combination.

RECOMMENDATIONS

☐ Vitamin B complex plus PABA injections are often effective.

☐ Vitiligo sometimes responds to the use of PABA and magnesium. Small spots of pigment will appear gradually, like freckles. The pigment merges until normal color is restored. Some vitiligo patients have premature gray or white hair. In a small percentage of these cases treated with PABA and magnesium, both skin and hair color returned to the original color.

CONSIDERATIONS

☐ An article in *Let's Live* magazine reported on a new treatment in which healthy pigment cells were transplanted. These transplants were successful in all but one case and none rejected the transplanting of healthy pigment cells to the affected area.

☐ Gerovital H-3 face cream (GH-3) from Rumania has given good results. There have been no known problems from using this cream, only satisfactory results. This face cream is for adult use only.

Warts

VENEREAL OR GENITAL WARTS

Venereal or genital warts are single or clusters of soft, cauliflower-like growths found in and around the vagina, anus, penis, groin, or scrotal areas. They are caused by the human papilloma virus (HPV). There are more than thirty-five types of HPV, and two have been associated with cancer of the cervix and genital area.

These rough, bumpy growths can be found by the vaginal opening and labia. They are sexually transmitted and are highly contagious. Males can also contract these warts on their genitals.

If venereal warts are suspected, women should immediately see a gynecologist and have a pap test. Men who suspect venereal warts should immediately see a doctor. Women who have been diagnosed with genital warts should have a vaginal and uterine pap smear every six months due to their increased risk for cancer. The incubation period for genital warts is usually three months or longer. Early detection is important because this virus can be spread before the carrier is even aware that he or she has it.

COMMON WARTS

These warts can be found on the hands, feet, forearms, and face and range in size from a pinhead to a small bean. They can also occur on the voice box or the larynx and cause hoarseness. They are rough, irregular skin growths, and are caused by a virus. Highly contagious, they can be spread by picking, trimming, biting, or touching them. They can also be spread on the face by shaving. Common warts most often occur on skin that is continuously exposed to friction, trauma, or abrasion. They may be flat or raised, dry or moist, and have a rough and pitted surface that is either flesh-colored or darker than the surrounding skin. They typically do not cause pain or itching and can be left to disappear on their own unless they become bothersome. See below for ways to control or eliminate these common types of warts.

NUTRIENTS

SUPPLEMENT	SUGGESTED DOSAGE	COMMENTS
Very Important		
Vitamin B complex	50 mg 3 times daily.	Important in normal cell multiplication.
Vitamin C	4,000–10,000 mg daily.	Has powerful antiviral capacity.
Important		
L-Cysteine (amino acid)	Use as directed on label.	Sulfur source. Needed for normal skin.
Vitamin A	100,000 IU for 1 month, decrease to 50,000 IU for 1 month, end with 25,000 IU.	Needed for normalizing skin and epithelial membranes (i.e., vagina).
Vitamin E capsules or oil	400–800 IU daily.	Can also be applied to common warts. Cut open a capsule or apply oil daily. Vitamin or enzyme cream can also be applied directly to common warts.
Zinc	50–80 mg daily.	Increases immunity against viruses.
Helpful		
Multivitamin and mineral complex	Use as directed on label.	For normal cell division.

RECOMMENDATIONS

☐ For removing common warts, some people have had good results with a crushed garlic clove placed directly on the warts. Cover with a bandage for twenty-four hours. Blisters will form and then the warts will fall off in about a week. Applying castor oil to the wart is also successful.

☐ Increase the sulfur-containing amino acids in the diet such as those found in asparagus, citrus fruits, eggs, garlic and onions, and desiccated liver tablets.

☐ The genital area should be kept dry if you have genital warts. After a bath use a hair dryer on low. Do not rub or irritate the area. Wear only cotton underwear.

☐ Adequate daily vitamin C is most important in maintaining effective immunity against warts.

☐ Do not have sexual intercourse until the genital warts are completely healed.

CONSIDERATIONS

☐ A new treatment of injecting natural interferon alpha, a powerful antiviral substance, directly into the genital warts has proven successful in 36 percent of the cases, and in 40 percent the warts decreased in size. However, treatment of large numbers of warts may be too uncomfortable and expensive (*The New England Journal of Medicine*, 1986 and *The Journal of the American Medical Association*, January, 1988).

☐ Some doctors have good results with the drug bleomycin. It is injected or applied locally.

☐ Freezing the warts with liquid nitrogen and fulguration with electrical cautery are other commonly used treatments for warts. Fulguration uses heat to destroy the warts.

Weakened Immune System

The immune system is most important to the body. It is the immune system that fights off disease-carrying germs and bacteria that enter the body. The antibodies and antitoxins of this system recognize these foreign bodies and attack them using leukocytes (white blood cells).

When the immune system weakens, infections can take over. You become more susceptible to colds, viruses, flus, and more serious illnesses. There are a number of substances (vitamins, minerals, enzymes, etc.) that are essential for the functioning of the human immune system.

- *Vitamin A* is the anti-infection vitamin. If used properly, vitamin A is rarely toxic and is very important in the body's defense system.

  Hans Neiper, M.D., the renowned European cancer specialist, recommends using high doses of beta-carotene, often in the form of carrot juice. Beta-carotene is the active ingredient in vitamin A. In addition, he suggests the use of emulsified vitamin A. Our experience would indicate the importance of vitamin A in the immune system.

- *Vitamin C*, with bioflavonoids, is essential to the formation of the adrenal hormones and in the production of lymphocytes, and has a direct effect on bacteria and viruses. Vitamin C may be the single most important vitamin for the immune system.

- *Vitamin E* interacts with vitamins A and C and selenium, acting as a primary antioxidant and scavenger of toxic free radicals. Vitamin E activity is an integral part of the body's defense system.

311

- *Kelp* in the form of giant red kelp, or brown kelp, has specific substances in it that are necessary for the immune system's functional integrity.

To strengthen the immune system, follow the program of supplements outlined below.

NUTRIENTS

SUPPLEMENT	SUGGESTED DOSAGE	COMMENTS
Helpful		
Acidophilus (Maxidophilus or Megadophilus)	As directed on label.	Restores important bacteria to the intestinal tract.
Coenzyme Q_{10}	100 mg daily.	Increases resistance to infectious organisms.
Garlic capsules (Kyolic)	2 capsules 3 times daily.	Odorless garlic that stimulates the immune system.
Germanium	200 mg daily.	Improves oxygen and promotes interferon production.
Kelp	8 tablets daily.	A balanced mineral food. Needed for immune system integrity. Use it instead of salt.
L-Cysteine and L-methionine and L-lysine and L-ornithine (amino acids)	500 mg each; take twice daily.	Destroys free radicals and viruses. Protects the glands, especially the liver.
Vitamin B_6 (pyridoxine) and vitamin B_{12} and folic acid and vitamin C	50 mg 3 times daily. 1,000 mcg 100 mg	Take on an empty stomach with juice and amino acids above. Amino acids need the presence of these nutrients for best absorption and for proper functioning of enzymes in the body. These supplements potentiate the amino acids.
Lecithin		Coats the cells and aids in their protection.
Multivitamin and mineral complex (high potency)	As directed on label.	Vitamins and minerals are essential for healing and defense.
Protein (free form amino acids)	As directed on label.	Free form amino acids are readily assimilated. Free form amino acids are protein "broken down" in a form that the body can use.
Proteolytic enzymes	2 tablets between meals and with meals.	Essential in protein digestion and immunity.
Raw thymus plus raw lymph and raw spleen concentrate and raw bone marrow	As directed on label.	All potentiate immune function.
Selenium	200 mcg daily.	Important free radical destroyers.
Superoxide dismutase (SOD) plus DMG (Gluconic from DaVinci Labs)	As directed on label.	Improves oxygen in the tissues.
Vitamin A plus beta-carotene	15,000 IU 10,000 IU	Needed for proper immune function.
Vitamin B complex	100 mg in tablet form. Injections may be necessary.	
Vitamin C plus bioflavonoids	3,000–10,000 mg daily divided up during the day.	*See* ASCORBIC ACID FLUSH in Part Three.
Vitamin E	400 IU daily.	Use A-E emulsion for easier assimilation.
Zinc chelate and copper	50–80 mg daily. 3 mg daily.	Zinc is very important for the immune system. However, in amounts over 100 mg, zinc can impair the immune response!

*These oral supplements are beneficial to the person undergoing chemotherapy. Additional vitamin B complex and vitamin E is suggested. All the nutrients listed are needed to strengthen a weak immune system whether it's damaged or not because of disease, poor living habits, chemotherapy, or a combination of all three.

HERBS

☐ Pau d'arco tea has an antibiotic effect. Also good are chlorophyll (a green drink needed daily), echinacea root, goldenseal, and red clover.

RECOMMENDATIONS

☐ Begin a diet of fresh fruits and vegetables, nuts, seeds, grains, and other foods that are high in fiber. Avoid eating animal products and processed foods, sugar, and soda.

☐ Mental depression results in a suppressed immune system response. A positive frame of mind is important in building up the immune system. *See* FASTING in Part Three and follow the program once a month to detoxify your body of poisons that can weaken the immune system.

☐ Check thyroid function (*see* HYPOTHYROID in Part Two to test for an underactive thyroid). An underactive thyroid results in immune deficiency.

☐ *See* CANDIDIASIS and ALLERGIES, both in Part Two.

CONSIDERATIONS

☐ Marijuana weakens the immune system. THC, the active ingredient in marijuana, alters the normal immune response, making the white blood cells 35 to 40 percent less effective.

☐ Mercury amalgam fillings have been linked to a weakened immune system. Toxic metals suppress the immune system. Hair analysis rules out heavy metal intoxication.

Weight Problems

See ANOREXIA NERVOSA; APPETITE, POOR; BULIMIA; OBESITY; UNDERWEIGHT.

Worms

Worms are parasites that live in the gastrointestinal tract. They are common in children. Types of worms include tapeworms, threadworms, hookworms, pinworms, or roundworms. They cause loss of appetite and weight, diarrhea, anemia, colon disorders, and rectal itching. Worm infestation also results in poor absorption of essential nutrients from the gastrointestinal tract. Causes include improper disposal of human waste, walking barefoot on contaminated soil, and ingestion of eggs or larvae from uncooked or partially cooked meat. Because the worms tend to come outside of the anus in the warmth of the bed, check this area of the child after he is asleep if you suspect he may have worms.

NUTRIENTS

SUPPLEMENT	SUGGESTED DOSAGE	COMMENTS
Important		
Garlic capsules (Kyolic)	2 capsules 3 times daily with meals.	Odorless garlic. For children, put fresh clove garlic in shoes to be absorbed through the skin.
Pumpkin extract		Contains zinc; aids in expelling the worms.

RECOMMENDATIONS

☐ Personal hygiene is very important. If you scratch the anus, the worm eggs can be transmitted to anything you handle.

☐ Use sodium chloride (a heavily salted diet) for children with pinworms for one to two weeks. Use areca nut (betel nut) for tapeworm. Drink male fern (aspidium) in a tea three times daily. Pinkroot, wormseed, and wormwood are good for all types of intestinal worms. Eat black walnut extract, pumpkin and sesame seeds, fig juice or figs, and chaparral tea or tablets on an empty stomach three times per day.

☐ Do not eat meats that are not fully cooked or meats that are left out of the refrigerator for too long. Avoid pork until the disorder is corrected.

☐ For severe infestation use high colonics. Use two per week for four weeks.

CONSIDERATIONS

☐ Children get roundworm more than other worms. Because of the associated nutritional deficiency, one must take large amounts of all supplements. A well-balanced diet is important.

X-Ray

See RADIATION POISONING.

Yeast Infection

When a fungus such as *Candida albicans* multiplies in the body, particularly in the vagina, the result is a yeast infection. Yeast infections are a common cause of vaginitis. Almost every woman will have a yeast infection at some time or another, and it is particularly common during pregnancy when the acidity and sugar content of a woman's vaginal secretions are altered. Using oral contraceptives can also lead to the development of a yeast infection. Because fungi such as *Candida albicans* thrive in the presence of sugar, women with diabetes will be more susceptible to yeast infections. In addition, those taking antibiotics may develop a yeast infection since antibiotics generally destroy the "good" bacteria in the body, upsetting the vaginal environment.

Common symptoms of a yeast infection include vaginal burning, itching, and discharge. The skin around the vagina may become sore and appear red.

NUTRIENTS

SUPPLEMENT	SUGGESTED DOSAGE	COMMENTS
Essential		
Garlic capsules (Kyolic)	2 capsules with meals or take 2 garlic-parsley capsules.	Odorless garlic that inhibits the infecting organism.
Vitamin C	2,000–5,000 mg daily.	Improves immunity.
Yeast-Gard vaginal suppositories	As directed on label.	Soothing to the vagina. Destroys the yeast organism (fungus).
Very Important		
Vitamin A and E emulsion	Take the recommended dosage or substitute with 50,000 IU vitamin A and 400 IU vitamin E daily.	Use emulsified form for quick assimilation. Powerful free radical scavengers that aid vaginal healing.
Helpful		
Acidophilus or Maxidophilus or Megadophilus	As directed on label.	Restores normal vaginal bacterial balance. Use milk-free type if allergic to milk.
Dioxychlor from American Biologics	5 drops in water twice daily.	Take this product if the infections are recurrent.
Protein (free form amino acids)	As directed on label.	Needed for repair of tissue. Free form is readily absorbed and assimilated.
Vitamin B complex (yeast free)	100 mg daily.	Candidiasis, a type of yeast infection, results in vitamin B deficiency.
Vitamin B$_6$ (pyridoxine)	50 mg 3 times daily.	
Vitamin D plus calcium and magnesium	As directed on label.	Women need extra amounts of these nutrients when the body fights infection.

HERBS

☐ Use pau d'arco.

RECOMMENDATIONS

☐ Include yogurt and soured products in your diet. Homemade yogurt may be the best treatment for this disorder. You may wish to purchase a yogurt maker—it is inexpensive and easy to use. Yogurt and soured products contain microorganisms called *lactobacilli*, normally present in the bowel and vagina, which actually destroy the fungus. Because the fungus multiplies in a sugary environment, reducing your intake of refined foods can alleviate symptoms.

CONSIDERATIONS

☐ You might try douching with two capsules of Kyolic (garlic) or with the juice of fresh garlic and water; alternate douching with acidophilus, which is described below. Keep the vagina clean and dry. To alleviate itching, open a vitamin E capsule and apply to the irritated area or apply an enzyme cream.

☐ You can also use acidophilus as an effective douche. This will help restore the normal balance of the bowel and vagina. Open two capsules of acidophilis and add them either to one quart of warm water or to plain yogurt. Apple cider vinegar is preferable to an over-the-counter product when douching.

☐ Many doctors prescribe Mycelex-G for a yeast infection. Ketoconazole is also used; no side effects to this drug have been documented.

☐ A new treatment for yeast infections is Terazol. Of the patients treated with Terazol, 95 percent have recovered within three days. Only a few reported any burning or itching.

☐ Cotton underwear may be preferable because it allows for free circulation of air.

☐ *See also* CANDIDIASIS and VAGINITIS in Part Two.

Conferring With Your Doctor Before Medical Tests

Many physicians recommend that you take diagnostic tests so that they can identify or rule out any medical problems before recommending treatment. Make sure that you are well-informed before testing. Discuss the following with your health care provider before you undergo testing:

1. Your allergies to foods, medications, anesthetics, or x-ray materials.

2. Instructions on what to do before the tests, such as discontinuing medication, refraining from smoking, and avoiding certain foods.
3. Pregnancy, if applicable.
4. Will there be a long wait and will you need help getting home after the tests?
5. The dangers and risks of the tests. Is there an alternative to the recommended test?

PART THREE

REMEDIES
AND THERAPIES

INTRODUCTION

In Part Two various treatment programs were recommended for each illness. Part Three explains how to implement each of the remedies and therapies. It describes when each treatment can be beneficial and offers instructions for effective use. You can choose from the more traditional remedies of juicing, fasting, and poultices or from the more conventional treatments of surgery and chelation therapy. These remedies can be used in conjunction with a healthy diet and supplementation program. After learning about the available treatments, you will be able to choose the option that is most suitable for you.

Ascorbic Acid Flush

Because vitamin C promotes the healing of wounds and protects the body from bacterial infection, allergens, and other pollutants, it is often beneficial to flush the body with ascorbic acid. Flushing the body with ascorbic acid can effectively treat chemical allergies and chemical poisoning, arsenic and radiation poisoning, influenza, and sprains, and can prevent a host of other illnesses, including cancer and AIDS.

PROGRAM FOR ADULTS

Place 1,000 milligrams (or one teaspoon) of ascorbic acid in a glass of water or juice. Take every half hour, keeping track of how much has been taken, until diarrhea results. Count the number of teaspoons that were needed to produce diarrhea. Subtract one from this amount. Take this resulting amount of ascorbic acid drinks every four hours for one to two days. Check to make sure that the stool remains at a "tapioca" consistency while taking the ascorbic acid. If it should become watery, decrease the dosage again. Use calcium ascorbate or another buffered product for the ascorbic acid flush.

PROGRAM FOR INFANTS AND CHILDREN

Place a quarter of a teaspoon of ascorbic acid in a glass of juice or water. Give this to the child every hour until a stool of "tapioca" consistency is produced. Calcium ascorbate may produce less diarrhea. If the child or infant is unable to produce this stool within twenty-four hours, increase the dose to half a teaspoonful every hour, and keep the child on this schedule for one or two days. Children should be given this treatment only under medical supervision.

CONSIDERATIONS

☐ A new form of vitamin C, called esterified vitamin C, is soon to be released on the market. It is significantly more active and remains in the system for a longer period. When this becomes available, use it in place of the ascorbic acid to flush the system.

Blood Purifier

This three- to five-day cleansing fast purifies the blood. Use distilled water, fresh lemon juice, beet juice, carrot juice, and dandelion teas and extract. Quality water is important. Drink at least eight glasses daily to aid in cleansing and to help carry toxins out of the body. Fresh lemon juice and distilled water are excellent purifiers.

Go on a raw vegetable diet for a few weeks, and include "green drinks." Lots of chlorophyll is needed in tablet form or in fresh juice. Wheatgrass or barley juice is good for the colon and for added chlorophyll. Alfalfa liquid is very good. Kyo-Green from Wakunaga of America Company contains both wheatgrass and barley grass. It is excellent as an aid to the immune system and for cleansing the blood.

To purify the blood, avoid white flour and all sugars. Also leave heated fats and oils out of the diet for one month.

NUTRIENTS

SUPPLEMENT	SUGGESTED DOSAGE	COMMENTS
Very Important		
Chlorophyll	Tablet form as directed or put in juice.	Cleanses the blood. Aids the immune system.
Important		
Cell Guard from Biotec Foods	As directed on label.	A good antioxidant.
Helpful		
Mainstream from New Moon Extracts	As directed on label.	Contains wheatgrass. Good for the liver.

HERBS

☐ Use goldenseal, red clover, dandelion, beriberi, Oregon grape, and pau d'arco. Echinacea is good for cleansing the lymph glands. Black radish, dandelion extract, and beet juice are good for the liver and aid in cleansing and healing. Burdock root helps eliminate toxins.

Improving Brain Function

Researchers are still attempting to unravel all of the brain's complexities. The brain is an amazing organ—

brain cells continue to die and are not replaced, but memories remain stored for a lifetime. The brain is made up of 100 billion nerve cells called neurons and can hold more information than all the books that have ever been published.

The brain manufactures hundreds of chemicals called neurotransmitters that affect moods, produce natural pain killers, natural tranquilizers, and a natural appetite suppressant. Neurotransmitters are made up of nutrients that allow information to pass from one circuit to another. This process allows all functions of the body to take place in proper sequence. All of these nutrients must be in balance or problems will occur. Linus Pauling, two-time Nobel Prize winner and world-renowned scientist, noted that nutrient concentrations may not always be high enough to supply all the organs and tissues, especially the brain. Many conditions that result from nutritional deficiencies alter mental states—in fact, changes in mood are often the first signs of a deficiency. Depression, memory loss, anxiety, and irritability are some of the signs.

The brain never sleeps and, overall, uses 20 percent of the body's energy. It requires constant oxygen, which it receives from the bloodstream, and uses approximately 25 percent of all oxygen inhaled. Therefore, proper oxygen is essential through a normal blood supply to the brain. The blood vessels supplying the brain with oxygen tend to clog as we age (see ARTERIOSCLEROSIS in Part Two). Without an adequate supply of oxygen and nutrients through the bloodstream, the brain will not function normally. Senility is one known result of loss of blood supply, and therefore oxygen, to the brain. When blood supply to any area of the brain is disconnected, or a hemorrhage from a blood vessel occurs, a stroke results.

The hypothalamus, a section of the brain, constantly monitors the blood sugar level by sending messages to the pancreas to release more insulin (which lowers blood sugar) and glucagon (which elevates blood sugar) into the bloodstream in order to normalize our sugar levels. The heart, liver, fat cells, muscles, and lungs all compete with the brain for blood sugar. In order to get sugar (glucose) fuel to the brain, you must have a correct diet and avoid simple sugars such as candy and soft drinks. Foods of this type trigger too much insulin release, which lowers blood sugar as in hypoglycemia, a condition that damages the brain. (See HYPOGLYCEMIA in Part Two.)

Many disorders stem from a malfunction of the central nervous system, which includes the brain and spinal cord. Nerve signals travel up and down the spinal cord, linking the brain to the rest of the body.

To function properly the brain daily requires four ounces of glucose, as well as sodium, potassium, unsaturated fatty acids, amino acids (protein), vitamins and minerals, and 400 calories.

Recent research has shown that excess fats and toxic "free radicals" forming in the bloodstream contribute to impaired brain function. Brain cells accumulate a form of cellular garbage called *lipofuscin*, a by-product of fats and free radicals. In excess, this garbage can damage and kill neurons. Antioxidants destroy free radicals and protect the brain against their by-product, lipofuscin.

NUTRIENTS

SUPPLEMENT	SUGGESTED DOSAGE	COMMENTS
Essential		
L-Glutamine (an amino acid)	As directed on label.	Improves mental and emotional stress. Very important in normal brain functioning.
Phenylalanine (an amino acid)	As directed on label.	Reduces appetite and depression. Do not use if pregnant, diabetic, or have high blood pressure.
Very Important		
Choline and inositol	10 g daily, under supervision only.	A deficiency produces memory loss and poor brain function.
DMG (Gluconic from DaVinci Labs)	As directed on label.	Improves tissue oxygen levels.
Ginkgo biloba extract	As directed on label.	An herb that improves cerebral oxygenation, and thereby brain function and memory.
High potency B complex with extra thiamine (B_1) and vitamin B_6 (pyridoxine) and niacinamide (B_3)		B vitamins are essential for normal brain function.
Vitamin A and E emulsion	As directed on label.	For easier assimilation. These are potent antioxidants.
Important		
Lecithin	1 capsule 3 times daily or 1 tbsp. 3 times daily.	Protects brain cells and improves memory and brain function.
Helpful		
Coenzyme Q_{10}	75 mg	Increases cerebral oxygen.
GABA (an amino acid)	450 mg taken on an empty stomach along with 50 mg vitamin B_6 and 500 mg vitamin C.	An important neurotransmitter.
L-Arginine plus L-lysine (amino acids)	Take on an empty stomach along with 50 mg vitamin B_6 and 500 mg vitamin C.	Important in maintaining a healthy immune system. L-Lysine is needed to avoid an imbalance.
L-Cysteine and glutathione (amino acids)	Take on an empty stomach along with 50 mg vitamin B_6 and 500 mg vitamin C.	Powerful detoxifiers needed for proper brain function.

L-Tyrosine (amino acid)	Take on an empty stomach along with 50 mg vitamin B$_6$ and 500 mg vitamin C.	Relieves depression and anxiety states.
Multimineral containing beta-carotene and zinc plus selenium	As directed on label. 200 mcg daily.	For essential minerals and important antioxidants.
RNA-DNA	As directed on label.	Do not use if you have gout or elevated serum acid. Aids in rebuilding and protecting cells.
SOD (Cell Guard from Biotec Foods)	As directed on label.	Contains 1.6 million units of SOD per capsule and is enteric coated. In a University experiment, after being given SOD, gerbils that were "brain dead" for 40 minutes and then revived had no signs of brain damage. Normally the animals survive only 4 minutes after blood flow is cut off from the brain.
Vitamin C	8,000 mg daily in divided doses.	An important antioxidant. Also improves circulation.

RECOMMENDATIONS

☐ Researchers have discovered that wheat, dairy products, chocolate, oranges, eggs, corn, soy, and grapes are behind many of the disorders associated with brain malfunctions. It is thought that these foods cause an allergic immune system reaction which results in inflammation in the brain. Monthly fasting appears to disrupt this allergic cycle. (See FASTING in Part Three.)

☐ A diet that will improve brain function should include whole grains, legumes, wheat germ, beans, peas, nuts, soybeans, fish, brewer's yeast, millet, cereal, brown rice, turkey, seaweed, lecithin, salmon, kelp, sardines, ginseng, and seeds.

☐ Exercise is very important. Walking is an excellent form of exercise.

☐ Learn to breathe deeply. This improves cerebral oxygen levels.

☐ Keep yourself in an environment that makes you use your brain. Don't let boredom, restlessness, or depression take hold. Always keep doing things that are satisfying and stimulating to the mind.

CONSIDERATIONS

☐ Two drugs used in Japan and Europe, Vinpocetine and Piracelam, appear to enhance brain function.

☐ Research has found that low-level lead exposure in

young children may be associated with impaired intellectual development and behavior problems. (Published in *Pediatric Research*, October 1983.)

Chelation Therapy

Chelating agents are used to bind with heavy toxic metals such as cadmium, lead, and mercury, and to excrete them from the body. These chelating agents are available in over-the-counter formulas that can be taken orally at home, or they can be administered intravenously under the supervision of a physician. Chelation (pronounced key-lay-shun) therapy has been used effectively to treat arteriosclerosis for more than forty years in the United States. This safe, nonsurgical remedy has also had beneficial results when used to treat cardiovascular disease, gangrene and other circulatory problems, myocardial infarction (heart attack), metal toxicities, as well as many other ailments.

Chelating agents can be used, for example, to bind with calcium and reduce the serum calcium level by excreting this mineral from the body through the kidneys. These chelating agents prevent calcium from accumulating in areas in which it does not belong.

ORAL CHELATING AGENTS

☐ Oral chelating agents offer a safe, convenient alternative to patients with serious circulation problems. Despite reservations voiced by the medical establishment about chelation therapy, many severely disabled and high-risk patients have reported dramatic improvement in arterial circulation after chelation treatment. The following chelating agents can be used to *prevent* many degenerative illnesses:

- Alfalfa, fiber, rutin, and selenium
- Calcium and magnesium chelate with potassium
- Chromium, kyolic, pectin, and potassium
- Coenzyme Q$_{10}$
- Copper chelate, iron, kelp, and zinc chelate

In addition, the following supplements can act as oral chelating agents to rid the body of excess minerals.

NUTRIENTS

SUPPLEMENT	SUGGESTED DOSAGE	COMMENTS
Alfalfa liquid or tablets	3 times daily with meals.	Detoxifies the liver and alkalizes the body. Chelates toxic substances from the body.

Coenzyme Q$_{10}$	100 mg daily.	Improves circulation and lowers blood pressure.
Kyolic (garlic tablets)	2 tablets with meals.	A good chelating agent and detoxifier.
L-Cysteine and L-methionine (amino acids)	500 mg twice daily, taken on an empty stomach with juice.	Vitamins B$_6$ and C can assimilate these amino acids, which contain sulfur.
L-Lysine (amino acid)	500 mg daily.	Aids in detoxifying harmful toxins and metals. Powerful free radical scavenger.
Rutin and apple pectin	As directed on label.	Binds with unwanted toxic metals and removes them from the body through the intestinal tract.
Selenium	200 mcg daily.	A powerful free radical scavenger.
Vitamin A	25,000–50,000 IU daily.	Aids in excreting toxic substances. Use emulsion formula for easier assimilation.
Vitamin B complex with extra B$_5$ (pantothenic acid) and B$_3$ (niacin) and B$_6$ (pyridoxine)	50 mg 3 times daily.	Aids in protection from harmful substances.
Vitamin C plus bioflavonoids	5,000–15,000 mg daily.	Powerful chelating agents and immunostimulants.
Vitamin E	600 IU emulsion formula or start with 600 IU capsule form, and increase slowly to 1,000 IU.	Removes toxic substances and destroys free radicals.

Recommendations

☐ In order to obtain necessary sulfur, eat plenty of legumes, eggs, garlic, and onions. A diet high in fiber is important. Obtain fiber from oat and wheat bran. Drink only steam-distilled water.

Considerations

☐ When using chelation therapy, make sure that essential minerals that might be displaced by chelating agents are replaced. Taking alfalfa, iron, kelp, and zinc to replace lost minerals is recommended.

☐ If you have arteriosclerosis and are interested in an oral chelation program, you can write to the following company for information:

Life Line Products
2554 Lincoln Boulevard
Suite 1111
Marina Del Rey, CA 90291

INTRAVENOUS CHELATION THERAPY

Intravenous therapy is often used to remove calcified, hardened plaque from the arterial walls, which in turn improves circulation. Most serious illnesses require intravenous chelation therapy in which repeated injections are necessary. When used under the care of a chelating physician, this safe procedure offers an alternative to vascular surgery; a coronary by-pass operation can be avoided in some cases.

EDTA (ethylene diamine tetraacetic acid), a synthetic amino acid, is the chelating agent that is administered intravenously to treat ailments such as high blood pressure and heart disease. EDTA is slowly released into the bloodstream; as it is transported through the arteries, it binds with the calcium that has deposited along the arterial walls and excretes it from the body through the kidneys. A strong chelating substance, EDTA attracts lead, strontium, and most divalent metals. Although there is controversy surrounding the use of this method, EDTA has not been found to be toxic when used correctly.

E. Cheraskin, M.D., D.D.S., of the University of Alabama calls EDTA a "homeostatic agent," asserting that it stabilizes cholesterol, hemoglobin, and kidney function. Cheraskin states that EDTA is not nephrotoxic, contrary to the claims of chelation opponents, but that it improves kidney function.

An IV infusion of three to four grams of EDTA should last at least four hours. Vitamins and minerals, particularly zinc, should be given to those who have had EDTA injections. Intravenous treatment should be given only under the supervision of a qualified physician.

Considerations

☐ There are over 150 doctors in the United States who are certified by the American Board of Chelation Therapy as approved chelation therapists. You can contact one of these two groups for information on those in your area:

The American College of Advancement in Medicine
23121 Verdugo Drive
Suite 204
Laguna Hills, CA 92653
(714) 586–7666 or (800) 532–3688

The American Board of Chelation Therapy
70 W. Huron Street
Chicago, IL 60610
(312) 787–2228

Colon Cleansing

A clean colon leads to improved health! Retained debris in the colon leads to absorption of toxins, resulting in "systemic" intoxication. *See* FASTING in Part Three and follow the program. This is the best way to remove toxins and waste from the body. *Also see* ENEMAS in Part Three and follow the instructions on the wheatgrass retention enema, or use chamomile tea, fresh lemon juice, garlic, or coffee retention enemas.

The following supplements will aid in cleansing the colon.

NUTRIENTS

SUPPLEMENT	SUGGESTED DOSAGE	COMMENTS
Very Important		
Fiber: Aerobic Bulk Cleanse (ABC) and glucomannan (guar gum) and brown rice and oat bran and psyllium husks	1 capsule 4 times daily or 1 tsp. 4 times daily.	Essential for a clean colon. Not habit-forming.
Important		
Aloe vera juice	½ cup 3 times daily.	George's is good. Heals colon inflammation.
Nondairy acidophilus or Bio Flora from New Moon Extracts	As directed on label.	Restores the normal "friendly" bacteria to the colon.
Helpful		
Apple pectin	As directed on label.	Source of quality fiber. Helps detoxify heavy metals.
Comfrey pepsin	2 capsules with meals.	Helps heal the colon. Do not take comfrey longer than 3 months in succession.
Green Magma (barley juice) or wheatgrass or Kyo-Green	As directed on label.	All these products assist in keeping the colon clear of toxic debris and aid in healing of the inflamed colon. Kyo-Green is a combination of barley juice and wheatgrass.
6-N-1 Cleanser from NCA or Sonne's Intestinal Cleanser (contains bentonite)	As directed on label.	

HERBS

☐ The following herbs should be rotated so as not to develop a reaction: cascara sagrada, goldenseal, senna leaf, comfrey, and pepsin.

☐ Lower bowel cleansers are fennel, barberry bark, cascara sagrada bark, and red raspberry. Slippery elm is good for inflammation of the colon and for excess. Use the regular slippery elm tea for an enema; it also brings quick relief.

☐ By mouth use: one tablespoon of bentonite mixed with one teaspoon of psyllium seed, a half cup of apple juice, and a half cup of steam-distilled water. Try adding a half cup of aloe vera juice and one teaspoon of Concentrace mineral drops from Trace Mineral Research for even better results.

RECOMMENDATIONS

☐ Implement a 50 percent raw foods diet, starting with two weeks of all raw foods, and then maintaining a diet of 50 percent raw foods.

☐ Eat fruit in the morning, along with plenty of fiber. This helps maintain a clean colon. Also, eat more sprouts and fresh vegetables. If a blood sugar problem is present, avoid sweet fruits.

☐ Avoid fats, oils, animal fats, dairy products, and fried foods until the colon has returned to normal and stools are normal. Use olive oil or essential fatty acids in moderation only.

Color Therapy: Coloring Your Inside World

The effects of color on our moods, health, and way of thinking have been studied by scientists for a number of years. Your preference of one color over another may have something to do with the way that color makes you feel.

Light is absorbed by the eye and converted to another form of energy, which enables us to see color. Photoreceptors in the retina of the eye, called the cones, translate these light waves into color vision. These sensory cells are effective only at higher light levels. Color vision requires different pigments, which are sensitive to blue, red, and green light.

According to Dr. Alexander Schauss, director of the American Institute for Biosocial Research in Tacoma,

Washington, these bonds of light energy stimulate the pituitary and pineal glands, which regulate hormones and other physiological systems in the body. These findings have been consistent even in those with visual handicaps and blindness. In addition, Dr. Schauss believes that color is a form of energy that produces physiological changes. These changes are not the result of psychological or cultural factors.

The color you choose for your surroundings can therefore effect changes in your body. For instance, red stimulates, excites, and warms the body. The color red increases the heart rate, brain wave activity, and respiration. Those who have poor coordination should avoid wearing the color red. In addition, those suffering from hypertension should avoid rooms with a red decor, which can cause their blood pressure to rise.

Pink has a soothing effect on the body. It can even relax the muscles. Because pink has a tranquilizing effect on aggressive and violent persons, it is often used in prisons, hospitals, and juvenile and drug centers. After only a few minutes in a pink room, a teenager suffering from drug-induced anxiety became calm and exhibited more rational behavior. After fifteen minutes in the pink room, the teenager fell asleep. Those suffering from anxiety or withdrawal symptoms would benefit from pink surroundings.

Orange is the choice color if you want to stimulate the appetite and reduce fatigue. Use this color to encourage the finicky eater or a child who refuses to eat. Try using orange tablecloths or placemats to pique the appetite of the undernourished. This color should be avoided by those who are trying to lose weight. If you are feeling tired or run down, wearing an orange garment can lift your energy level.

If you want to stimulate the memory, yellow is the preferred color. If you want to remember something, jot it down on yellow paper. Yellow is the most memorable of all the colors. It also raises the blood pressure and increases the pulse rate, but to a lesser degree than red does. As the color of sunshine, yellow has an energizing effect; it can help your depression by lifting your spirits.

Green is the color of spring and new beginnings. This color has a soothing and relaxing effect on the body as well as the mind. Green is appealing to the dieter. Those who are depressed or anxious can benefit from green surroundings. Green also helps the aging.

If you want to relax, blue might be a good choice. Blue has a calming effect on the body; it lowers the blood pressure, heart rate, and respiration. In a hot, humid environment, blue has a cooling effect. In another study, children prone to tantrums and aggressive behavior became calmer after being in a classroom painted blue. Interestingly, both blind and sighted children reacted the same to the blue surroundings. These findings support Dr. Schauss's theory that color responses are physiological rather than psychological or cultural. Light is transferred to the hypothalamus, where it is interpreted with the help of the pineal and pituitary glands. As a result, physiological changes in the body are effected.

Enemas

There are two types of enemas, cleansing and retention. The cleansing enemas are not retained or held in the body; they are used to flush out the colon. You will need to use steam-distilled water and an enema bag.

COFFEE ENEMA

Coffee used in this way has a different effect on the body than if it were ingested orally. When used in an enema, it does not go through the normal digestion process. It is beneficial in treatment when used properly because it stimulates the liver to throw off toxins. Coffee enemas are used in cases of degenerative disease to help stimulate the liver to excrete toxins or "poison bile." This kind of enema is called a retention enema because it is held in or retained for fifteen minutes.

To make the solution for a coffee enema, place two quarts of steam-distilled water in a pan and add six heaping tablespoons of ground coffee (don't use instant or decaffeinated). Boil for fifteen minutes, cool, and strain. Use only one pint of coffee at a time—save the rest in a jar.

As well as treatment for liver toxins, coffee enemas are used while fasting to relieve headaches caused by the build-up of toxins during detoxification.

Coffee enemas should not be abused. Use once daily while following the program for your disorder or occasionally when needed. Don't use petroleum jelly on the tip of the enema—instead, use a 200 IU capsule of vitamin E to lubricate the end. Stick a pin in the end of the capsule and squeeze the liquid onto the tip. This will also have a healing effect on the anus and the lining inside the colon if these areas are inflamed.

Excessive use of coffee enemas over a period of time (six months or longer) may precipitate anemia. This can be overcome with dessicated liver tablets or liver injections, which should be used if you are taking the enema daily over long periods. Limit the amount of coffee enema used to a half a pint and use only once daily unless you are being treated for cancer. Cancer patients may need up to three enemas a day.

Coffee enemas may also deplete some of the B vitamins and minerals. For cancer or AIDS patients, or others with severe illnesses, 1 cc of B complex or 2 cc of injectable liver can be added. One dropper full of liquid kelp or sea water concentrate (found in health food stores) should be added to replace the minerals that are lost. Try to retain the enema for fifteen minutes. Used daily, this will replace any lost B vitamins and will help to rebuild the liver and give an extra boost of energy. Five drops of either Aerobic 07 from Aerobic Life Products or Dioxychlor from American Biologics may also be added to the enema to kill unwanted bacteria in the colon.

LEMON JUICE ENEMA

This is not a retention enema. Use two quarts of steam-distilled water and the juice of three lemons. Do not use water that is too cold or too warm—use lukewarm water. Two droppers of liquid kelp can be added to the enema for minerals. The best position to use when receiving the enema is "head down and rear up." After completing the fluid insertion, lie on your right side, then rotate onto your back, and finally roll over and lie on your left side. As you are doing this, massage your colon. This helps loosen all fecal matter.

If you have trouble with constipation, use this lemon enema alternately with coffee enemas twice a week. The bowels will shortly move on their own, the colon will be clean, and the stool will not be foul-smelling.

If you are allergic to lemons, use wheatgrass, garlic, or plain steam-distilled water. You can also open three capsules of Natural Relief or use a half a teaspoon of Cameo Classic Facial. Both of these are from Whole Natural Earth Products. Because the facial is a natural clay product, it is beneficial when used this way.

Pure water contains a pH of seven, which is in balance with the body's pH. The EPA (Environmental Protection Agency) says that *pure* water is water that is bacteriologically safe, but studies have shown that the pH of tap water can range from one to fourteen. Water in the Northeastern and Northwestern United States is more acidic than in other parts of the country. If the water you use does not have a pH of seven, you can add three capfuls of Natural Relief in a quart of water. This will balance the pH. You can have your water tested to find out what the pH is. For more about water, *see* WATER in Part Three.

L. BIFIDUS RETENTION ENEMA

This enema should be used only three to six times a year. Use it for cases of candidiasis, severe gas and bloating, all yeast infections, when high colonics have been used, and when antibiotics have been used over long periods of time. This enema is used to replace intestinal flora ("friendly" bacteria) that have been removed or destroyed. The severely ill patient should take this enema.

The formula consists of six ounces of Eugalen Topfer Forte (found in natural foods stores) mixed in one quart of warm distilled water. The Eugalen Topfer Forte comes in dairy- or vegetable-based formulas— use the vegetable type if you have a sensitivity to dairy products. Mix until the formula is dissolved. Implant as much of the mixture as you can retain, and hold for one hour or longer. If you take a plain water enema first, it will be easier to retain. Do not retain the plain water enema.

This implant is good for severe gas, and gives relief within minutes. Powdered forms of acidophilus may also be used. Neo-Flora and Primadophilus are non-dairy forms. However, the Eugalen Topfer Forte works best.

Fasting

Fasting is an effective and safe method of detoxifying the body. The body needs a periodic rest from the chemicals and toxins that are in the environment. Fasting should always be monitored by a health professional.

Fasting is not starvation! It is a technique that wise men have used for centuries to heal the sick. To understand the principles of fasting is to understand one's own body.

Fasting is recommended for almost any illness because our bodies need rest. The body goes through high and low cycles, as does everything in the universe, including the sun, the moon, the stars, and the tides. Even insects and animals have cycles.

Help your body during its low phase; don't put a heavy load on it by eating. If you learn to "go with the flow" of the cycle, and accept it and help your body through the low phase, you will feel better, and your lows won't last as long. After a period of time, the body builds up toxins from chemicals, pollution, and overindulgences. It is during this low phase that the body is ridding itself of all toxins. This is a "normal detoxification phase."

During these low or "down" times, you may develop headaches, diarrhea, or depression. Doesn't it sound reasonable to help the body get rid of the toxins instead of letting the toxins build up? Fast when your body is at a low phase and help it detoxify itself. Then you will experience the "up" phase of the cycle, when you go through a period of feeling great. It is because the body is clean again. However, we start to pollute our bodies again, and in time toxins build up and we have our "down" days.

Fast regularly and help the body heal itself and stay well. Give all of your organs a rest. Fasting can help reverse the aging process, and if we use it correctly, we will live longer, happier lives. Just three days a month will do it. Each time you complete a fast, you will feel better. Your body will have a chance to heal and rebuild its immune system by regular fasting. You can fight off illness and the degenerative diseases so common in this chemically polluted environment we live in. When you feel a cold or any illness coming on, or are just depressed—*fast!*

A person can extend his life by several years through fasting. You heal faster, give your organs a rest, clean your liver and kidneys, purify your blood, cleanse your colon, lose unnecessary weight, get rid of toxin build-up in tissues, clear the eyes and tongue, cleanse the breath, and lose excess water. Remember: Proper diet and supplements, exercise, and fasting will more than double your energy and keep you well and happy.

A three-day fast helps the body get rid of toxins. A five-day fast starts the healing process. A ten-day fast should take care of most problems before they arise—a fast this long is good twice a year. Do *not* fast on water alone! Fasting over three days should be supervised by a qualified health professional. For a longer fast, continue until the tongue is cleared of its coating, the breath is sweet, and you are very hungry. Then come off the fast. Continue to work while on the fast.

Diabetics should never fast unless under a doctor's supervision. Hypoglycemics should never fast without also using a quality protein supplement. Spirulina is a good choice—it is a near-perfect food. Make sure the spirulina is of good quality, has been laboratory tested, and has been cleaned before processing.

Fasting should become a part of your life. Fast at least three days a month.

RECOMMENDATIONS

☐ Eat only raw foods for two days before starting the fast, and only raw foods for two days coming off the fast. The desired effects of the fast may be ruined by eating cooked foods immediately following the fast.

☐ If you must have something to eat, eat a piece of watermelon. Always eat watermelon alone. You can also try fresh applesauce made in a blender or food processor. Leave the skins on the apples.

☐ Do not chew anything, such as gum, while on the fast. The digestive process starts with chewing—enzymes are secreted into the gastrointestinal tract. With no food in the stomach for these enzymes to digest, trouble occurs.

☐ Spirulina can be used by anyone on a fast. It is high in protein and has all the vitamins and minerals the body needs, plus chlorophyll for cleansing. Take tablets or powder, five tablets three times daily or one teaspoon three times daily in juice.

☐ Extra fiber must be a part of the daily diet. Use bran; oat bran is good. Also good is Aerobic Bulk Cleanse (ABC), a colon cleanser, mixed with half George's Aloe Vera Juice and half natural cranberry juice. This mixture adds fiber and has a healing and cleansing effect also. Psyllium seed or glucomannan are other quality fiber products.

☐ When using glucomannan or any fiber capsule, be certain to drink a large glass of water, because the fiber capsules expand. It may be best not to take supplements of wheat bran, because this may be irritating to the colon wall.

☐ Drink only steam-distilled water—dilute juices with it. Use pure juices only, and avoid those with sweeteners or additives. Do not drink orange or tomato juice. The best juices to use are fresh lemon juice; cabbage, beet, carrot, celery, grape, and apple juice; and "green drinks," which are juices made from green leafy vegetables. "Green drinks" are excellent detoxifiers. Raw cabbage juice is good for ulcers, cancer, and all colon problems. Do not store cabbage juice, because as it sits, it loses its vitamin U content.

☐ To aid in rebuilding the immune system, drink pau d'arco and echinacea herb teas mixed with one-third unsweetened cranberry juice, four times a day. Herb teas are good while fasting. Drink rose hips, dandelion, red clover, alfalfa, and chamomile, if you are not allergic to ragweed. Slippery elm is excellent for inflammation of the colon and also gives fast relief when used in an enema.

☐ The following is an excellent fresh juice and broth: three carrots, two stalks of celery, one turnip, two beets, a half head of cabbage, a quarter of a bunch of parsley, a quarter of an onion, and a half clove of garlic. This could be the best juice on our planet for healing many illnesses.

☐ You can also use a pure vegetable broth with no seasoning added. Gently boil any fresh vegetable, including onions and garlic. Drink the broth 2–3 times during the day.

☐ Garlic capsules (Kyolic) aid in the healing process. Take two capsules twice a day. Kyolic oil is good, too, if you prefer that rather than capsules. Kyo-Green is excellent while fasting. It contains all the nutrients needed to aid in the healing process.

☐ Clinics have reported using the low sodium Concentrace, which are trace mineral drops, in the following manner: put one teaspoon in apple, grape, or papaya juice. As an internal cleanser, use Concentrace mineral drops, one and a half cups of juice, one and a half cups of water, two teaspoons of psyllium husk powder, and a half cup of aloe vera juice. Or, use another fiber in place of the psyllium husk, or even bentonite.

☐ Use a coffee or lemon juice enema (*see* ENEMAS in Part Three).

☐ Try dry-brush massages to help rid the skin of toxins and dead cells. Always brush toward the heart—wrist to elbow, elbow to shoulder, ankles to knees, knees to hips, etc. Use a *natural* bristle brush, and make sure it has a long handle so that you can reach your back. Large amounts of dead skin will be flaked away as the pores are freed of impediments. This will greatly improve circulation and the skin's excretion of poisons. Those who have acne, eczema, or psoriasis should avoid brushing. Do not brush areas that are broken or recently scarred, or that have protruding varicose veins.

☐ Some people, especially the elderly, need certain vitamins and minerals daily. If you are one of these people, you should continue to take vitamins while on the fast. When you are drinking juices, reduce the dosage of supplements that you take.

☐ A final word of advice: It took years to wear your body down, and it will take time to build it back up to its peak. But believe us, it can be done. Remember, when you start to feel badly, and in a "down" cycle, help yourself to come back up. Fast and feel better!

Glandular Therapy

Although glandulars have been used by European physicians since the turn of the century, they have more recently been made available in the United States. Glandular therapy involves the use of glandular and organ substances to promote the functioning ability of an individual's organs or glands. The theory behind the use of a specific glandular is that it will help those cells in the body that are similar to it. For example, a patient having adrenal failure will take raw adrenal concentrate because its inherent qualities support the adrenal function of the recipient in a way that no other nutritional supplements or dietary factors can. Diabetic and hypoglycemic patients, as well as individuals suffering from chronic fatigue, are sometimes given adrenal concentrate as part of their treatment program.

Raw concentrates of glandular and organ tissue have been made available in tablet form. These nutritional food supplements contain concentrated amounts of protein derived from a particular gland or organ of an animal. Studies have shown that these glandular substances are organ-specific rather than species-specific. Using radioactive isotope tracing, it was discovered that glandular tissues were absorbed by the bloodstream and deposited for use in the corresponding glands of the recipient. This discovery was documented by Dr. A. Kment in German medical publications of 1958 and 1972. In other words, when an individual eats raw cellular material from a bovine liver, it will be picked up by the bloodstream and carried to the individual's liver. Raw liver concentrate can thus promote liver function in those suffering from liver diseases. It can help liver problems associated with alcoholism, hepatitis, jaundice, and toxemia. Even cooked liver has beneficial effects if the animal source was raised on feed that was not treated with pesticides, as is the case in Argentina.

Although the use of glandulars may seem unappealing at first glance, it was actually practiced to some degree when man consumed animal as a food source. Most "primitive" people ate all animal parts, including its glands, organs, and muscle tissues. Because each part of the animal contained different levels of different nutrients, eating the whole animal was one way of maintaining a balanced diet. Not too long ago most American families regularly included heart, stomach, and other organ meats in their diets. Most Americans today have acquired a distaste for organ meats, preferring the flavor of muscle meats. They do not know how to cook organ meats properly. Organ meats are now considered a French delicacy.

Glandular therapy was first used in 1931 to treat a patient suffering from muscle spasms after her thyroid was removed and damage to her parathyroid gland was incurred. Dr. Niehans removed a young calf's parathyroid glands and injected the patient with these glandular substances. She reacted positively to the injection and lived for more than thirty-five years without suffering a relapse.

When used in conjunction with a well-balanced diet, vitamins, and other nutritional supplements, glandular therapy is an effective and safe treatment that can be used for an organ or gland that has been operating inadequately since birth, that has been functioning at a decreased capacity due to illness, or that has been progressively deteriorating in functioning ability from aging.

In addition to the glandulars described above, thymus concentrate has been administered by many physicians to build stronger immune systems. Raw kidney concentrate is used to help combat kidney damage that is sometimes incurred with cadmium toxicity, high blood pressure, kidney infections, and kidney stones. Raw spleen, thymus, heart, and pituitary concentrates are also available in health food stores, or can be ordered from various companies.

Hair Analysis

Hair analysis provides an accurate assessment of the concentration of minerals in the body—those that are toxic in any amount, those that are essential, and those that are necessary in small amounts, but toxic in larger amounts. This noninvasion technique readily determines exposure to toxic substances such as mercury, lead, and cadmium. The correlation between mineral concentrations in the internal organs of the body and levels in the hair is much more reliable than the correlation between intracellular mineral concentration and the levels found in serum and urine specimens. Normal trace element concentrations, as detected in the serum or urine, may be quite variable; however, hair analysis gives accurate readings of the intracellular concentrations of these substances.

A small amount of hair is removed from the nape of the neck for hair analysis. Because harsh chemical treatment of the hair from coloring, bleaching, and perming may result in possible inaccuracies, a pubic hair specimen may be used instead.

Judge Brian of the Federal District Court at Alexandria, Virginia, tried a case challenging the accuracy and reliability of hair analysis. In January 1985 he determined that hair analysis is a reliable indicator of essential and toxic elements and minerals contained in the body as a whole. Given the evidence that was presented concerning multielemental spectral hair analysis, Judge Brian concluded that the procedure was a "useful guide in the hands of a health care professional." He further added that when "used along with other relevant information in the treatment, the results of this procedure can help in prescribing nutritional supplements and in the caring for a specific patient where a chemical imbalance in the body is suspect."

Before hair analysis, medical practitioners who were interested in the concentration of trace elements in the body had to rely on urine and serum sampling. Unfor-

tunately, these tests have been shown to be inaccurate because they do not measure the intracellular concentration of minerals.

In addition to being accurate and easily performed, hair analysis provides a relatively permanent record of mineral concentrations. Computerized information can analyze the correlation between various elements in the hair. A treatment program can then be designed for identified disease states. After hair analysis has determined the intracellular mineral content of the body, the initial results can be compared with follow-up hair analyses to determine the effects of treatment.

Prior to the onset of symptoms indicative of metal toxicity, significant health information can be obtained using hair analysis. Heavy metal intoxication, especially lead poisoning, is far more common than what has been reported in the media. Hair analysis allows early detection of these potentially toxic elements, often before the patient manifests serious symptoms. Treatment of the problem, using chelation therapy and other programs, can therefore be started before the condition becomes irreversible.

The following table lists the minerals that can be measured through hair analysis. Next to each element is its symbol. In addition, the way in which a mineral interacts with other elements is also given in the table. In the sulfur entry, note that the presence of sulfur promotes the action of molybdenum. Also listed are the elements whose actions are inhibited in the presence of sulfur: calcium, copper, and selenium. In addition, the last column names the elements that will inhibit the action of the mineral in the initial column entry. Zinc is listed in the sulfur entry as the element that inhibits the action of sulfur.

INTERACTION OF MINERALS

Mineral Name	Elements Promoted by Mineral	Elements Inhibited by Mineral	Inhibitors of the Mineral
Aluminum (Al)	P	F	
Arsenic (As)	Co, I	Se	
Beryllium (Be)		Mg	
Cadmium (Cd)		Cu	Zn
Calcium (Ca)	Fe, Mg, P	Cu, F, Li, Mn, Zn	Cr, Pb, S
Chlorine (Cl)*			
Chromium (Cr)		Ca	
Cobalt (Co)	As, F	Fe, I	
Copper (Cu)	Fe, Mo, Zn	P	Ag, Ca, Cd, Mn, S
Fluorine (F)		Mg	Al, Ca
Iodine (I)	As, Co, G		
Iron (Fe)	Ca, Cu, K, Mn, P		Co, Mg, Pb, Zn
Lead (Pb)		Ca, Fe, K	Se, Zn
Lithium (Li)		Na	Ca
Magnesium (Mg)	Ca, K, P	Fe	Mn
Manganese (Mn)	Cu, Fe, K, P	Mg	Ca

Mercury (Hg)*			
Molybdenum (Mo)	Cu, S	P	N
Nickel (Ni)*			
Nitrogen (N)		Mo	
Phosphorus (P)	Al, Be, Ca, Fe, Mg, Mn, Zn	Na	Cu, Mo
Potassium (K)	Fe, Mg, Mn, Na		Pb
Selenium (Se)		Cd, Pb	As, S
Silver (Ag)		Cu	
Sodium (Na)	K		Li, P
Sulfur (S)	Mo	Ca, Cu, Se	Zn
Zinc (Zn)	Cu, P	Cd, Fe, Pb, S	Ca

*Mineral interactions have not been documented.

Juicing

The fresh juices mentioned in this book are, ideally, juiced in your kitchen and consumed immediately. Juicing is beneficial because it takes little energy to digest juice, and your body is getting plenty of necessary elements from the juice. Fruits and vegetables that are free of pesticides (organically grown) will provide optimum nutrition.

To make your own juices, you must first obtain a juicer. There are several good juicers on the market, from inexpensive models to those that cost over a thousand dollars.

Fresh fruit and vegetable juice is an excellent way to get vitamins, minerals, enzymes, purified water, proteins, carbohydrates, and chlorophyll. Many fruits and vegetables can be juiced with the peel still on to ensure that all of the vitamins and minerals go into the juice. Juices should not be stored, because they slowly lose their nutrients.

Juices can roughly be placed into three categories:

1. *Green juices or "green drinks."* Green juices stimulate cells and rejuvenate the body. They also build red blood cells. Green juices made from sprouts contain chlorophyll, which heals and cleanses the body. "Green drinks" can also be made by adding chlorophyll, purchased at your natural foods store, to juice. Green juices are made from spinach, celery, cabbage, dandelion greens, alfalfa sprouts, and other similar vegetables.
2. *Vegetable juices.* Fresh vegetables are restorers and builders. They help remove excesses of protein, fat, and acid wastes from the body. Vegetable juices help build the immune system and guard against illness.
3. *Fruit juices.* Fruit juices are cleansers. One favorite is watermelon juice. The seeds, rind, and fruit can be juiced; most juices extract the pulp and leave you with clean, delicious juice. Watermelon juice is an excellent cleanser. Apples are delicious when juiced, as are citrus fruits and berries. Fruit juices are wonderful combined, too.

Fruit juices are best taken in the morning. Vegetable juices are best taken in the afternoon.

Music Therapy

Music seems to have an effect on our moods and health in much the same way color does. Soft music, when combined with some relaxation techniques, has been used to alleviate stress and relax muscles. Music touches the spirit and can be very relaxing and healing. Researchers suggest that music promotes the production of pain-killing hormones called endorphins in the brain. It generates the relaxation response. Music therapy has produced some good results in those undergoing cardiac rehabilitation or alcohol and drug rehabilitation; those suffering from asthma, depression, high blood pressure, migraines, and ulcers; and the mentally retarded. Although soft music can be soothing, discordant types of hard rock music have an adverse effect on the mind and body!

Pain Control

Pain is a message from the body that you are having trouble in a particular area. Without pain you would remain unaware of any health problems and would never know when the body needed help repairing itself. Disease, injury, and strenuous activity may cause pain in the affected body part, signaling that damage has been incurred. It also signals you to rest the injured area so that tissues can be repaired and so that additional damage can be prevented. Pain motivates you to seek treatment as well. Some people are born with a rare neurological disorder that makes them insensitive to pain. Unfortunately, they do not experience pain when they incur various injuries such as burns, cuts, and fractures, or if they bite their tongue. Because they are unaware of their pain, they cannot prevent damage or seek fast treatment.

Pain may result from a combination of physical and mental problems. Some people can tolerate pain better than others. In some people, pain is cyclical; pain produces anxiety and this anxiety intensifies the pain. Fear of the physical problem and anticipation of the pain can also heighten the pain. Those with an uneasy mind will suffer more from chronic pain. If the patient knows why he is experiencing pain, he can better tolerate it.

There are various techniques that can be used to alleviate pain. One method often used to relieve pain is heat therapy. By increasing the temperature in a selected area of the body, heat will enhance blood circulation and increase mobility in that area. Chronic musculoskeletal problems are best treated with heat therapy. For basic aches and pains, first apply heat to the affected area. Moist heat from a warm shower or hydrocollator can reduce stiffness and relax muscles. A hydrocollator is a unit in which a gel is contained within a cotton or canvas sack. Prepare the hydrocollator by heating it in hot water and wrapping it in a towel. Apply it to the painful area for approximately twenty minutes. Also try a poultice for heat therapy (see POULTICE in Part Three). When using heat therapy, be careful about overdoing it. Monitor the intensity of the heat and the duration and frequency of treatment. After heat has been applied, firmly rub or massage the affected area; this will also relieve tension. Do not massage if the area is inflamed or if a serious injury has been incurred. Those with phlebitis or other vascular problems should not use massage.

Because heat may increase swelling, some injuries respond better to cold therapy. Applying ice will numb the nerve endings in the affected part by reducing the activity of the body cells in that area. Acute strains, sprains, and muscle pulls should be treated with ice to relieve pain and swelling. Prepare an ice pack and rub it on the painful area using a circular motion for five to seven minutes.

An ice rub for lower back pain can be very therapeutic. If you are unable to reach all of the aching areas of the lower back, you can try another form of physical therapy that relieves tension in the same way as a massage. Place two tennis balls on the floor and position them under the small of the back, one on each side of the spine, so that you are able to slide your back over them easily. Relax your body and then slowly work the tennis balls up and down the back. Doing some easy stretching exercises beforehand is recommended.

Alternating hot and cold treatments may work well for some injuries. A warm shower can relieve tension in a stiff neck. After the shower, you can further sooth the muscles by carefully rubbing the area in small circles with the three middle fingers. An ice massage can be very therapeutic for sore neck muscles as well. A sitz bath also uses the principals of heat and cold therapies (see SITZ BATH in Part Three).

Many headaches are caused by sinus congestion. Applying pressure to specific areas of the head can open up the sinuses and ease tension. Rub the area surrounding the bones just above and below the eyes, and massage the cheeks directly in line with these points. Hang the head down to facilitate sinus drainage. Applying heat to the sinuses is also beneficial.

In addition to massage and hot and cold therapies, some medications can provide relief from pain. Ben-Gay and Icy Hot analgesics are counterirritants that stimulate blood flow to the affected area. Always take precautionary measures when using a counterirritant. Do not apply a heating pad or cover the area with anything except everyday clothing if a counterirritant has been applied. Using a heating pad on top of the counterirritant could increase the medication's rate of absorption into the skin and cause serious damage to the skin. In addition, some products such as DMSO (dimethylsulfoxide) could cause the counterirritant to be absorbed into the bloodstream if used with any of these rubs. If any pain or injury persists, consult your physician.

Over-the-counter drugs that can relieve pain include those that contain acetaminophen, aspirin, and ibuprofen. Advil, Mediprin, and Nuprin are some of these products. Never give children aspirin, especially if they have flu-like symptoms. Vitamin C taken with aspirin makes the effects of the analgesic last longer.

Natural pain relievers include germanium and DL-phenylalanine, an amino acid. There are also certain herbs that lessen pain. (See HERBS in Part One.) See also COLOR THERAPY, MUSIC THERAPY, and SURGERY in Part Three for other pain control techniques.

How to Use a Poultice

The benefits of heat and cold therapies were described in PAIN CONTROL in Part Three. When heat is applied to a certain section of the body, the capillaries become dilated and blood flow is consequently increased. Moist heat is often used to relax tense areas, soothe inflamed parts, or draw toxins from the infected area. Like hydrocollators, poultices often use heat to relieve tension and alleviate pain. Agents used in poultices also act as counterirritants. A poultice is made up of a substance that is usually heated, mixed to the consistency of a paste, and then spread on either gauze, muslin, linen, or other white cotton material large enough to cover the affected area completely. The poultice is applied directly to the area; sometimes a pin or other fastener is used to secure it in place. Another cotton layer is generally wrapped around the poultice to reduce heat loss.

Poultices can relieve pain and inflammation associ-

Types of Poultices

Herbs commonly used in poultices and their benefits are listed below.

- A *chaparral* poultice is often used in addition to dandelion and yellow dock root for skin disorders such as acne, eczema, psoriasis, rashes, and itchy or dry skin.
- *Comfrey*, which can be used in combination with pau d'arco, ragwort, and wood sage, gives good results when used as a poultice for tumors and external cancers.
- *Dandelion root*, like chaparral and yellow dock root, is very therapeutic for skin disorders such as acne, eczema, rashes, psoriasis, and itchy or dry skin.
- *Echinacea root* is excellent for lowering fever, which often occurs with amoebic infections.
- An *elderberry* poultice can relieve the pain associated with piles and hemorrhoids.
- *Fenugreek and flaxseed powder* can be used with equal parts of slippery elm bark powder to make a poultice for inflammations.
- *Goldenseal* is good for inflammations of all kinds.
- A poultice made of *lobelia* and charcoal, which is available in a health food store, is very beneficial for insect bites, bee stings, and almost all wounds. It can also be used with slippery elm bark powder for rheumatism, blood poisoning, and abscesses.
- A poultice of *mullein leaves* is recommended for ulcers, inflamed piles, mumps, inflammation of the tonsils, sore throat, and lung disorders. Use four parts mullein leaves to one part hot vinegar and one part water.

- *Mustard* is good for swelling, lung congestion, and inflammation, and can help relax tense muscles. When an irritant plant, such as mustard, is used to make a plaster, it is best to use the paste between two pieces of cloth.
- *Onion* poultices are good for ear infections and boils and sores that have difficulty healing. Use between a piece of cloth and not directly on the area.
- *Pau d'arco* can be beneficial for tumors and external cancers.
- *Poke root* is good for an inflamed or sore breast.
- *Ragwort* has therapeutic value when used to treat tumors and external cancers.
- *Sage*, like poke root, can help to relieve breast inflammation and soreness.
- *Slippery elm* can be used in combination with flaxseed powder and fenugreek for swelling. Mix equal parts of each with water to make a paste and apply to the inflamed area. Slippery elm can also be used alone for inflamed and gangrenous sores (often associated with diabetes) and leg ulcers. Use of a slippery elm poultice upon appearance of sores and ulcers can help to prevent gangrene. Lobelia can also be used with slippery elm for rheumatism, blood poisoning, and abscesses.
- *Yellow dock root* can be used with chaparral and dandelion for skin disorders such as acne, eczema, psoriasis, rashes, and itchy or dry skin.

---

ated with abscesses; boils; carbuncles; fibrocystic disease; fractures; enlarged glands such as the neck, breast, or prostate; leg ulcers; sprains; sunburn; tumors; and ulcerated eyelids. Many natural substances can be used for the poultice. Herbs are a popular choice for poultices. Comfrey, echinacea, goldenseal, mullein leaves, poke root, turmeric, and yellow dock are very therapeutic.

If you are using herbs for your poultice, it is best to grind the herbs to a powdered or granulated form. Herbs that are ground can be used in a poultice by adding water until the mixture is the consistency of a thick paste. If you are using a granulated form, add a small amount of ground flaxseed or cornmeal and mix until it is the consistency of a thick paste. Spread this paste on a piece of fresh white cotton so that it is a quarter of an inch thick, and cover the area completely. Wrap a towel around the poultice to prevent heat loss. If you choose fresh herbs for your poultice, simmer two

ounces of the herb in half a pint of water for approximately two minutes. Do not drain. Pour the entire mixture into a cheesecloth. It is best to cleanse the area first with hydrogen peroxide before applying the poultice. Apply the herb poultice directly to the affected area, making sure that it covers the area completely. A second layer should be added to retain heat.

The duration of treatment with poultices will vary according to the type of injury and the type of substances chosen for the poultice. Poultices using herbs are generally used for six to eight hours. You should generally apply fresh poultices when the one being used cools and loses its effectiveness. Once a poultice has been used, do not reheat. Wash the skin thoroughly after removing the poultice. If the amount of pus from a sore increases when using a poultice, discontinue use.

Not all poultices use heat for therapy. A cold clay poultice can be used to relieve sunburn pain. Clay is used in poultices to treat sprains and fractures as well.

Sitz Bath

As a form of hydrotherapy, the sitz bath increases blood flow to the pelvic and abdominal area. This remedy alternates cold and heat therapies in order to treat many disorders including cystitis, hemorrhoids, and prostate problems.

To prepare a sitz bath, fill the bathtub so that the water covers the hips and reaches the middle of the abdomen. The temperature of the water will vary with your condition and the type of illness you are treating. If a small tub is available to contain your body, you can bathe the feet simultaneously in a separate pail or tub. The temperature of the water in the foot bath should always be a few degrees greater than the temperature of the sitz bath. You may wish to cover your body with a sheet or blanket to increase comfort and protect the body.

Fill the bathtub with relatively hot water, making sure that the temperature of the water does not exceed 120°F. You might want to first bathe in water from 90°F to 100°F, and then gradually increase the temperature to 110°F. The feet should be immersed in slightly hotter water. Applying a cold compress to the forehead may also help. When using the sitz bath to treat an illness, you should generally soak in it for twenty to forty minutes. After this moist heat has soothed the body, you can further stimulate the body by contrasting with cooler water. You may wish to shower or splash your body with some cooler water before drying off. Make sure that the sitz bath, cold compress, and foot bath are all prepared ahead of time.

Epsom salts and the use of certain herbs can be used in combination with the sitz bath to produce the best results.

Surgery

Millions of surgical operations are performed annually in the United States, many of which may be unnecessary. Before deciding on surgery, explore all other means of treating the problem. Make sure that any surgical recommendation is given by a board certified surgeon; you want to feel confident that the surgeon is qualified to perform the type of surgery you need. Getting a second opinion is advisable. You will be better able to decide on the best form of treatment if you are well-informed. Don't be afraid to ask your doctor

questions. Your physician should address the following concerns:

- What are my chances of survival *without* the operation?
- Are there other forms of treatment that have had good results?
- What are the risks of surgery?
- What percent of the operations performed of this type have been successful?
- What physical changes will result from this operation and what improvements can I expect?
- How long is the recovery period?
- What is the cost of the operation and how much of it will my insurance cover?
- Are there any activities that I will not be able to do after the operation?
- Who will administer the anesthesia?

After you have been informed of all your options and feel that surgery is the only viable alternative, you can use the nutritional guidelines given in the chart to prepare for the surgery. Supplying your body with the nutrients below can assist in the healing process and lessen your discomfort and pain after surgery. If you are overweight and have sufficient time to diet before surgery, work off some weight and make sure your diet is well-balanced and healthy. Nutrition is an important factor because how well you recover from surgery is affected by your general health before surgery.

The following supplements will help you prepare for and recover from surgical procedures.

NUTRIENTS

SUPPLEMENT	SUGGESTED DOSAGE	COMMENTS
Acidophilus (in high potency powdered form)	3 times daily.	To stabilize the intestinal bacterial flora.
Coenzyme Q$_{10}$ and	60 mg daily.	Two free radical destroyers that improve tissue oxygenation. Germanium also relieves pain.
germanium	100 mg daily.	
Free form amino acids (protein supplement)	As directed on label.	Aids in collagen synthesis and wound healing. Free form amino acids are a readily available form of protein, easily absorbed and assimilated in the body.
Garlic capsules (Kyolic)	2 capsules 3 times daily.	Kyolic is an odorless, natural antibiotic that enhances immune function.
L-Cystine (amino acid)	500 mg twice daily.	Speeds healing of wounds.
Multivitamin complex containing beta-carotene and vitamin A	As directed on label.	For necessary minerals. Vitamin A is needed for protein utilization such as in tissue repair, and is also a free radical scavenger.

Unsaturated fatty acids	As directed on label.	Good sources are MaxEPA and salmon oil.
Vitamin C (buffered)	6,000–10,000 mg daily in divided doses.	Aids in tissue repair and healing of wounds. Vital in immune function.
Vitamin E	After the stitches are removed, cut open a vitamin E capsule and apply to the incision.	Promotes healing and reduces scar formation. *Warning:* Avoid vitamin E the week before surgery. It thins the blood. However, be sure to take it the day after surgery.
Vitamin K	As directed on label.	This important vitamin is needed for blood clotting. Food sources of vitamin K include alfalfa, blackstrap molasses, and all leafy green vegetables.
Zinc plus	80 mg daily.	Important for tissue repair.
calcium and	1,500 mg daily.	
magnesium	1,000 mg daily.	

HERBS

☐ Herb teas are recommended, including echinacea, goldenseal, pau d'arco, and rose hips.

RECOMMENDATIONS

☐ Ask your surgeon if there is anything that you can do to prepare for the surgery. In addition to the surgeon's recommendations, you should omit vitamin E, aspirin, and all compounds containing aspirin two weeks prior to surgery. These substances have a tendency to thin the blood.

☐ Many operations require that the patient be shaved. If this is necessary, tell the surgeon that you prefer to be shaved the day of surgery. Studies show that the infection rate is lower for patients who are shaven the day of surgery when compared with those who are shaven the night before. Make sure your doctor and those who will care for you are aware of any allergies that you may have to drugs, chemicals, or foods.

☐ Check with your surgeon before using any treatments at home. If the surgeon concurs, take two cleansing enemas using the juice of a fresh lemon before entering the hospital. It is important to have a clean colon. Taking a half glass of George's Aloe Vera Juice in the morning and before bedtime will help keep your colon clean. Take a bottle of this remedy with you to the hospital. It tastes like spring water and needs no refrigeration.

☐ Add fiber to the diet. It insures better intestinal tract function.

☐ Don't overwork your body by eating highly processed foods after surgery. Try to consume at least eight glasses of liquids each day, including distilled water, herb teas, juices, and protein drinks.

CONSIDERATIONS

☐ Some foods interfere with medications. Milk, dairy products, and iron supplements may interfere with some forms of antibiotics. Acidic fruits, such as oranges, pineapples, and grapefruits, can inhibit the action of penicillin and aspirin. Avocados, bananas, cheese, chocolate, colas, and aged and fermented foods can interfere with monoamine oxidase, a drug used to treat depression and hypertension. A drug used to treat Parkinson's disease will also be rendered ineffective in the presence of vitamin B_6. Because alcohol interferes with the action of many drugs, it should be avoided when taking any medication. In addition to these food restrictions, you should avoid fatty foods before and after surgery; these will slow the digestion process. *See* DRUG ADDICTION in Part Two for a list of the nutrients that are lost with the use of different drugs.

☐ Remember: It will take the body a few weeks to recover from the trauma of surgery. Hormonal imbalances will be corrected and the rate of metabolism will be adjusted during this period. Most incisions close within two days and heal within a week to the point that the skin will hold together under normal stress and body movement. You must exercise caution, however, when engaging in strenuous activity such as lifting. Make sure you obtain your doctor's approval before beginning to exercise. Light exercise will help circulation and speed your physical recovery and healing. Calcium is lost when the body is inactive and should be replaced. Vitamin C and protein are needed by the body to form collagen; these help promote healing.

☐ Blood transfusion might be required during surgery. Consider the benefits of storing your own blood before surgery for use during the operation. Using your own blood helps prevent infection and avoids the risk of contracting hepatitis or the AIDS virus. Blood transfusions may be a factor in the development of tumors as well. In *The Conquest of Cancer*, Virginia Livingston Wheeler, M.D., documented the presence of cancer-causing microbes, called progenitor cryptocides, in the blood. Liquid blood can be stored for forty-two days; frozen blood can be stored for a longer period. Consult with your surgeon about the preparation needed. You may need to take iron supplements a week before the first blood collection. Arrange the appointments so that the last time you give blood is at least four days before surgery.

☐ Post-surgical depression is not uncommon. A healthy dietary program will help depression.

☐ Nicholas Cavarocchi, M.D., of Temple University recommends that heart patients be given 2,000 IU capsules of vitamin E twelve hours prior to heart surgery. This amount of vitamin E lowers free radical levels in the blood.

Therapeutic Foods and Liquids

The benefits of raw fruits and vegetables were described in NUTRITION, DIET, AND WELLNESS in Part One. Two easy-to-make recipes that derive their healthful benefits from raw potatoes are given below. These foods are high in potassium and should be made fresh daily. When purchasing potatoes, choose ones that do not have a green tint. The chemical solonine is created by light and gives the potato its green tint. Solonine can interfere with nerve impulses and cause diarrhea, vomiting, and abdominal pain.

Potato Peeling Broth

3 potatoes, cut in halves
1 carrot, sliced
1 celery stalk, sliced
onion or garlic

1. Scrub potatoes well and cut out the eyes.
2. Cut potatoes in half. Cut the peel from the potato, making sure to keep about ½ inch of potato with the peel. Discard the remaining potato center.
3. Slice carrot and celery.
4. Place potatoes and carrot and celery slices in a pot, cover with water, and boil for about ½ hour, adding onion and garlic to taste.
5. Cool and strain. Serve.

Raw Potato Juice

potatoes, cut in halves
high quality water

1. Scrub potatoes well and cut out the eyes.
2. Cut potatoes in half. Cut the peel from the potato, making sure to keep about ½ inch of potato with the peel. Discard the remaining potato center.
3. Put potatoes through a juicer. A pound of potatoes will yield about 4–6 ounces of juice.
4. Combine potato juice with an equal amount of water or with other fresh juices. Add a carrot or stalk of celery to your drink, if desired.
5. Drink immediately—do not allow to stand.

APPENDIX

GLOSSARY

absorption. A process by which nutrients are absorbed through the intestinal tract into the bloodstream to be used by the body. If the nutrients are not absorbed, the body becomes deficient in building and healing substances.

acids. Compounds often found in plant tissues (especially fruits) that prevent secretion of fluids and shrink tissue. Nine important acids are:

1. *Acetic acid*. An inorganic acid of which a 5 percent solution and water makes vinegar.
2. *Ascorbic acid*. An organic acid; vitamin C. Used as a cosmetic and antioxidant.
3. *Citric acid*. An organic acid in citrus fruits, often used in cosmetics to lower the pH of a product.
4. *Hyaluronic acid*. An organic acid known as the most effective natural moisturizer. It is present in human skin, and is able to hold 500 times its own weight in water.
5. *Hydrochloric acid*. A strong corrosive inorganic acid that can cause burns and produce toxic vapors. Produced in the stomach for digestion.
6. *Lactic acid*. An inorganic acid present in skin and human tissue that is a natural moisturizing agent.
7. *Retinoic acid*. The active ingredient of the Retin-A skin treatment.
8. *Sorbic acid*. An organic acid and food preservative.
9. *Sulfuric acid*. A highly corrosive inorganic acid that is used in batteries and other industrial appliances. It can cause severe burns.

adaptogen. Derived from the Greek words *adapto*, which means to adjust and make suitable, and from the suffix *gen*, which means producing. An adaptogen, therefore, is a substance that produces suitable adjustments in the body. Adaptogens tend to regulate body functions and when the job is completed, they are eliminated or incorporated into the body without side effects. Adaptogens such as the herbs garlic, ginseng, echinacea, ginkgo, goldenseal, and taheebo are natural substances that benefit the body.

AIDS (acquired immune deficiency syndrome). An immune system deficiency disorder that suddenly alters the body's ability to defend itself. The AIDS virus invades the T-cells and multiplies, causing a breakdown in the body's immune system, eventually leading to overwhelming infection and/or cancer, with ultimate death.

allergen. A substance that is capable of producing an allergic response in the body.

allergy. A reaction anywhere in the body's tissue caused by a specific substance.

Alzheimer's disease. A disease of the middle-aged and elderly. Characterized by progressive dementia and diffuse cerebral cortical atrophy, and microscopically by the loss of neurons and the presence of plaques and neurofibrillary tangles.

amino acid. An organic acid containing nitrogen chemical building blocks that aid in the production of protein in the body. Eight of the twenty-two known amino acids are considered "essential," and must be obtained from dietary sources because they cannot by synthesized by the body.

anabolic compounds. Allow the conversion of nutritive material into complex living matter in the constructive metabolism.

analgesic. Medication that relieves pain.

anemia. A condition resulting from an unusually low number of red blood cells or too little hemoglobin in the red blood cells.

anemia, pernicious. Anemia caused by a vitamin B_{12} deficiency.

angina pectoris (angina). Chest pain with sensations of suffocation caused by temporary reduction of oxygen to the heart muscle through narrowed diseased coronary arteries.

antacid. Neutralizes acid in the stomach, esophagus, or first part of the duodenum.

antibiotic. Medication that helps the body fight infection by neutralizing or destroying bacteria.

antibody. A protein molecule from the immune system that counteracts the effects of invading organisms and other foreign substances.

antigen. Any substance that can elicit the formation of an antibody specific for that substance when introduced into a foreign species.

antihistamine. Prevents histamine from acting on body tissues. *See* histamine.

antioxidant. A substance that slows oxidation (see oxidation). Examples include vitamins C and E, the minerals selenium and germanium, superoxide dismutase (SOD), coenzyme Q_{10}, catalase, and some amino acids.

arteriosclerosis. A common arterial disorder. Characterized by calcified yellowish plaques, lipids, and cellular debris in the inner layers of the walls of large and medium-sized arteries.

artery. Blood vessel that carries blood away from the heart to the organs, glands, and tissues.

ascorbate. A mineral salt of ascorbic acid (i.e., vitamin C) that aids in the absorption of both vitamin C and the mineral.

autoimmune disease. Occurs when the body's immune system reacts to and damages its own tissues and organs. Examples include multiple sclerosis, rheumatoid arthritis, systemic lupus, Bright's disease, and diabetes.

autologous transfusion. A transfusion of one's own blood that has been preserved for later use. This stored personal blood is a protection against AIDS, hepatitis, and other communicable diseases.

bacteria. Microscopic germs. Some bacteria are "harmful" and can cause disease, while other "friendly" bacteria protect the body from harmful invading organisms.

benign. Refers to cells that are not cancerous. Literally means innocent; not malignant.

beta-carotene. A derivative of vitamin A. Widely accepted today as a cancer preventative.

bile. A substance released by the liver into the intestines for the digestion of fats.

bioflavonoid (vitamin P). Any of a group of colored flavones (crystalline compounds) found next to the peel in many fruits. Essential for the stability and absorption of ascorbic acid.

biopsy. Excision of tissue from a living being for diagnosis.

blood count. The number of red and white blood cells and platelets in a sample of blood.

carcinogen. Any agent that is cancer-causing.

cardiac. Pertaining to the heart.

cardiac arrhythmias. Abnormal heart rate or rhythm.

carotene. Converted into vitamin A in the body from a yellow pigment that has several forms (i.e., alpha-, beta-, and gamma-carotene).

CAT scan (computerized axial tomography scan). A scanning procedure using x-rays and a computer to detect abnormalities of the body's organs.

cell. All living tissues are composed of cells, which are very small complex units consisting of a nucleus, cytoplasm, and a cell membrane.

cellulose. A nondigestible carbohydrate found in the outer layers of fruits and vegetables .

chelation. Chelation therapy uses EDTA or other supplements that carry out heavy metals like lead, cadmium, and arsenic, as well as other foreign substances, from the body. In the process of chelation, a larger protein molecule surrounds or encloses a mineral atom. The purpose of chelation is to increase the flow of blood to the vital organs and tissues of the body by reducing calcium deposits in the arteries and blood vessels.

chemotherapy. A treatment of disease by any chemicals. Used most often to refer to the chemical treatments used to combat cancer cells.

cholesterol. A crystalline substance, consisting of various fats, that is naturally produced by all vertebrate animals and humans. Cholesterol is widely distributed and manufactured in the body and facilitates the transport and absorption of fatty acids.

clotting factors. Substances in the bloodstream, especially vitamin K, that are important in the process of blood clotting. Prolonged bleeding is produced when these substances are absent.

cobalt 60. Used widely in radiation therapy; a radioactive isotope of the element cobalt.

co-carcinogen. An environmental agent that acts with another to cause cancer.

coenzyme. A heat stable molecule that must be associated with another enzyme for the enzyme to perform its function in the body. It is necessary in the utilization of vitamins and minerals.

cold-pressed. A method used to process oils from food without heat to preserve the nutrients.

colonoscope. An instrument for examining the colon.

complex carbohydrate. Includes indigestable molecules of fiber (e.g., starch and glycogen). Slowly releases sugar into the bloodstream and also adds the fiber.

contraceptive. Device, substance, or method used to prevent pregnancy.

contusion. A bruise; an injury in which the skin is not broken.

convulsion. Uncontrollable contraction of the voluntary muscles that results from abnormal cerebral stimulation.

cruciferous. A group of vegetables named for their cross-shaped blossoms (e.g., broccoli, Brussels sprouts, cabbage, cauliflower, turnips, and rutabagas), which may help prevent colon cancer.

cystoscope. An instrument for examining the urinary bladder.

dementia. An acquired progressive impairment of intellectual function. Marked compromise exists in at least three of the following mental activity spheres: memory, language, personality, visuospatial skills, and cognition (i.e., abstraction and calculation).

detoxification. The process of reducing the body's toxic build-up of various poisonous substances.

disorientation. The loss of a normal relationship to one's surroundings (i.e., the inability to comprehend time, people, and place).

diuretic. Increases urine flow, causing the kidneys to excrete more than the usual amount of sodium, potassium, and water.

DNA (deoxyribonucleic acid). The substance in the cell nucleus that genetically codes amino acids and their peptide chain pattern, and determines the type of life form into which a cell will develop.

edema. Fluid retention in the body resulting in swelling.

EDTA (ethylene diamine tetraacetic acid). An organic molecule used in chelation therapy.

EEG (electroencephalogram). A test measuring brain wave activity.

EKG or ECG (electrocardiogram). A test that shows a tracing of the electrical conduction of the heart.

electrolyte. A chemical substance with an available electron in its structure that enables it to transmit electrical impulses when dissolved in fluids.

ELISA (enzyme-linked immunosorbent assay). A test that detects the presence of the AIDS virus antibody.

emulsion. A substance that shares the chemical characteristics of water and oil (the liquids will not mix). It promotes mixing and dispersion between the two compounds (e.g., lecithin).

endemic. Used to refer to a disease that constantly occurs in any particular geographical region.

endorphins. Natural polypeptide opiate-like substances in the brain. One function of endorphins is the suppression of pain.

endoscope. Instrument for examining the interior of a hollow organ.

enzymes. Specific protein catalysts that increase chemical reaction time in the body without being consumed.

epidemic. Describes a disease occurring in extensive outbreaks, or with an unusually high incidence at certain times and places.

Epstein Barr virus (EBV). A virus that causes infectious mononucleosis and that is possibly capable of causing other diseases in immunocompromised hosts.

essential fatty acids. Substances that the body cannot manufacture and therefore must be supplied in the diet. *See* fatty acids.

essential nutrient. Any single substance of the forty-five different nutrients needed by the body for building and repairing.

excision. Surgical cutting away and/or taking out.

fatty acids. Nutritional substances found in nature (fats and lipids), which include cholesterol, triglycerides, fatty acids, prostaglandins, and stearic, palmitic, linoleic, linolenic, eicosapentaenoic (EPA), and decohexanoic acids. Important nutritional lipids include lecithin, choline, gamma-linoleic acid, and inositol.

FBS (fasting blood sugar). Blood is drawn before breakfast (i.e., after fasting), then the glucose (sugar) in the blood is measured.

flatulence. Distention of the stomach or other intestinal tract parts with air or other gases.

free radical. A free radical is an atom or group of atoms that has at least one unpaired electron. Because another element can easily pick up this free electron and cause a chemical reaction, these free radicals can effect dramatic and destructive changes in the body. Free radicals are activated in heated and rancid oils and by radiation in the atmosphere, among other things.

free radical scavenger. A substance that removes or destroys free radicals.

fungus. One-celled organisms belonging to the plant kingdom. Its members contain a number of species including *Candida albicans*, which are capable of causing severe disease in immunocompromised hosts.

gastritis. Inflammation of the stomach lining.

gastroenteritis. Inflammation of the stomach and the intestines.

gastrointestinal. Pertaining to the stomach, small and large intestines, colon, rectum, liver, pancreas, and gallbladder.

genetic. Individual characteristics that are inherited.

gingivitis. Inflammation of the gums surrounding the teeth.

gland. An organ that excretes materials and manufactures substances not needed for its own metabolic function.

hair analysis. A painless and easy way to test for levels of toxic and essential minerals. A small amount of hair is taken from the nape of the neck and the mineral content of the hair is determined. A computerized analysis reveals the person's condition for the last three months.

helper T-lymphocyte. A lymphocyte subtype active in the process and stimulation of immunity. This cell is the one principally infected and killed by the AIDS virus.

hemicellulose. An indigestible carbohydrate resembling cellulose, found in the plant's outer layer, which absorbs water.

hemoglobin. A molecule of which iron is an essential component. Necessary in the red blood cells' transport of oxygen.

hepatitis. Inflammation of the liver usually resulting in jaundice.

herbal therapy. Uses various herbal combinations for healing as well as cleansing purposes. Herbs are used in the form of tablets, capsules, tinctures, extracts, and herbal baths with poultices. Herbs are a valuable adjunct to many therapies.

heterosexual. Attraction to the opposite sex.

histamine. A chemical in the body tissues that constricts the smooth bronchial tube muscles, dilates small blood vessels, allows fluid leakage to form itchy skin and hives, and increases secretion of stomach acid.

HIV (human immunodeficiency virus). The causative agent of AIDS, it is considered synonomous with HTLV-III/LAV.

Hodgkin's disease. Cancer of the lymphatic system and lymph nodes.

homeopathy. A system of medicine based on the belief that the cure of disease can be effected by minute doses of substances that, if given to a healthy person in large doses, would produce the same symptoms as are present in the disease being treated. Homeopathy employs natural substances in small doses to stimulate the body's reactive process to remove toxic waste and bring the body back into balance.

homosexual. Attraction to the same sex.

hormone. An essential substance produced by the endocrine glands that regulates many bodily functions.

host. An organism in which another microorganism lives and from which the invading microorganism obtains nourishment.

hydrochloric acid (HCl). An inorganic acidic compound, excreted by the stomach, that aids in digestion.

hypercalcemia. Abnormally high calcium levels in the blood.

hypertension. High blood pressure.

hypoallergenic. A substance that has a low capacity for inducing hypersensitivity (i.e., an allergic reaction).

hypocalcemia. Abnormally low calcium levels in the blood.

hypotension. Low blood pressure.

immune system. A combination of cells and proteins that assists in the host's ability to fight (i.e., resist) foreign substances such as viruses and harmful bacteria. The liver, spleen, thymus, bone marrow, and lymphatic system are interrelated in the immune system's normal function.

immunity. The condition that enables a living organism to resist and overcome disease or infection.

immunodeficiency. Any immune reaction deficiency involving antibody or cell-mediated immunity.

immunology. The science dealing with the specific mechanism by which living tissues react to foreign biological material in a way that may enhance resistance or immunity.

immunotherapy. Techniques used to stimulate or strengthen a patient's own immune system.

impotence. An inability to maintain an erection of the penis.

infection. The invasion of a host by organisms such as viruses, protozoa, fungi, or bacteria with resultant disease.

insomnia. The inability to sleep.

insulin. An essential hormone produced by the pancreas. It regulates the metabolism of sugar in the body.

interaction. Occurs when a substance is introduced in the body and reacts with an already present substance. Interactions occur between drugs and other drugs, and vitamins, herbs, and foods. Vitamins may interact with other vitamins, minerals, herbs, and foods. Minerals may also interact with other minerals, foods, and herbs, as can herbs with other herbs.

interferon. A protein formed by the cells of the immune system in the presence of a virus, etc. It prevents viral reproduction, and is capable of protecting noninfected cells from viral infection. Several kinds of interferon exist including alpha, beta, and gamma.

intestinal flora. The "friendly" bacteria present in the intestines that are essential for the digestion and metabolism of certain nutrients.

IV (intravenous infusion). A small needle placed in a vein to assist in fluid replacement or the giving of medication.

lactase. An enzyme that aids the body in converting lactose to glucose and galactose. It is also necessary for digestion of milk and milk products.

laser. An instrument used in surgical procedures.

lecithin. A mixture of phospholipids that is composed of fatty acids, glycerol, phosphorus, and choline or inositol. Lecithin can be manufactured in the body. All living cell membranes are largely composed of lecithin.

leukemia. Cancer of the lymph glands and bone marrow resulting in overproduction of white blood cells (related to Hodgkin's disease).

lipid. Fat or a fatty substance.

lipoprotein. A conjugated protein that, with lipids, forms an integral part of a molecule. Lipoproteins act as agents of lipid transport in the lymph and blood.

lymph. A clear fluid that flows through lymph vessels and is collected from the tissues throughout the body. Its function is to nourish tissue cells and return waste matter to the bloodstream. The lymph system eventually connects with and adds to venous circulation.

lymph glands. Located in the lymph vessels of the body, these glands trap foreign material and produce lymphocytes. These glands act as filters in the lymph system, and contain and form lymphocytes and permit lymphatic cells to destroy certain foreign agents.

lymphadenopathy. A lymph gland enlargement in response to any foreign substance or disease.

lymphocyte. A type of white blood cell found in lymph, blood, and other specialized tissue such as bone marrow and tonsils. B- and T-lymphocytes are crucial components of the immune system. The B-lymphocytes are primarily responsible for antibody production. The T-lymphocytes are involved in the direct attack against invading organisms. The helper T-lymphocyte, a subtype, is the main cell infected and destroyed by the AIDS virus.

lymphokines. Substances produced by the cells of the immune system when exposed to antigens. These substances are *not* antibodies, but they play a vital role in the on-board defense system.

lymphoma. Any tumor of the lymphatic tissues.

macrobiotics. A lifestyle and diet adapted from the Far East and made known in America by Michio Kushi. The principles of the diet consist of balancing the yin and yang energies of foods. In brief, yin foods, such as water, are expansive, while yang foods, such as salt or meat, are constrictive. For the most part, the diet consists of whole grain cereals, millet, rice, soups, and vegetable dishes, with beans and supplementary foods depending on the individual and the condition. Different types of cancers are considered either yin or yang, and the macrobiotic program must be adapted to each individual.

malabsorption. Lack of nutrient absorption from the intestinal tract into the bloodstream.

malignant. Dangerous. Mainly used to describe a cancerous growth—when used this way, it means that the growth is cancerous and predisposed to spreading.

mammography. An x-ray examination of the breast.

melanoma. A malignant tumor originating from pigment cells in the deep layers of the skin.

menopause. A decrease in the production of female hormones and the cessation of menstruation. Usually occurs after age forty-five or when the female organs are removed.

metabolism. The chemical processes of living cells in which energy is produced in order to replace and repair tissues and maintain a healthy body. Responsible for the production of energy, biosynthesis of important substances, and degradation of various compounds.

microgram. 1/1,000 of a milligram in weight.

milligram. 1/1,000 of a gram by weight.

MRI (magnetic resonance imaging). A technique used in diagnosis that combines radio waves and magnetic forces to produce detailed images of the internal structures of the body.

mucous membranes. The membranes, such as the mouth, nose, anus, and vagina, that line the cavities and canals of the body which communicate with the air.

naturopathy. Medical practice using herbs and other various methods to produce a healthy body state by stimulating innate defenses without the use of drugs.

neuropathy. A group of symptoms caused by abnormalities in motor or sensory nerves. Symptoms include tingling or numbness in hands or feet followed by gradual, progressive muscular weakness.

neurotransmitter. Any chemical that results in the transmission of nerve impulses between neurons in the brain and nerves.

nucleic acid. A chemical compound found in all viruses and plant and animal cells. RNA and DNA are the two principal types.

nutrients. Substances needed by all living cells to maintain life.

occult blood test. A test used in screening for cancer that identifies bodily excretion of blood (i.e., stool, sputum, urine).

oncology. The study of cancer.

oncologist. A cancer specialist.

orotate. An oratic acid salt (nucleic acid); an effective molecule for transporting minerals through cellular membranes. Functions as an essential part of every living cell.

osteopathy. A school of healing that teaches that the body is a vital mechanical organism whose structural and functional integrity are coordinated and interdependent, and that the abnormality of either constitutes disease. Its major contribution to treatment is manipulation.

osteoporosis. Softening of the bones.

oxidation. A chemical reaction that occurs when oxygen is added, resulting in a chemical transformation.

pau d'arco herb tea. A South American tea made from tree bark that is generally found in Brazil or Argentina. The tea is said to have anti-cancer properties.

Pap test. Microscopic examination of cells collected from the vagina and cervix to test for uterine cancer.

parasite. An organism that lives off of another organism.

pellagra. A disease caused by a deficiency of thiamine (B_1), usually occurring in alcoholics or in persons with malabsorption disorders.

peroxides. Free radicals that are by-products formed in our bodies when molecules of fat react with oxygen.

phenylketonuria. An inherited disease caused by a lack of an enzyme necessary for converting phenylalanine into a form the body can use.

placebo. A pharmacologically inactive substance. Often used to compare clinical responses against the effects of pharmacologically active substances in experiments.

polyunsaturated fats. Originate from vegetables and are liquid at room temperature. These oils are a good source of the unsaturated fatty acids. They include flaxseed with added vitamin B_6 (pyridoxine), sunflower oil, safflower oil, and primrose oil.

precancerous lesions. Abnormal tissue that is not yet malignant.

prognosis. A forecast as to the outcome of disease.

prostaglandin. A potent hormone—similar in structure to an unsaturated fatty acid—that acts in extremely low concentrations on local target organs; first isolated from the prostate.

protein. Complex compound formed from nitrogen and found in all animal and vegetable tissues. Essential in the body, protein is used for growth and repair. Proteins from animal sources contain the essential amino acids. Proteins are changed to amino acids in the body.

proteolytic enzymes. Enzymes that are able to break down certain proteins, yet do not attack the beneficial proteins that make up the normal cells of the body. These proteolytic enzymes are said to have great value in fighting cancer as well as many other diseases. If the body were always capable of producing adequate proteolytic enzymes, it is possible that cancer would not develop. In theory, cancer cells have a type of protein coating that is destroyed by these proteolytic enzymes. When this protein is destroyed, the body's white cells are able to attack the cancer cells and destroy them.

radiation. The emission and transmission of energy. Often used to refer to what is actually radioactivity, which is, basically, the release of energy and particles by unstable isotopes.

radiation therapy. Usually refers to treatment of cancer with ionizing radiation, including Roentgen rays, radium, or other radioactive substances.

RDA. Recommended daily allowance of vitamins or other nutrients as determined by the FDA.

remission. Abatement of disease.

retrovirus. A class of viruses with RNA as its core nucleic acid. Within this group is the causative agent of AIDS and other viruses that cause immunodeficiency and cancer in animals.

RNA. A ribonucleic acid found in plant and animal cells; a complex protein chemical. Important in the coding of genetic information with DNA carrying information from the nucleus of the cell into the cytoplasm.

saturates. Solid fats of animal origin.

sero-negativity. The absence of antibody positivity.

sero-positivity. Synonymous with antibody positivity.

serotonin. A neurotransmitter present in nerve tissue. Considered essential for relaxation, sleep, and concentration.

serum. The cell-free fluid of the bloodstream. Appears in a test tube after the blood clots.

simple carbohydrate. A simple form of sugar: glucose, lactose, fructose, etc. This type of sugar is rapidly absorbed into the bloodstream.

stroke. A sudden severe attack, usually caused by arteriosclerosis, that results in brain damage.

symptom. A reaction to a bodily disorder.

syndrome. A group of signs and symptoms that, when considered together, are known or presumed to characterize a disease.

synergism. An interaction between two or more nutrients in which the action of the nutrients is greater when they are taken together than when taken individually.

T-cell. A type of lymphocyte crucial to the immune system and involved in the direct attack upon invading organisms.

therapy, alternative. The treatment of disease using techniques supplementing surgery, radiation, and chemotherapy.

thrush. A fungal infection from *Candida albicans*. Occurs most often in infants, immunocompromised patients, and AIDS victims. Characterized by small whitish spots on the tongue and inside of the cheeks.

toxicity. A poisonous reaction in the body that impairs bodily functions and/or damages cells. Caused from ingesting an amount of a substance that is higher than one's level of tolerance.

toxin. A poison to the body that impairs bodily functions.

tremor. Involuntary trembling.

triglyceride. A compound consisting of glycerol and a fatty acid. Triglycerides are fat storage molecules and are the major lipid component of the diet.

vaccine. A preparation administered to induce immunity against a specific agent. It may be a suspension of living or dead organisms, or a solution of pollens or viral-bacterial antigens. Intended to induce immunity by antibody production without producing the disease itself.

virus. Any of a vast group of minute structures composed of a protein coat and a core of DNA and/or RNA that reproduces in the cells of the infected host. Capable of infecting all animals and plants, causing devastating disease in immunocompromised individuals. Viruses are not affected by antibiotics, and are totally dependent on the cells of the infected host for the ability to reproduce.

vital signs. Pulse, breathing, blood pressure, and temperature.

vitamin. Approximately fifteen essential nutrients that the body cannot manufacture and that need to be supplied for life and health.

water-soluble. Dissolves in water.

western blot. A test designed to detect the AIDS virus exposure by assessing the presence of the AIDS virus antibody.

withdrawal. Termination of a habit-forming substance. *See also* detoxification.

yeast. Yeast is a single-cell organism that may cause infection in the mouth, vagina, gastrointestinal tract, and any or all bodily parts. Common yeast infections include candidiasis and thrush.

MANUFACTURER AND DISTRIBUTOR INFORMATION

Specific products mentioned in this book have no connection with the production of the book. They are mentioned because they are high-quality products. Addresses and telephone numbers are provided for some of the manufacturers and distributors of the products so that you may order or obtain information from them. The addresses and telephone numbers are subject to change. For your convenience, the products distributed by the companies and some of the services provided have also been listed below. The supplement recommendations in this book are for adults only, except where otherwise indicated.

Abkit, Inc.
1160 Park Avenue
Dept. HP-10
New York, NY 10128
(212) 860-8358
CamoCare Cream

Aerobic Life Products, Inc.
9811 Ferguson Road
P.O. Box 28802
Dallas, TX 75228
(214) 328-3159 or (800) 798-0707

Alboher, Pamela Ray, Ph.D.
5888 E. 82nd Street
Indianapolis, IN 46250
(317) 462-2004
Cytotoxic Allergy Testing

Allergy Research Group
400 Preda Street
San Leandro, CA 94577

American Biologics
P.O. Box 1880
San Ysidro, CA 92073
1-(800) 227-4458 or 1-(619) 429-8200
Proteolytic Enzymes: Inflazyme Forte

Amni
21019 Alexander Court
Hayward, CA 94545
Candidiasis

Auro Trading Group
Alive Energy
18 A Hanger Way
Watsonville, CA 95076
1-(800) 225-6111
Products for the Next Millennium

Bio-Strath
14851 N. Scottsdale Road
Scottsdale, AZ 85254
1-(800) 528-4499

Biotec Foods
2600 S. King Street, Suite 203
Honolulu, HI 96826
1-(800) 331-5888
Cell Guard
Ageless Beauty
Superoxide Dismutase (SOD)

Bowstick Tea Distributor
Roy Kupsinel, M.D.
P.O. Box 550
Oviedo, FL 32765

Cardiovascular Research, Ltd.
1061-B Shary Circle
Concord, CA 94518
1-(800) 888-4585
Caprystatin (Candidiasis)
Ecological Formulas

Carlson Laboratories, Inc.
15 College Drive
Arlington Heights, IL 60004
(312) 255-1600

Dash Products
P.O. Box 2888
Tuscaloosa, AL 35403
1-(800) 367-9599
Products for Athletes

DaVinci Laboratories
20 New England Drive
Essex Junction, VT 04352
DMG Gluconic

Doctors Mutual Service, Inc.
18722 Santee Lane
Valley Center, CA 92082
Sublingual Glandulars

Earthrise Company
P.O. Box 1196
San Rafael, CA 94915
1-(800) 233-6520 ext. 11
Spirulina

Efamol Research
P.O. Box 818
Kentville, Nova Scotia
Canada, B4N4H8
(902) 678-5534

Enzymatic Therapy
P.O. Box 1508
Green Bay, WI 54302

Essential Organics
P.O. Box 325
Organic Park
Derry, NH 03038
Hypoallergenic Vitamins
Aller Guard

Esteem Products, Ltd.
1 Evergreen Plaza
Box 40327
Bellevue, WA 98004
(206) 562-1281 or (800) 255-7631

Ethical Nutrients
20370 N. Rand Road
Palantine, IL 60074
1-(312) 438-9420

Freeda Pharmacy and Vitamins
36 East 41st Street
New York, NY 10017
1-(212) 685-4980

Futurebiotics
48 Elliot Street
Brattleboro, VT 05301
1-(800) 367-5433

HMS-Pep Products, Inc.
3155 N. Commerce Court
P.O. Box 715
Castle Rock, CO 80104
(303) 688-6633 or (800) 324-42620
Manufacturer of Pep Products

Janssen Pharmaceuticals, Inc.
40 Kingsbridge Road
Piscataway, NJ 08854
(201) 524-9143
Nizoral Tablets

Kroeger Herb Products
1122 Pearl Street
Boulder, CO 80302
(303) 443-0261 or (800) 225-8787

Life Extension
1142 W. Indian School Road
Phoenix, AZ 85013-9985
Products and Newsletter Update

Livingston-Wheeler Clinic
3232 Duke Street
San Diego, CA 92110
(619) 224-3515

Merit Pharmaceuticals
2622 Humboldt Street
Los Angeles, CA 90031

Michael's Naturopathic Programs
7040 Alamo Downs Parkway
San Antonio, TX 78238

Miller Pharmacal Group, Inc.
245 W. Roosevelt Road, #8-51
Box 279
West Chicago, IL 60185
1-(800) 323-2935
Proteolytic Enzymes

Montana Naturals International, Inc.
19994 Highway 93
P.O. Box 1
Arlee, MT 59821
(800) 872-7218

Natren, Inc.
10935 Camarillo Street
North Hollywood, CA 91602
(800) 992-3323 or (800) 992-9393
Megadophilus
Bifido Factor/Life Start Two
Life Start
Bulgaricum I.B.

NatureMost of New England, Inc.
50 Walnut Street
P.O. Box 721
Middletown, CT 06457
1-(203) 346-8991 or (800) 234-2112

Nature's Bounty
90 Orville Drive
Bohemia, NY 11716
(516) 567-9500 or (800) 645-5412
Vitamin B_{12} Nasal Gel

Nature's Concept, Inc.
18165 Napa Street, No. 8
Northridge, CA 91325
(818) 772-6590 or (800) 999-1006

Nature's Plus
10 Daniel Street
Farmingdale, NY 11735

Nature's Pride
19569 N.E. 10th Avenue
N. Miami Beach, FL 33197
EPA Pure/700

New Dimensions Distributors
16548 E. Laser Drive A-7
Fountain Hills, AZ 85268
Linseed Oil

New Moon Extracts, Inc.
601 South Grove
Barrington, IL 60010
Nondairy Acidophilus and Herbs

Nutri-Cell, Inc.
1038 N. Tustin Street, Suite 309
Orange, CA 92667
(714) 953-8307

Nutri-Dyn Products, Inc.
2470 Wisconsin Street
Downers Grove, IL 60515
1-(800) 332-3130

Professional Specialties
1803-132nd Avenue, N.E.
Bellevue, WA 98005
Capricin

Profitable Nutrition Distributors
2920 Skokie Road
Highland Park, IL 60035
1-(800) 541-4720

Pulsebeat Enterprises
2600 Netherland Avenue
Bronx, NY 10463
Chronic Bowel and Digestive Problems Self-Test

Quality Longevity Medical Center
2642 Gotes Avenue
Irving, CA 92714
Cytotoxic Testing Kits

Quest Vitamins
140 Arrowood Lane
San Mateo, CA 94403
(415) 349-1233
Germanium and Coenzyme Q_{10}

Rainbow Light Nutritional Systems
207 McPherson Street
P.O. Box 3033
Santa Cruz, CA 95063
(408) 429-9089 or (800) 635-1233
Herbal Spirulina

Randal Nutritional Products
1595 Hampton Way
P.O. Box 7328
Santa Rosa, CA 95407
(800) 331-4967 or (800) 221-1697
Vimco Vitamins

Salus of America, Inc.
158 Business Center Drive
Corona, CA 91720
Floradix Formula

Solaray Products
2815 Industrial Drive
Ogden, UT 84401
1-(800) 669-8877

Source Naturals
P.O Box 2118
Santa Cruz, CA 95063
1-(800) 538-0740
*Coenzyme Q_{10} and Germanium
(Distributors Only)*

TerraMaxa
3301 W. Central Avenue
Toledo, OH 43606
Herbs

U.A.S. Laboratories
9201 Penn Avenue S., Suite 10
Minneapolis, MN 55431
DDS Products

Vital Health Products
P.O. Box 158
Hales Corners, WI 53130
Peroxy Gel

Vitamin Research Products
Organic Park, Box 325L
Derry, NH 03038
Hypoallergenic Supplements

Wakunaga of America Company, Ltd.
23510 Madero
Mission Viejo, CA 92691

Warren Laboratories, Inc.
12603 Executive Drive, Suite 806
Stafford, TX 77477
George's Aloe Vera Juice

HEALTH ORGANIZATIONS

Allergy Research Group
400 Preda Street
P.O. Box 480
San Leandro, CA 94577
(800) 545-9960

ALS Society of America
(Amyotrophic Lateral Sclerosis)
15300 Ventura Boulevard
Suite 315
Sherman Oaks, CA 91403
(818) 990-2151

Alzheimer's Disease and Related Disorders Association
70 East Lake Street
Chicago, IL 60601
(312) 853-3060

American Anorexia Nervosa Association, Inc.
133 Cedar Lane
Teaneck, NJ 07666
(201) 836-1800

American Holistic Medical Association
2727 Fairview Avenue East No. G
Seattle, WA 98102

American Medical Association
535 N. Dearborn Street
Chicago, IL 60610

American Nutrition Society
9337 Shoslane Avenue
Northridge, CA 91324
(818) 345-4365

Association of Heart Patients
P.O. Box 54305
Atlanta, GA 30308
(404) 523-0826

The Epilepsy Foundation of America
4351 Garden City Drive
Landover, MD 29785

Hearing and Tinnitus Help Association
32A S. Main Street (Route 32)
New Hope, PA 18938
(215) 862-3475

Help Anorexia, Inc.
P.O. Box 2992
Culver City, CA 90231
(213) 558-0444

Hypoglycemia Association, Inc.
2643 Liberty Parkway
Baltimore, MD 21222
International Association for Medical Assistance
to Travelers
736 Center Street
Lewiston, NY 14092
(716) 754-4883

National Neurofibromatosis Foundation
141 Fifth Avenue, Suite 7S
New York, NY 10010
(212) 460-8980 or (800) 323-7938 (outside New York)

The Stroke Foundation, Inc.
898 Park Avenue
New York, NY 10021
(212) 734-3434

HOSPITALS AND CLINICS

Contact the following hospitals and clinics for information and services. Specialty areas of the hospitals are provided in some cases for easy reference.

Advanced Health Center
2691 Richter
Suite 127
Irvine, CA 92714
Cytotoxic Test Kits

American Biologics
Mexico S.A. Medical Center
15 Azucenas Street
Tijuana, B.C.
Mexico
1-(800) 227-4458 or 1-(619) 429-8200
Live Cell Therapy and Metabolic/Nutritional Treatment for Degenerative Diseases (Cancer, AIDS)

C.T. Smith, M.D., Ph.D.
(I.C.B.R.)
P.O. Box 898
Bridgeton, MO 63044
Live Cell Therapy

Desert Arthritis Medical Clinic
13-630 Mountain View Road
Desert Hot Springs, CA 22240

Genesis West, Inc.
241 Hazel Avenue
Redwood City, CA 94060
1-(800) 227-8823
Live Cell Therapy

International Foundation for Homeopathy
2366 Eastlake Avenue East
Suite 301
Seattle, WA 98102
(206) 324-8230
Provides a List of Classical Homeopaths

Livingston-Wheeler Clinic
3232 Duke Street
San Diego, CA 92110
1-(619) 224-3515

Quality Longevity Medical Center
2642 Gotes Avenue
Irving, CA 92714
Cytotoxic Testing Kits

Stanford University Hospital
Department of Dietics
Room P1070
Stanford, CA 94305-5223
1-(415) 723-6904
All Services Available

The UCLA Medical Center/Mark Taper Center for Health Treatment
950 Veteran Avenue
Los Angeles, CA 90024
1-(213) 825-9791
Diet, Stress, Exercise, Behavior Programs

Wildwood Sanitarium and Hospital
Wildwood, GA 30757
1-(404) 820-1493
Offers Cleansing Fasts, Water Therapy, Diet, Exercise, Stress Control

HEALTH AND MEDICAL HOT LINES

The hot lines listed below provide information, help, and support for those with various illnesses and for those in emergency situations. Hot lines can provide you with the most current medical information, and all calls are confidential.

AIDS Hot Line. Explains symptoms, means of transmission, and high-risk categories. Call (800) 342-AIDS, or call collect (202) 245-6867 if in Alaska or Hawaii.

Alzheimer's Association. Provides free literature and referrals to local chapters. Call (800) 621-0379, or call (800) 572-6037 if in Illinois.

American Association on Mental Deficiency. Call (800) 424-3688, or call (202) 387-1968 if in Washington, D.C.

American Council for the Blind. Call (800) 424-8666, or call (202) 833-1251 if in Alaska, Hawaii, or Washington, D.C.

American Diabetes Association. Call (800) 232-3472, or call (703) 549-1500 if in Virginia or Washington, D.C.

American International Hospital and Clinic in Zion, Illinois. Offers information about alternatives for the diagnosis and effective treatment of cancer. Call (800) FOR-HELP, or call (312) 872-8722 if in Illinois.

American Kidney Fund. Assists kidney patients unable to pay for treatment. Call (800) 638-8299, or call (800) 492-8361 if in Maryland.

Cancer Information Service. Provides information on cancer treatment research and physicians. Call (800) 4-CANCER, or call (202) 636-5700 if in Washington, D.C.

Cystic Fibrosis Foundation. Sends information on cystic fibrosis and services available. Call (800) 638-8815, or call (301) 881-9130 if in Maryland.

Heartlife. Provides information on heart disease, pacemakers, medication, and nutrition. Call (800) 241-6993, or call collect (404) 523-0826 if in Alaska or Georgia.

Impotence Foundation. National organization that provides public information, advice, and referrals for impotence and male and female dysfunctions. Call (800) 221-5517.

The Living Bank. Provides information and maintains a registry for people to donate their organs, tissues, bones, or body for transplants or research. Call (800) 528-2971, or call collect (713) 528-2971 if in Texas.

Medic Alert Foundation. Maintains individual files on computer to provide information on the person with the medical bracelet in case of an emergency. Call (800) 344-3226. If in California, call (800) 468-1020. If in Alaska or Hawaii, call (209) 668-3333.

National Association for Speech and Hearing Action. Call (800) 638-TALK, or call (301) 897-8682 if in Alaska, Hawaii, or Maryland.

National Child Abuse Hot Line. A 24-hour service that offers counseling facilities and provides reporting agencies for child abuse. Call (800) 422-4453.

National Cocaine Hot Line. Provides referrals to hospitals, counseling centers, and doctors specializing in cocaine treatment. Call (800) COCAINE, or call (201) 522-7005 if in Alaska or Hawaii.

National Down's Syndrome Society. Call (800) 221-4602 outside New York. If in New York, call (212) 460-9330.

National Health and Information Clearinghouse. Provides information and referrals. Answers health and disease-related questions. Call (800) 336-4797, or call (703) 522-2590 if in Alaska, Hawaii, Virginia, or Washington, D.C. Call collect if necessary.

National Institute on Drug Abuse. For drug abuse prevention programs, call (800) 638-2045. If in Alaska, Hawaii, or Maryland, call (301) 443-2450.

National Jewish Center's Lung Line. Call (800) 222-5864, or call (303) 355-5864 if in Colorado.

National Parkinson Foundation. Call (800) 327-4545. Call (800) 433-7022 if in Florida, or (305) 547-6666 if in Miami.

National Pesticide Telecommunications Network. Provides information on health hazards of pesticides, safety precautions, how to obtain lab analysis, toxicity levels in soil, garments, carpets, etc. Call (800) 858-7378, or call (512) 399-5352 if in Alaska or Hawaii.

National RP Foundation Fighting Blindness. Provides information on retinitis pigmentosa and other inherited retina degeneration. For donor program, referrals, and information on specialists and research centers, call (800) 638-2300. If in Maryland, call collect (301) 655-1011.

Non-Emergency Surgery Hot Line. Free referrals for second opinions. For free brochure "Thinking of Having Surgery?" write to Surgery, HHHS, Washington, D.C. 20201. Call (800) 638-6833, or call (800) 492-6603 if in Maryland.

Pride Action. For information on drug abuse and effects of specific drugs, call (800) 241-7946.

Runaway Hot Line. Accepts calls from runaways. Offers free bus ride home, forwards messages to home, and offers referrals for medical aid and shelter. Call (800) 231-6946, or call (800) 392-3352 if in Texas.

Spina Bifida Association. For referrals to local chapters, call (800) 621-3141. If in Illinois, call collect (312) 663-1562.

V.D. Hot Line. For consultation, information, and clinic referral on all aspects of sexually transmitted diseases, call (800) 227-8922.

SUGGESTED READING

A suggested reading list is provided for those who wish to explore an individual topic further. The following list of books was compiled to provide you with further sources of information.

Airola, Paavo. *Cancer Causes, Prevention, and Treatment: The Total Approach*. Phoenix, AZ: Health Plus Publishers, 1972.

Airola, Paavo. *How to Get Well*. Phoenix, AZ: Health Plus Publishers, 1974.

Airola, Paavo. *How to Keep Slim, Healthy, and Young With Juice Fasting*. Phoenix, AZ: Health Plus Publishers, 1971.

Airola, Paavo. *Hypoglycemia: A Better Approach*. Phoenix, AZ: Health Plus Publishers, 1977.

Aladjem, Henrietta. *Understanding Lupus: What It Is, How to Treat It, How to Cope With It*. New York: Scribner, 1986.

Appleton, Nancy. *Lick The Sugar Habit*. Garden City Park, NY: Avery Publishing Group, 1989.

Astor, Stephen. *Hidden Food Allergies*. Garden City Park, NY: Avery Publishing Group, 1989.

Atkins, Robert C. *Dr. Atkins' Nutritional Breakthrough: How to Treat Your Medical Condition Without Drugs*. New York: William Morrow & Co., 1981.

Barnes, Broda O. and Galton, Lawrence. *Hypothyroidism: The Unsuspected Illness*. New York: Cromwell, 1976.

Becker, Robert O. and Selden, Gary. *Body Electric: Electromagnetism and the Foundation of Life*. New York: William Morrow & Co., 1987.

Bland, Jeffrey. *Medical Applications of Clinical Nutrition*. New Canaan, CT: Keats Publishing, 1983.

Bland, Jeffrey. *Your Health Under Seige: Using Nutrition to Fight Back*. Greene, 1982.

Blauer, Stephen. *The Juicing Book*. Garden City Park, NY: Avery Publishing Group, 1989.

Bliznakov, Emile and Gerry Hunt. *The Miracle Nutrient: Coenzyme Q*$_{10}$. New York: Bantam Books, 1987.

Brighthope, Ian. *The AIDS Fighters*. New Canaan, CT: Keats Publishing, 1988.

Brinkley, Ginny, Linda Goldberg and Janice Kukar. *Your Child's First Journey*. Garden City Park, NY: Avery Publishing Group, 1989.

Buist, Robert. *Food Chemical Sensitivity*. Garden City Park, NY: Avery Publishing Group, 1988.

Buist, Robert. *Food Intolerance*. Garden City Park, NY: Avery Publishing Group, 1989.

Check, William A. and Ann G. Fettner. *The Truth About AIDS: Evolution of an Epidemic*. New York: Holt, Rinehart & Winston, 1985.

Clare, Sally and David. *Creative Vegetarian Cookery*. Bridport, England: Prism Press, 1988.

Crook, William G. *The Yeast Connection: A Medical Breakthrough*, rev. ed. New York: Vintage Books, 1986.

Davidson, Paul. *Are You Sure It's Arthritis?* New York: Macmillan Publishing Co., 1985.

Davis, Adelle. *Let's Eat Right to Keep Fit*. New York, NY: Harcourt Brace Jovanovich, Inc., 1970.

de Haas, Cherie. *Natural Skin Care*. Garden City Park, NY: Avery Publishing Group, 1989.

Donsbach, Kurt W. *Dr. Donsbach's Guide to Good Health*. Long Shadow Books, 1985.

Editors of *East West Journal*. *Shopper's Guide to Natural Foods*. Garden City Park, NY: Avery Publishing Group, 1988.

Edwards, Linda. *Baking for Health*. Garden City Park, NY: Avery Publishing Group, 1988.

Erasmus, Udo. *Fats and Oils*. Vancouver: Alive Press, 1987.

Feingold, Ben F. *Why Your Child Is Hyperactive*. New York: Random House, 1985.

Feingold, Helene and Ben. *The Feingold Cookbook for Hyperactive Children and Others With Problems Associated With Food Additives and Salicylates*. New York: Random House, 1979.

Fink, John. *Third Opinion*. Garden City Park, NY: Avery Publishing Group, 1988.

Fujita, Takuo. *Calcium and Your Health*. Tokyo: Japan Publications, 1987.

Germann, Donald R. *The Anti-Cancer Diet*. New York: Wyden Books, 1977.

Gregory, Scott J. and Leonardo, Bianca. *They Conquered AIDS!* True Life Publications, 1989.

Heidenry, Carolyn. *Making the Transition to a Macrobiotic Diet*. Garden City Park, NY: Avery Publishing Group, 1988.

Heinerman, John. *Aloe Vera, Jojoba & Yucca*. New Canaan, CT: Keats, 1982.

Howard, Mary Ann. *Blueprint for Health*. Grand Rapids, MI: Zondervan Publishing House, 1985.

Howell, Edward. *Enzyme Nutrition*. Garden City Park, NY: Avery Publishing Group, 1987.

Kushi, Aveline and Wendy Esko. *The Macrobiotic Cancer Prevention Cookbook*. Garden City Park, NY: Avery Publishing Group, 1987.

Kushi, Michio. *The Macrobiotic Approach to Cancer*. Garden City Park, NY: Avery Publishing Group, 1989.

Kushi, Michio. *The Macrobiotic Way*. Garden City Park, NY: Avery Publishing Group, 1986.

Lance, James W. *Migraine and Other Headaches*. New York: Scribner, 1986.

Lerman, Andrea. *The Macrobiotic Community Cookbook*. Garden City Park, NY: Avery Publishing Group, 1989.

Levitt, Paul and Elissa Guralnick. *The Cancer Reference Book*. New York: Paddington Press, 1979.

Livingston-Wheeler, Virginia and Edmond G. Addleo. *The Conquest of Cancer: Vaccines and Diet*. New York: Franklin Watts, 1984.

Olkin, Sylvia Klein. *Positive Pregnancy Fitness: A Guide to a More Comfortable Pregnancy and Easier Birth Through Exercise and Relaxation*. Garden City Park, NY: Avery Publishing Group, 1987.

Ott, John N. *Light, Radiation, and You: How to Stay Healthy*. Old Greenwich, CT: Devin-Adair Publishers, 1982.

Passwater, Richard A. *Supernutrition*. New York: Dial Press, 1985.

Passwater, Richard A. and Cranton, Elmer. *Trace Elements, Hair Analysis and Nutrition*. New Canaan, CT: Keats Publishing, 1983.

Pauling, Linus. *Vitamin C and the Common Cold*. San Francisco, CA: W.H. Freeman & Co., 1970.

Pearsall, Paul. *Superimmunity: Master Your Emotions and Improve Your Health*. New York: McGraw-Hill, 1987.

Pfeiffer, Carl. *Nutrition and Mental Illness: An Orthomolecular Approach to Balancing Body Chemistry*. Rochester, VT: Inner Traditions, 1988.

Pfeiffer, Carl. *Zinc and Other Micro-Nutrients*. New Canaan, CT: Keats, 1978.

Phillips, Robert H. *Coping With Osteoarthritis*. Garden City Park, NY: Avery Publishing Group, 1989.

Randolph, Theron G. *Human Ecology and Susceptibility to the Chemical Environment*. Charles C. Thomas, Publisher, 1981.

Rapp, Doris J. *Allergies and the Hyperactive Child*. New York: Sovereign Books, 1979.

Sayce, Valerie and Fraser, Ian. *Exercise Can Beat Your Arthritis*. Garden City Park, NY: Avery Publishing Group, 1989.

Shannon, Sara. *Diet for the Atomic Age*. Garden City Park, NY: Avery Publishing Group, 1987.

Shelton, Herbert M. *Fasting Can Save Your Life*, rev. ed. Natural Hygeine, 1981.

Shute, Wilfrid. *Dr. Wilfrid E. Shute's Complete Updated Vitamin E Book.* New Canaan, CT: Keats Publishing, 1975.

Smith, Lendon. *Feed Your Kids Right: Dr. Smith's Program for Your Child's Total Health.* New York: McGraw–Hill, 1979.

Stern, Gai. *International Whole Meals.* San Leandro, California: Prism Press, 1987.

Todd, Gary Price. *Eye Talk.* 1988.

Treben, Maria. *Health from God's Garden: Herbal Remedies for Glowing Health and Glorious Well-Being.* Rochester, VT: Thorsons Publishers, 1987.

Wade, Carlson. *Carlson Wade's Amino Acids Book.* New Canaan, CT: Keats Publishing, 1985.

Walker, Morton. *The Chelation Way.* Garden City Park, NY: Avery Publishing Group, 1990.

Weber, Marcea. *Macrobiotics and Beyond.* Garden City Park: Avery Publishing Group, 1989).

Weber, Marcea. *Whole Meals.* Dorset: Prism Press, 1983.

Weiner, Michael A. *Maximum Immunity.* Boston, MA: Houghton Mifflin Co., 1986.

Wigmore, Ann. *Be Your Own Doctor: A Positive Guide to Natural Living,* rev. ed. Garden City Park, NY: Avery Publishing Group, 1983.

Wigmore, Ann. *Recipes for Longer Life.* Garden City Park, NY: Avery Publishing Group, 1982.

Wigmore, Ann. *The Wheatgrass Book.* Garden City Park, NY: Avery Publishing Group, 1985.

Wigmore, Ann. *Why Suffer?*, rev. ed. Garden City Park, NY: Avery Publishing Group, 1984.

Williams, Roger J. and Dwight K. Kalita. *A Physician's Handbook on Orthomolecular Medicine.* New Canaan, CT: Keats Publishing, 1979.

Williams, Xandria. *What's in My Food?* Bridport, England: Prism Press, 1988.

Wlodyga, Ronald R. *Health Secrets From the Bible.* Triumph Pub., 1979.

Woessner, Candace, Judith Lauwers, and Barbara Bernard. *Breastfeeding Today.* Garden City Park, NY: Avery Publishing Group, 1988.

Ziff, Sam. *Silver Dental Fillings: The Toxic Timebomb.* Aurora Press, 1984.

ABOUT THE AUTHORS

Dr. James Balch is a graduate of Indiana University's School of Medicine. He completed his surgical residency at Indiana University Medical Center, specializing in urology. Following a two-year tour of duty in the United States Navy, Dr. Balch established a private practice as a urologist. He is presently a member of the American Medical Association, is board certified in the American Board of Urology, and is a fellow in the American College of Surgeons.

During the past ten years, Dr. Balch has helped patients to assume a portion of responsibility for their own well-being. This philosophy is reflected in his newspaper column and his radio broadcast. Through the years, Dr. Balch has appeared on numerous television and radio shows throughout this country.

Dr. Balch works with his wife, Phyllis Balch, who is a certified nutritional consultant. Phyllis Balch, who received her certification from the American Association of Nutritional Consultants, has been a nutritional counselor for over a decade. She serves as nutritional consultant in her husband's practice, and also contributes to his health column. Her interest in natural foods led to the establishment of a health foods store, *Good Things Naturally.*

In addition to the experience she has gained working with her husband, Phyllis Balch has studied nutritionally-based therapies, procedures, and treatments abroad.

INDEX

Index